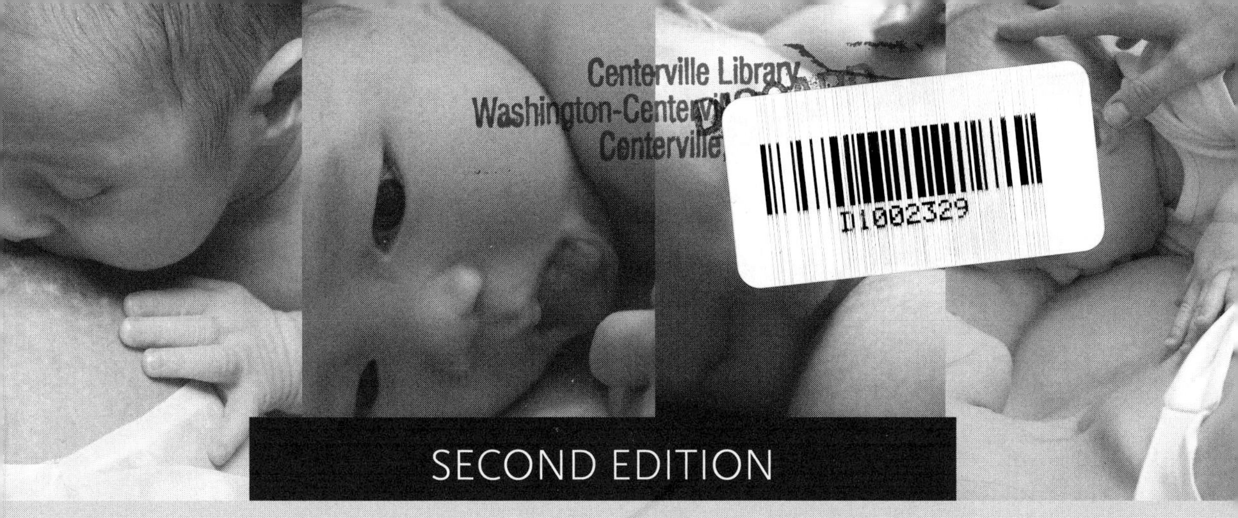

SECOND EDITION

SUPPORTING SUCKING SKILLS in Breastfeeding Infants

Edited by
Catherine Watson Genna, BS, IBCLC
Woodhaven, New York

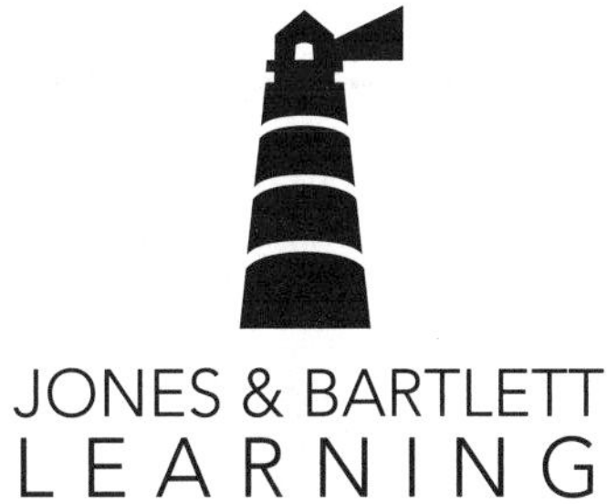

JONES & BARTLETT
LEARNING

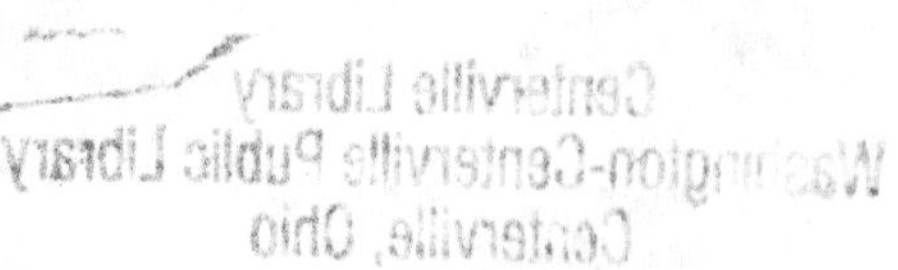

World Headquarters
Jones & Bartlett Learning
5 Wall Street
Burlington, MA 01803
978-443-5000
info@jblearning.com
www.jblearning.com

Jones & Bartlett Learning books and products are available through most bookstores and online booksellers. To contact Jones & Bartlett Learning directly, call 800-832-0034, fax 978-443-8000, or visit our website, www.jblearning.com.

Substantial discounts on bulk quantities of Jones & Bartlett Learning publications are available to corporations, professional associations, and other qualified organizations. For details and specific discount information, contact the special sales department at Jones & Bartlett Learning via the above contact information or send an email to specialsales@jblearning.com.

Production Credits
Publisher: Kevin Sullivan
Acquisitions Editor: Amanda Harvey
Editorial Assistant: Sara Bempkins
Production Manager: Carolyn F. Rogers
Associate Marketing Manager: Katie Hennessy
V.P., Manufacturing and Inventory Control: Therese Connell
Composition: Shawn Girsberger
Cover Design: Kristin E. Parker
Cover Images: clockwise from top left: © niderlander/ShutterStock, Inc.; © Catherine Watson Genna, BS, IBCLC; © SvetlanaFedoseyeva/ShutterStock, Inc.; © Hemera/Thinkstock
Printing and Binding: Malloy, Inc.
Cover Printing: Malloy, Inc.

Library of Congress Cataloging-in-Publication Data
Supporting sucking skills in breastfeeding infants / [edited by] Catherine Watson Genna. — 2nd ed.
p. ; cm.
Includes bibliographical references and index.
ISBN 978-1-4496-4736-0 (pbk.)
I. Genna, Catherine Watson.
[DNLM: 1. Breast Feeding. 2. Infant, Newborn. 3. Lactation—physiology. WS 125]

649'.33—dc23

2011048357

6048

Printed in the United States of America
16 15 14 13 12 10 9 8 7 6 5 4 3 2 1

Contents

CHAPTER 7 Breastfeeding Preterm Infants 171

Kerstin Hedberg Nyqvist

CHAPTER 8 The Influence of Anatomic and Structural Issues on Sucking Skills 197

Catherine Watson Genna

FOREWORD

Diane Wiessinger

If we were writing a handbook on bicycle riding for extraterrestrials, we would first study bicycling in all its complexity—how to mount, balance, turn, and stop. The first edition of our book would probably include considerable detail about what a bicycle is and how it works. That would be followed by precise instructions on, for instance, the exact placement of the ball of the left foot on the pedal as the right leg is swung over the bicycle. A few determined ETs would be able to put together a general picture from our mountain of minutiae (and our limited number of graphics and nonexistent film footage) and actually learn to ride; most would make clumsy attempts, feel defeated by our thoroughness, and quit.

Our second edition would emphasize certain aspects as being important, while leaving many of the details to the reader to work out with practice. This would be a much more useful book, but its continued emphasis on many steps would prevent most readers from gaining the grace and perspective of the average human 10-year-old bicyclist. Our third edition, I hope, would appear in two volumes: one for instructors, and one for would-be bicyclists. The instructors' volume would retain all the steps, but there would be no expectation that the bicyclists themselves would need to learn them all. For the bicyclists who needed extra help, a few brief and well-timed suggestions would allow them to be off and away without ever understanding exactly how they were doing it. The understanding part could be left to the instructors, whose modest but aptly chosen interventions were based on a thorough knowledge of all the small steps.

Breastfeeding is biology. Therefore, some mothers and babies have always needed help and will always need help, just as some of us need glasses or a math tutor. In our zeal to help those mothers and babies, we have spent decades dissecting breastfeeding and carefully detailing all of its parts: the anatomy and physiology of mother and baby, the angles of neck and mouth, the positions of arms and legs, the variations in breasts and nipples. Sometimes it seemed that the more we knew, the more trouble women had. Today, in addition to the familiar cry that "I wanted to breastfeed but I didn't have enough milk," we too often hear "I wanted to breastfeed but my baby never latched." The reasons for this apparent shift are numerous, but we are beginning to recognize that our rigorous attending to every detail, and our eagerness for mothers to do the same, is sometimes part of the problem.

Time for a change. Mothers and babies, as you'll see in this book, already possess an advanced understanding of breastfeeding, provided we don't intervene unnecessarily. At the same time, mothers are perhaps more lacking in confidence than they have ever been—confidence in their bodies generally, confidence in their babies' abilities, and confidence in their inherent "mothering wisdom." Books for mothers are just beginning to portray the larger, right-brained picture of breastfeeding, with less emphasis on a rigid, left-brained list of steps and more emphasis on the innate abilities of mother and baby. But that leaves the instructors with perhaps a greater-than-ever need to know the supporting details for those mothers and babies who need them.

This book is for us, the instructors, to help us recognize when certain steps in the breastfeeding balance have gone awry, to provide detailed ideas on correcting them, and to give us deep enough knowledge over a broad enough area that we can choose the right level of intervention and leave the rest of the process alone.

It is not enough, of course. Only as we become a breastfeeding culture will the final pieces fall into place. Right now, our friend the extraterrestrial comes to an earth on which only a few people ride bicycles. Most of the advertising, most of the language, most of the images are of easy-to-learn, readily available tricycles. But imagine the ET who comes to earth and sees everyone around him riding bicycles! He tries and falls, but he keeps trying. Eventually he sails off, steady and confident. Why did he succeed? Not only because he read a general guide that provided him with the big picture. Not only because his instructor had a nice, thick book of potentially helpful interventions. But because he saw around him, everywhere he went, people of all sizes and shapes and ages on bicycles. He learned to his very core that this is what people do, that this is what people enjoy, and that, if all of them can do it, then he can do it too. Maybe with just a little bit of help.

Foreword

Nancy Mohrbacher

No matter how skilled we are, if we work with breastfeeding families long enough, we all eventually encounter a baby immune to our usual interventions. What do we do after we've exhausted our entire bag of tricks? That's when I give thanks for this book and its incredible editor, Catherine Watson Genna, who has compiled a multidisciplinary masterpiece that enables all of us who work with infants to broaden our insights beyond the limits of our field.

As a lactation consultant, this book provides me with access to practical wisdom from occupational therapy, speech-and-language pathology, neurology, physical therapy, neonatology, family counseling, and many other specialties. And it offers far more than just strategies to improve breastfeeding effectiveness. Equally important, it describes how we can convey information in ways that enhance a mother's emotional connection to her baby and her self-efficacy. With the help of this book, I can be more than the sum of my lactation training for mothers desperate for a miracle.

This amazing resource also serves as a bridge from other disciplines to the field of lactation. Many healthcare professions focus primarily on pathology and abnormality. Breastfeeding requires a different mindset because like walking and talking, it is a normal human behavior. Healthcare providers uncertain about how to evaluate breastfeeding can turn to this book's detailed descriptions of normal feeding and sucking. If a baby is not breastfeeding normally, it also explains why this deserves their attention. Because breastfeeding is a normal and essential part of early life, "its absence means something is fundamentally wrong with the infant's world."

Genna's medical training and interest in genetic disorders give her unique insights into the respiratory, cardiac, musculoskeletal, gastrointestinal, metabolic, and neurological issues that can underlie breastfeeding problems. In some cases, feeding issues may be the first sign of a condition in need of treatment. Her research on tongue tie and her years spent working with babies with oral anatomical variations have helped her determine those strategies that best facilitate breastfeeding.

Yet this book is far more than a treatise on unusual conditions. It also includes the latest research on basic breastfeeding dynamics. Since its first edition, we have made giant leaps forward in our understanding of the role gravity plays in early breastfeeding and the effects of feeding position on baby's inborn feeding reflexes. These recent paradigm shifts are described brilliantly by some of the top minds in the field.

Also since this book's first edition, the risk to mothers when breastfeeding fails is now better understood. A growing body of research links lack of breastfeeding and early weaning to the number one killer of women, cardiovascular disease, as well as to breast and ovarian cancers, metabolic syndrome, Type-2 diabetes and many other life-threatening health problems. Because early weaning has significant negative effects on women's health—even decades later—no one can afford to be cavalier about breastfeeding outcomes.

What should you do if, despite all good intentions, your breastfeeding reach sometimes exceeds your grasp? Keep this book within easy reach. Use it to expand your knowledge and skills. Then, as I do, thank Catherine Watson Genna for compiling this outstanding work.

INTRODUCTION

Catherine Watson Genna

Breastfeeding is *normal* infant feeding. All that most infants need to breastfeed are a receptive state and the correct sequence of environmental signals. Infants placed on their mother's abdomen after unmedicated births are able to crawl up to the breast, attach deeply, and suck correctly. If those infants were either exposed to narcotic medications or separated from their mother for even a few minutes, they have greater difficulty finding the breast, and if they were both drugged and separated most fail even to attempt the normal seeking behavior.

The normal ability to self-attach, although strongest immediately after birth, does not become extinct for several months. It has been used successfully with older infants to overcome their learned resistance to attempting to latch. However, the older and more savvy an infant becomes, the more important cognitive processes become to feeding. Giving the right signals when an infant is in a receptive state can allow the neurobehavioral feeding program to overcome the infant's frustration with trying to get the breast to "work."

Understanding how infants expect to encounter the breast, the movement patterns that help them navigate and find their way, and the relationships to gravity that facilitate attachment to the breast helps the lactation consultant assist in cases where the dyad has not yet made breastfeeding work. Paradigms have shifted from infant helplessness models that required the mother to hold the baby's head, restrain the hands, and RAM baby onto the breast to facilitating mother-infant instinctual interactions and using gravitational stability as a base for infant competence. The information on latch in this edition has been completely revised to encompass research on biological nurturing and clinical experience in integrating these techniques into a clinical toolbox for dyads experiencing latch difficulties. Many more photos illustrate the latch techniques as well.

Inability to breastfeed is a red flag for further infant problems; breastfeeding is an essential component of normal infant life and its absence means something is fundamentally wrong with the infant's world. Minor anatomical variations such as ankyloglossia (tongue-tie) and recessed or small mandible can make breastfeeding more challenging. Breastfeeding management can often be modified to allow an infant with these conditions to feed successfully. Infants with respiratory issues such as laryngomalacia or tracheomalacia can usually be successful breastfeeders, with positional and temporal modifications.

Infants who are unable to breastfeed with proper management need careful examination of their cardiac, respiratory, musculoskeletal, gastrointestinal, metabolic, and neurological functioning. Any medical illness that causes pain can interfere with an infant's state control and neurobehavioral organization and make feeding more difficult. Some ill infants can work toward breastfeeding, some infants will not be capable for some time or at all, and their mothers can be supported to provide their milk in whatever way the infant can feed.

This edition contains a new chapter on biomechanics, an emerging frontier of lactation. Conditions which cause imbalance in muscle tone or restrict joint range of motion are often amenable to body work. A new chapter by pediatric chiropractor Sharon Vallone gives some basic information on ways that different practitioners can assist infants with musculoskeletal limitations.

This book is for any healthcare professional who works with infants. It is deliberately multidisciplinary because many different professionals work with new families and need to understand normal feeding, normal sucking, and how to help infants with problems. Specialization, although necessary, fragments knowledge, and teamwork is then required to assemble a whole picture. This book is intended to provide the information each team member needs about normal infant feeding to facilitate that teamwork, and to assemble in one volume many of the strategies that assist infants in sucking and feeding correctly.

Each profession has maxims that have been passed down through the generations without scrutiny. The authors of this work have endeavored to return to the research to try to share the most reliable information possible. Unfortunately, much of the research on infant feeding confuses cultural and biological norms. The text draws on both clinical experience and empirical evidence, and endeavors to differentiate clearly between the two.

I encourage you to read the book in order, and then return and re-read the assessment section at the end of Chapter 1 to help consolidate the information in a complete framework for breastfeeding evaluation.

Acknowledgments

Thanks to all the readers of the first edition who gave me feedback and shared your own expertise and experience—you've made this a stronger book:

Speech pathologists, occupational therapists, and feeding therapists who are at the forefront of helping infants with medical challenges achieve normal feeding.

Mothers of babies with rare disorders who shared details about how they made breastfeeding work with their children

The "tribe" of breastfeeding helpers who share information at conferences; on Lactnet, PPLC, and LactSpeak; and through mother-to-mother support group Leader/ Counselor networks and study groups. Thanks for your generosity, wise women and gentlemen.

My fellow members of the International Affiliation of Tongue-Tie Professionals, who generously share techniques and collaborate on research across disciplines so we can refine our understanding of normal and our judgment on when and how to intervene.

Medical, midwifery, and nursing professionals worldwide who understand that breastfeeding is so much more than just nutrition, and continue to facilitate normal birth, parenting and feeding on behalf of their tiny patients.

I am grateful to my contributors, and honored to have your participation in this book. Every one of you is a shining star in your field, with many demands on your time. Thank you for updating your chapters with the latest research and newest clinical skills.

Thanks to Diklah Barak, Karen McGratty, Rachel Myr, Lisa Amir, and Nina Berry for their research assistance. How wonderful to have friends on many continents who are able to retrieve articles that would otherwise be unavailable. Jennifer Petersen, thank you for your help with the chapter on bodywork.

A project of this magnitude would be impossible to add to my already busy life without support and practical help from my family. Thank you Dave for your love and support, and my Alyssa for taking over many of the little daily tasks that suck up time but are so essential for family life. And to all my family and friends, thank you for the emotional support and patience with my reduced availability. And special gratitude to Kathy M., Kathy W., Donna, and Angela for ensuring that moms in Queens got great lactation help when I needed to prioritize this book.

Finally, thanks to my "people" at Jones & Bartlett Learning: Sara Bempkins for doing all the boring editorial stuff with patience and grace; Jeanne Hansen for the extremely careful job of copyediting; and Carolyn Rogers for shepherding the book through production again.

And once again, thanks to my clients for trusting me with your precious children. You and they are my best teachers.

CONTRIBUTORS

Diklah Barak, BOT, IBCLC
Development and Feeding Therapist
Brooklyn, NY

Nils Bergman, MB, ChB, MPH, DCH, MD
Health Systems Research Unit, Medical Research Council of South Africa (Affiliate)
Professional Advisory Boards: LLL South Africa, Breastfeeding Associations of South Africa, International Lactation Consultant Association
Cape Town, South Africa

Elizabeth V. Coryllos, MS(s), MD, FAAP, FACS, FCCP, FAASP, FRCS(s), IBCLC
Associate Professor, Department of Surgery
Stony Brook University Medical Center of the State University of New York
Emeritus Director, Department of Pediatric Surgery
Winthrop University Hospital
Mineola, NY

Judy LeVan Fram, MEd, PT, IBCLC
Private Practice Lactation Consultant
Brooklyn, NY

Robin Glass, MS, OTR, IBCLC
Assistant Professor
Department of Rehabilitation Medicine
University of Washington
Seattle Children's Hospital
Seattle, WA

Rebecca Glover, RN, RM, IBCLC
Private Practice Lactation Consultant
Perth, Western Australia

*Kerstin Hedberg Nyqvist, RN, PhD, IBCLC**
Associate Professor in Pediatric Nursing
Department of Women's and Children's Healt
Uppsala University
Uppsala, Sweden

*Chele Marmet, BS, MA, IBCLC**
Director and Co-Founder, Lactation Institute
Los Angeles, CA

Lisa Sandora, MA, CCC-SLP, IBCLC
Speech-Language Pathologist and Lactation Consultant
TriHealth Bethesda North Hospital
Cincinnati, OH

*Ellen Shell, MA, IBCLC**
Co-founder, Lactation Institute
Encino, CA

Christina Smillie, MD, FAAP, FABM, IBCLC
Medical Advisory Board, La Leche League International
Medical Director, Breastfeeding Resources
Stratford, CT

Linda J. Smith, MPH, BSE, FACCE, IBCLC
Director of Perinatal Policy, American Breastfeeding Institute
Bright Future Lactation Resource Centre Ltd.
Dayton, OH

Sharon A. Vallone, DC, FICCP
Private Practice, KIDSPACE Adaptive Play, LLC
Postgraduate Faculty, Palmer College of Chiropractic, Davenport, IA and New Zealand College of Chiropractic, Auckland, NZ
Chair of the Board, Kentuckiana Children's Center, Louisville, KY
Vice Chair, International Chiropractors Association Council on Chiropractic Pediatrics

---

* Retired, not recertified

Diane Wiessinger, MS, IBCLC
Common Sense Breastfeeding
Ithaca, NY

Nancy Williams, MA, CCE, MFT, IBCLC
Private Practice, Marriage, Family, and Child Therapist
Consultant for Care Net Pregnancy Centers
Adjunct Faculty, Psychology Department, Brandman (Chapman) University, Santa Maria Campus, CA
Assistant Area Professional Liaison Leader, La Leche League of Southern California/Nevada

Lynn Wolf, MOT, OTR, IBCLC
Assistant Professor
Department of Rehabilitation Medicine
Seattle Children's Hospital
University of Washington
Seattle, WA

Photo Credits

CHAPTER 1

Figure 1-1: Courtesy of Brian Palmer, DDS.
Figure 1-2: © Catherine Watson Genna, BS, IBCLC
Figure 1-3: Courtesy of Peter Mohrbacher.
Figures 1-4 through 1-40: © Catherine Watson Genna, BS, IBCLC

CHAPTER 3

Figure 3-1: © Catherine Watson Genna, BS, IBCLC
Figure 3-2: Reprinted with permission by Linda J. Smith and Dennis Smith.

CHAPTER 4

Figures 4-1 through 4-5: © 2007, 2010, Christina M. Smillie, Ivy Makelin, and Kittie Frantz. Used with permission. Adapted from the DVD, C.M. Smillie, MD, *Baby-Led Breastfeeding: The Mother-Baby Dance*, available from GeddesProduction.com.

CHAPTER 5

Figure 5-1: Courtesy of La Leche League of Hong Kong.
Figure 5-2A: Courtesy of Karl B. Walker.
Figure 5-2B: Courtesy of Julie Nathanielsz.
Figure 5-2C: © Suzanne Colson
Figure 5-3: Courtesy of Scott Pryor.
Figure 5-4: Courtesy of Rebecca Glover.
Figure 5-5: Courtesy of Rebecca Glover.
Figure 5-6: Courtesy of John Wiessinger.
Figure 5-7: Courtesy of Rebecca Glover.

Figure 5-8: Courtesy of Rebecca Glover.
Figure 5-9: Courtesy of Rebecca Glover.
Figure 5-10: Courtesy of Shaughn Leach.
Figure 5-11: Courtesy of Rebecca Glover.
Figure 5-12: Courtesy of Rebecca Glover.
Figure 5-13A, B: Courtesy of Shaughn Leach.
Figure 5-14: Courtesy of Rebecca Glover.
Figure 5-15: Courtesy of Rebecca Glover.
Figure 5-16: Courtesy of Rebecca Glover.
Figure 5-17A, B, C, D: Courtesy of Rebecca Glover.
Figure 5-18A, B, C: Courtesy of Rebecca Glover.
Figure 5-19: © Catherine Watson Genna, BS, IBCLC
Figure 5-20A: Courtesy of Diane Wiessinger.
Figure 5-20B: Courtesy of Rebecca Glover.
Figure 5-20C: Courtesy of Barbara Wilson-Clay.
Figure 5-21: © Catherine Watson Genna, BS, IBCLC
Figure 5-22: Courtesy of Shaughn Leach.
Figure 5-23: Courtesy of Shaughn Leach.
Figure 5-24: Courtesy of Rebecca Glover.
Figure 5-25A, B: Courtesy of Diane Wiessinger.
Figure 5-26: Courtesy of Diane Wiessinger.
Figure 5-27: © Catherine Watson Genna, BS, IBCLC
Figure 5-28A, B, C, D: Courtesy of Diane Wiessinger.

CHAPTER 6

Figure 6-1: Reprinted with permission from Wolf, L. S., & Glass, R.P. (1992). *Feeding and swallowing disorders in infancy: Assessment and management*. Austin, TX: Pro-Ed.
Figure 6-2: © Catherine Watson Genna, BS, IBCLC
Figure 6-3: Reprinted with permission from Wolf, L. S., & Glass, R.P. (1992). *Feeding and swallowing disorders in infancy: Assessment and management*. Austin, TX: Pro-Ed.
Figure 6-4: Reprinted with permission from Wolf, L. S., & Glass, R.P. (1992). *Feeding and swallowing disorders in infancy: Assessment and management*. Austin, TX: Pro-Ed.
Figure 6-5: © Catherine Watson Genna, BS, IBCLC

CHAPTER 7

Figures 7-1 through 7-8: Reprinted with permission by Kerstin Hedberg Nyqvist, RN, PhD, IBCLC.

CHAPTER 8

Figures 8-1 through 8-56: © Catherine Watson Genna, BS, IBCLC

CHAPTER 9

Figures 9-1 through 9-12: © Catherine Watson Genna, BS, IBCLC

CHAPTER 10

Figure 10-1: Photograph by J. Petersen, 2009.
Figure 10-2A, B: Photograph by J. Petersen, 2008.
Figure 10-3: Photograph copyright permission granted by P.J. Harrison, Vancouver, Washington, 2006.
Figure 10-4: Photograph copyright permission granted by R. A. Bowen, Department of Biomedical Sciences, ARBL Colorado State University, Fort Collins, CO, 1994.
Figure 10-5: Photograph copyright granted by Sutherland Cranial Teaching Foundation.
Figure 10-6: Photograph copyright permission granted by the Craniosacral Therapy Educational Trust.
Figure 10-7: Photograph by J. Petersen, 2008.
Figure 10-8: Copyright Robert S. Pope, PhD, Department of Neurobiology and Anatomy, West Virginia University.

CHAPTER 11

Figures 11-1 through 11-12: © Catherine Watson Genna, BS, IBCLC

CHAPTER 12

Figures 12-1 through 12-10: © Catherine Watson Genna, BS, IBCLC
Figure 12-11A, B, C: Reprinted with permission by Mellanie Sheppard, BS, IBCLC.
Figures 12-12 through 12-48: © Catherine Watson Genna, BS, IBCLC

CHAPTER 13

Figures 13-1 through 13-31: Used with permission of the Lactation Institute/Chele Marmet.

CHAPTER 14

Figure 14-1: Courtesy of Nancy Williams, MA, IBCLC.

COLOR PLATES

Plates 1 through 7: © Catherine Watson Genna, BS, IBCLC

Plate 8: Reprinted with permission from "Morphological analyses of the human tongue musculature for three-dimensional modeling" by Takemoto, H., Journal of Speech, Language, and Hearing Research, 44, p. 105. Copyright 2001 by American Speech-Language-Hearing Association. All rights reserved.

Biological Nurturing® is a registered trademark of The Nurturing Project, Ltd. in the United States and other countries.

CHAPTER

1

Breastfeeding: Normal Sucking and Swallowing

Catherine Watson Genna and Lisa Sandora

Normal Sucking

All mammals share a neurobehavioral program for sucking. They are competent to get to the teat—without maternal assistance—attach to it, and transfer milk. Humans are no exception. When born without labor medications and placed immediately on mom's abdomen, a human infant goes through the following behavioral sequence leading to breastfeeding (Ransjo-Arvidson et al., 2001):

1. Hand-to-mouth movements
2. Tongue movements
3. Mouth opening
4. Focusing on the nipple
5. Crawling to the nipple
6. Massaging the breast to evert the nipple
7. Licking
8. Attaching to the breast

Labor medications and separation from mother disrupt this sequence and can lead to incorrect sucking patterns (Righard & Alade, 1990). A later return to skin-to-skin contact can reestablish the original behavioral sequence and allow the infant to learn to attach (see Chapter 4).

Much of the difficulty with inducing infants to breastfeed is due to failure to understand their behavioral sequence and the environmental triggers for each behavior. Human infants expect positional stability; complete prone positioning against mom's abdomen or chest allows the infant better neck control and refined jaw and tongue movements. The gravitational input from being prone on a semireclined mother optimizes feeding-related reflex behaviors, facilitating latch and breastfeeding (Colson, Meek, & Hawdon, 2008). When infants self-attach, they extend their neck and lead with their chin. When the chin contacts the breast, the baby starts seeking the nipple. When the nipple contacts the philtrum (the ridge between the nose and upper lip), the baby gapes widely and grasps the nipple and the surrounding tissue with the tongue, seals to the breast, and begins to suck. Infants use tactile (touch) and olfactory (smell) cues to help them identify the nipple (Porter & Winberg, 1999). An infant who has difficulty locating the nipple with the face or mouth may use the hands to assist the search (Genna & Barak, 2010).

One can use these expectations to assist babies who have difficulty latching on. The infant helplessness model leads moms to try to do too much for the baby, and many mothers handle their breast like a bottle, trying to center the nipple in the baby's mouth. Healthy, neurotypical infants simply need snug support against mom's ribcage and tactile proximity to the breast, preferably so the nipple is at the philtrum and the chin is on the breast, and they are able to open well, bring the tongue down, lunge forward, and grasp the breast. When infants are unable to self-attach, special techniques can be used to assist them. These are covered in Chapter 5.

Although a neurobehavioral program guides the initial attachment and sucking experiences, rapid learning occurs. Human infants are able to experiment with different sucking pressures and different lip, tongue, and jaw movements to maximize the amount of milk they obtain or to reduce an uncomfortably fast flow. Some of these compensations will be adaptive for the infant and comfortable for the mother, but some will not and will require intervention. This book focuses on interventions that have proven helpful in practice.

In order to intervene in any process, it is important that normal be well understood. Ideally, the infant orients to the nipple (rooting response), opens the mouth widely (gape response), and brings the tongue down to the floor of the mouth and extends it over the lower lip to grasp the breast. As the mouth closes, the anterior tongue cups the breast, and the body of the tongue grooves to conform to and hold the breast. The breast is enclosed between the grooved tongue, cheeks, and palate, forming a teat. The nipple is as far back in the mouth as possible, generally to the posterior hard palate (Jacobs, Dickinson, Hart, Doherty, & Faulkner, 2007).

After attachment, the infant holds the breast with the anterior and mid-tongue, and the lips assist. The soft palate hinges downward and contacts the back of the tongue. The soft palate, grooved tongue, lips, and cheeks make a sealed chamber around the nipple. The baby then drops the back of the tongue and lower jaw to produce negative (suction) pressure (Geddes, Kent, Mitoulas, & Hartmann, 2008). The tongue is still grooved from front to back, which allows the milk that sprays from the nipple to gather in a small pool, or bolus. The soft palate elevates, and the pharyngeal walls contract to meet it in order to close off the nasopharynx, or nasal air space. Finally, the vocal folds are closed by the arytenoid cartilages approximating (moving together), the epiglottis tilts down to direct milk around the vocal folds, the suprahyoid muscles pull the larynx upward to shorten the pharynx, and the tongue uses positive pressure to push (Kennedy et al., 2010) the bolus of milk into the pharynx for transit to the esophagus during swallowing.

Anatomy

The newborn human mouth is particularly well designed for sucking (**Figure 1-1**). The tongue is large in relation to the size of the oral cavity. When the mouth is open, the tongue

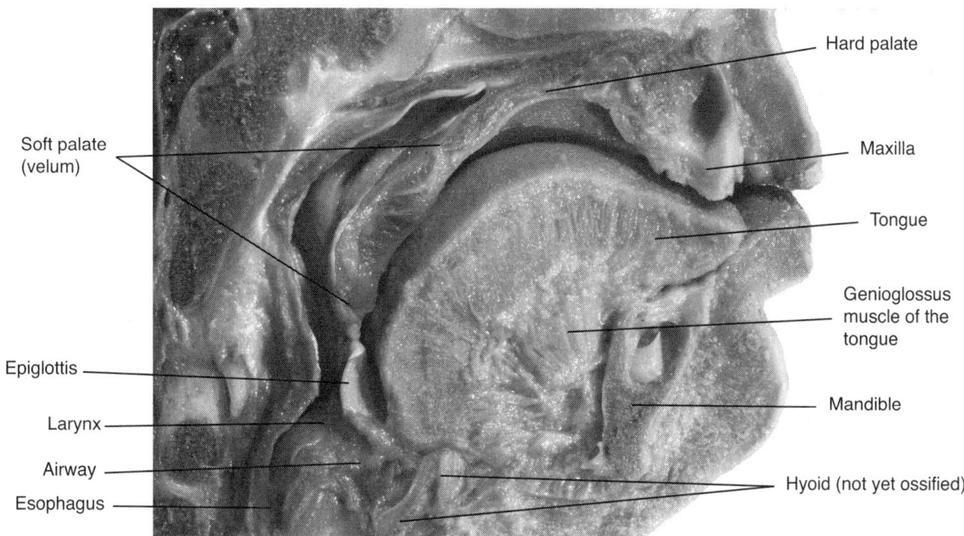

Figure 1-1 Midsaggital section, oral anatomy of a 7-month fetus.

and breast fill it completely, providing stability to the tongue and jaw movements. The normal resting position of the tongue is with the tip over the lower lip, where it can easily contact the breast.

The cheeks contain fat pads that add to the thickness of the cheek wall and help guard against collapse of the cheeks when the oral cavity is enlarged by tongue depression (**Figure 1-2**). If the cheeks collapse, the oral cavity becomes smaller and the negative pressure decreases. Ultrasound studies have demonstrated that the negative pressure in the mouth is vital to milk transfer (Ramsay & Hartmann, 2005) and that milk flows from the breast when the posterior tongue is down and the suction pressure is highest (Geddes et al., 2008). The fat pads of the cheeks also provide lateral (side) borders to keep the tongue in midline during sucking. Although newborns can perform lateral (side-to-side) tongue movements, these are generally not used during feeding until solids are begun after 6 months of age. The *buccinators* are the muscles of the cheek, which compress the cheeks when activated to maintain contact between the

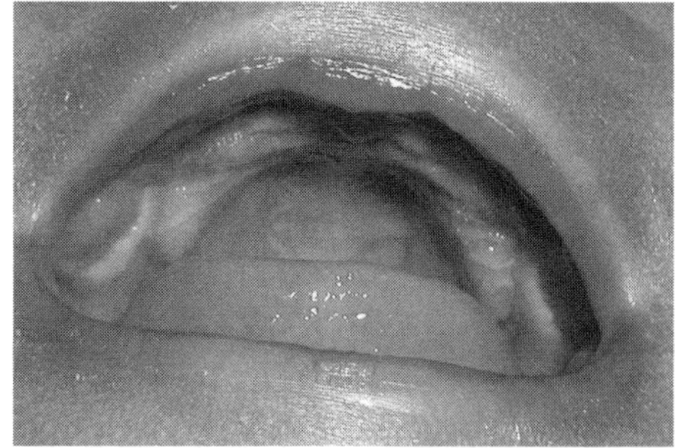

Figure 1-2 Buccal fat pads provide lateral stability to the tongue in newborns.

cheek and breast during breastfeeding and to keep food in contact with the teeth during chewing. The buccinators are innervated by the facial nerve.

The lips are soft and flexible, and the lower lip is generally flanged outward on the breast, allowing contact with the soft mucous membrane. The upper lip is usually in a more neutral position when attachment is correct. (An overly turned-out upper lip is a sign of a shallow latch and can favor excessive use of the lips to press milk out of the breast.) Around the outside of the soft lips is a complex circular muscle made up of many fibers, named the *orbicularis oris*. Partial contraction of this muscle helps maintain the lips' seal on the breast. The mentalis muscle at the base of the lower lip elevates and protrudes the lip, and it is very active during breastfeeding. These muscles are innervated by the facial nerve.

The mandible (lower jaw) is usually short in newborns, due to the position of the chin on the chest in utero, which may mechanically restrict jaw growth. The infant's predominant flexor muscle tone pattern, which favors jaw opening over closing, may help compensate for the short mandible. Poor grading of movement (fine control over the speed and amount) also favors a large gape. The masseter muscle on the outside of the jaw and the medial pterygoid on the inner side relax to depress the mandible, and they contract to elevate the mandible during sucking. Both sides working together allow symmetrical jaw movement during sucking; unilateral action of the masseter and lateral pterygoid causes the sideways jaw movements of chewing. The temporalis muscle closes the mandible during sucking. The fibers of the muscles of mastication (chewing) are more similar to cardiac muscle than normal skeletal muscle, allowing for faster functioning and less fatigue (Korfage, Koolstra, Langenbach, & van Eijden, 2005a; Korfage, Koolstra, Langenbach, & van Eijden, 2005b). These muscles of mastication are innervated by the trigeminal nerve's third (mandibular) branch.

Tongue and jaw motions are linked through mutual attachments to the hyoid bone to make it easier for the infant to use the tongue and jaw in concert during sucking. The mandible raises to help generate positive pressure during swallowing, and the mandible drops during suction (negative pressure). The tongue is a complex structure made of interdigitated muscle layers. In the past, a distinction was made between extrinsic and intrinsic tongue muscles, but careful dissections using advanced staining techniques have revealed that fibers from muscles that were thought to arise outside the tongue become incorporated into the body of the tongue (Hiiemae & Palmer, 2003; Takemoto, 2001). It is helpful to think of intrinsic muscles as changing the shape of the tongue and extrinsic muscles as connecting the tongue to other structures to help it move in concert with those structures (such as the soft palate and hyoid).

The intrinsic muscles of the tongue include the genioglossus, which pulls the tongue down during the negative pressure phase of sucking; the superior longitudinal muscles, which lift the tongue tip; the inferior longitudinals, which lower the tongue tip and help move it from side to side; the vertical muscles, which help thin the tongue; and the transverse muscles, which along with the genioglossus and the extrinsic muscles help to groove the tongue (**Figure 1-3**). Most of the fibers of the intrinsic tongue muscles are fast responding,

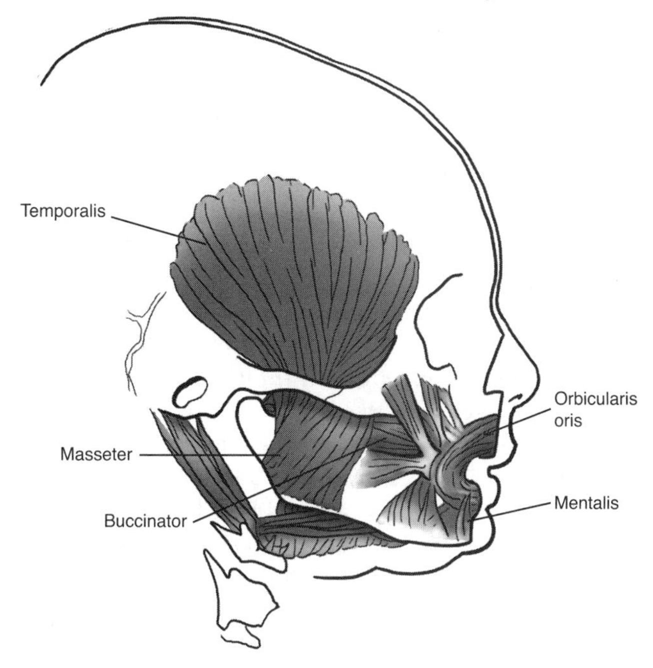

Figure 1-3 Facial muscles involved in feeding.

allowing rapid changes in tongue configuration (Stal, Marklund, Thornell, De Paul, & Eriksson, 2003). The extrinsic muscles include the palatoglossus, which helps elevate the back of the tongue and brings the soft palate down to seal the back of the mouth; the styloglossus, which helps pull the tongue up and back; and the hyoglossus, which retracts and pulls the tongue down low in the mouth. All the tongue muscles except the palatoglossus are innervated by the hypoglossal nerve (XII); the palatoglossus is innervated by the vagus nerve (X). An understanding of the arrangement and relationships of the tongue muscles allows facilitation of correct sucking in infants with difficulties. See **Plate 8** for a three-dimensional representation of the arrangement of the muscles of the tongue, courtesy of Hironori Takemoto, PhD.

In humans, the airway and food passages cross, creating a *biological timeshare* (Cichero, 2007). Air passes from the nasopharynx through the pharynx and into the larynx through the vocal folds to the trachea, bronchi, and lungs. Food passes from the oropharynx through the pharynx, around the epiglottis, and to the esophagus. To reduce passage of air to the stomach, the cricopharyngeus muscle remains contracted to close the top of the esophagus unless a swallow is occurring. To keep food out of the airway, the larynx elevates and the true and false vocal folds close, and the epiglottis tips over the airway. The muscles of the airway and food passages are innervated by the vagus nerve (X).

Newborns have unique anatomical airway protection to help compensate for their immature laryngeal closure. At birth, the hyoid bone is still cartilage and not yet mineralized. The larynx is high, reducing the amount of space the bolus needs to travel. The epiglottis is high and elongated; it touches or overlaps the soft palate at rest, and the upper airway is very short. This helps to direct milk to the esophagus and reduces the risk of aspiration. This airway configuration also encourages the infant to extend the neck, which reduces resistance to airflow in the airway and brings the small mandible forward to have as much contact with the breast as possible. Tongue and mandible contact with the breast needs to be as complete as possible for proper mechanical advantage during sucking.

Suckling or Sucking: Differences Between Suckling at the Breast and Sucking at the Bottle

Older literature on feeding posits that suckling (the front-to-back, wavelike movement of the tongue) changes to sucking (a straight up-and-down movement of the tongue and jaw) at around 3 months of age. A Japanese study (Iwayama & Eishima, 1997) of breastfed and bottle-fed infants, which used bottles, showed a transition to a sucking pattern in infants older than age 3 months, but this might have been due to mechanical differences between breast and bottle or growth of the oral cavity in relation to the static artificial nipple. Electromyography (EMG) studies have confirmed that muscle activation is different between breastfeeding and bottle feeding, with less use of the mentalis and masseter muscles and more use of the buccinator and orbicularis oris muscles in bottle feeding (Gomes, Trezza, Murade, & Padovani, 2006; Inoue, Sakashita, & Kamegai, 1995; Nyqvist, 2001). Lactation consultants have long been skeptical of the idea that there are two age-dependent forms of sucking at the breast. The author's ultrasound suck research has shown that breastfeeding children up to 4 years old use the same sucking pattern reported by Geddes, Kent, Mitoulas, and Hartmann (2008) and Miller and Kang (2007). For this reason, the term *suckling* shall be used to mean the act of feeding at the breast, and the term *sucking* will be used to describe the oral motor activity that transfers milk, with the understanding that breastfeeding is the biological norm for human beings, and normal sucking is the sucking that occurs at the breast.

Deglutition (Swallowing)

For professionals working with children who have feeding issues, there are two terms that are useful to understand: feeding and swallowing. *Feeding* refers to what takes place during the *oral preparatory phase*, from sucking up to bolus formation, and the *oral phase*, propelling the bolus posteriorly in the mouth. In contrast, *swallowing* encompasses all four phases: the oral preparatory, oral, pharyngeal, and esophageal phases from when the milk enters the mouth until it enters the stomach. The primary focus of the lactation consultant is to assess the feeding aspects (the oral preparatory and oral phases); however, it is important to understand the entire process and how posture and positioning affect swallowing. Generally, evaluation of the pharyngeal and esophageal phases are carried out through instrumental tests, such as the videofluoroscopic swallow study (VFSS) and fiberoptic endoscopic evaluation of swallowing (FEES) discussed later in this chapter. **Figure 1-4** shows the appearance of the upper digestive tract of an older infant on a VFSS. Tests are typically ordered by a physician and performed and interpreted by speech-language pathologists or occupational therapists.

The anatomical structures used for feeding are also used for breathing and speech production. An infant is faced with the challenge of using these structures in a highly orchestrated way in order to maintain oxygenation and acquire adequate intake to grow.

Sucking is the initial stage of a four-part swallowing process (Corbin-Lewis, Liss, & Sciortino, 2005; Logemann, 1998). Swallowing has four phases that must take place in a synchronous, organized fashion for safe feeding to occur.

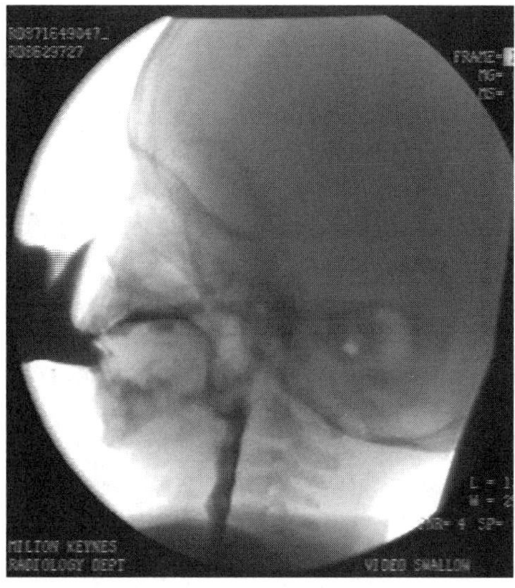

Figure 1-4 VFSS of a toddler drinking from a sippy cup. The dark liquid outlines the path milk takes during swallowing.

Although both sucking and swallowing occur prenatally, they do not necessarily occur together. In utero, both sucking and swallowing have been observed in fetuses as early as 12.5 weeks of age. Color Doppler sonography reveals amniotic fluid flow consistent with mature swallow in some fetuses starting at 29 weeks gestation and in a larger proportion by 37–38 weeks (Grassi, Farina, Floriani, Amodio, & Romano, 2005). A full-term fetus swallows 450 ml of amniotic fluid in a day (Bosma, 1986). This volume is greater than early postnatal daily intake. This discrepancy may be due to the need for the neonate to coordinate sucking, swallowing, and breathing. The high viscosity and low volume of colostrum make it a safer food for an inexperienced newborn, and the fact that it is less fluid than the baby is accustomed to may increase motivation to breastfeed often and stimulate maternal milk production. Indeed, more frequent breastfeeding (Chen, Nommsen-Rivers, Dewey, & Lonnerdal, 1998; Bystrova et al., 2007) and more efficient milk removal (Morton et al., 2009) in the first days of life lead to increased milk production even weeks later. Conversely, birth interventions, maternal obesity, and mother–infant separation also delay copious milk production and reduce colostrum and milk intake (Chantry, Nommsen-Rivers, Peerson, Cohen, & Dewey, 2011; Matias, Nommsen-Rivers, Creed-Kanashiro, & Dewey, 2010; Nommsen-Rivers, Chantry, Peerson, Cohen, & Dewey, 2010). See Chapter 3 for more information.

Healthy human infants rapidly improve their coordination of swallowing and breathing over the first few days (Weber, Woolridge, & Baum, 1986) and weeks of life, even when held in awkward (supine) positions for breastfeeding to allow comparison with bottle-fed infants (Kelly, Huckabee, Jones, & Frampton, 2007; Weber et al., 1986). With increasing age, newborns are more likely to breathe out right after swallowing during breastfeeding than bottle feeding (Kelly et al., 2007), which provides another layer of protection against aspiration. Older infants who are breastfeeding and growing normally swallow with each suck cycle during the mother's milk ejection (Geddes, Chadwick, Kent, Garbin, & Hartmann, 2010) and vary the location of the swallow in the respiratory cycle (D. T. Geddes, personal communication, July 2008).

Neural Control of Sucking and Swallowing

Cranial nerves in the brainstem provide the sensory and motor fibers that innervate and provide feedback to the face, mouth, pharynx, larynx, and stomach. Two sets of specialized nerve tracts in the brainstem, referred to as the swallowing centers, direct movements for swallowing. Sensory fibers from the cerebral cortex, cerebellum, and brainstem influence coordination of swallowing (Morris & Klein, 2000, p. 47). Functional magnetic resonance imaging (MRI) studies of brain activation during voluntary swallows in adults have shown that brain regions involved in controlling the swallow include the somatosensory and motor cortex areas, the cerebellum, thalamus, putamen, cingulate gyrus, and insula (Cichero & Murdoch, 2006; Malandraki, Sutton, Perlman, Karampinos, & Conway, 2009). Infants with neurological deficits are therefore at risk of dysphagia (swallowing abnormalities).

Reflexive Control of Sucking and Swallowing

The newborn infant depends primarily on reflexes for feeding. Reflexes are prewired templates for life-sustaining movements in the infant that gradually become integrated into voluntary movement patterns (**Table 1-1**) or become inhibited by higher brain centers as these mature.

The *rooting* reflex is stimulated by touch to the face and mouth. It causes the infant to turn toward the breast, open the mouth, depress and extend the tongue, and grasp the breast.

The *transverse tongue* reflex occurs when the lateral edge of the tongue is stroked. The infant's tongue should move toward the source of stimulation. *Tongue protrusion* occurs when the anterior tongue is touched. The *phasic bite* reflex is not elicited during sucking unless the infant retracts the tongue and exposes the gum ridge to stimulation. These reflexes diminish by around age 6 months in preparation for the introduction of solid foods.

Like sucking, *swallowing* is not a simple reflex; it encompasses complex, highly orchestrated sensory and motor events that are under both voluntary and involuntary control (Arvedson & Brodsky, 2002).

The *cough* reflex is of great importance to feeding because it allows the infant to expel material that has entered the airway and/or has been aspirated. This protective reflex is triggered by sensory receptors (chemoreceptors) in the larynx, causing the vocal folds to snap shut and a cough to propel the foreign material out of the airway (Arvedson & Lefton-Greif, 1998). In preterm infants, the laryngeal chemoreflex is not as mature, and the infant may experience the apnea component (to avoid breathing in the fluid that has penetrated the larynx) and bradycardia (slow heart rate) but not cough to expel the fluid. Since normal breathing does not resume until after the cough clears the airway, preterm infants are at risk of stopping breathing if they fail to swallow safely. As vagus myelination improves with maturity and feeding experience, these issues resolve (Becker, Zhang, & Pereyra, 1993; Newman 1996).

Table 1-1 Oral–Motor, Cranial Nerve, and Reflex Evaluation

Reflex	Stimulus	Behavior	Cranial Nerves Involved	Present At
Protective Reflexes				
Cough	Fluid in larynx or bronchi	Upward movement of air to clear the airway	X Vagus	35–40 weeks gestation
Gag	Touch back of tongue	Mouth opening, head extension, floor of mouth depresses	IX Glossopharyngeal X Vagus cortex	26–27 weeks gestation
Adaptive Reflexes				
Phasic bite	Stimulate gums	Rhythmic up and down jaw movement	V Trigeminal	28 weeks gestation
Transverse tongue	Stroke sides of tongue	Tongue moves toward side of stimulus (lateralizes)	XII Hypoglossal	28 weeks gestation
Tongue protrusion	Touch tongue tip	Tongue protrudes from mouth	XII Hypoglossal	38–40 weeks gestation
Rooting	Stroke cheek or near mouth	Infant senses stimuli and localizes toward source, opens mouth (gapes), extends and depresses tongue to grasp breast, creates seal against breast	V Trigeminal VII Facial XI Accessory XII Hypoglossal	32–37 weeks gestation (MMP*)
Sucking	Touch to junction of hard/soft palate	Wavelike tongue movement coordinated with up and down jaw movement	V Trigeminal VII Facial IX Glossopharyngeal XII Hypoglossal	

*Majorie Meyer Palmer, NOMAS Certification Course, 2006.
Source: Adapted from Hall, 2001.

The *gag* reflex is the other protective reflex that prevents the infant from swallowing a solid object or a bolus larger than the pharynx can handle.

The Four Phases of Swallowing

In order to develop an understanding of the four phases of the swallow, a listing of the phases and the structures involved in each phase are as follows (Stevenson & Allaire, 1991):

Oral preparatory phase:

- Lips
- Tongue/mandible
- Cheeks
- Hard palate

Oral transitory phase:

- Tongue/mandible

Pharyngeal phase:

- Soft palate (velum)
- Pharyngeal muscles surrounding the throat
- Epiglottis
- Laryngeal muscles
- Arytenoid mass (made up of the false vocal folds, true vocal folds, and arytenoid cartilages; the arytenoid cartilages sit on top of the true vocal folds posteriorly, and they open the airway during breathing and close the airway during swallowing)
- Upper esophageal sphincter

Esophageal phase:

- Esophagus

How the Four Stages of Deglutition Work

Oral Preparatory Phase

Rooting, attachment, and sucking comprise the beginning of the oral preparatory phase. During sucking, the tongue forms a central trough or groove for channeling the milk

Is It Tongue Stripping (Positive Pressure) or Suction (Negative Pressure) That Removes Milk?

Studies have described infants as using a stripping, wavelike tongue motion (Bosma, Hepburn, Josell, & Baker, 1990; Hayashi, Hoashi, & Nara, 1997; Newman, 1996; Weber et al., 1986) during feeding. Geddes (née Ramsay) (Geddes, Kent, Mitoulas, & Hartmann, 2008; Ramsay & Hartmann, 2005) indicate that milk is not removed by the stripping motion of the tongue. These ultrasound studies indicate that milk flows due to the creation of suction (negative pressure) when the tongue and jaw drop during sucking.

The movements that appear to be tongue stripping may in reality be the tongue modulating pressure changes to create the positive pressure that pushes the bolus toward the esophagus during swallowing. As research continues, the mechanisms for milk removal from the breast will be further elucidated.

posteriorly. The lateral edges of the tongue seal to the palate to keep the bolus organized (Cichero & Murdoch, 2006; Yang, Loveday, Metreweli, & Sullivan, 1997). Milk is delivered onto the tongue as the back of the tongue drops to create negative pressure in the mouth.

Oral Transitory Phase

Wavelike mechanical movements and pressure changes (positive pressure) created by the tongue propel the bolus to the back of the oral cavity.

Pharyngeal Phase

In newborns, the presence of the bolus at the valleculae at the base of the tongue triggers the swallow. The following mechanisms for protection of the airway are engaged (Arvedson & Brodsky, 2002; Mendell & Logemann, 2007; Moriniere, Boiron, Alison, Makris, & Beutter, 2008):

1. The breathing stops.
2. The soft palate (velum) elevates to close off the nasal cavity and prevent the bolus from going into the nose (nasopharyngeal reflux), and the outer layer of pharyngeal muscles contract to shorten the pharynx.
3. The true and false vocal folds (cords) come together to close over the trachea.
4. The hyoid moves up and anteriorly.
5. The larynx (suspended from the hyoid by muscles and cartilage) is elevated by this same upward movement, compressing the upper airway.
6. As the tongue moves the food posteriorly by creating positive pressure, the epiglottis also moves back and downward over the larynx to divert the bolus laterally and back toward the esophagus.
7. The pressure of contractions of the inner layer of pharyngeal muscles moves the bolus to the esophagus.
8. The upper esophageal sphincter opens, and the bolus enters the esophagus.

What Is Peristalsis?

Peristalsis is defined as "progressive contraction down a muscular tube." This is the activity seen in the esophagus as the bolus is progressively moved toward the stomach. Logemann (1998) points out that it is inaccurate to use this term in reference to the movement of the bolus in the oral and pharyngeal phases of the swallow because anatomically they are not muscular tubes. Rather, there are pressure changes propelling the bolus. This can be seen by the rolling wave of the tongue in the oral cavity creating positive pressure, which move the bolus over the base of the tongue (Logemann, 1998). Therefore, the term *peristalsis* will be used in this text to describe what occurs in the esophageal phase, and tongue movements involved in swallowing will be described as *wavelike*.

It is important that the pharyngeal phase of the swallow be well coordinated because this is the phase during which there is the greatest risk of aspiration. The infant's ability to propel the bolus to the tongue base (valleculae) is important for setting the pharyngeal phase in motion and signaling the onset of the cascade of movements that protect the airway and direct the bolus to the esophagus (Arvedson & Brodsky, 2002).

Esophageal Phase

The bolus moves through the esophagus (food tube) toward the stomach, consisting of the following stages:

1. Peristaltic movement of the bolus through the esophagus
2. Opening of the lower esophageal sphincter to allow the bolus to enter the stomach

Dysphagia

Dysphagia, or swallowing disorder, can range from mild to severe. The feeding specialist, a speech-language pathologist or occupational therapist, sometimes in cooperation with a specialist physician, assesses the swallowing mechanism during the oral and pharyngeal phases. The clinical examination involves observing oral movements in isolation and while the infant is feeding. If a swallowing problem is suspected, instrumental procedures are carried out to identify the source of the swallowing disorder and which phase or phases are disrupted. **Table 1-2** shows the evaluation procedures that are used to identify dysphagia. For a more extensive discussion of these instrumental procedures, refer to Arvedson and Brodsky (2002).

Feeding Assessment

Feeding assessment is a complex process that involves observation of oral structure and oral motor functioning, as well as observation of the global body condition including muscle tone, energy level, appropriate arousal, and aerobic capacity. All body systems participate in feeding, not just the gastrointestinal and renal systems, whose involvement is obvious. Feeding is aerobic exercise for the human infant, so the heart, lungs, and

Table 1-2 Instrumental Procedures for Identifying Dysphagia

Instrumental Procedure	Parts of Swallow Studied
Upper gastrointestinal study (upper GI)	Esophagus, stomach, duodenum
Videofluoroscopic swallow study	Oral preparatory, oral, pharyngeal, upper esophageal phases of swallowing Identifies cause of dysphagia and aspiration
Ultrasound	Oral preparatory and oral phases of swallowing
Cervical auscultation (CA)	Sounds of breathing and swallowing in pharyngeal phase
Fiber-optic endoscopic evaluation	Looks at pharyngeal and laryngeal structure of swallowing (FEES) before and after the swallow

Cervical Auscultation

Listening over the neck or under the chin with a stethoscope is an easy, useful way for lactation consultants to scrutinize swallowing sounds. Normal swallowing sounds like a crisp, rapid biphasic click (Vice, Bamford, Heinz, & Bosma, 1995; Vice, Heinz, Giuriati, Hood, & Bosma, 1990). Wet, bubbling sounds can indicate air passing through an incompletely cleared pharynx (Bosma, 1986), and short, discrete bouts of stridor during the swallow can indicate that fluid has leaked into the larynx (laryngeal penetration). In addition, delayed initiation of the swallow, inefficient swallowing (multiple swallows needed to clear the pharynx), and slower than normal swallowing (a drawn-out click that represents a small bolus) can be identified (Cichero & Murdoch, 2002). The integration of swallowing and breathing can clearly be heard because inspiration and expiration each have characteristic sounds. Feeding-induced apnea or breath-holding (several swallows without an intervening breath) becomes obvious, as do stressed swallows. Infants with clinical symptoms due to dysphagia (repeated respiratory infections, feeding refusal) that do not resolve with management changes (prone feeding to assist bolus handling, applying pressure on the breast near the areola to obstruct some ducts during rapid milk flow, feeding from a partially pumped breast, treatment of tongue-tie if indicated, calibration of milk supply to meet infant need if hyperlactation is responsible) should be referred for VFSS to determine whether oral feeding is safe. Exclusively breastfed infants rarely have repeated respiratory infections even if they are aspirating because human milk is less irritating to the human respiratory epithelium than other foods. In this case, breastfeeding with interventions to improve handling of flow can continue, but caution is warranted when weaning begins (feeding any liquid or food other than human milk).

circulatory system are vital for providing the oxygen necessary for the work of feeding. The musculoskeletal system participates both in providing stability for the infant and in performing specific movements that allow milk to be transferred from the breast to the infant's mouth and into the GI tract while excluding it from the respiratory passages. Cellular respiration (mitochondrial enzymes) provides the energy for each cell from the metabolism of blood-borne glucose, which is maintained by the liver and pancreas and the hormonal systems of the body. The nervous system must work properly to direct the activities of all the other systems.

A healthy infant, given a normal environment, can perform the necessary functions to maintain life and health, one of which is feeding. As mammals, human infants have the ability to move to, attach to, and remove milk from the mammae, or breasts. Conversely, if a newborn in a normal environment cannot breastfeed, the index of suspicion is increased that all is not well. Healthy infants indicate hunger by feeding behaviors, which include lip smacking, tongue movements, hands to mouth, squirming, and scanning with the cheeks and moving themselves from an adult's shoulder down to the breast (or from mom's belly up to the breast using the stepping reflex). These behaviors were once seen as hunger cues, but now it is understood that they are functional behaviors that are part of the competent infant's feeding sequence. When mothers are educated to work with these normal behaviors, attachment to the breast becomes far easier.

This section will provide a framework for evaluating the infant's feeding behaviors at the breast. The purpose is to provide the reader with a system for evaluating the dynamics of feeding and swallowing from a breastfeeding perspective so an intervention plan can be developed.

Most infants seen by lactation consultants have minimal or mild disorders. These may be transient problems, such as incoordination of suck–swallow–breathe due to inexperience or poor feeding secondary to labor medications, or they may be persistent, such as the abnormal tongue movements from a tight lingual frenulum. These infants may have difficulty transferring milk at the breast but may be able to functionally bottle feed, offering false reassurance. Abnormal tongue movements may persist without intervention. In contrast, infants with moderate to severe problems are likely to have difficulty with both breastfeeding and bottle feeding and are more easily identified. Tracheomalacia or laryngomalacia may first become apparent as feeding volumes increase over the first few days of life. Lactation consultants (LCs) may therefore be the first to identify the short sucking bursts and stressed respiration typical of a respiratory anomaly. It is important for all members of the healthcare team to work together in the baby's best interest. Breastfeeding is usually an achievable goal, given practice, milk expression to support milk production, and supplementation in a manner supportive of normal feeding skills.

Breastfeeding promotes normal physiological development and optimal growth and function of the orofacial structures. Each step in normal development depends on the step before, and though the child may be able to function using compensatory strategies, these compensations do not promote optimal development. Therefore, early intervention may avoid the need for more extensive therapy later.

Ideally, a *feeding team* addresses significant feeding and/or swallowing issues. A feeding team is a group of specialists who work together to develop an individualized feeding program for the infant or child. A pediatrician or neonatologist may serve as the medical coordinator. A speech–language pathologist, occupational therapist, nurse, and dietitian are included in the basic team. Other team members may include a social worker, psychologist, physical therapist, gastroenterologist, neurologist, otolaryngologist, pulmonologist, allergist, endocrinologist, and dentist. Team members evaluate the infant's skills from their professional perspective and report the results to the team. For example, the otolaryngologist may assess the integrity of the infant's oral, pharyngeal, and laryngeal structures through endoscopy and report to the team any abnormalities in anatomy and physiology along with suggestions for treatment. The feeding team devises a plan of action that will address the infant's needs (Arvedson & Lefton-Greif, 1998; Morris & Klein, 2000). In order to participate as a feeding team member, the LC should have an understanding of normal feeding, techniques for assessing problems, and interventions for facilitating development of feeding skills.

Factors Affecting Feeding

Gestational Age

In order to assess the infant's feeding behavior, the clinician should have an understanding of how the infant develops and what to expect in terms of reflexive oral behaviors, state, endurance, and coordination of sucking, swallowing, and respiration. The younger the gestational age of the infant, the more his or her feeding skills are likely to be disrupted by lower aerobic capacity, lower muscle tone, lower energy, and decreased neurological maturity.

Preexisting Medical Diagnosis

Information about medical conditions that affect feeding competence will shed light on the infant's capabilities, challenges, and behaviors. It is useful to keep the diagnosis in mind but approach the infant as an individual with his or her own set of feeding skills. It is helpful to know if and how the medical condition typically affects feeding and swallowing, while realizing that there is always a contiriuum of effects and the individual may be mildly, moderately, or severely affected in each area.

Screening Tools Versus Assessment Tools

A *screening tool* identifies individuals at risk for feeding and swallowing problems by a rapid observation of signs and symptoms. An *assessment tool* provides more in-depth information as to the nature of the problem so that a plan of corrective or facilitative action can be taken (Logemann, 1998).

Current breastfeeding assessments are technically screening tools that have been devised primarily to identify which breastfeeding behaviors are present in the mother and infant and if the potential for breastfeeding to occur is present. These are predominantly observational scales where the LC or nurse indicates the presence or absence of behaviors associated with breastfeeding. These screening tools have primarily been designed for use in the early postpartum period and may be viewed as a signal that breastfeeding is not getting off to a good start. Dyads identified as at risk can then be referred for further assessment and intervention to protect the mother's milk production in the sensitive calibration phase and ensure the infant's nutrition.

Examples of breastfeeding screening tools that can be used with term infants are as follows:

- Infant Breastfeeding Assessment Tool
- Latch Assessment Documentation Tool
- Via Christi Breastfeeding Assessment Tool
- Mother-Baby Assessment Tool

The Preterm Infant Breastfeeding Behavior Scale (Nyqvist, Rubertsson, Ewald, & Sjöden, 1996) is an observational tool for use with preterm infants to identify prebreastfeeding and early breastfeeding behaviors.

For a complete in-depth description of these and other breastfeeding scales, consult Walker (2006, pp. 116–126).

Other Oral Motor Assessment Tools

Speech pathologists and occupational therapists have used observational feeding tools to observe infant bottle feeding behaviors in the preterm and term population. The Neonatal Oral-Motor Assessment Scale (NOMAS) was developed to assess bottle feeding, though the author states that it can be used with breastfeeding infants as well (Palmer, 2006). The NOMAS is used to rate tongue and jaw movements during both nonnutritive and nutritive sucking. Infants with problems are diagnosed with disorganized sucking if they have deficiencies of rate and rhythm, or they are diagnosed with dysfunctional sucking if they display abnormal tongue or jaw movements that interrupt the feeding (Palmer, 1998).

Another observational tool, the Early Feeding Skills (EFS) Assessment (Thoyre, Shaker, & Pridham, 2005), is a cue-based approach to feeding assessment and intervention in preterm hospitalized infants. The EFS is a checklist for determining infant readiness and tolerance for feeding based on infant physiologic, motor, and state regulation; oral-motor abilities; and coordination of suck-swallow-breathe.

Facilitation Versus Compensation

Techniques for assisting with feeding issues fall under two categories:

- *Facilitative strategies:* Techniques that encourage normal development
- *Compensatory strategies:* Techniques that allow for more optimal feeding but do not change the underlying problem

Examples of facilitative strategies used with breastfeeding babies include the following (adapted from treatment strategies in Hall, 2001):

- Skin-to-skin contact with the mother to increase arousal and interest in the breast
- Regulation of suck-swallow-breathe bursts (also called external pacing) with clinician-imposed pauses prior to coughing, drooling, or color changes in the infant, either by removing the baby from the breast or by pressing on the breast to block some ducts to reduce milk flow
- Oral stimulation to increase feeding readiness

Examples of compensatory strategies used with breastfeeding babies include the following:

- Approaching the infant when he or she is alert and ready to breastfeed
- Maintaining a quiet environment conducive to attending to feeding
- Attempting alternative positioning to compensate for infant or maternal anatomical variations
- Cuddling and flexing the infant when stress cues are exhibited
- Using a nipple shield when the infant has difficulty grasping the breast due to tongue-tie
- Using a nipple shield when the infant is preterm and cannot maintain attachment
- Providing cheek support when the baby has low tone, carefully observing for the ability to handle flow rate
- Providing jaw support for wide jaw excursions to prevent loss of attachment

These strategies are just a few examples of ways to improve feeding skills. The determination of what strategies are appropriate for an individual infant can be made when a complete assessment is carried out.

Clinical Breastfeeding Assessment

An in-depth breastfeeding assessment will give the clinician more specific information about the infant's feeding ability at the breast. A detailed assessment facilitates the formulation of a care plan for alleviating the problem. According to Arvedson and Lefton-Greif (1998), there are two basic questions asked during a feeding and swallowing evaluation: What is the cause of the problem? and How can it be fixed? This approach can also be adapted to the clinical breastfeeding assessment.

The steps of a clinical breastfeeding assessment are as follows:

1. Determine whether the breastfeeding problem is the result of
   a. basic positioning or attachment issues;
   b. an underlying anatomical problem in the infant (or a problematic interaction with the mother's anatomy);
   c. an underlying neurological problem in the infant.
2. Analyze the steps needed to alleviate the problem:
   a. Correct basic attachment, positioning, and management.
   b. Identify and implement compensatory techniques for anatomical problems and/or refer to another professional for further evaluation and treatment (e.g., frenotomy).
   c. Identify and implement facilitative techniques to improve neurological development and/or refer to another professional with specific expertise in this area.

3. Collaborate with the parents on an individualized plan for them to follow at home to meet their breastfeeding goals with both short-term and long-term objectives.
4. Provide education, anticipatory guidance, demonstration, and return demonstration of the techniques to be followed.
5. Arrange for follow-up.

Morris and Klein stated, "Assessment and treatment are sides of the same coin. Each assessment contains treatment probes to discover the most effective approaches to remediating the difficulties that have brought the child and family for the evaluation" (2000, p. 174). This perspective can also apply to the clinical breastfeeding evaluation, where compensatory and facilitative techniques can be incorporated by the clinician. Both compensatory and facilitative techniques should be practiced during the assessment to determine their effectiveness in enhancing feeding skills. If successful, they can be incorporated into the feeding plan.

The clinical assessment consists of several areas of evaluation. Some clinicians carry out all of the following areas, whereas some focus only on specific areas:

- Oral-motor observation of the infant and digital suck examination
- Breast examination of the mother
- Breastfeeding assessment of the infant and mother, including assessment of milk transfer
- Assessment of feeding using compensatory techniques, facilitative techniques, and alternate feeding devices (when appropriate)
- Milk expression (when appropriate)

Global Observations of the Infant

As part of the initial portion of the assessment, it is useful to globally observe the following characteristics related to the infant's neurological and physiological functioning:

- Tone
- Grading of movement
- Symmetry
- State and level of arousal or alertness
- Respiratory pattern
- Color

This information will be used as a baseline for comparison when the infant is engaged in feeding. A global assessment is useful because it can yield information that will contribute to the clinician's understanding of what may be happening during a feeding. The following information provides some guidelines.

Tone

An infant with low muscle tone may let the extremities hang, recruit accessory muscles to help maintain stability, or use fixing to help compensate (see Chapter 11). There may be hypotonia in the facial area where the infant appears expressionless. At the breast, the hypotonic infant may lose suction and spill milk from the mouth. A hypertonic infant may exhibit arching when put to the breast and have a retracting jaw when sucking. Hypertonic infants may seem stiff and may have difficulty opening the mouth wide (gaping) and initiating sucking bursts. These effects and compensations are usually easily visible, as are excessive excursions (downward movement) of the mandible that cause the lip seal to be disrupted. See **Figures 1-5 through 1-7** for examples of infants with hypotonia and normal muscle tone.

Infants may increase their tone in response to stress. The facial expression (wide or narrowed eyes, furrowed forehead) will usually help differentiate a stressed infant from a hypertonic one.

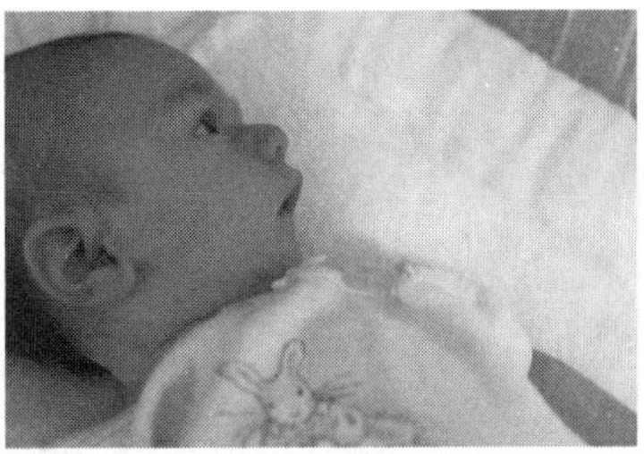

Figure 1-5 Infant with benign neonatal hypotonia. Note that the mouth hangs open and arms fall to the side of the body.

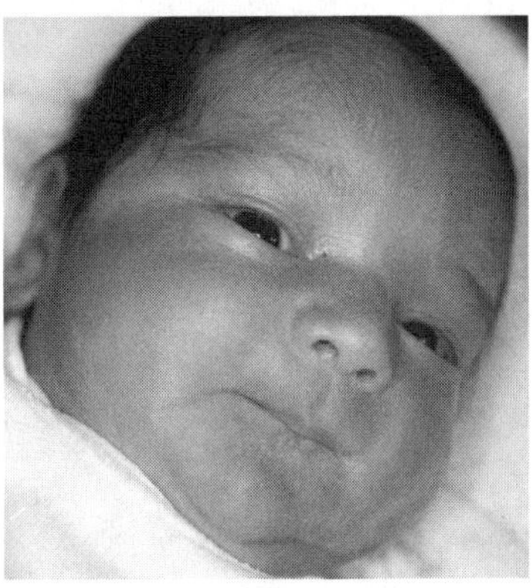

Figure 1-6 Infant with normal muscle tone. Note the crisp creases from normal contraction of the muscles of facial expression.

Grading of Movement

Infant grading (smoothness) of motion generally depends on stability. Neurologist Amiel-Tison noted that head and neck support improved fine motor control in neonates (Gosselin, 2005). When prone on the semireclined mother's trunk or abdomen, infants are capable of remarkably accurate movement (Colson et al., 2008). A head lift cannot generally be maintained more than a second or two, but that is long enough for the baby to bob his or her way to the breast. The quality of grading will also be apparent in the jaw movement. The movements should be smooth and equal, in midline, with a slight pause or bounce or accentuation of the downward jaw excursion as the baby maintains negative pressure in the mouth and draws milk from the breast.

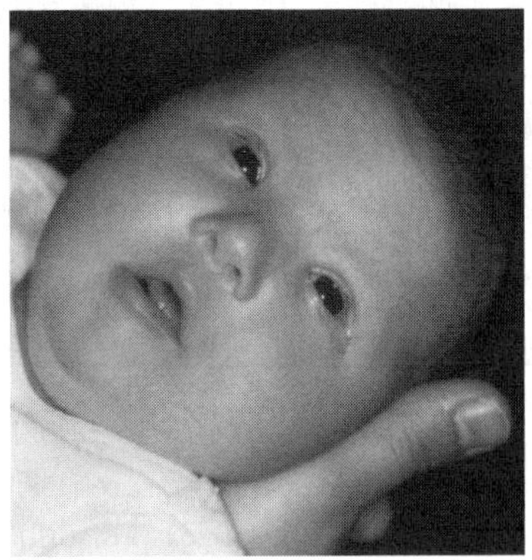

Figure 1-7 Infant with hypotonia due to Down syndrome. Note the expressionless look due to low tone of facial muscles.

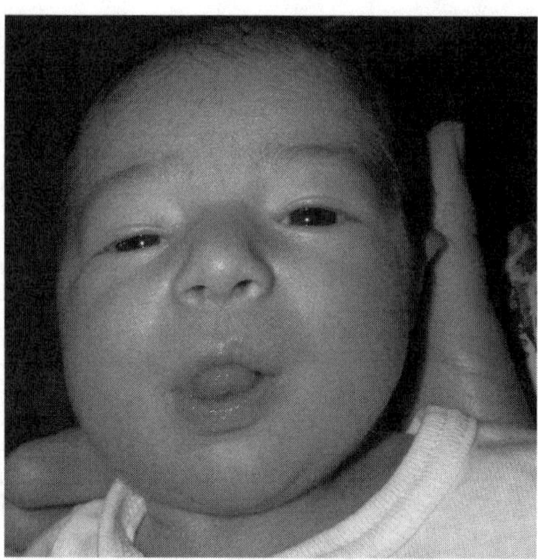

Figure 1-8 Facial and neck asymmetry from torticollis.

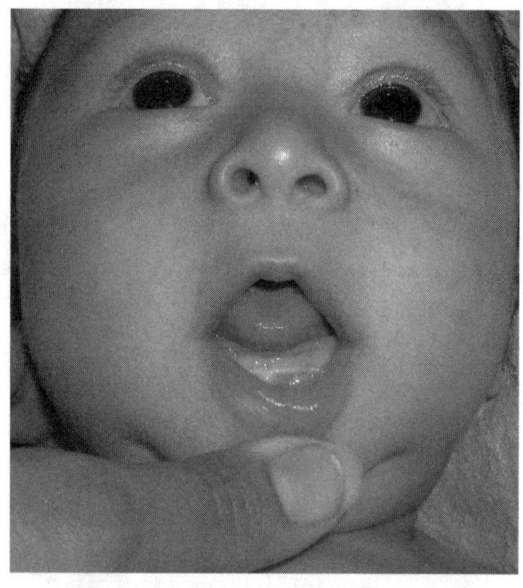

Figure 1-9 Normal symmetry.

Symmetry

Symmetry across the midline is an indication of equal nerve and muscle activity on each side of the body. Nerve palsies, birth injuries, and adverse effects of restricted in utero positioning, such as torticollis, may all cause asymmetry and feeding difficulties (**Figures 1-8 and 1-9**).

State and Level of Arousal (Alertness)

Infants who are transferring milk are usually alert, with open eyes and an intent facial expression. As the feeding progresses and the baby becomes sated, the fingers generally relax and open, the eyes close, and the muscle tone softens. Infants who are hyperaroused may cry or be unable to inhibit rooting and move on to the next step of attachment. Most LCs have seen infants who shake their heads furiously, trying to identify the nipple when it is already in the mouth. Sliding the baby's body toward mom's contralateral breast and bringing the lower lip and tongue closer to the areolar margin (and farther from the nipple) will often allow the tongue to contact the breast and the baby to attach. Using gravity (using a semi-reclined maternal position) so the infant's chin digs into the breast may achieve the same goal. Infants who are underaroused may fall asleep before attaching. Infants who find feeding threatening or stressful will show motoric, behavioral, and autonomic signs, including color changes, increased respiratory rate, tone changes, yawning, tuning out, and crying (see Chapter 10).

Respiratory Pattern

An infant's respiratory rate (RR) must be slow enough to coordinate with sucking and swallowing (**Table 1-3**). Though most infants are not able to feed with an RR over 80, if the infant is willing to breastfeed, he or she is probably capable of doing so. It is normal

Table 1-3 Respiratory Pattern

Resting Respiratory Rates for Infants	Breaths per Minute
Term infant	30–40
Preterm infant	40–60 (reflects cardiorespiratory immaturity)
Ill infant	60–80

Source: Adapted from Hough, 1991 (as cited in Arvedson & Lefton-Greif, 1998).

for RR to increase during respiratory pauses in feeding, but it should stabilize again before the infant begins another sucking burst. Respiratory effort should remain normal through the feeding; overuse of chest or throat muscles during breathing indicate excessive work of respiration. Short sucking bursts with long respiratory pauses may indicate cardiorespiratory immaturity or instability.

Color

Changes in skin color can reflect reduced oxygenation due to cardiorespiratory problems or autonomic instability secondary to stress. These are most apparent around the mouth, eyes, and nipples, and in the hands and feet. Mottling usually reflects a chilled infant. Pallor, duskiness, and cyanosis (blueness) are signs of reduced tissue oxygenation. Flushed and ruddy colorations are usually a sign of autonomic instability. A gray infant may have a cardiac problem. (See **Plates 1 and 3** for photos of cyanosis.)

Neurological Screen of the Infant

Probing the infant's reflexes reveals valuable information about the infant's neurological status. **Table 1-1** on page 9 summarizes the information necessary to assess the cranial nerves and reflexes the infant uses in feeding (adaptive reflexes) and airway protection (protective reflexes). An alert infant who does not exhibit adaptive behaviors may have a neurological deficit.

Oral Assessment of the Infant

A visual examination of the infant's oral structures will provide useful information regarding the structures at rest and in isolated movements. The clinician may also want to do a digital examination of the infant sucking nonnutritively to assess the tongue's range of motion. Sucking behavior is better assessed when fluid (a few drops of expressed milk from a dropper or syringe) is used during a digital suck exam. This allows evaluation of sequential tongue movements, adaptability to different flow conditions, and coordination of sucking, swallowing, and breathing. It is normal for infants to modulate sucking pressure in response to milk flow. During nonnutritive sucking, the hungry neurotypical infant keeps increasing the sucking pressure in an attempt to get milk and will decrease sucking pressure when milk is delivered.

Offering a finger across the baby's lips both shows respect for the infant's personhood and prepares him or her to suck. When the baby opens the mouth, allow the gloved finger to touch the tip of the tongue and observe whether the infant draws the finger in or not. If the tongue retracts, note this and try to stimulate the front of the lower gum to see if the baby will extend the tongue. When the baby draws the finger in, note how well the tongue grooves around the finger and the strength of the tongue movements. When the fingertip is near the junction of the hard and soft palate, the infant will generally begin to suck. Note how well the baby maintains contact with your finger during the suck. After assessing the nonnutritive suck, give some drops of expressed milk and note any changes in the sucking pattern. The baby should be able to keep the anterior tongue grooved around your finger while the posterior tongue and jaw drop to create negative pressure. The sucking should be deep, drawing, and rhythmic. If the anterior or midtongue loses contact with the finger, the baby may lose the latch; if the tongue retracts, allowing the tooth-bearing surface of the lower gum ridge to contact the finger, the baby will bite or chew. Note any sliding of the tongue. If this occurs on the finger, it will likely be worse on the breast because the mouth is more open while breastfeeding than finger sucking, providing more challenge to tongue mobility. A forceful posterior tongue elevation or high vacuums are other compensations that can be identified on a digital suck exam. Some infants hold the breast with the anterior tongue flat, rather than grooved, which requires more muscular effort and pressure to maintain a stable mouthful. This compensation for lack of tongue grooving will be apparent on a digital suck exam as well.

Tongue

A well-coordinated tongue that has full range of motion is of great importance in feeding and the oral preparatory and oral stages of swallowing. Note the tongue's appearance, any anatomical variations, and symmetry or asymmetry of movements. The clinician can observe tongue movements while interacting with the infant or elicit them with a gloved finger. The following movements can be observed or elicited, and any inabilities or limited abilities to perform the movements can be recorded along with possible causes:

- Ability to protrude or extend tongue (during quiet alert state interactions or when the lower gum ridge is stimulated with the clinician's fingertip; see **Figure 1-10**)
- Ability to lateralize tongue (when the outer gum ridge is stroked from the center to the side by the clinician's digit; see **Figure 1-11**)
- Ability to elevate tongue (observe for elevation of the tongue tip to the palate if the infant cries or attempt to stimulate this action by touching the upper gum ridge with a gloved finger; see **Figure 1-12**)

Anatomical Variations of the Tongue. The relative tongue length may impact feeding skills. A short tongue may restrict the ability to attach to the breast, and a long tongue may be held on the palate and may not develop normal coordination. A submucosal frenulum may retract the tongue and make it appear short (see Chapter 9), but a truly short tongue will have normal mobility. Asymmetry of the tongue can be structural or can result from an underlying neurological problem, in which case the tongue deviates to the stronger side (**Figure 1-13**). A

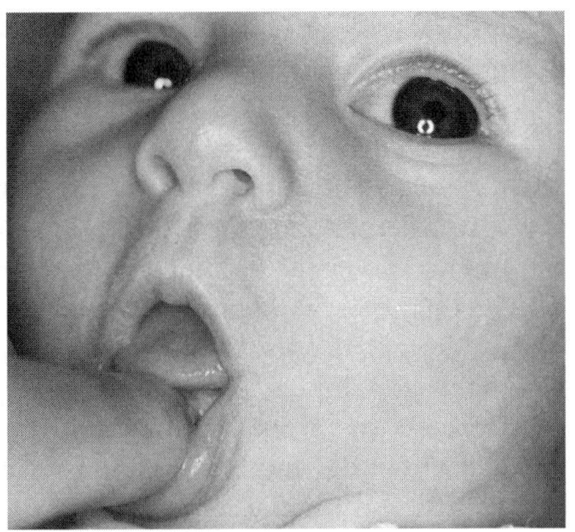

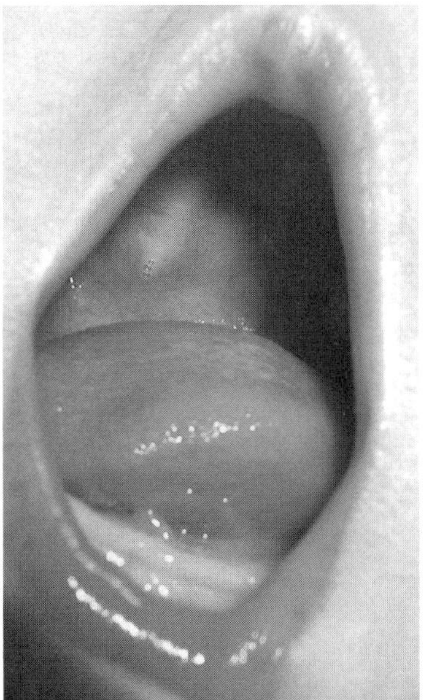

Figure 1-10 (Above) Normal tongue extension.

Figure 1-11 (Top right) Normal lateralization.

Figure 1-12 (Right) Normal elevation.

Figure 1-13 (Bottom left) Asymmetrical tongue movement due to tongue-tie.

Figure 1-14 (Bottom right) Flat tongue due to both tongue-tie and hypotonia.

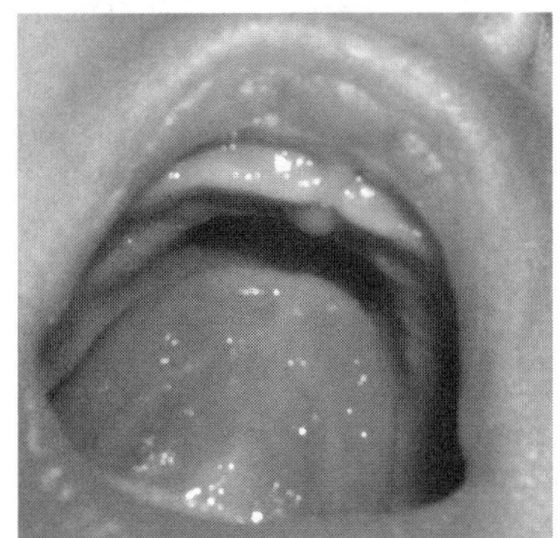

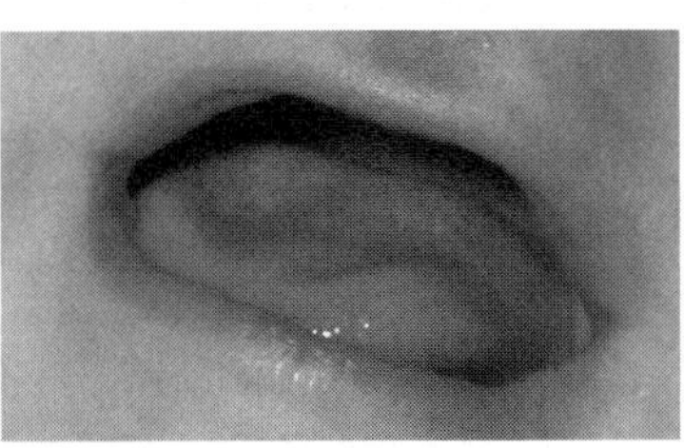

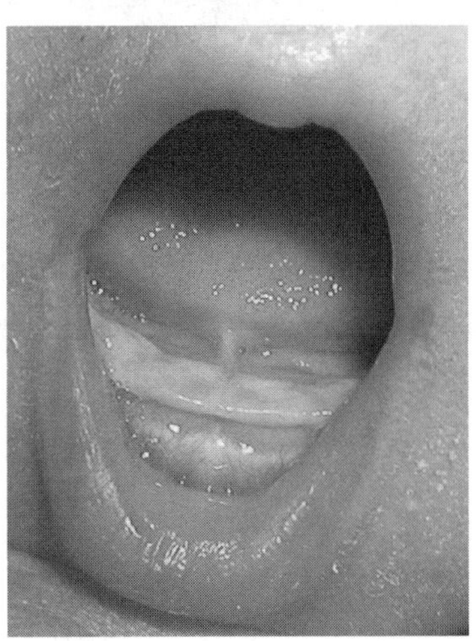

flat tongue may indicate low tone or a severe tongue-tie (**Figure 1-14**). Infants with decreased muscle tone, an excessively large tongue, or a small mandible may also protrude their tongue at rest. Preterm infants may adopt an open-mouth posture with the tongue protruded in an effort to open the airway when there are respiratory issues. Tongue tip elevation in a preterm infant indicates stressed respiratory status and unreadiness to feed. (See **Plate 7** for a photo of an infant fixing the tongue to the palate.) Changing the infant's position to reduce respiratory stress (particularly placing the baby skin to skin with the mother) may improve feeding readiness.

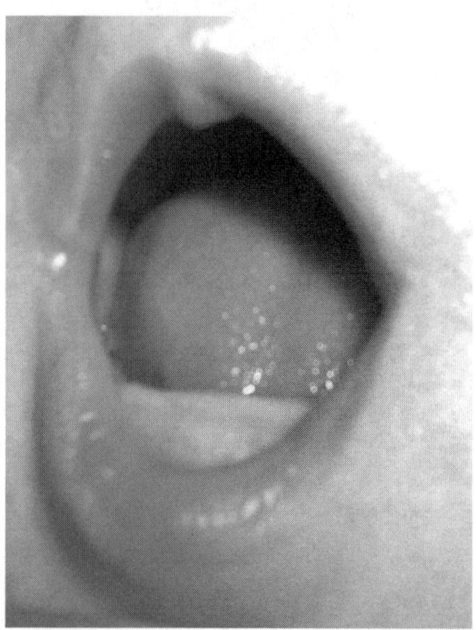

Figure 1-15 Tongue retraction and posterior elevation (humping) due to tongue-tie.

An infant with posterior tongue elevation (humping) at rest will block the oral cavity and make attachment difficult (**Figure 1-15**). A tongue with a thick, bunched configuration that distributes its muscle mass posteriorly when retracting is usually restricted by a tight lingual frenulum. Tongue retraction also prevents the tongue from grasping the breast and is a common cause of latch failure. It is often postulated that infants who have had unpleasant oral experiences will use the tongue to block access to the mouth. Although this is not proven, infants are sentient beings and deserve to be treated with respect.

Range of motion is perhaps the most important factor in an infant's ability to breastfeed with tongue-tie. A thin, elastic frenulum will generally impact tongue movement less than a thick, fibrous one. Elasticity of the floor of the mouth may partially compensate for a restrictive lingual frenulum. If the floor of the mouth is tight and the frenulum is short and inelastic, the infant is at risk for very poor tongue function. The extent of the lingual frenulum along the underside of the tongue is another important determinant of function, with a longer attachment generally restricting tongue elevation and extension more than a shorter one of equal thickness and elasticity.

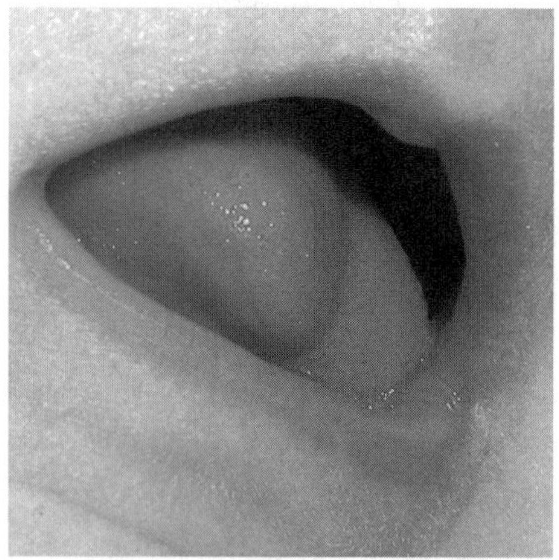

Figure 1-16 Bunched tongue due to tongue-tie. Note how the entire length of the tongue is pulled down in midline by the frenulum.

A severely restrictive lingual frenulum will usually keep the tongue behind the gum line, especially as the mouth opens. The tongue will appear flat or bunched into an unusual configuration (**Figure 1-16**). Touching the future tooth-bearing

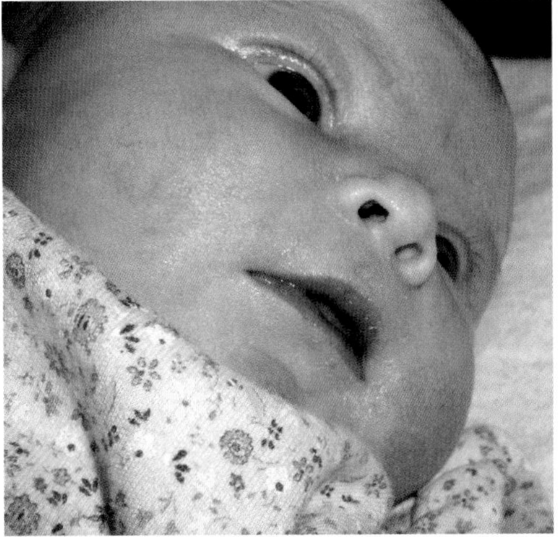

Plate 1 Circumoral and periorbital cyanosis.

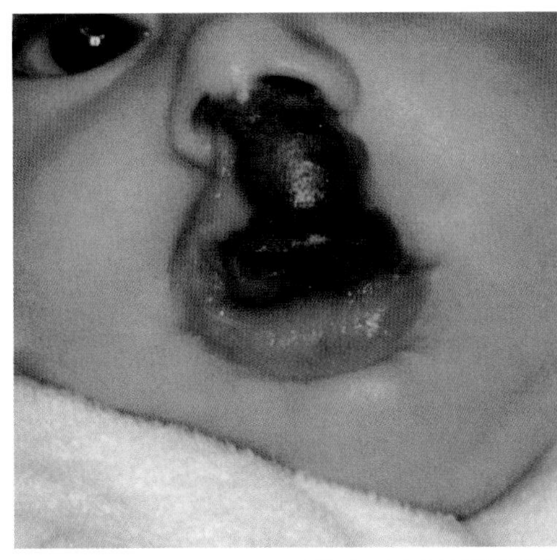

Plate 2 Ulcerated hemangioma.

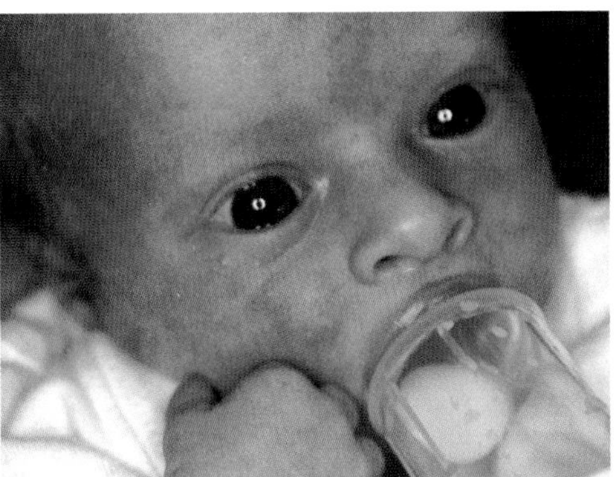

Plate 3 Fixation of the orbicularis oris causes mild cyanosis around the mouth.

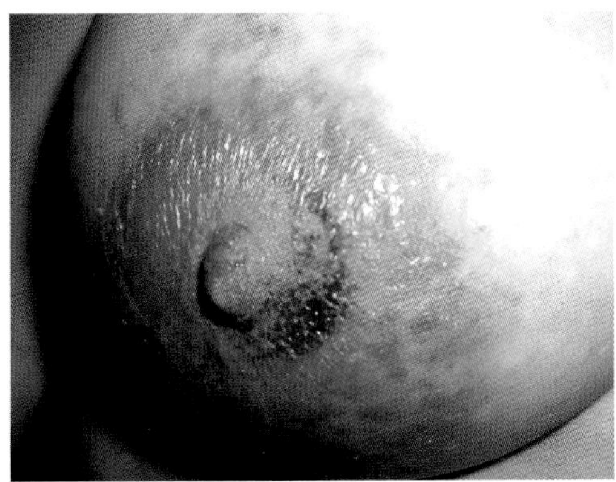

Plate 4 Breast injury from sliding of the tongue and jaw in a micrognathic infant. Increased head extension changed sucking mechanics and allowed spontaneous healing.

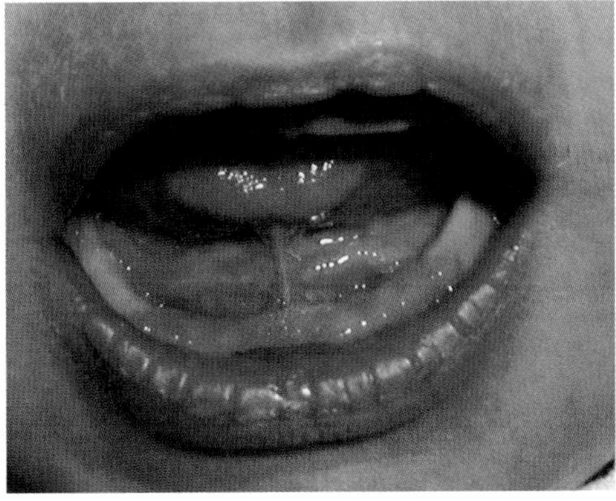

Plate 5 Blanching of the tongue tip on attempted elevation in a severely tongue-tied infant.

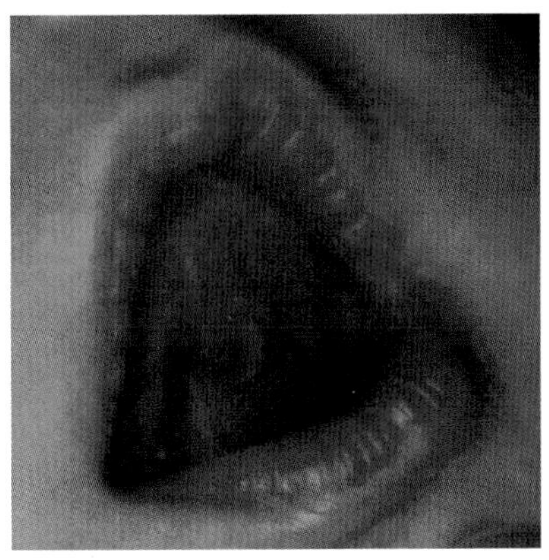

Plate 6 Tongue tip elevation in an infant with a shorter than average mandible.

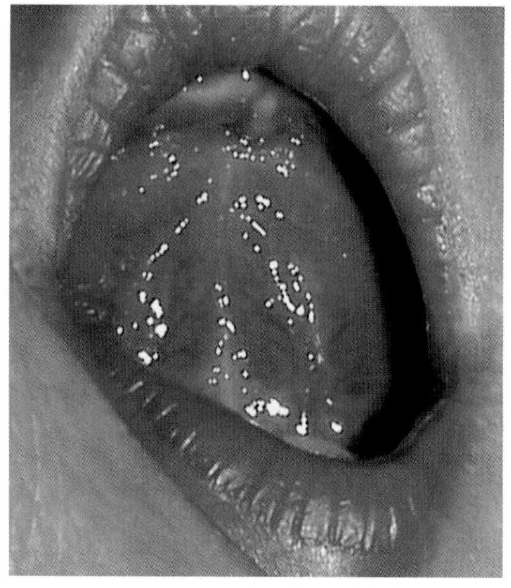

Plate 7 Tongue tip fixing to stabilize the airway in a micrognathic infant. Note the muscular tension in the tongue.

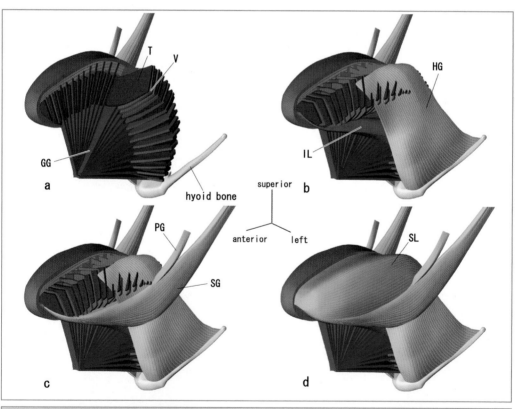

"Extrinsic" Muscles		"Instrinsic" Muscles	
GG genioglossus	SG styloglossus	SL superior longitudinal	V vertical
PG palatoglossus	HG hyoglossus	IL inferior longitudinal	T transverse

Plate 8 Spatial arrangement of muscle fibers in human tongue.

surface of the exposed lower gum ridge triggers reflexive biting, which is normally inhibited by the presence of the tongue tip. The combination of inability to elevate the tongue to grasp the breast and the triggering of the normal phasic bite reflex causes these infants to chew at the breast.

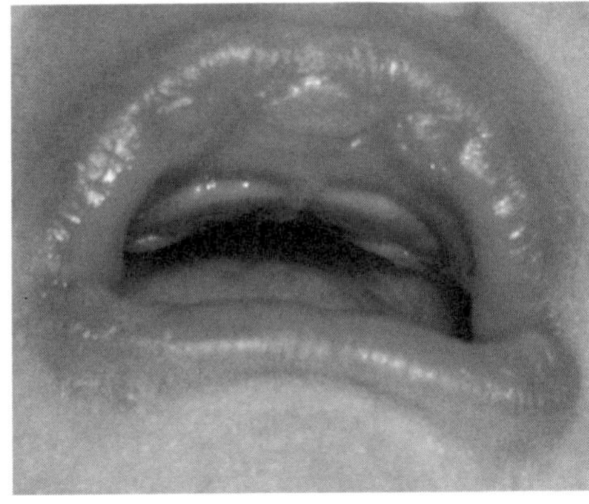

Figure 1-17 Tight labial frenulum. Note the large blister on the center of the upper lip.

Fasciculations or Tremors of the Tongue and/or Mandible. Neurologically immature or impaired infants can exhibit tremors during activity or at rest due to insufficient muscle activation by the brain (see Chapter 11). Muscle fasciculations can also occur due to fatigue in tongue-tied infants who recruit accessory muscles and use less ergonomic compensatory sucking strategies. This a reliable sign that the infant is working too hard to feed. Oral anatomy and oral motor function should be thoroughly assessed when tremors occur, and growth should be followed closely.

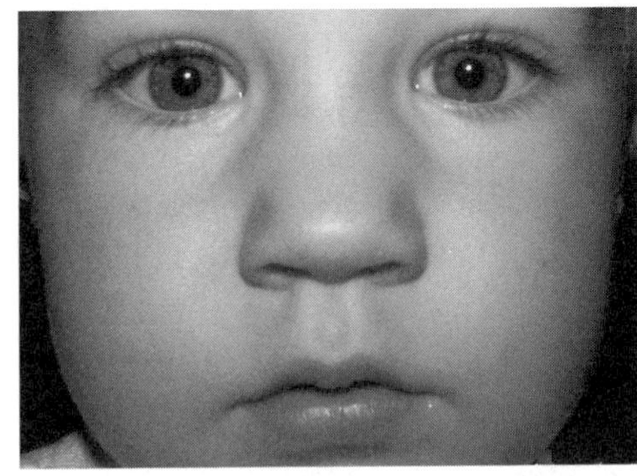

Figure 1-18 Gull wing sign and paranasal bulge in a toddler with soft palate dysfunction.

Lips

Lips are gently applied to the breast with the lower lip flanged completely outward and the upper lip neutral to lightly flanged. A tight superior labial frenulum can produce sucking blisters on the mucosal surface of the upper lip (**Figure 1-17**) and can make it more difficult to maintain latch. Infants with restrictive tongue attachments may use sweeping motions of the upper lip during sucking, causing a large sucking blister on the vermillion border of the upper lip. Observe the lips and note any anatomical variations. Make note of any asymmetry, which is often due to nerve damage and muscle weakness that causes the lip to deviate (pull) toward the stronger side. Increased or decreased tone can occur with neurological deficits.

An indentation of the upper lip vermillion (gull wing sign), especially when paired with a paranasal bulge, can indicate the presence of an occult submucosal cleft (Stal, 1998) (**Figure 1-18**). A cleft of the lip may or may not influence the infant's ability to breastfeed, depending on the existence of a concomitant submucous cleft of the palate and how well the mother's breast tissue fills the defect.

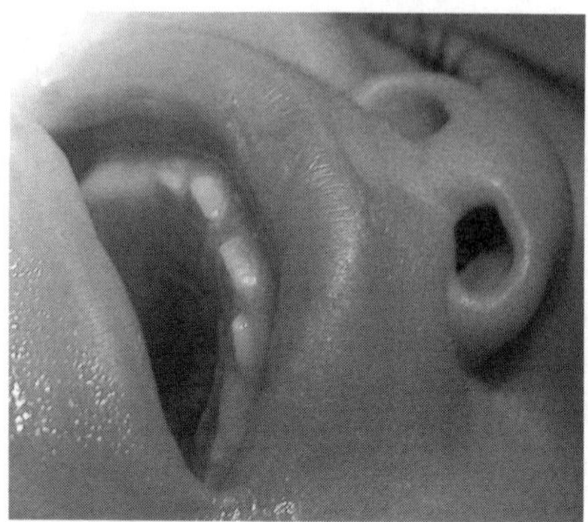

Figure 1-19 Flared nostrils.

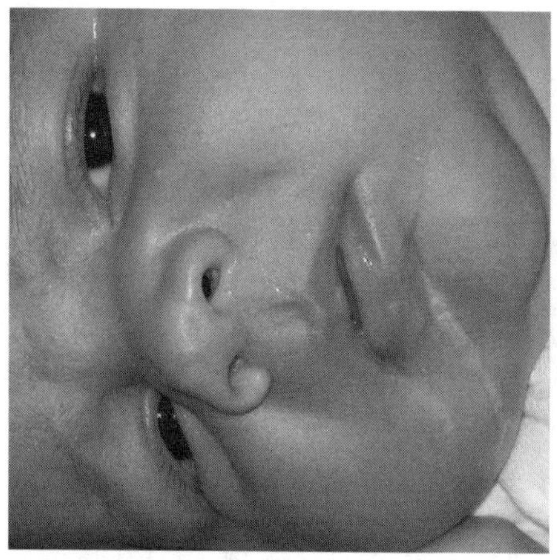

Figure 1-20 Simultaneous regurgitation from mouth and nose.

Nose

The nose should be symmetrical, and the infant should be able to breathe at rest without flaring the nares (nostrils). Flared nares (**Figure 1-19**) indicate increased effort of breathing. Note any congestion, discharge, sounds of effortful nasal respiration, and the presence of nasal regurgitation (**Figure 1-20**), which can indicate soft palate dysfunction.

Cheeks

Full-term infants have fat pads within the buccal muscles that give them their full, rounded appearance. Their purpose is to provide lateral stability during the first few months. Preterm infants, depending on gestational age, may not have fully developed fat pads and may suffer cheek collapse during sucking that reduces their ability to create intraoral negative pressure. Record any anatomical variations, asymmetries, or tonal differences between the cheeks.

Jaw

Tongue and jaw movements are linked and synchronized during sucking. Infants typically have a receded jaw, but one that is unusually receded can reduce the mechanical advantage of the jaw during sucking. Reduced alignment of the maxilla and mandible can reduce milk transfer. It is unusual for an infant to have a protruded jaw. Asymmetry of the jaw opening may indicate congenital torticollis (Wall & Glass, 2006) (**Figure 1-21**). Other signs of torticollis include the infant's head turning to one side with a flattened occiput on that side (plagiocephaly) and the head tilting toward the opposite side with neck shortening and limited range of movement. The skin creases at the base of the neck on the infant's back will be asymmetrical. Additional signs include asymmetrical placement of the eyes and ears, with one eye appearing larger than the other (**Figure 1-22**). The ear on the compressed side is usually cupped outward, and the contralateral ear is flattened to the skull. The unilateral upward tilt of the lower jaw and alveolar ridge in infants with torticollis contributes to feeding difficulty. Severe torticollis may result in increased tone and rotation of the body all the way down the affected side. Infants with torticollis require immediate referral for occupational or physical therapy or other effective bodywork.

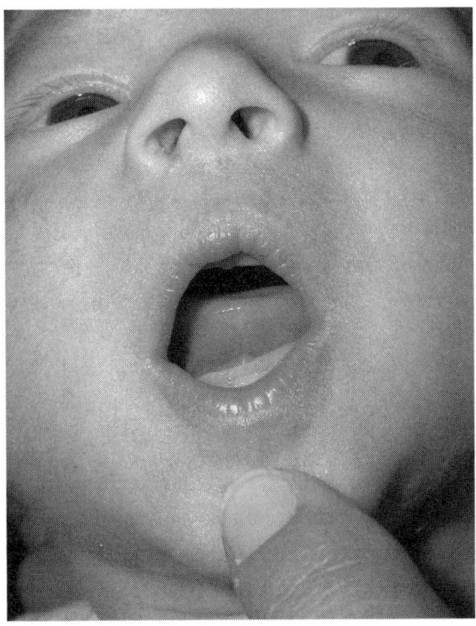

Figure 1-21 Mandibular asymmetry due to congenital muscular torticollis.

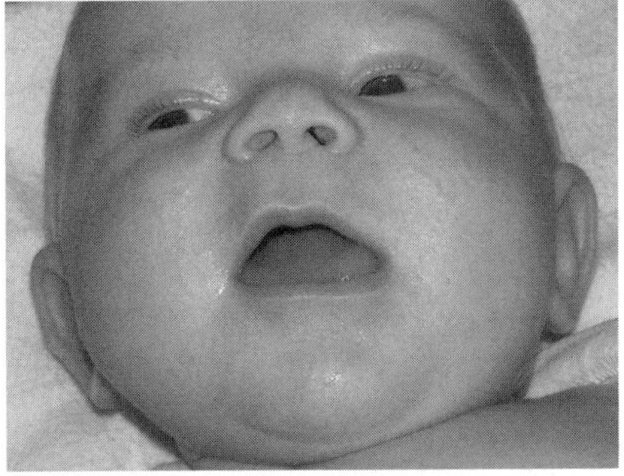

Figure 1-22 Subtle asymmetry in infant with feeding difficulties.

Wide jaw excursions that disrupt the attachment or clenching where the jaw moves minimally are problematic. The disorganized infant with immature sucking abilities may have inconsistent jaw movements, arrhythmic movements, or difficulty initiating movements (**Figure 1-23**).

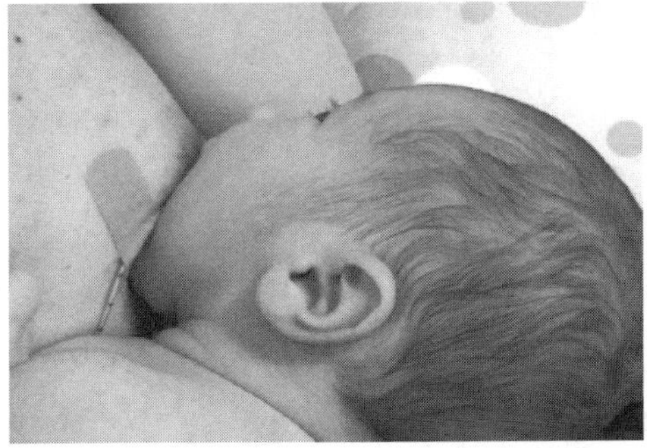

Figure 1-23 Excessive jaw excursion causes the infant to lose contact with the breast with his tongue and upper lip.

Hard and Soft Palates

The hard palate is continuous with the alveolar (gum) ridge in the front and the soft palate (the movable portion) positioned posteriorly. The movement of the soft palate may be noted if a gag reflex is elicited or when the infant cries. Clefts are the most obvious deviation affecting the palates (**Figure 1-24**). Even a submucosal cleft may affect the infant's ability to produce suction and effectively breastfeed (see Chapter 8). It is difficult to see the soft palate in a young infant, because the tongue fills the mouth. Strategies for better visualizing the posterior palate include digital photography, using a tongue depressor, and stimulation of the gag reflex at the soft palate with a cotton swab. Asymmetries in soft palate movements (just as in the tongue) can indicate a neurological deficit.

A highly arched or narrow hard palate is an indication of abnormal or restricted tongue movement (**Figures 1-25 and 1-26**). The tongue normally shapes the palate, widening it into a broad U shape. It is unclear if there is any contribution of a high palate to breastfeeding

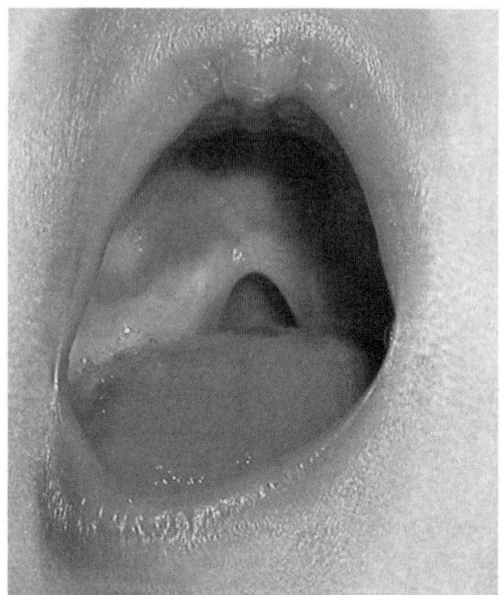

Figure 1-24 Cleft of the soft palate.

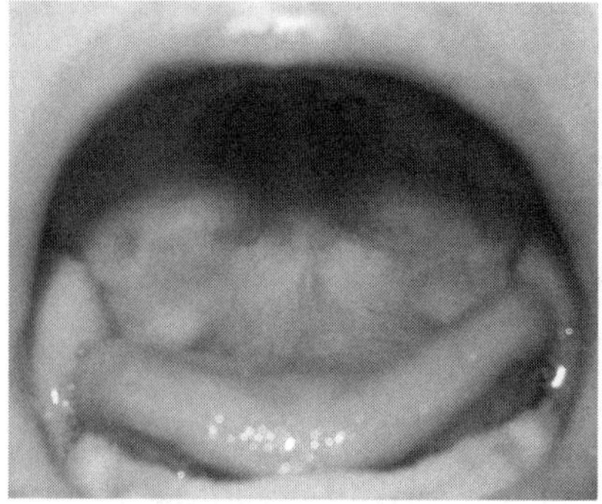

Figure 1-25 High arched, narrow palate due to tongue-tie.

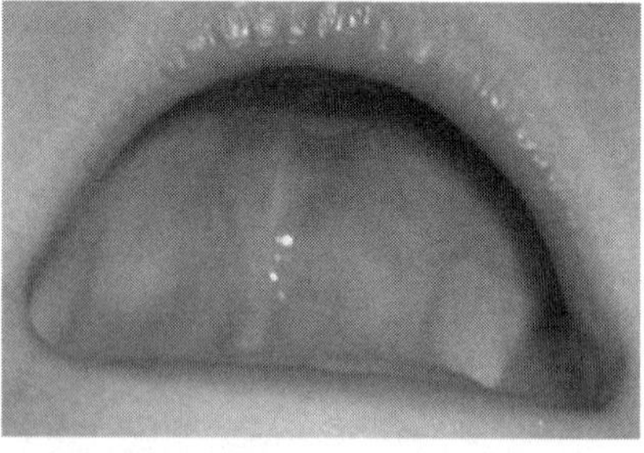

Figure 1-26 High arched, unusually shaped palate caused by a genetic deletion syndrome (Phelan-McDermid syndrome).

difficulty in and of itself, and in the author's research, narrow infant palates due to tongue-tie have spontaneously broadened in the month after frenotomy. A high, narrow palate may be hypersensitive to stimulation due to lack of tongue contact in utero. The resultant hyperactive gag reflex may make the infant reluctant to accept the breast deeply into the mouth and may interfere even more with the acceptance of firmer objects.

A preterm or ill infant whose history includes intubation or orogastric tube feedings may have a channel palate from the pressure of the narrow tube. Infants who have experienced repeated invasive oral procedures may develop hypersensitivity and aversion that may influence their willingness to accept anything into their mouth. Infants who have required intensive care may also be fearful of being held. They may need gentle desensitization, starting with holding in a way that they can accept (perhaps back toward the mother) and moving gradually toward a breastfeeding position.

Breast Assessment of the Mother

The focus of this text is the infant; however, breastfeeding requires a dyad. Anatomical mismatches between the mother and the infant influence the infant's feeding abilities. Look at the mother's breasts to see how well the infant's limitations may be accommodated.

Breast Characteristics

Mild breast hypoplasia may be less problematic with a vigorous infant than a challenged one. Increased intermammary spacing (more than 1.5 inches) increases the index of suspicion for decreased glandular development in the breasts, as does breast asymmetry (**Figures 1-27, 1-28, 1-29**). Persistent maternal Tanner stage 4 breasts (bulbous areolas) may improve feeding ability for some infants and be disadvantageous for others. Flat or inverted nipples (**Figures 1-30, 1-31**) will be more challenging for

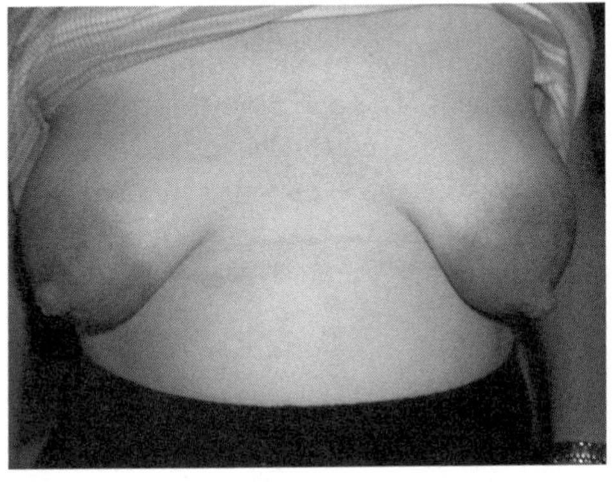

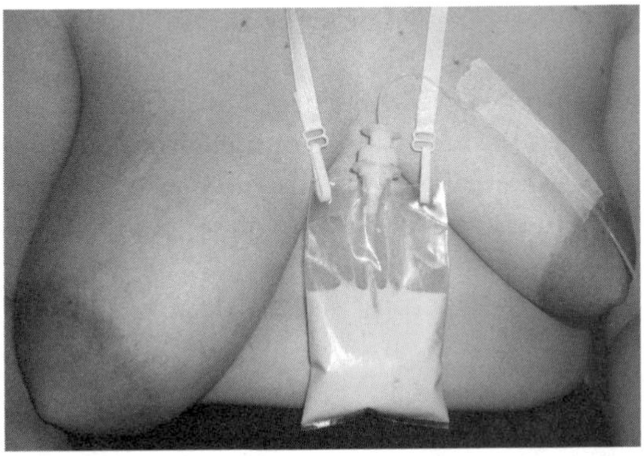

Figure 1-27 (Top left) Mild hypoplasia with wide intramammary space.

Figure 1-28 (Top right) Breast asymmetry, with use of a Lact-Aid nursing trainer due to lower milk production in the smaller breast.

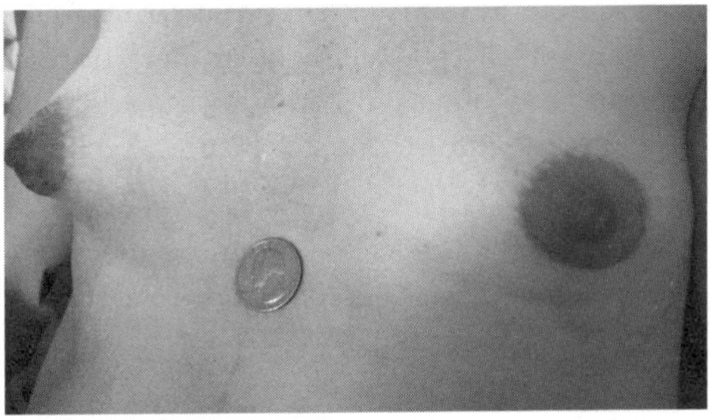

Figure 1-29 (Right) Severe breast hypoplasia.

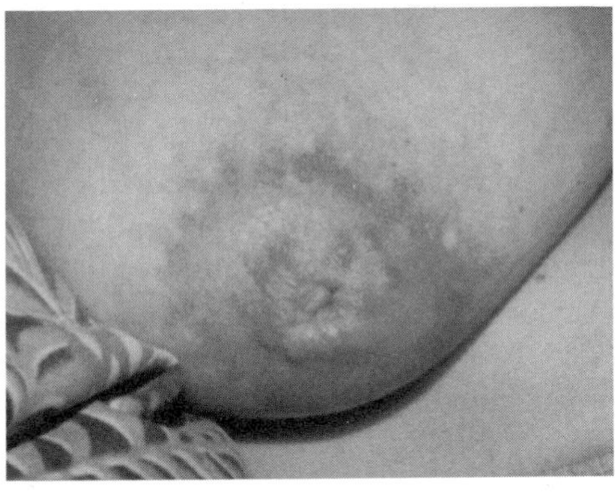

Figure 1-30 (Left) Inverted nipple.

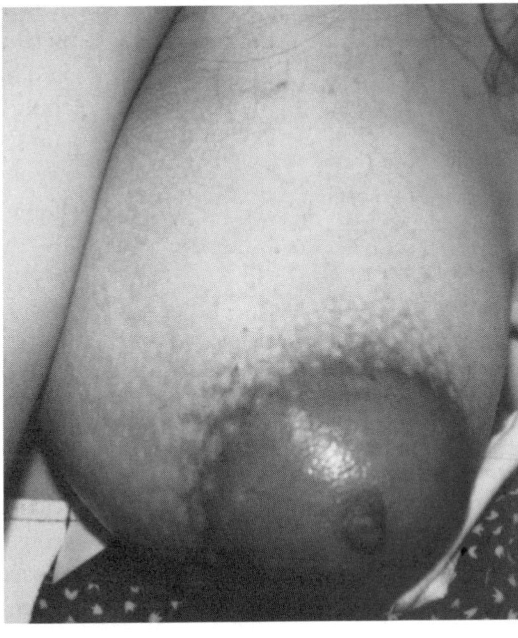

Figure 1-31 (Right) Breast engorgement flattens the nipple and makes attachment difficult.

a tongue-tied or hypotonic infant to grasp, whereas long nipples may be difficult for a child with a hyperactive gag. Wide, inelastic nipple tissue may make feeding ineffective for infants with small mouths until they grow into them. The placement of the nipple on the breast will determine what positions will be most effective for the individual dyad. Maternal motor skills and previous breastfeeding exposure and experience all contribute to the support she can offer her infant.

Breastfeeding Assessment

Tools

When sucking problems exist, pre- and postfeeding weights need to be measured in the same clothing on a sensitive digital scale designed for test weighing. A penlight or otoscope is helpful in visualizing oral structures. A neonatal stethoscope is helpful for cervical auscultation (listening at the neck or underside of the chin) to assess swallowing sounds and coordination of swallowing and breathing. A digital camera or camcorder helps to preserve information for future reevaluation, and photos or videos may be provided to the mother as teaching tools or to the infant's physician as documentation. Even experienced clinicians may notice important details that were initially missed when reviewing such documentation.

Observation

Attachment and positioning are essential to infant performance at the breast. Look at infant support and alignment; complete contact between mother's body and infant's chin, chest, trunk, and abdomen; hip flexion around the mother's side; and maternal ergonomics and comfort (**Figures 1-32 and 1-33**). Note how much assistance the mother requires to provide optimal support for her infant. Biological nurturing (laid-back or semireclined) maternal positions improve ergonomics, gravitational support, and reflex behaviors in both partners (Colson, 2007a; Colson, 2007b).

Stimuli that best trigger the inborn neurobehavioral feeding program in human infants include skin-to-skin contact with the mother, chin contact with the breast, and nipple contact with the philtrum (ridge between upper lip and nose). When given these cues, a hungry infant will gape widely, extend and depress the tongue, grasp the breast and seal to it with the tongue and lips, and begin sucking.

Compensatory Strategies

Based on the assessments, the following techniques could be employed to enhance breastfeeding given the anatomical limitations of the mother and/or baby:

- Positioning to enhance support and maximize attachment
- Nipple shield to make nipple or areola more graspable
- Reverse pressure softening (RPS) (Cotterman, 2004) or brief prepumping to soften the nipple and areola area to make it more elastic
- Using a nipple everter device, such as a Supple Cup (www.supplecups.com), before feeding to make the nipple more prominent and graspable
- At-breast supplementation to improve milk transfer

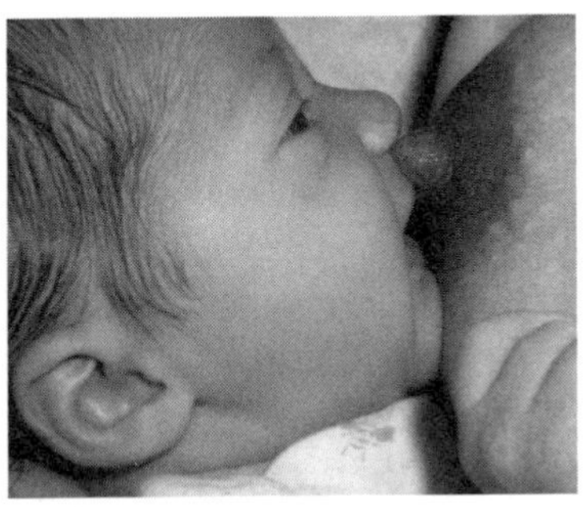
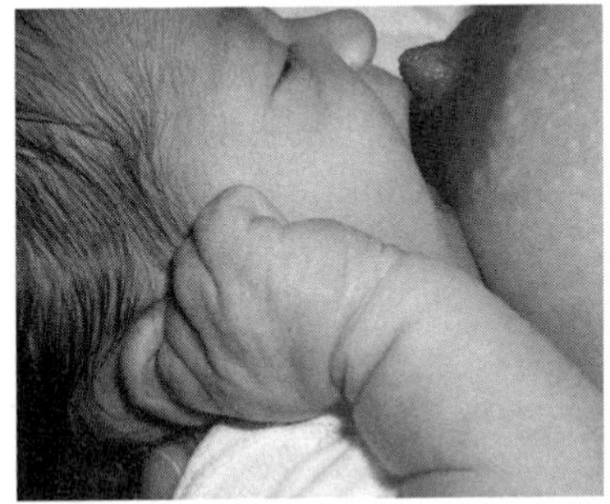
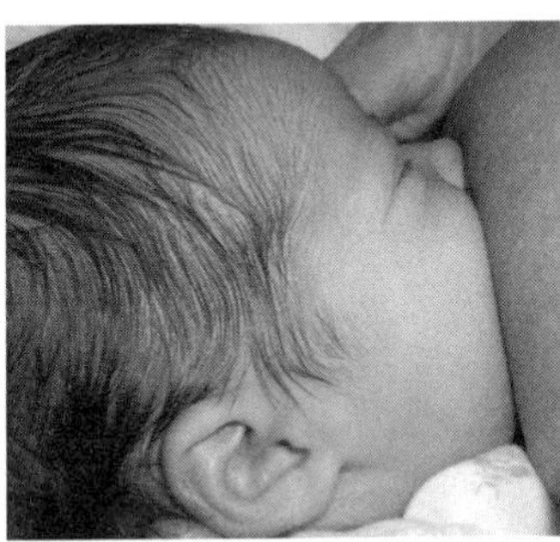

Figure 1-32 Good alignment allows the infant to self-attach to the breast.

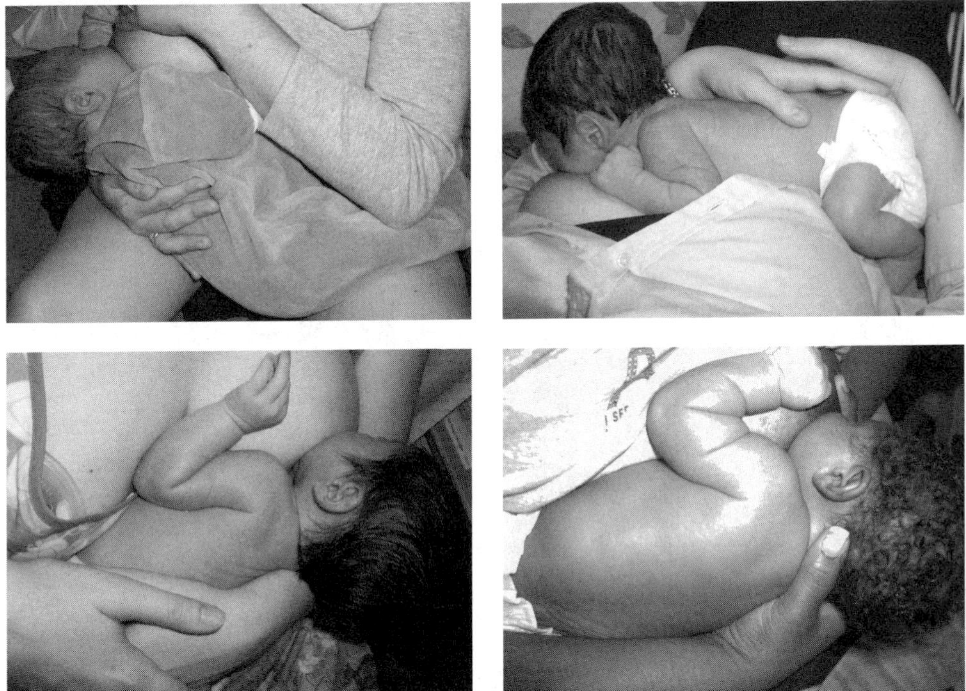

Figure 1-33 Placement of the infant where the breast naturally falls, and supporting him against the mother's body, is usually more ergonomic for the mother and gives the infant optimal stability.

Tongue

The infant's tongue position during approach to the breast is one of the most important factors in successful attachment. The tongue is down in the mouth over the lower gum or lip. At the point of latch, the anterior portion of the tongue lifts upward to contact the

If the Infant Initiates Sucking Before Attaching and Is Unable to Latch

Facilitative strategy: Ask the mother to wait until the infant stops sucking and then begin again. Because sucking is reflexive in the first few months, the infant may persist in the pattern without assistance from the mother.

breast as the tissue is drawn into the mouth. Optimal attachment is vital to filling the mouth and stabilizing the tongue so it can function as well as possible.

Ankyloglossia (tongue-tie) usually has a negative effect on feeding. Although some tongue-tied infants are able to latch and transfer milk (Geddes et al., 2010), most are less efficient than their peers with unrestricted tongue motion (Geddes, Langton et al., 2008; Ramsay, Langton, Jacobs, Gollow, & Simmer, 2004). Others are unable to attach to the breast at all (**Figure 1-34**). Some infants attach but fail to transfer enough milk to sustain growth and stimulate maternal supply, or they may cause maternal nipple or breast damage due to repetitive stress from abnormal movements of the tongue. Ask the mother about her sensations during feeding. Pinching or biting sensations may be due to excessive positive pressure from the tongue or jaws; friction (often described as feeling like sandpaper or a cat's tongue on the nipple) may be due to compensatory in-out (sliding) movements of the tongue; and

If the Tongue Tip Elevation Obstructs Attachment

When the infant is not lowering the tongue tip, try the following strategies to encourage the infant to lower it.

Facilitative strategies:

- Allow the infant more time to organize oral movements and drop the tongue to begin nuzzling and licking the breast.
- Tickle down the tongue tip with an adult finger immediately before attachment, which might help if the infant does not spontaneously drop the tongue.
- Briefly fingerfeed some expressed milk. Fingerfeeding can be useful for habitual tongue tip elevation by teaching the baby that food belongs on top of the tongue.
- Watch for rapid respirations to determine if the infant is able to feed. The infant needs to be able to spare time in the respiratory cycle to close the airway for a safe swallow. Rapid respiration implies difficulty meeting oxygen needs at rest; oxygen needs are greater during feeding.

Compensatory strategies:

- A silicone nipple shield may provide stronger tactile input and allow the infant to slide the tongue under the teat during the learning period.
- Supplementary oxygen (provided by nasal cannula or "blow by") during feeding for infants with tongue tip elevation secondary to rapid respiration.

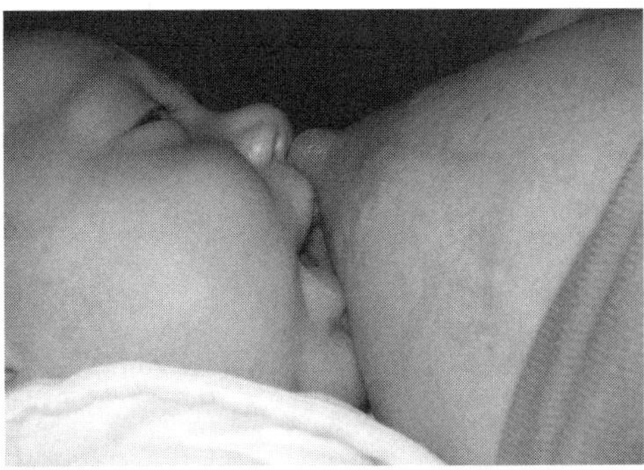

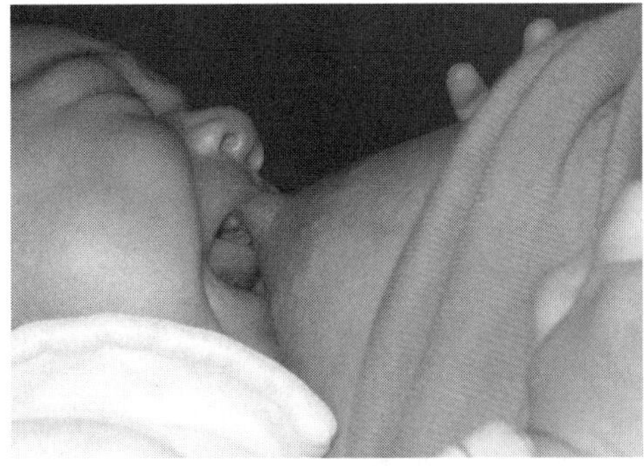

Figure 1-34 This infant with tongue-tie cries in frustration from the absence of his expected cue (tongue tip on breast), which causes his tongue to elevate and block the mouth.

feeling percussive movement against the nipple may be due to excessive posterior tongue elevation (humping; see Chapter 8). Pain without evidence of damage may be from nipple base compression (Geddes, Langton et al., 2008) or from excessive negative (suction) pressures during sucking (McClellan et al., 2008). Excessive pressures during sucking can be ameliorated with the use of a nipple shield (D. Geddes, personal communication, May 2007).

If the Tongue Is Retracted or Unable to Grasp the Breast

Facilitative strategy: Massage the anterior tongue with a fingertip until it extends over the lower gum. Finger feed for one or more feedings.

Lips

Hoover (1996) found that breastfeeding was pain-free if the infant's lip angle was 130 to 160 degrees. In young infants, the angle of the lips will often be hidden by the cheeks, which contact the breast and remain rounded. The nasolabial crease should remain soft, and the upper lip should be neutral to slightly everted on the breast and should be relatively immobile during sucking. Older infants and toddlers generally do not touch the breast with their cheeks during breastfeeding. Their lip angle should be at least 130 degrees to ensure maternal comfort. See **Figure 1-35** for an example of ineffective latch and **Figure 1-36** for an example of optimal latch.

Overuse of the upper lip is associated with large sucking blisters, which is easily visible as a sweeping motion of the lip during feeding. It may be associated with the in-and-out movement of the breast.

Facilitative strategy: Increase the depth of attachment, check for tongue-tie, and work on strengthening the tongue movements.

If the Tongue Tip Is Humped or Blocking the Infant's Oral Cavity

Facilitative strategy: Massage the posterior tongue. Finger feed with counterpressure to the humped area of the tongue.

If the Tongue Tip Is Elevated or Blocking the Infant's Oral Cavity

Facilitative strategy: Tickle the tongue tip down, and calm the infant.

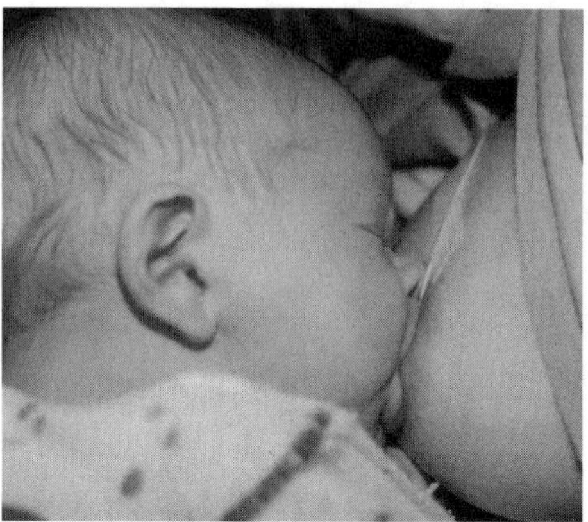

Figure 1-35 An overly flanged upper lip is a sign of shallow attachment or overuse of the lip to compensate for tongue immobility. This infant's head is flexed, bringing his nose into the breast and the chin away, reducing mechanical advantage.

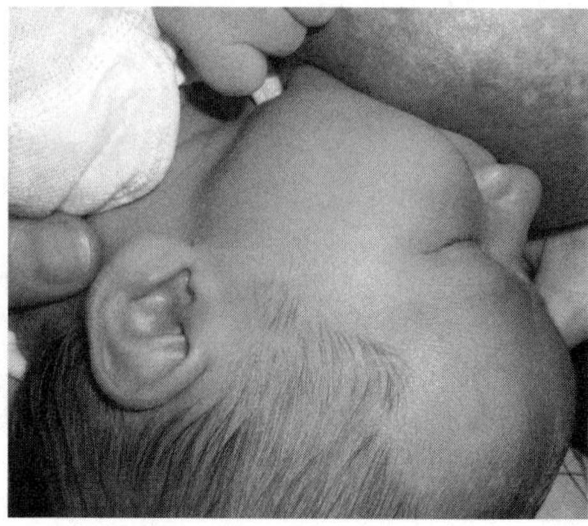

Figure 1-36 Optimal latch for a young infant. The upper lip is neutral, cheeks are rounded, head is slightly extended, chin is on the breast, and nose is free.

Jaw

Latching infants need to open widely to grasp enough breast tissue to efficiently transfer milk. The jaw movements should be smooth, with a slight pulse on the downward component and a slight pause with the jaw open as the mouth fills with milk. Grading of jaw opening and closing should be smooth. Infants displaying jerky movements, snapping at the temporomandibular joint, or sideways or circular jaw movements should be referred for speech therapy.

Cheeks

In newborns, the cheeks should press against the breast, hiding the lower lip, which is completely everted. The cheeks should remain smooth during sucking. Shallow attachment will cause a tight everted upper lip, excessive movement of the upper lip, tight nasolabial creases, and dimpling of the cheek during sucking (**Figures 1-37 and 1-38**). Dimpling of the cheek could also indicate buccinator (cheek muscle) weakness and instability or failure of the anterior tongue to elevate and groove to hold the breast in the mouth.

Feeding at the Breast

Sucking speed is inversely proportional to milk flow. Before the milk ejection reflex (MER), the infant may suck rapidly, with two sucks per second and infrequent swallows. The sucks are shallower, with less jaw excursion than sucking after the MER. During rapid milk flow, the infant generally sucks about once per second, with a 1:1:1 suck-swallow-breathe ratio. During slower but still significant milk flow, the ratio can be 2:1:1. A ratio of 3:1:1 is

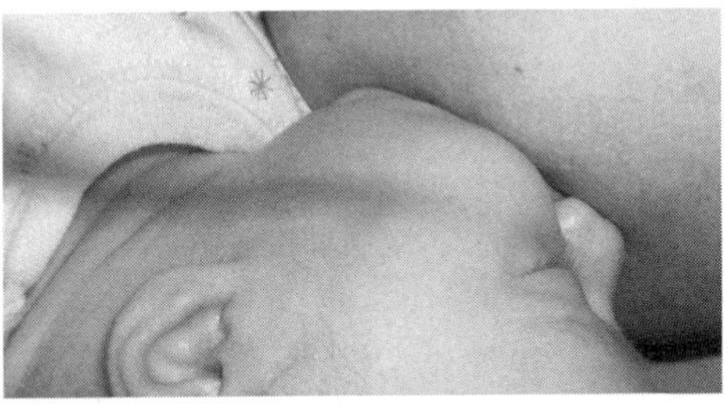

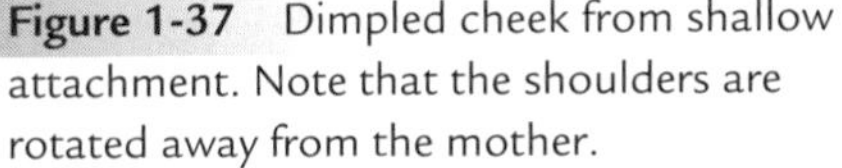

Figure 1-37 Dimpled cheek from shallow attachment. Note that the shoulders are rotated away from the mother.

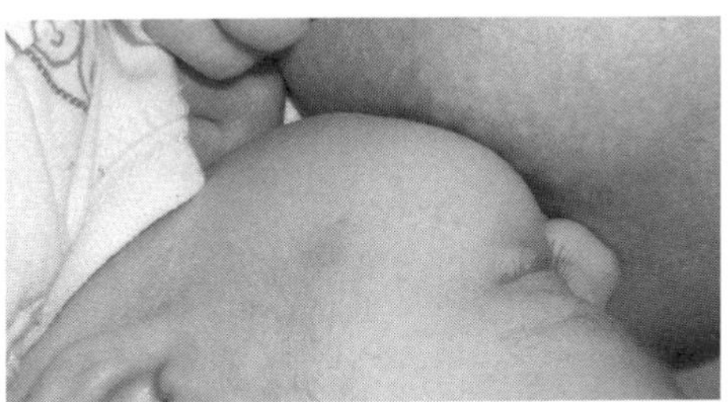

Figure 1-38 Same infant, better alignment and attachment.

considered the break-even point, where energy expended in feeding equals calories taken in. Larger numbers of sucks between swallows generally indicate little milk transfer. However, at the end of a normal feeding, the infant may "linger over dessert," ingesting very high-fat milk, and ideally should *not* be taken off the breast. A sated infant will release the breast voluntarily and rest on mother's body. An infant who comes off the breast and is squirming around generally wants to take the other breast in search of a faster milk flow.

Normal sucking bursts consist of 10 to 30 suck–swallow–breathe triads, followed by a 3- to 5-second respiratory pause. Breathing is initially rapid during the respiratory pause, and when it returns to baseline, the infant resumes sucking. Swallowing sounds are normally subtle, with a quiet "cuh" sound representing the soft palate closing off the nasopharynx to prevent milk from entering the nose. As the baby adjusts to a new milk ejection, swallowing may become slightly louder. Gulping sounds (hard swallows) represent stressed or difficult swallowing and may counterintuitively be associated with small boluses.

Observation of the infant's burst pause pattern can reveal cardiorespiratory instability—the sucking bursts will be short, consisting of 3–5 sucks with prolonged respiratory pauses. Immature infants may use a transitional sucking pattern consisting of 5–8 sucks and swallows with breathing mostly between sucking bursts (Palmer, 1993). Difficulty coordinating sucking, swallowing, and breathing can manifest as gulping, coughing, color changes, aerophagia (air swallowing), and short bursts of stridor (high-pitched breathing, in this case occurring as the vocal folds snap shut to keep milk out of the airway during a poorly timed swallow). The difficulty can stem from maternal hyperlactation and rapid milk flow or, more frequently, from the infant's inability to handle a normal flow. Infants with mild difficulties will usually respond to being removed from the breast briefly for a respiratory pause or feeding in a prone or side-lying position. Steady pressure on the breast with the side of the mother's hand during the first and strongest milk ejection will block off the flow in the occluded ducts and slow the flow. The mother's hand should be placed as close to the areolar margin as possible without disrupting the infant's latch, since many of the large ducts are superficial and branch close to the nipple (Geddes, 2007; Geddes, 2009). Infants with severe difficulties with flow may refuse to feed or become fussy during feeding, especially as they approach 3 months of age, when feeding becomes more volitional and less reflexive.

Ineffective Sucking or Low Maternal Milk Flow?

Ask the mother to express milk for a few minutes. If several ounces are obtained, the problem is likely with the infant. If several milliliters are obtained, the problem may be with the mother, or the supply may have responded to the infant's inability to drive it.

A periodontal (curved-tip) syringe or syringe and feeding tube can be used diagnostically at the breast in such cases to see how the baby suckles with a better milk flow. If the baby does well with the additional flow, supplementing at the breast preserves breastfeeding while the supply is rebuilt.

If the infant is still not capable of transferring milk, the milk production will falter if expression does not occur frequently—approximately eight times per day (Hill, Aldag, & Chatterton, 2001). Feeding with expressed milk and brief breastfeeding for practice may be a better use of the dyad's energy.

Respiratory Pattern

Infants take breathing breaks whenever they need to in order to maintain normal blood oxygen levels, as long as the flow of milk is under their control. It was once thought that infants could swallow and breathe simultaneously, due to the anatomical proximity of the soft palate and epiglottis. Although this arrangement does help protect them from aspiration, intricate coordination is still required between swallowing and breathing, as the paths for food and air cross in the pharyngeal region. Therefore, swallowing requires a brief interruption of breathing. Breastfed infants frequently swallow after inspiration or expiration is completed (Kelly et al., 2007; Mizuno & Ueda, 2006; Prieto et al., 1996), limiting the potential for aspiration.

Colostrum is viscous and present in relatively low volumes, probably allowing a training period for safer practice of this coordination. Weber et al. (1986) identified improvements in coordination of breathing and feeding in breastfed infants during the first 5 days of life.

Respiration during sucking pauses should be quiet, unlabored, and usually slightly more rapid than breathing during the sucking bursts. Infants with high baseline respiratory rates or increased work of breathing might not be able to afford the respiratory pauses of frequent swallowing. They will generally use short sucking bursts and longer respiratory pauses to meet their conflicting needs for nutrition and oxygen, respectively. No attempts should be made to prod the infant. When the respiratory rate returns to baseline, the infant will begin to suckle again. This ability to self-regulate is one of the reasons that physiologic stability is greater during breastfeeding than during bottle feeding. Infants with reduced aerobic capacity generally need to be fed more frequently to make up for their longer pauses and reduced work capacity.

Signs of respiratory difficulties include the following:

- Rapid, panting respiration during pauses
- Stridor or other respiratory noises (may be due to airway instability)
- Harsh and wet respiratory sounds (may be due to nasopharyngeal backflow, velopharygneal insufficiency, or aspiration)
- Increased effort of breathing (retractions of the chest or in the suprasternal notch)
- Mouth breathing (nasal blockage or deviated septum) (**Figure 1-39**)
- Short sucking bursts
- Loss of milk through the lips or nose
- Apnea, bradycardia, and desaturation
- Color changes
- Panting or purring (cardiac issue causing pulmonary hypertension)

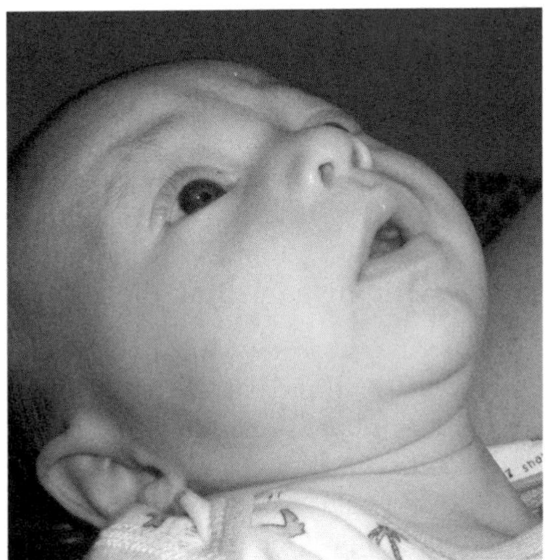

Figure 1-39 Infant with upper respiratory obstruction displays mouth breathing and worried facial expression.

If the infant does not have the aerobic capacity to breastfeed, prompt medical assessment is warranted. Evolving cardiac issues (aortic stenosis, transposition of the great vessels) become life threatening as the ductus arteriosus closes.

Indications of Satiety

In addition to pre- and postfeeding weight, observation of infant body language will provide clues that the infant has taken sufficient milk. When sated, a young infant will release the breast, rest his or her face on mom's breast, and go to sleep (**Figure 1-40**). In addition, the hands generally relax from a fisted posture to gentle flexion of the fingers as the baby is satisfied. Older infants will let go of the breast and woo mom into interaction. During the more distractible stages of development (4–6 months) the baby may come on and

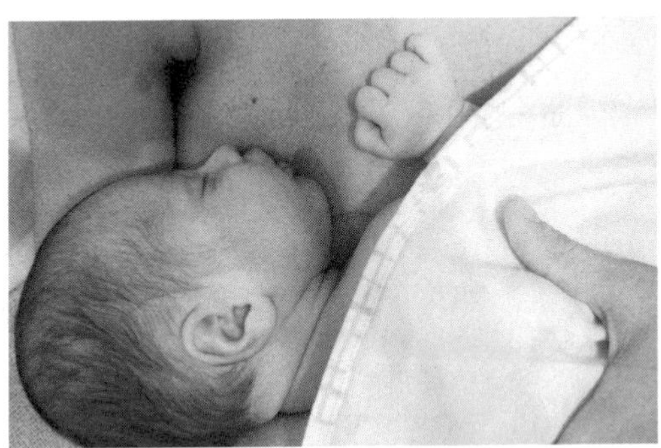

Figure 1-40 Infants remove themselves from the breast when satiated.

off the breast, alternating eating with engaging mom's attention or paying attention to other interesting environmental happenings.

Infants who regularly fall asleep at the breast without removing themselves might not be getting sufficient milk, particularly if they protest or begin to suckle again when attempts are made to remove them or put them down. Breastfeeding that typically takes more than 40 minutes per session is a potential red flag that the infant is feeding ineffectively.

Developing a Feeding Plan with the Mother

Careful assessment with attention to the infant's structure and functioning, the feeding skills that are present, and those that are yet to develop provides a framework for choosing interventions. The feeding plan provides compensations and facilitations to ensure the infant's present nutrition while building future feeding skills.

Basic management issues are easily solved with maternal education and practice with improved positioning and attachment. More complex feeding problems require a multi-step plan. Some possible components of the plan include the following:

- Referral to physicians if anatomical or neurological issues are suspected
- Alternative feeding methods while working toward transition to exclusive breastfeeding
- Maintaining or increasing milk production by pumping with a hospital-grade, metal piston-driven breast pump at least eight times each day
- Encouraging skin-to-skin contact and comfort sucking at the breast when the infant is not hungry to maintain interest in breastfeeding
- Positioning and attachment techniques based on the results of evaluation
- Determining whether oral exercises are appropriate; specific oral exercises are selected to reduce maladaptive movements and encourage correct ones

New procedures should be demonstrated, and the parents should return the demonstration to assure that the techniques are understood. Written instructions should be provided. Provisions for follow-up should be made. Progress can be followed by telephone, video conferencing, or email with return visits when the plan needs to be revised or updated.

> A firm background in both the individual components and the gestalt of normal feeding is required for lactation consultants working with infants who have sucking difficulties. Providing normal cueing in the form of ideal positioning and skin-to-skin contact with the mother is the first step to promoting normal feeding. Next, compensatory and facilitative strategies are applied as probes and added to the feeding plan if they are effective and well tolerated by both mother and infant. If normal feeding is not restored by these interventions, the infant should be referred to a feeding team for further evaluation.

References

Arvedson, J. C., & Brodsky, L. (2002). *Pediatric swallowing and feeding: Assessment and management* (2nd ed.). Albany, NY: Singular Thomson Learning.

Arvedson, J. C., & Lefton-Greif, M. A. (1998). *Pediatric videofluoroscopic swallow studies: A professional manual with caregiver guidelines.* San Antonio, TX: Therapy Skill Builders (Harcourt).

Becker, L. E., Zhang, W., & Pereyra, P. M. (1993). Delayed maturation of the vagus nerve in sudden infant death syndrome. *Acta Neuropathologica (Berlin), 86*(6), 617–622.

Bosma, J. F. (1986). Development of feeding. *Clinical Nutrition, 5,* 210–218.

Bosma, J. F., Hepburn, L. G., Josell, S. D., & Baker, K. (1990). Ultrasound demonstration of tongue motions during suckle feeding. *Developmental Medicine and Child Neurology, 32*(3), 223–229.

Bystrova, K., Widström, A.-M., Matthiesen, A.-S., Ransjö-Arvidson, A., Welles-Nyström, Vorontsov, I., Uvnäs-Moberg, K. (2007). Early lactation performance in primiparous and multiparous women in relation to different maternity home practices: A randomised trial in St. Petersburg. *International Breastfeeding Journal, 2*(9). Retrieved from http://www.internationalbreastfeedingjournal.com/content/2/1/9

Chantry, C. J., Nommsen-Rivers, L. A., Peerson, J. M., Cohen, R. J., & Dewey, K. G. (2011). Excess weight loss in first-born breastfed newborns relates to maternal intrapartum fluid balance. *Pediatrics, 127,* e171–e179.

Chen, D. C., Nommsen-Rivers, L., Dewey, K. G., & Lonnerdal, B. (1998). Stress during labor and delivery and early lactation performance. *The American Journal of Clinical Nutrition, 68,* 335–344.

Cichero, J. (2007, May). Suck:swallow mechanisms: Listening to swallowing sounds and suck-swallow-breathe coordination: Case studies. Talk given at *Seeking Suckling Success: Recent Research, Proven Practice,* sponsored by the College of Lactation Consultants of Western Australia, Freemantle, Australia.

Cichero, J. A., & Murdoch, B. E. (2002). Acoustic signature of the normal swallow: Characterization by age, gender, and bolus volume. *The Annals of Otology, Rhinology, and Laryngology, 111,* 623–632.

Cichero, J. A. Y., & Murdoch, B. E. (2006). *Dysphagia: Foundation, theory and practice.* Chichester, England: John Wiley & Sons.

Colson, S. (2007a). Biological nurturing (1). A non-prescriptive recipe for breastfeeding. *The Practicing Midwife, 10*(9), 42, 44, 46–47.

Colson, S. (2007b). Biological nurturing (2). The physiology of lactation revisited. *The Practicing Midwife, 10*(10), 14–19.

Colson, S. D., Meek, J. H., & Hawdon, J. M. (2008). Optimal positions for the release of primitive neonatal reflexes stimulating breastfeeding. *Early Human Development, 84,* 441–449.

Corbin-Lewis, K., Liss, J. M., & Sciortino, K. L. (2005). *Clinical anatomy and physiology of the swallowing mechanism.* Clifton Park, NY: Thompson.

Cotterman, K. J. (2004). Reverse pressure softening: A simple tool to prepare areola for easier latching during engorgement. *Journal of Human Lactation, 20*(2), 227–237.

Geddes, D. T. (2007). Inside the lactating breast: The latest anatomy research. *Journal of Midwifery and Women's Health, 52,* 556–563.

Geddes, D. T. (2009). Ultrasound imaging of the lactating breast: Methodology and application. *International Breastfeeding Journal, 4*(4). Retrieved from http://www.internationalbreastfeedingjournal.com/content/4/1/4

Geddes, D. T., Chadwick, L. M., Kent, J. C., Garbin, C. P., & Hartmann, P. E. (2010). Ultrasound imaging of infant swallowing during breast-feeding. *Dysphagia, 25,* 183–191.

Geddes, D. T., Kent, J. C., McClellan, H. L., Garbin, C. P., Chadwick, L. M., & Hartmann, P. E. (2010). Sucking characteristics of successfully breastfeeding infants with ankyloglossia: A case series. *Acta Paediatrica, 99*(2), 301–303.

Geddes, D. T., Kent, J. C., Mitoulas, L. R., & Hartmann, P. E. (2008). Tongue movement and intra-oral vacuum in breastfeeding infants. *Early Human Development, 84*, 471–477.

Geddes, D. T., Langton, D. B., Gollow, I., Jacobs, L. A., Hartmann, P. E., & Simmer, K. (2008). Frenulotomy for breastfeeding infants with ankyloglossia: Effect on milk removal and sucking mechanism as imaged by ultrasound. *Pediatrics, 122*, e188–e194.

Genna, C. W., & Barak, D. (2010). Facilitating autonomous infant hand use during breastfeeding. *Clinical Lactation, 1*, 15–21.

Gomes, C. F., Trezza, E. M., Murade, E. C., & Padovani, C. R. (2006). Surface electromyography of facial muscles during natural and artificial feeding of infants. *Jornal de Pediatria, 82*(2), 103–109.

Gosselin, J. (2005). The Amiel-Tison neurological assessment at term: Conceptual and methodological continuity in the course of follow-up. *Mental Retardation and Developmental Disabilities Research Review, 11*(1), 34–51.

Grassi, R., Farina, R., Floriani, I., Amodio, F., & Romano, S. (2005). Assessment of fetal swallowing with gray-scale and color Doppler sonography. *American Journal of Roentgenology, 185*, 1322–1327.

Hall, K. D. (2001). *Pediatric dysphagia resource guide.* San Diego, CA: Singular.

Hayashi, Y., Hoashi, E., & Nara, T. (1997). Ultrasonographic analysis of sucking behavior of newborn infants: The driving force of sucking pressure. *Early Human Development, 49*(1), 33–38.

Hiiemae, K. M., & Palmer, J. B. (2003). Tongue movements in feeding and speech. *Critical Reviews in Oral Biology and Medicine, 14*(6), 413–429.

Hill, P. D., Aldag, J. C., & Chatterton, R. T. (2001). Initiation and frequency of pumping and milk production in mothers of non-nursing preterm infants. *Journal of Human Lactation, 17*(1), 9–13.

Hoover, K. (1996). Visual assessment of the baby's wide open mouth. *Journal of Human Lactation, 12*(1), 9.

Inoue, N., Sakashita, R., & Kamegai, T. (1995). Reduction of masseter muscle activity in bottle-fed babies. *Early Human Development, 42*(3), 185–193.

Iwayama, K., & Eishima, M. (1997). Neonatal sucking behaviour and its development until 14 months. *Early Human Development, 47*(1), 1–9.

Jacobs, L. A., Dickinson, J. E., Hart, P. D., Doherty, D. A., & Faulkner, S. J. (2007). Normal nipple position in term infants measured on breastfeeding ultrasound. *Journal of Human Lactation, 23*, 52–59.

Kelly, B. N., Huckabee, M. L., Jones, R. D., & Frampton, C. M. (2007). The first year of human life: Coordinating respiration and nutritive swallowing. *Dysphagia, 22*, 37–43.

Kennedy, D., Kieser, J., Bolter, C., Swain, M., Singh, B., & Waddell, J. N. (2010). Tongue pressure patterns during water swallowing. *Dysphagia, 25*, 11–19.

Korfage, J. A., Koolstra, J. H., Langenbach, G. E., & van Eijden, T. M. (2005a). Fiber-type composition of the human jaw muscles—(part 1) origin and functional significance of fiber-type diversity. *Journal of Dental Research, 84*, 774–783.

Korfage, J. A., Koolstra, J. H., Langenbach, G. E., & van Eijden, T. M. (2005b). Fiber-type composition of the human jaw muscles—(part 2) role of hybrid fibers and factors responsible for inter-individual variation. *Journal of Dental Research, 84*, 784–793.

Logemann, J. A. (1998). *Evaluation and treatment of swallowing disorders* (2nd ed.). Austin, TX: Pro-Ed.

Malandraki, G. A., Sutton, B. P., Perlman, A. L., Karampinos, D. C., & Conway, C. (2009). Neural activation of swallowing and swallowing-related tasks in healthy young adults: An attempt to separate the components of deglutition. *Human Brain Mapping, 30*, 3209–3226.

Matias, S. L., Nommsen-Rivers, L. A., Creed-Kanashiro, H., & Dewey, K. G. (2010). Risk factors for early lactation problems among Peruvian primiparous mothers. *Maternal and Child Nutrition, 6*, 120–133.

McClellan, H., Geddes, D., Kent, J., Garbin, C., Mitoulas, L., & Hartmann, P. (2008). Infants of mothers with persistent nipple pain exert strong sucking vacuums. *Acta Paediatrica, 97*, 1205–1209.

Mendell, D. A., & Logemann, J. A. (2007). Temporal sequence of swallow events during the oropharyngeal swallow. *Journal of Speech, Language, and Hearing Research, 50,* 1256–1271.

Miller, J. L., & Kang, S. M. (2007). Preliminary ultrasound observation of lingual movement patterns during nutritive versus non-nutritive sucking in a premature infant. *Dysphagia, 22*, 150–160.

Mizuno, K., & Ueda, A. (2006). Changes in sucking performance from nonnutritive sucking to nutritive sucking during breast- and bottle-feeding. *Pediatric Research, 59*, 728–731.

Moriniere, S., Boiron, M., Alison, D., Makris, P., & Beutter, P. (2008). Origin of the sound components during pharyngeal swallowing in normal subjects. *Dysphagia, 23*, 267–273.

Morris, S. E., & Klein, M. D. (2000). *Prefeeding skills* (2nd ed.). San Antonio, TX: Therapy Skill Builders.

Morton, J., Hall, J. Y., Wong, R. J., Thairu, L., Benitz, W. E., & Rhine, W. D. (2009). Combining hand techniques with electric pumping increases milk production in mothers of preterm infants. *Journal of Perinatology, 29*, 757–764.

Newman, L. A. (1996). Infant swallowing and dysphagia. *Current Opinion in Otolaryngology and Head and Neck Surgery, 4,* 182–186.

Nommsen-Rivers, L. A., Chantry, C. J., Peerson, J. M., Cohen, R. J., & Dewey, K. G. (2010). Delayed onset of lactogenesis among first-time mothers is related to maternal obesity and factors associated with ineffective breastfeeding. *The American Journal of Clinical Nutrition, 92*, 574–584.

Nyqvist, K. H. (2001). Early oral behaviour in preterm infants during breastfeeding: An electromyographic study. *Acta Paediatrica, 90*(6), 658–663.

Nyqvist, K. H., Rubertsson, C., Ewald, U., & Sjöden, P.-O. (1996). Development of the Preterm Infant Breastfeeding Behavior Scale (PIBBS): A study of nurse-mother agreement. *Journal of Human Lactation, 12*(3), 207–219.

Palmer, M. M. (1993). Identification and management of the transitional suck pattern in premature infants. *Journal of Perinatal and Neonatal Nursing, 7*(1), 66–75.

Palmer, M. M. (1998). A closer look at neonatal sucking. *Neonatal Network, 17*(2), 77–79.

Palmer, M. M. (2006, January). NOMAS® certification course. Raleigh, NC.

Porter, R. H., & Winberg, J. (1999). Unique salience of maternal breast odors for newborn infants. *Neuroscience and Biobehavioral Reviews, 23*, 439–449.

Prieto, C. R., Cardenas, H., Salvatierra, A. M., Boza, C., Montes, C. G., & Croxatto, H. B. (1996). Sucking pressure and its relationship to milk transfer during breastfeeding in humans. *Journal of Reproduction and Fertility, 108*, 69–74.

Ramsay, D. T., & Hartmann, P. E. (2005). Milk removal from the breast. *Breastfeeding Review, 13*(1), 5–7.

Ramsay, D. T., Langton, D., Jacobs, L., Gollow, I., & Simmer, K. (2004). Ultrasound imaging of the effect of frenulotomy on breastfeeding infants with ankyloglossia. *Abstracts of the Proceedings of the 2004 ISRHML Conference.*

Ransjö-Arvidson, A.-B., Matthiesen, A.-S., Lilja, G., Nissen, E., Windström, A.-M., & Uvnäs-Moberg, K. (2001). Maternal analgesia during labor disturbs newborn behavior: Effects on breastfeeding, temperature, and crying. *Birth, 28*(1), 5–12.

Righard, L., & Alade, M. O. (1990). Effect of delivery room routines on success of first breast-feed. *Lancet, 336*(8723), 1105–1107.

Stal, P., Marklund, S., Thornell, L. E., De Paul, R., & Eriksson, P. O. (2003). Fibre composition of human intrinsic tongue muscles. *Cells, Tissues and Organs, 173*(3), 147–161.

Stal, S. (1998). Classic and occult submucous cleft palates: A histopathologic analysis. *The Cleft Palate–Craniofacial Journal, 35*(4), 351–358.

Stevenson, R. D., & Allaire, J. H. (1991). The development of normal feeding and swallowing. *Pediatric Clinics of North America, 38*(6), 1439–1453.

Takemoto, H. (2001). Morphological analyses of the human tongue musculature for three-dimensional modeling. *Journal of Speech Language and Hearing Research, 44*(1), 95–107.

Thoyre, S. M., Shaker, C. S., & Pridham, K. F. (2005). The early feeding skills assessment for preterm infants. *Neonatal Network, 24*(3), 7–16.

Vice, F. L., Bamford, O., Heinz, J. M., & Bosma, J. F. (1995). Correlation of cervical auscultation with physiological recording during suckle-feeding in newborn infants. *Developmental Medicine and Child Neurology, 37*, 167–179.

Vice, F. L., Heinz, J. M., Giuriati, G., Hood, M., & Bosma, J. F. (1990). Cervical auscultation of suckle feeding in newborn infants. *Developmental Medicine and Child Neurology, 32*, 760–768.

Walker, M. (2006). *Breastfeeding management for the clinician: Using the evidence.* Sudbury, MA: Jones and Bartlett.

Wall, V., & Glass, R. (2006). Mandibular asymmetry and breastfeeding problems: Experience from 11 cases. *Journal of Human Lactation, 22*(3), 328–334.

Weber, F., Woolridge, M. W., & Baum, J. D. (1986). An ultrasonographic study of the organisation of sucking and swallowing by newborn infants. *Developmental Medicine and Child Neurology, 28*(1), 19–24.

Yang, W. T., Loveday, E. J., Metreweli, C., & Sullivan, P. B. (1997). Ultrasound assessment of swallowing in malnourished disabled children. *The British Journal of Radiology, 70*, 992–994.

CHAPTER

2

Breastfeeding and Perinatal Neuroscience

Nils Bergman

Introduction

Breastfeeding is a brain-based behavior of the newborn, an inborn ability that is regulated by the limbic system of the brain. Newborns are born with the behavioral capability to breastfeed. However, this capability is fragile and requires the uninterrupted presence of the mother, with specific stimuli at early critical periods working to reinforce the inborn ability. The behavior can easily be modified, modulated, or abolished. The normal innate behavior that the newborn exhibits at the breast, which develops and matures in the first day, is breastfeeding. One of its components is suckling, but breastfeeding is far more: it is the total occupation of the newborn. The restoration of this behavior is the objective of the authors of this book.

I shall use the terms *suckle* or *suckling* to refer to the somatic behavior of the infant on the breast. Accepting the word *sucking* as an activity for breastfeeding may cause confusion and reinforces the cultural myth that bottle feeding and breastfeeding are equivalent. There is no science or research supporting the safety of bottle feeding; it simply is assumed to be normal.

Likewise, many labor ward routines and hospital practices are not supported by scientific research or evidence-based medicine (Smith & Kroeger, 2010). Numerous assumptions concerning fetal and newborn brain development have been derived to justify our practices, rather than the other way around. Recent neuroscience has very dramatically shifted, leaving most of our practices without justification. These practices cause a host of behavioral problems in babies, not least evidenced by breastfeeding problems and failure of newborns and infants to suckle normally.

I will summarize the main points of this new neuroscience in this chapter.

Early Developmental Mechanisms

Genes and DNA

After conception, there is a very rapid differentiation and development of the fetal brain. For the first 10–14 weeks, development is determined by heredity, by genes expressed from the DNA of the fetus. At 20 weeks gestation, all anatomical parts of the brain are in place, and the DNA has put in place the template that makes development possible, like an unformatted hard disk. The primary element in subsequent development is experience.

Neural Cells

The functional cell of the brain for our purposes is the neuron. Neurons form in the brain until 28 weeks of gestational age, and not beyond (with few exceptions). After they are formed, they migrate to other parts of the brain, and in the process they connect to sensory organs. They are sensitive cells, and when they are sensitized, they trigger an action potential, or fire. Various sensations will make various cells fire. That firing causes first budding and then axon formation on one end and dendrite formation on the other. Ongoing firing makes more branches, and at the ends of branches synapses form, which when fired repeatedly result in stabilization of the synapse, or wiring. Ultimately almost all the neurons of the brain will be connected to one another in a network. Shatz (1992)—with unusual brevity for a neuroscientist—summarizes thus: "Cells that fire together, wire together" (p. 64).

Neuronal Plasticity

Genetic determination does continue after 14 weeks, but its importance in the development process is overtaken by two more important processes, the first of which has been described; the second can be described as *use it or lose it*.

From very early in gestation, there is a parallel process of programmed cell death and elimination of redundancy, or pruning. By 40 weeks of gestational age, half the precious neurons that were formed have been lost! Some neurons undergo programmed cell death and are dismantled and removed. A suboptimal level of stimulation results in fewer branches and poorer connections in the remaining neurons. A certain critical repetition of firing is needed to stabilize the synapse, which is then immune from elimination or removal. This process continues throughout development (McCain & Mustard, 1999).

Neuronal plasticity, therefore, relates to the interplay between firing and wiring of neurons and removing those that are not used (Teicher, 2002). From 28 weeks the number of neurons is maximal, from 40 weeks the number of synapses peak, and from there on neuronal plasticity refers to pruning and removing neurons and their synapses. (This is also called *sculpting*, in that the end result comes from removing unwanted parts.) The parts of the brain that now capture the stimuli become pathways, and they may or may not myelinate, which makes them faster and more complex pathways. The end result of this process is a hardwired brain. It used be thought that the brain could regenerate and repair because an amazing recovery in function is observed in many cases. However, this is a misconception; though a very young brain can wire new pathways with residual neural cells, this ability is rapidly lost. The brainstem (which controls breathing and heart rate, etc.) is hardwired at the time of birth. The limbic system of the brain, which controls basic autonomic functions, moods, emotions, and self-control, is hardwired by the age of 3 years. The cerebral cortex (and the cerebellum) retains a degree of neuronal plasticity into adult life, and cortical synapses continue to form as needed (McCain & Mustard, 1999).

Essentially, the genes set in motion a process that establishes the scaffolding of the brain, but the final result as to what cells remain and how cells are connected is determined by experience, the result of neuronal plasticity (Teicher, 2002). This is in sharp contrast to the belief that most medical professionals have derived from their training: if brain development is genetic, then it does not matter too much if some experience along the way is poor. Although the growth in absolute brain size after birth is clearly seen, the assumption that new neurons are added is false.

Developmental Competence

Throughout the developmental sequence, whether embryo, fetus, newborn, or infant, the organism is regarded from a biological perspective as complete for that stage (Alberts, 1994; Als et al., 1994). A fetus succeeds very well in the uterus, where its behaviors ensure well-being and development. These behaviors are actually neurobehaviors because they are governed by the developing midbrain and limbic system. The organism is not designed to succeed outside the uterus while it is a fetus. It may seem a bit obvious, but the key principle is that each stage of development is completely dependent on being in the right place.

Developmental competence requires the successful accomplishment of the requirements of each stage in order to be able to work toward competence at the next level (National Research Council Institute of Medicine, 2000). In many school systems you have to pass the current grade if you are to have the background skills to pass the next grade. Likewise, suboptimal development at any stage of the organism will impact the development trajectory in a negative way.

Throughout this development, it is the experience of the organism that drives the development. This experience translates to sensory stimuli sent to the brain, which is first and foremost a sensory organ. The fetus has extraordinary sensory discrimination. Various sensory systems are activated during the second trimester; by the beginning of the third trimester its discrimination in terms of kinesthesia, smell, and sound are greater than at any other time in life (Graven, 2004; Philbin, 2004; Schaal, Hummel, & Soussignan, 2004). In effect, the brain makes sense of sensations. However, the brain is primarily a social organ; the sense the brain makes of its experience is about relationships.

Neurobehavior

The newborn behavior arises from the limbic system and expresses itself through three main systems: the autonomic nervous system, the hormonal system, and the somatic (or muscular) system. Although these can be studied separately, and parts of each can be studied in detail, what is essential to appreciate is that there is a program that integrates autonomic, hormonal, and somatic expression, and it is the program as a whole that achieves the required homeostasis, well-being, and development. The term *homeorrhesis* refers to homeostasis along a developmental trajectory; homeostasis alone would put development on hold.

There are three such programs, and they are mutually exclusive, meaning that the body cannot operate more than one at a time. Each has its own set of hormones, its own autonomic wiring, and its own muscular or somatic functions (Despopoulos & Silbernagl,

1986). The analogy to computer software is apt. A computer operates in a single environment at a time, be it word processing, spreadsheet, or database.

The *nutrition* program is the default setting. This is mainly governed by a parasympathetic or vagal nervous system (with sympathetic counterbalance) and ensures that the body keeps balance and homeostasis and that food is digested and temperature controlled. There are many hormones, including insulin and growth hormone.

The *defense* program actively and immediately switches off other programs. It is governed mainly by the sympathetic nervous system, its hormones include adrenaline and cortisol, and its somatic expression is summarized in the well-known phrase *fight or flight*. This can, however, be overwhelmed, and then a more primitive parasympathetic program takes over, expressed as freeze then dissociation.

The *reproduction* program is sensitive, uses both parts of the autonomic nervous system, and has a host of hormones depending on the circumstances, including estrogen and oxytocin.

It is critically important to understand that the place or habitat determines which of the programs will operate. Biologists use the term *habitat* for place, and habitat determines the neurobehavior of the organism. This behavior is focused on ensuring well-being through the fulfillment of basic biological needs. The habitat that the organism occupies provides these needs, so *niche* refers to the behaviors appropriate to the habitat (Alberts, 1994). Thus the fetus acts successfully in the uterus to ensure balance and homeostasis and to achieve oxygenation, warmth, nutrition, and protection. These are termed *basic biological needs*.

At birth, mammals experience a habitat transition. What is evident from biological studies is that the newborn is in control of its destiny, and that control depends entirely on being in the right habitat. Newborn rats will, without maternal assistance, move toward mother's belly to find warmth, to suckle, and to ensure protection (Alberts, 1994). In the process, they will evoke or elicit caregiving behaviors from their mother.

Timetables

Another important factor determining brain development is time and timing. The ongoing presence of the mother is part of the essential experience for the developing organism. The sound of mother's heartbeat gives an ongoing awareness of time (Rivkees, 2004). The mother's daily rhythms and routines imprint themselves on the developing brain. Maternal biorhythms influence the developing fetus (Browne, 2004). The infant's brain develops sleep cycling during the last trimester, with cycles lasting from 60 to 90 minutes. These become more differentiated and developed after birth and are important for the wiring of the brain (Rivkees, 2004). Lastly, DNA and genes initiate development, and experience continues it, but there is also an underlying timetable. Timing is embedded in innate or genetic timetables, a kind of biological clock that creates a developmental agenda (McCain & Mustard, 1999). These have also been described as "brain expectations" (Schaal et al., 2004, p. 270).

Critical Periods

This development agenda or timetable has critical periods, which are defined as "windows of opportunity in early life when a child's brain is exquisitely primed to receive sensory input in order to develop more advanced neural systems" (Shore, 1997). The timetable primes particular parts of the brain in the specific sequence required to achieve a higher level of function and therefore structure. During such times, the brain is "exquisitely susceptible to adverse factors," and these can both "positively and negatively impact the structural organization of the brain" (Schore, 2001a, p. 12). Neuroscientists have in fact identified this by studying adult brain pathology and tracing back in time, and they conclude that "alterations in the functional organization of the human brain . . . [is] correlated with the absence of early learning experiences. Social stressors are far more detrimental than nonsocial aversive stimuli" (Schore, 2001b, p. 206). The infant's immature brain is "exquisitely vulnerable to early adverse experiences, including adverse social experiences" (Schore, 2001b, p. 208; see also Teicher, 2002).

In the study of such early experiences and critical periods, there is generally a salient stimulus, a particular stimulation required along a specific pathway to fire and wire over a particular period (McCain & Mustard, 1999). However, "the wiring of the brain's pathways is best supported when it can integrate quality sensory input through several pathways at once, particularly during critical periods of development" (McCain & Mustard, 1999, p. 27).

Many physicians and researchers do not accept that the concept of a critical period, as described in animals, applies to humans. In lower-order animals, such periods may be extremely short and transient, and it is believed that humans develop far more slowly and therefore this does not apply. This assumption is, however, just that: an assumption without proof. The term *sensitive period* is often more accepted.

The Critical Period of Birth

For any mammal, the transition from uterine to extrauterine life is a critical period in more ways than one. The fetus is suddenly transposed from placental nutrition in a liquid environment to a new means of nutrition in an air environment. There are critical adaptations the organism must achieve, and for many species there is significant mortality in the process. However, from a neurological use of the term, birth is the ultimate critical period. The events of the innate timetable have been converging to prepare for birth. From an evolutionary perspective, this was an extremely dangerous event, and there is an extremely precise series of steps and events that must be accomplished very rapidly for survival. At birth, all the senses of the newborn are exquisitely primed to receive new stimuli, and the infant feels everything maximally, without filters. (Filters develop quickly, an early form of learning, as synapses are pruned.) Each of the senses have a key role to ensure that pathways are fired, which in turn will enable subsequent higher levels of functioning.

Skin-to-Skin Contact and Smell

The salient stimuli that the newborn timetable requires at birth are mother's smell (perhaps reassuring of continuity) and skin-to-skin contact, which will provide touch, warmth, stability, and movement. Essentially, the rich parasympathetic and sympathetic innervation of the skin allows the maternal and newborn autonomic nervous systems to communicate directly. In this way the baby learns what normal is, and the physiological set points are regulated. Further, the nerve fibers of smell and touch lead directly to the amygdala (seat of emotional memory and fear conditioning) (Schore, 2001a). The amygdala then fires and wires a pathway to the left frontal lobe, activating the approach center of the brain (pre-fronto-orbital tract) (Amodio, Master, Yee, & Taylor, 2008; Schore, 2001a). The earlier default was a right-sided avoid center, so now the amygdala can appropriately signal an approach to good emotions and expectations of a reward and an avoidance of bad emotions to avoid punishment. This is the platform for future emotional and social intelligence. This takes 8 weeks to hardwire optimally (Schore, 2001a); mother's continuous presence is needed to achieve the optimal pathway. Notice that it was the same skin-to-skin contact that achieved regulation in the newborn body that also led to emotional and social intelligence. However, all the senses make a package of "quality sensory input through several pathways at once" (McCain & Mustard, 1999, p. 27) that reinforce the pathway and connect it to others. These stimulations will fire and wire the brain and create the first beginnings of vital pathways, which need ongoing stimulation to establish and hardwire. Clearly, there is only one place where this package exists: mother. And at birth, the baby needs the full exposure of these stimuli without filters.

Self-Attachment

All mammals at birth behave in very specific stereotyped ways, unique to their species, involving movements toward the mother and the nipple, with subsequent suckling. In many mammals this is immediately evident at birth. The human being is a mammal, and as such is no different from other mammals. Due to relative biological immaturity, the human newborn requires approximately an hour of undisturbed time (Widstrom et al., 1987) for the infant to begin suckling; a longer time can be required in other mammals.

The reproductive program is operative at this critical time, in both mother and newborn. The salient stimuli required of the particular pathways in the critical period stimulate specific areas of the limbic system. This makes the autonomic nervous system adjust or regulate to achieve homeostasis, the required hormones are produced, and the appropriate somatic or body movements take place. It is only the latter that we can observe as behavior, but that behavior is dependent on the autonomic and hormonal events.

Given the labor ward routines developed in the past 100 years, this was unknown until the work of Winberg, Widstrom, Righard, and others in the late 1970s (Righard & Alade, 1990). The observed behavior is generally termed *self-attachment*. The suckling observed at the end of self-attachment is evidence that the requirements of the particular critical period have been achieved.

It is, however, not the complete picture, which is greatly more complex. The next grade follows immediately. Neurons need repetitive firing in order to stabilize and wire into pathways. The salient stimuli should continue. After successful self-attachment, the newborn will go into a sleep cycle. Sleep cycling is now recognized as an absolute requirement for healthy brain development. It is involved in all stages of neuronal development, pathway formation, and circuit maintenance for memory and learning (Peirano, 2003). One important part of the sleep cycle is quiet sleep, when short-term sensory memory is fired through the amygdala and hippocampus for long-term memory (Graven, 2006), and another is at the end of the cycle when new synapse connections are observed. Healthy sleep cycles occur only when the salient stimuli—those ensuring maternal presence—remain in place. Newborns will wake spontaneously after 4 to 6 hours on average. In separated newborns, the postnatal sleep may be 12 hours or more. Separated infants experience chaotic sleep patterns and may not achieve the wiring that came from the firing.

We noted earlier that the place determines behavior, and stimuli activate the autonomic nervous system and the hormones and make muscles do the right thing. The purpose of these behaviors is to ensure the basic biological needs of the organism (Alberts, 1994):

- Oxygenation
- Warmth
- Nutrition
- Protection

When these needs are met, the infant will continue to function (breastfeed), which will ensure that these needs continue to be met, which further ensures that the brain structure continues to develop, which provides for both better breastfeeding and for the ability to function at subsequently more complex levels.

It is more than this, however. For example, other critical pathways have been stimulated, which may not have been evident in observable muscular behaviors. The metabolic (autonomic and hormonal) adjustment of achieving cardiorespiratory balance and thermal regulation and other homeostasis in general requires approximately 6 hours of continued mother–infant skin-to-skin contact after birth (Bergman, Linley, & Fawcus, 2004). Other evidence of critical period sensitivity is that a single dose of glucose given to newborns at 3 hours of age had a negative impact on the breastfeeding rate at 3 months of age (Martin-Calama et al., 1997). The psychoimmune axis is activated at this early stage, and skin-to-skin contact in the first day improved immunity during the first year of life (Sloan, Camacho, Rojas, & Stern, 1994; Syfrett & Anderson, 1993). Stettler et al. (2005) reported that in American infants bottle-fed with formula, the amount of weight gained in the first week of life accurately predicts their obesity at 30 years of age.

Bonding

Klaus and Kennell (1976) described major differences in maternal behavior following early continuous contact. At an early stage, Anderson (1989) described the mother–infant dyad as "mutual caregivers" (p. 196). Mammalian research clearly shows that the newborn has as great an affect on the mother as vice versa. The pair should be regarded a single psychobiological organism. Mammalian research also elucidates the purpose of this critical period; it is to establish the breastfeeding program. Mammals that are disturbed during such critical periods fail to establish breastfeeding and die. Mammalian young (and primates in particular) generally wean of their own volition. Our Western culture weans early and does not recognize the need to breastfeed for 2 years or more; our researchers would not imagine looking for such an outcome.

Based on comparative mammalian biology and neuroscience, I believe the self-attachment previously described results in a neurological synergistic process that equates to the mammalian term *bonding*. The brain processes involved here are at the level of the old mammalian brain embedded in the limbic system and the midbrain. Further, I regard this as quite distinct from attachment, which in neurological terms is related to cerebral cortical pathways and may be uniquely human. Bonding greatly enhances the quality of attachment, but it also results in long-term behavioral differences, such as increased duration of breastfeeding. These effects are determined at the level of the limbic system.

Where early contact is missing, critical period bonding will not occur, but attachment can make compensations for this. Attachment will become the key factor in sculpting the brain, and it is a cerebral cortical process, rather than a limbic system process. Without the optimal limbic wiring, the attachment may not be optimal for the mother–infant dyad. The attachment may be wholly good and optimal, but the neural pathways for breastfeeding are not cortical, they are limbic. Attachment cannot achieve prolonged breastfeeding, bonding can. Obviously cortical choices and external circumstances have major influences, which makes teasing out the relative contributions difficult!

Human beings are generally not regarded as behaving by instinct, as in the meaning of an animal behavior over which there is no control. We are uniquely human in that we are able to make a cerebral cortical conscious choice. However, the old mammalian brain is in accord and synchrony with our biology and our well-being, and it has an impeccable evolutionary track record. When cerebral choice goes against the old mammalian brain, we may be "straining mother–infant dyads beyond their limits of adaptability" (Lozoff, Brittenham, Trause, Kennell, & Klaus, 1977, p. 1), and we are likely doing harm.

There is ongoing debate as to how long mother and newborn should stay together after birth. The World Health Organization (WHO) and UNICEF, in the Baby-Friendly Hospital Initiative (BFHI), initially recommended 30 minutes and subsequently extended it to 60 minutes. The question should in fact be the opposite; the debate should be about when separation of mother and infant should take place, if at all. From a neurological point of view, separation should not take place at all. It is purely our Western culture and entrenched hospital practices, unsupported by any kind of science or research, that assumes separation is required or normal.

Later Developmental Mechanisms

In the first weeks of life a number of new neurological processes are important in understanding the newborn and in supporting its development and breastfeeding.

State Organization

State organization refers to the infant's ability to appropriately control the levels of sleep and arousal (Ludington-Hoe & Swinth, 1996). This is also related to sleep cycling. The organism will cycle through various states, and each state has a specific purpose and specific risks (Graven, 2006). In the first 90 minutes of life, a healthy, undrugged newborn will be in the active awake state, and this corresponds with the critical period: a conscious and aware absorption of sensory stimuli. Thereafter regular cycling enhances development (Lehtonen & Martin, 2004), and extremes of deep sleep and hard crying should be avoided (Schore, 2001b).

Attention

Als and colleagues (1989) identified the ability to achieve attentive control as the key agenda or achievement in the first weeks of life. The human being is above all a social being, and the ability to relate starts with this capability. This is an important achievement toward attachment.

Attachment

Mothers (and other family members) behave in very specific ways to newborns; for example, they speak in a particular kind of voice and seek out eye contact. The response from the infant creates a kind of reverberation, or a two-way game. The result is attachment. It starts on the first day and continues in ever more complex and variable forms through the first few years of life.

In the first months of life, attachment is the primary driving force in sculpting the brain of the infant into its final configuration (Teicher, 2002).

Through the processes in neuronal plasticity, the pathways for optimal right brain development will be laid down (Schore, 2001a). Breastfeeding is the basic and fundamental activity or behavior that ensures continuity and a sense of well-being that will optimize the result of the brain sculpting. It also provides species-specific and unique nutritional requirements designed for brain growth.

Touch and contact facilitate "the flow of affective information from the infant . . . to the mother. The language of mother and infant consists of signals produced by the autonomic nervous system of both parties" (Schore, 2001a, p. 32). A feature of human development is that the autonomic nervous system (which regulates heart rate and breathing and all homeostasis) is wired to the cranial nerves. Thus mother's face and movements and emotional face play registers through the infant's cranial nerves to the autonomic and hormonal homeostasis of the baby, and vice versa (Porges, 2001).

From years of study, Myron Hofer concludes:

> The mere presence of the mother not only ensures the infant's well-being, but also creates a kind of invisible hothouse in which the infant's development can unfold. This is a private realm of sensory stimulation constructed by the mother and infant from numberless exchanges of subtle clues. For a baby the environment is the mother. What seems to be a single physical function, such as grooming or nursing, is actually a kind of umbrella that covers stimuli of touch, balance, smell, hearing and vision, each with a specific effect on the infant. Through "hidden maternal regulators" a mother precisely controls every element of her infant's physiology, from its heart rate to its release of hormones, from its appetite to the intensity of its activity. (Gallagher, 1992)

The key developmental mechanism that sustains the "invisible hothouse" is the neurobehavior called suckling. This behavior is place dependent, and for the first weeks of life it requires continuous mother–infant skin-to-skin contact.

Conclusion

"The mammalian brain is designed to be sculpted into its final configuration by the effects of early experiences" (Teicher, 2002, p. 397). These experiences are embedded in the attachment relationship.

Separation Behaviors

Protest–Despair Response

In the first section of this chapter, three limbic system programs were described. Further, it is the habitat that determines which of those programs control the body. The reproduction and nutrition programs have been described, and the habitat that elicits them is the mother's chest, or mother–infant skin-to-skin contact. At birth and in the weeks beyond, the human organism recognizes only two habitats: mother or other.

Separation from the mother to any other habitat will immediately elicit the defense program. This has been extensively studied in animals since the 1950s (Bowlby, 1969; Harlow, 1958), and it is described as *protest–despair*. The organism knows its life and survival depend on the right habitat, and the first response is sympathetically mediated protest, shown by crying and by extensor activity. The crying is intended to alert the primary caregiver of the crisis and threat to life and health. Protest as such is not necessarily harmful, and may even be necessary for optimal development of resilience, unless it is repetitive and prolonged (Schore, 2001b). When protest does not give the desired result, the parasympathetically mediated despair phase follows. The sequence is regarded as a single neurological behavior, or program. In despair, the organism shuts down all metabolic systems for prolonged survival, conserving calories by lowering the temperature and heart rate, with inhibition of crying and immobilization, feigning death.

At birth, the protest–despair behavior is easily demonstrated. In my own research, separation in the first hour of life results in a very brief protest response followed by a profound parasympathetic despair response, evidenced by a slower heart rate and a drop in core temperature of 1 or 2 degrees Celsius within 5 minutes (faster than possible by evaporative and radiative cooling).

The reason for this may lie in the development stages of the autonomic nervous system (Porges 1998). At birth, the human has developed only the first part of the autonomic nervous system, the unmyelinated or primitive vagus nerve, which provides the parasympathetic nervous system pathway to the body. In nutrition mode it governs the body metabolism; in defense mode it shuts down metabolism completely and causes dissociation or immobilization. At 8 weeks of age the second part, the sympathetic nervous system, becomes active. When activated, this system produces a muscular response, the well-known fight or flight. At 6 months of age a third stage appears, the myelinated vagus. This is the part that connects to the cranial nerves and higher cerebral centers and allows the organism to make social choices and choose between immobilization or fight or flight, or it can choose from complex alternatives determined by interpretation of the social relationships in the stress situation.

Hyperarousal Dissociation

For many years, the medical establishment regarded the human being as exalted and unique in nature, and no parallels to protest-despair were drawn from or researched in mammal studies. This is ironic because Harlow (Bowlby, 1969) started his research on monkeys after observations of human orphans in Germany after the Second World War.

However, in the 1990s major research on the human brain took place in a variety of disciplines, including psychiatry and psychopathology (Schore, 2001a, 2001b). Without reference to mammalian studies, the exact parallels are reported, only in different words. Protest is called *hyperarousal*, and despair is called *dissociation*. The research shows that in hyperarousal the brain is hypermetabolic, with massive activation of the sympathetic nervous system. In dissociation, the sympathetic system remains maximal, but the parasympathetic system is equally massively activated and tries to make the brain hypometabolic. This creates "a chaotic biochemistry in the developing brain" and a "toxic neurochemistry" (Schore, 2001b, p. 212). The massive firing of the stress pathways reinforces them to the point where they rapidly become exempt from elimination and so are hardwired. The result is that more adaptive and alternative pathways do not get the opportunity to develop, and the organism is left with primitive, monotonous, and simplistic responses to stress and an inefficiently regulating right brain, which impacts future psychiatric and somatic health across the life span. Potential pathways that would have been conducive to health, waiting for stimuli in critical periods, will now atrophy and may be removed altogether. The exact biochemical mechanisms for how this happens have been described. Schore (2001b) defines infant mental health as the ability to vary response to stress, and this depends on an efficiently regulated right brain. Hyperarousal-dissociation retards the development of this ability.

Modern neuroscience also emphasizes the importance of the critical period. The absence of positive stimulation at such a time may be as harmful as the presence of a negative stimulus. Insofar as negative experiences result in hardwired pathways persisting into adult life, neuroscientists conclude that adverse social experiences have worse effects than "aversive nonsocial stimuli" (Schore, 2001b, p. 206) such as hypoxia, intracranial bleeds, or chemicals. In the early developing brain, neural precursor cells are able to replace damaged cells to some extent, and the long-term outcome is potentially better than that of an equivalent injury later in life. When bad pathways are hardwired, the good pathways are dismantled and removed, and long-term permanent problems result.

> Schore writes, "Neuroscience is currently exploring early beginnings of adult brain pathology . . . [and showing] alterations in the functional organization of the human brain . . . correlated with the absence of early learning experiences" (2001b, p. 204).

The fetal metabolic programming or Barker hypothesis (Barker, Eriksson, Forsen, & Osmond, 2002) comes from epidemiological studies of birth records followed through to adult life and provides further support. If the uterine environment has been suboptimal in any way, this can hardwire the brainstem and limbic system in ways that will adversely impact health across the life span. The WHO has recognized a new pandemic dubbed syndrome X or metabolic syndrome—a combination of hypertension, obesity, and diabetes. It is possible that the early pathways for autonomic control of blood pressure and hormonal control of fat cells and glucose metabolism were laid down under stress conditions in the perinatal period. These persist and set the future adult on a trajectory of a thrifty limbic regulation of metabolism, which, in an environment of plenty, results in syndrome X.

Practice Recommendations

What are the implications of this new knowledge? One of the primary axioms of the medical profession is *primum non nocere*, or *first do no harm*. What we really want to do is prevent things from going wrong in the first place. Mothers and infants should never be harmed by being separated; their bonding and attachment should be supported. The behaviors described in this chapter will then emerge, and they can be supported and encouraged according to the circumstances.

When some serious circumstances should arise, and for some overriding reason separation is necessary, then our knowledge of neuroscience should guide the rehabilitation of the neurobehavior of suckling, and restoration to the mother or another primary caregiver should be achieved as soon as possible.

After things have gone wrong, very specific management and skills are needed, as described in this book. But these do require some basic fundamentals to be in place, if we want to elicit the limbic neurobehavior of breastfeeding, so we must restore the infant's habitat.

Space does not permit detailed discussion on this topic, but the next chapter of this book summarizes research that has been done on current labor ward routines and makes suggestions consistent with a better understanding of modern neuroscience. Separation causes stress in the mother and infant. Maternal anxiety has adverse effects, including potentially decreased milk production. But her stress is evident also to the baby, and it reinforces baby's hyperarousal–dissociation. Chapter 3 contains more information on the effect of birth interventions on infant neurobehavior.

The present reality is that most newborns experience prolonged separation. The kinds of questions that need to be answered are as follows:

- How much separation can the newborn tolerate?
- How long does it take for the newborn organism to recover from separation?

When the newborn infant is separated, autonomic and hormonal systems rapidly achieve dissociation. One hormone in particular is worthy of mention: somatostatin (Uvnas-Moberg, 1989). This hormone is the antagonist to growth hormone, and it acts directly on the gut with a powerful inhibitory action on the 20 or more hormones described that regulate every aspect of gut function. Its own direct effects are to inhibit gastrointestinal secretion, inhibit gut motility, and reduce blood flow to the gut and absorption from the gut. The result of this is gastric retention, vomiting, and constipation. This will occur even if mother's milk is put into the gut.

Somatostatin is relatively easy to measure. It has been found that after restoration of the right habitat, it takes at least 20 and probably 30 minutes to eliminate somatostatin from the system. It is probable that other dissociation hormones behave in the same way, but they have yet to be measured. Autonomic effects are likely to recover more quickly. The advice, therefore, is that for any intervention or therapy, the first 30 minutes should start with doing absolutely nothing, apart from placing baby on mother's chest and making them both comfortable. If after 30 minutes both are sleeping, therapy should await their spontaneous awakening.

There are reports of warm baths having a positive effect on restoration. This may well enhance the quality of the restored maternal–infant environment, evoking memories in the child. This is perhaps more effective if the infant is some weeks old and has mastered state and attentional behaviors and therefore can engage more directly. There may be other measures that are supportive in restoring the mother–infant connection and foster attachment.

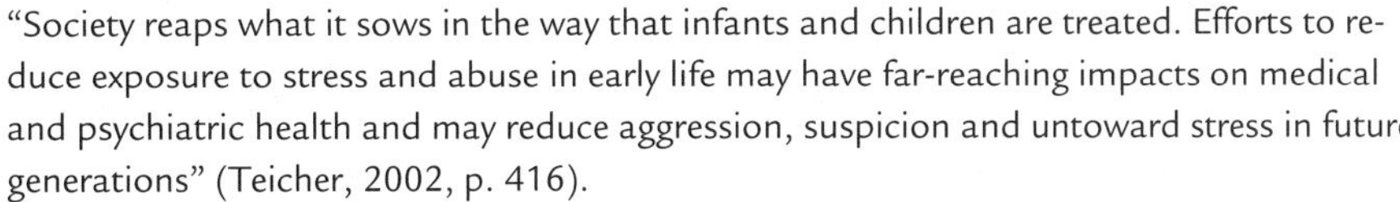

"Society reaps what it sows in the way that infants and children are treated. Efforts to reduce exposure to stress and abuse in early life may have far-reaching impacts on medical and psychiatric health and may reduce aggression, suspicion and untoward stress in future generations" (Teicher, 2002, p. 416).

References

Alberts, J. R. (1994). Learning as adaptation of the infant. *Acta Paediatrica, 397*(Suppl.), 77–85.

Als, H., Lawhon, G., Duffy, F. H., McAnulty, G. B., Gibes-Grossman, R., & Blickman, J. G. (1994). Individualized developmental care for the very low-birth-weight preterm infant. Medical and neurofunctional effects. *JAMA: The Journal of the American Medical Association, 272*(11), 853–858.

Amodio, D. M., Master, S. L., Yee, C. M., & Taylor, S. E. (2008). Neurocognitive components of the behavioral inhibition and activation systems: Implications for theories of self-regulation. *Psychophysiology, 45*, 11–19.

Anderson, G. C. (1989). Risk in mother-infant separation postbirth. *Journal of Nursing Scholarship, 21*(4), 196–199.

Barker, D. J., Eriksson, J. G., Forsen, T., & Osmond, C. (2002). Fetal origins of adult disease: Strength of effects and biological basis. *International Journal of Epidemiology, 31*(6), 1235–1239.

Bergman, N. J., Linley, L. L., & Fawcus, S. R. (2004). Randomized controlled trial of skin-to-skin contact from birth versus conventional incubator for physiological stabilization in 1200- to 2199-gram newborns. *Acta Paediatrica, 93*(6), 779–785.

Bowlby, J. (1969). *Attachment and loss. Volume 1: Attachment.* New York, NY: Basic Books.

Browne, J. V. (2004). Early relationship environments: Physiology of skin-to-skin contact for parents and their preterm infants. *Clinics in Perinatology, 31*(2), 287–298.

Despopoulos, A., & Silbernagl, S. (1986). *Color atlas of physiology* (3rd Rev. ed.). Stuttgart, Germany: Georg Thieme Verlag.

Gallagher, W. (1992, July/August). Motherless child. *The Sciences, 32*, 12–15.

Graven, S. N. (2004). Early neurosensory visual development of the fetus and newborn. *Clinics in Perinatology, 31*(2), v, 199–216.

Graven, S. (2006). Sleep and brain development. *Clinics in Perinatology, 33*, 693–706.

Harlow, H. F. (1958). The nature of love. *American Psychologist, 13*, 673–685.

Klaus, M. H., & Kennell, J. H. (1976). *Maternal-infant bonding.* St Louis, MO: C. V. Mosby.

Lehtonen, L., & Martin, R. J. (2004). Ontogeny of sleep and awake states in relation to breathing in preterm infants. *Seminars in Neonatology, 9*(3), 229–238.

Lozoff, B., Brittenham, G. M., Trause, M. A., Kennell, J. H., & Klaus, M. H. (1977). The mother-newborn relationship: Limits of adaptability. *Journal of Pediatrics, 91*(1), 1–12.

Ludington-Hoe, S. M., & Swinth, J. Y. (1996). Developmental aspects of kangaroo care. *Journal of Obstetric, Gynecologic, and Neonatal Nursing, 25*(8), 691–703.

Martin-Calama, J., Buñuel, J., & Valero, M. Labay, M., Lasarte, J., Valle, F., & de Miguel, C. (1997). The effect of feeding glucose water to breastfeeding newborns on weight, body temperature, blood glucose and breastfeeding duration. *Journal of Human Lactation, 13*(3), 209–213.

McCain, M. N., & Mustard, J. F. (1999). *Reversing the real brain drain: Early years study final report.* Toronto, Canada: Ontario Children's Secretariat.

National Research Council Institute of Medicine. (2000). *From neurons to neighborhoods.* Washington, DC: National Academy Press.

Peirano, P., Algar, C., & Uauy, R. (2003). Sleep-wake states and their regulatory mechanisms throughout early human development. *Journal of Pediatrics, 143*(4), S70–S79.

Philbin, M. K. (2004). Planning the acoustic environment of a neonatal intensive care unit. *Clinics in Perinatology, 31*(2), viii, 331–352.

Porges, S. W. (1998). Love: An emergent property of the mammalian autonomic nervous system. *Psychoneuroendocrinology, 23*(8), 837–861.

Porges, S. W. (2001). The polyvagal theory: Phylogenetic substrates of a social nervous system. *International Journal of Psychophysiology, 42*(2), 123–146.

Righard, L., & Alade, M. O. (1990). Effect of delivery room routines on success of first breast-feed. *Lancet, 336*(8723), 1105–1107.

Rivkees, S. A. (2004). Emergence and influences of circadian rhythmicity in infants. *Clinics in Perinatology, 31*(2), 217–228.

Schaal, B., Hummel, T., & Soussignan, R. (2004). Olfaction in the fetal and premature infant: Functional status and clinical implications. *Clinics in Perinatology, 31*(2), 261–285, vi–vii.

Shatz, C. (1992). The developing brain. *Scientific American, 267*(3), 60–67.

Schore, A. N. (2001a). Effects of a secure attachment relationship on right brain development, affect regulation, and infant mental health. *Infant Mental Health Journal, 22*(1–2), 7–66.

Schore, A. N. (2001b). The effects of early relational trauma on right brain development, affect regulation, and infant mental health. *Infant Mental Health Journal, 22*(1–2), 201–269.

Shore, R. (1997). *Rethinking the brain: New insights into early development.* New York, NY: Families and Work Institute.

Sloan, N. L., Camacho, L. W., Rojas, E. P., & Stern, C. (1994). Kangaroo mother method: Randomised controlled trial of an alternative method of care for stabilised low-birthweight infants. Maternidad Isidro Ayora Study Team. *Lancet, 344*(8925), 782–785.

Smith, L. J., & Kroeger, M. (2010). *Impact of birthing practices on breastfeeding* (2nd ed.). Sudbury, MA: Jones and Bartlett.

Stettler, N., Stallings, V. A., Troxel, A. B., Zhao, J., Schinnar, R., Nelson, S. E., . . . Strom, B. L. (2005). Weight gain in the first week of life and overweight in adulthood. *Circulation, 111*, 1897–1903.

Syfrett, E. B., & Anderson, G. C. (1993, November). *Early and virtually continuous kangaroo care for lower-risk preterm infants: Effect on temperature, breastfeeding, supplementation and weight.* Paper presented at the biennial conference of the Council of Nurse Researchers, American Nurses Association, Washington, DC.

Teicher, M. H., Andersen, S. L., Polcari, A., Anderson, C. M., & Navalta, C. P. (2002). Developmental neurobiology of childhood stress and trauma. *The Psychiatric Clinics of North America, 25*(2), 397–426.

Uvnäs-Moberg, K. (1989). Gastrointestinal hormones in mother and infant. *Acta Paediatrica Scandinavica, 351*(Suppl.), 88–93.

Widström, A. M., Ransjö-Arvidson, A. B., Christensson, K., Matthiesen, A. S., Winberg, J., & Uvnäs-Moberg, K. (1987). Gastric suction in healthy newborn infants. Effects on circulation and developing feeding behaviour. *Acta Paediatrica Scandinavica, 76*(4), 566–572.

CHAPTER

3

Why Johnny Can't Suck: Impact of Birth Practices on Infant Suck

Linda J. Smith

Introduction

For breastfeeding to succeed the baby must be able to feed (cue, find the breast, attach, suck, swallow, and breathe smoothly); the mother must be producing milk normally and willing to bring her baby to her breast many times a day; breastfeeding must be comfortable for both; and the surroundings must support the dyad. If the newborn is unable to breastfeed, and/or if lactogenesis is delayed or impaired, and/or if the mother is unwilling to bring her baby to her breast many times a day and night, then the baby will be fed a human milk substitute, which increases the risk of sickness and death and undermines the mother's goals. Any practice, intentional or unintentional, that causes or contributes to infant immaturity, birth injury, pharmacological influence, central nervous system function, delayed lactogenesis or adverse breast condition, and/or impaired maternal-infant bonding puts the mother and baby at higher risk of poorer health outcomes.

The effects of immaturity, medications, and mechanical interventions are cumulative and synergistic. There is a paucity of research that addresses any direct relationship of birth practices to breastfeeding outcomes. A 2002 systematic review of unintended effects of epidurals included only two articles that specifically address breastfeeding outcomes (Lieberman & O'Donoghue, 2002). Jordan and colleagues (Jordan, Emery, Bradshaw, Watkins, & Friswell, 2005) describe the dilemma of establishing cause and effect:

> Because "failure to breastfeed" is not recognized as a possible harmful effect of medication, there are few methodological precedents in this area. The complex, but under researched, physiological process of establishing lactation is not generally considered vulnerable to pharmacological influences. The transitory nature and "ordinariness" of "switching to bottle feeding" render the usual algorithms for identifying adverse drug reactions inadequate, inapplicable or even irrelevant. Susceptibility to bottle feeding is often regarded as determined exclusively by socio-cultural factors. The possibility of an additional dose-related impact of medication has not previously been explored in this context (p. 931).

Professional segmentation is a major barrier to accurately evaluating breastfeeding-related outcomes of birth practices, despite the fact that "mothers and babies form an inseparable biological and social unit" (World Health Organization [WHO] & UNICEF, 2003, p. 3). During pregnancy and breastfeeding, professional specialties tend to focus on either the mother or the baby, rarely both (Smith, 2010). Obstetricians and anesthesiologists are rarely involved in helping mothers establish successful breastfeeding in the early hours and days postbirth. Pediatricians are rarely involved in decisions regarding labor management and may not even be notified of pregnancy-related complications that affect breastfeeding. Anesthesiologists are even further removed from postbirth and pediatric outcomes than obstetricians. Midwives in many countries provide continuity of care but may lack in-depth education about breastfeeding in general and infant suck issues in particular (Marzalik, 2004). In many places, communication channels are inadequate between prebirth and postbirth care providers, leaving the establishment of breastfeeding to fall through the cracks. Mechanisms and tools for identifying infant sucking problems are inconsistently applied.

Infant Maturity

Infant maturity is one indicator or trigger of spontaneous onset of labor (Vidaeff & Ramin, 2008). Simply put, when the baby is ready for extrauterine life, labor begins on its own. If compelling medical reasons indicate a significant advantage to inducing labor artificially, then by definition the baby is unlikely to be fully mature. Elective induction of labor before 41 weeks of gestation is a risk for poor outcomes for mother and baby (Beebe, Beaty, & Rayburn, 2007; Glantz, 2005). Immaturity itself, alone and in combination with other consequences of induction, affects the infant's ability to feed. Prematurity is a well-known complication to breastfeeding initiation for the baby and mother. (See Chapter 7 for more on preterm birth.)

Induction of labor, especially prior to 39 completed weeks of gestation, is associated with an increased risk of infant death (Kramer et al., 2000). Medical reasons for induction include prolonged rupture of membranes without labor; postdates (greater than 42 completed weeks of gestation); maternal hypertension; maternal health problems such as diabetes; chorioamnionitis (intrauterine infection); and intrauterine growth restriction. Elective inductions for primigravidas may increase the risk of cesarean surgery. Induction of labor may be performed with drugs (e.g., oxytocin), hormones (e.g., several forms of prostaglandin), mechanical stimulation (e.g., stripping or artificial rupture of membranes), or ingested substances (e.g., castor oil). Artificial rupture of membranes to induce or augment labor increases the risk of intrauterine infection, which is a risk factor for cerebral palsy and a host of other consequences, and it only slightly shortens labor. Induction with oxytocin increases the risk of infant jaundice and is implicated in a rising number of babies with kernicterus, or bilirubin staining of the brain, causing severe neurological impairment and even death. Bhutani and colleagues studied a cluster of babies with kernicterus and found five common risk factors (Bhutani, Donn, & Johnson, 2005; Johnson, Bhutani, Karp, Sivieri, & Shapiro, 2009):

- Oxytocin use to induce labor
- Vacuum extractor use at delivery
- Less than 38 weeks gestation
- Large for gestational age (LGA)
- Maternal desire to exclusively breastfeed

Exclusive breastfeeding did not cause these infants' injuries; rather, immature, injured infants were unable to effectively breastfeed and inadequate lactation support resulted in severe underfeeding of vulnerable infants.

Induction of labor is sometimes done for less than compelling medical reasons, resulting in a late preterm or borderline baby with immature or disorganized feeding abilities and a higher risk of readmission to the hospital (Boies, Chantry, Howard, & Vaucher, 2004; Wang, Dorer, Fleming, & Catlin, 2004). Some lactation professionals have reported an impression of a weaker milk ejection after a long induction. Elective induction of labor with prostaglandin E_1 (PGE_1, misoprostol, Cytotec), commonly used to soften the cervix during induction of labor, is inadequately researched for safety and associated with hyperstimulation of the uterus and increased risk of uterine rupture (Hofmeyr, Gulmezoglu, & Pileggi, 2010). Babies of mothers who received oxytocin during labor were twice as likely to have sucking problems in the first hours and days after birth (Wiklund, Norman, Uvnas-Moberg, Ransjo-Arvidson, & Andolf, 2009).

When a decision is made to induce labor, regardless of the reason, a cascade of interventions is triggered, which usually includes the following:

- Unnaturally strong, closely spaced uterine contractions that cause increased pressure on the baby's head (presenting part) and leave less time for the infant to recover between contractions
- Increased maternal pain, which triggers a desire/need for more chemical pain relief
- Early and continuous epidural, resulting in maternal immobility, intravenous hydration and even overhydration, a longer and slower labor, increased maternal and infant fever because of the epidural, and reduced maternal and infant endorphins
- High likelihood of assisted delivery by forceps or vacuum-extraction devices, which cause infant pain, bruising, injury, and possibly disruption of central nervous system structures
- Increased risk of cesarean surgery (Kaul et al., 2004)

Thus, when labor is induced, the infant is more likely to be immature, drugged, injured, and separated from the mother at birth. Each of those factors, individually and collectively, impairs the mother–baby dyad, compromises the initiation of breastfeeding, and makes the transition into external gestation (Montagu, 1986) more challenging.

Chemicals and Drugs: Direct Effects on Sucking, Swallowing, and/or Breathing

All drugs administered to a pregnant or laboring woman reach the fetus/baby. This is not a new issue. Five decades ago, Apgar introduced a scoring system for newborn conditions to evaluate anesthetic treatment of laboring women and urged caution on the use of labor anesthetics (Apgar, 1953). The Apgar score measures **a**ctivity (muscle tone), **p**ulse (heart rate), **g**rimace (reflex irritability), **a**ppearance (skin color), and **r**espiration (breathing). However, Apgar scores do not measure the infant's feeding ability.

Drugs administered during labor appear in umbilical cord blood within a few seconds to a few minutes (Loftus, Hill, & Cohen, 1995). Labor anesthetics and narcotics are chosen for their effect on sensory nerves, with an effort to find drugs that do not affect motor nerves and with the least likely effect on the child. "An ideal anesthetic for childbirth blocks only those nerves subserving pain, leaving all other functions intact. No current drug or technique has that degree of selectivity. Among available methods, however, a properly managed epidural anesthetic comes closest" (Caton, Frolich, & Euliano, 2002, p. 3). Although various combinations of drugs have been studied, no one single protocol or combination is consistently used, reported, or evaluated for breastfeeding outcomes.

Narcotics and anesthetic drugs given by intravenous injection have long been known to depress respiratory function, thereby compromising the infant's ability to coordinate sucking, swallowing, and breathing (Nissen et al., 1995). Regardless of the route of administration, the effects on the infant are dose related. Drugs given by epidural versus IV require a larger absolute dose for effect. The pediatric half-life of some narcotics is far longer than the maternal half-life; therefore, the drugs continue to affect the baby long after the mother has metabolized the drugs. For example, the pediatric half-life of bupivacaine and mepivacaine is 8.1 hours and 9 hours, respectively. The half-life of fentanyl is dose related and can be up to 18 hours or more. Drugs are cleared via infant metabolism, taking about five half-lives for approximately 97% of the drug to clear. Sepkoski, Lester, Ostheimer, and Brazelton (1992) documented the effects of bupivacaine using the Neonatal Behavioral Assessment Scale, reporting that deficits in motor (sucking) and orientation (cueing) were dose related and persisted for at least 30 days. Measurement ceased at 30 days, so the duration of any potential negative effects remains unknown.

There is mounting evidence that narcotics, especially those administered into the epidural space, affect the infant's neurobehavior, including ability to suck, swallow, and breathe in a coordinated manner. Ransjo-Arvidson et al. (2001) documented that "several types of analgesia given to the mother during labor may interfere with the newborn's spontaneous breast-seeking and breastfeeding behaviors and increase the newborn's temperature and crying" (p. 5). Radzyminski (2005) correlated low neurobehavioral scores with poorer breastfeeding behaviors. Baumgarder, Muehl, Fischer, and Pribbenow (2003) reported that "labor epidural anesthesia had a negative impact on breast-feeding in the first 24 hours of life even though it did not inhibit the percentage of breast-feeding attempts in the first hour" (p. 7). In other words, the babies had the *opportunity* to breastfeed but were *unable* to latch and suck.

Direct evidence that narcotics compromise breastfeeding is accumulating. Jordan et al. (2005) reported that "intrapartum fentanyl may impede establishment of breastfeeding, particularly at higher doses" (p. 927). Beilin et al. (2005) reported that among experienced breastfeeding mothers, dose-related administrations of fentanyl were associated with stopping breastfeeding before 6 weeks. Wiklund et al. (2009) reported that infants exposed to epidural anesthesia were nearly four times less likely to suckle the breast in the first 4 hours after birth and were nearly half as likely to be exclusively breastfed at hospital discharge.

When narcotic pain relief is administered, especially via epidural injection, other drugs are commonly used as well. Synthetic oxytocin is often administered to augment contractions and speed up labor, and it interferes with both mother's and baby's emerging innate behaviors (Jonas et al., 2009; Jonas, Nissen, Ransjo-Arvidson, Matthiesen, & Uvnas-Moberg, 2008).

Intravenous fluids are administered to prevent supine hypotension. Overhydrated mothers may experience more breast edema, causing difficulty in breastfeeding (Cotterman, 2004). Intravenous hydration is associated with excess weight loss in newborns, leading to excess formula supplementation (Chantry, Nommsen-Rivers, Peerson, Cohen, & Dewey, 2010). Maternal IV hydration is also associated with infant hypoglycemia, hyponatremia, and jaundice (Singhi, 1988; Singhi, Chookang, Hall, & Kalghatgi, 1985).

When the mother has an epidural catheter in her back, her mobility is restricted, causing her to remain supine, which further retards the progress of labor and is associated with increased fetal malpresentation with resultant abnormal pressures on the infant skeleton and longer labor (Lieberman, Davidson, Lee-Parritz, & Shearer, 2005). The risk of instrument use and cesarean surgery is increased (Cheng, Shaffer, & Caughey, 2006), resulting in increased risk to the infant of abnormal mechanical pressures and injury.

Epidural drugs reduce the infant's ability to cope with pain. Epidural drugs inhibit maternal β-endorphins produced during labor (Goland, Wardlaw, Stark, & Frantz, 1981) and the levels of β-endorphins in colostrum and milk (Zanardo et al., 2001). Skin-to-skin contact and breastfeeding are comforting (Gray, Miller, Philipp, & Blass, 2002; Gray, Watt, & Blass, 2000), and human milk itself is analgesic (Shah, Aliwalas, & Shah, 2006). Therefore, the infant's ability to suck is compromised by epidural drugs, the pain-relieving components in milk are reduced, and the baby is more likely to be separated from the mother. The likely result is an infant who suffers more pain and is unable to relieve that pain through normal breastfeeding.

Physics and Forces: Mechanical Effects of Birth Practices and Procedures

Normal birth requires molding of the fetal skull with associated shifting of the four segments of the occiput, both parietal bones, and three segments of each temporal bone (Netter, 1989). The parietal bones override the basilar portion of the occiput and the two

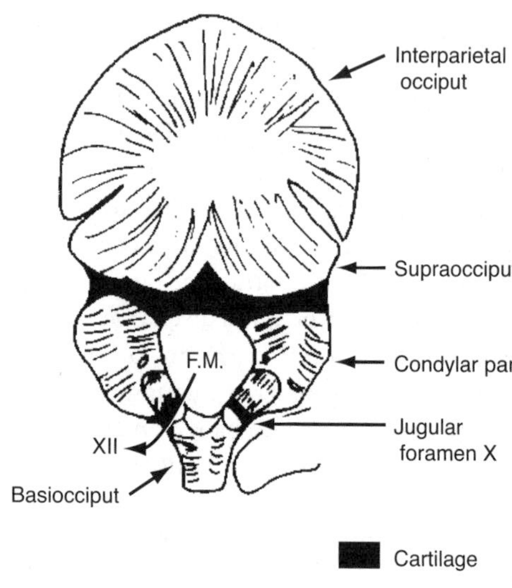

Figure 3-1 External view of occiput at birth.

halves of the frontal bone, allowing the fetal head to corkscrew through the maternal pelvis (**Figure 3-1**).

The hypoglossal nerve (XII) controls tongue movement, including the patterns necessary for latching and sucking. In the infant, cranial nerve XII lies in the space between segments of the occipital bone that later fuse to form the hypoglossal canal in adults. Disruption of the occipital segments could lead to nerve entrapment of the hypoglossal nerve(s), which in turn could cause or contribute to ineffective, mispatterned, and/or disorganized contraction patterns in the tongue muscle group. During cesarean surgery, the surgeon's hands lift on the condylar segments, possibly disrupting the cranial base and altering alignment and function of the hypoglossal nerve, which could affect milk transfer (Evans, Evans, Royal, Esterman, & James, 2003).

Three cranial nerves and the jugular vein pass through the jugular foramen, which lies between the occipital segments and the temporal bones:

- Glossopharyngeal nerve (IX), with sensory fibers in the posterior palate and tongue, which, among other functions, triggers the gag response
- Vagus nerve (X), with sensory fibers to the heart, lungs, trachea, bronchi, larynx, pharynx, gastrointestinal tract, and external ear, and motor fibers to the larynx, heart, lungs, trachea, liver, and gastrointestinal tract
- Spinal accessory nerve (XI) innervates the trapezius and sternocleidomastoid (SCM) muscles, which stabilize the infant's head and maintain airway patency
- Jugular vein, affecting venous return and fluid balance in the cranium

Mechanical analysis of the forces of labor on the fetal skull confirms clinicians' observations of the effects of molding (Lapeer & Prager, 2001). After birth, sucking and crying help expand the cranial vault and allow the bones to gradually move back into alignment during the first 1–2 weeks postbirth (Ward, 2003).

Cranial asymmetry of the occipital, temporal, and/or parietal bones is often accompanied by disrupted alignment of the cranial base (Frymann, 1966). In the first 1–3 days of life, cranial asymmetry is associated with primiparity, assisted delivery, and long labor. Early posterior cranial flattening or other unusual head shapes can progress to deformational plagiocephaly (asymmetry without suture fusing). Cranial asymmetry is more common in males, twins, and on the right side, and it may be associated with torticollis (shortening of the SCM muscle). Cephalohematoma is a well-known risk factor for posterior deformational plagiocephaly. Multiple births and uterine constraints have been reported as risk factors for plagiocephaly but not for true synostosis (premature fusion of the sutures) (Peitsch, Keefer, LaBrie, & Mulliken, 2002).

Excessive pressures to the fetal head, which can be caused by uterine tetany, forceps delivery, or excessive external fundal pressure, can increase fetal intracranial pressure (Amiel-Tison, Sureau, & Shnider, 1988). The use of a vacuum extractor substantially increases the amount of force applied to the occipital segments and entails a documented risk of complications. Hall et al. (2002) reported that "data strongly suggests that success of breastfeeding is associated with events in the first two weeks of life, if not the first 3 to 5 days" (p. 659). Vacuum vaginal delivery was a strong predictor of early cessation of breastfeeding (Hall et al., 2002). The FDA's 1998 Public Health Advisory warns of increased risk for two major life-threatening complications: subgaleal hematoma (subaponeurotic hematoma) and intracranial hemorrhage (brain bleeds) (U.S. Food and Drug Administration, 1998).

Babies with poor suck may have cranial, postural, and/or jaw asymmetry. Wall and Glass (2006) reported that of 11 babies with mandibular asymmetry and torticollis seen in a Seattle lactation clinic, "10 of the 11 mothers had complications of labor and birth, including prolonged labor in 6 cases, resulting in 1 forceps-assisted birth and 4 Cesarean births" (p. 329).

More definitive research on the effect of mechanical (physical) forces of labor on the infant's ability to suck, swallow, and breathe needs to be conducted. Asymmetry in any part of the infant's body, especially the head and neck, may be one indication of significant abnormalities that contribute to poor suck.

Birth Injuries and Insults

Injuries to the baby's head, face, or upper body can interfere with the baby's ability to suck, swallow, and breathe comfortably. Lacerations can occur during forceps use or cesarean surgery, forceps or vacuum extractors can cause significant bruising and even wounds, and mechanically difficult births are associated with cranial and facial asymmetry. Stellwagen, Hubbard, Chambers, and Jones studied asymmetries in newborns, reporting that "moderate facial asymmetry was associated with a longer second stage of labour, forceps delivery, a bigger baby and birth trauma. Moderate cranial and mandibular asymmetries were associated with birth trauma. More than one significant asymmetry was found in 10% of newborns" (2008, p. 829). Wall and Glass reported that facial asymmetry and torticollis are associated with impaired sucking ability in newborns (2006).

Instrument delivery with forceps causes lateral compression of the parietal and three segments of each temporal bone. Forceps use can cause bruising and nerve damage to the sides of the infant's cranium, causing the jaw to deviate to the paralyzed side when the mouth is open (Tappero & Honeyfield, 1993).

Suctioning an otherwise vigorous baby is associated with oral aversion, injury to the posterior oropharynx, removing normal immunologically important mucus, and failing to prevent meconium-aspiration pneumonia, even in babies born through meconium-stained amniotic fluid (Vain et al., 2004).

Circumcision, especially if performed without analgesia and/or before breastfeeding is well established, causes significant infant pain and interferes with mother-infant interactions (Howard, Howard, & Weitzman, 1994; Marshall et al., 1982). No studies have specifically investigated breastfeeding outcomes of infant circumcision.

Bruising from instruments can increase risk for jaundice and even kernicterus. Treatment for jaundice leads to separation from mother, and formula supplementation often interferes with breastfeeding. A baby with bruises or lacerations on the head may be unable to feed in positions that put pressure on the wounded areas.

Brachial plexus injuries cause the infant significant pain, especially when held in certain positions and postures that mothers might unknowingly adopt during breastfeeding (A. C. Blair & Smith, 2007; Mollberg, Hagberg, Bager, Lilja, & Ladfors, 2005). Cephalhematoma; head, shoulder, arm, or facial fractures; dislocation of triangular cartilage of the nasal septum; nerve injuries; subgaleal hemorrhage; intracranial bleeding; and other physical injuries to the infant are more common in mechanically difficult births, instrument-assisted births, and cesarean birth. Poor feeding may be a sign of intracranial hemorrhage (Avrahami, Frishman, & Minz, 1993).

Consequences of Separation

In utero, the fetus is literally bathed—internally and externally—in the mother's body and receives food, oxygen, flavors from family foods, food preferences, oxygen, immunities unique to the family, comforting touch, random passive movement, sound, and even visual stimulation. The mother is the baby's entire environment. The baby swallows *and* breathes amniotic fluid, which matures the lungs and provides protein and tactile experiences in the gut. Some babies suck their fingers, which may be practice for coordinating suck, swallow, and breathe patterns later.

At birth, the baby's internal and external environment drastically and permanently changes. Suddenly sound and light are unmediated; the baby must coordinate sucking, swallowing, and breathing to obtain food and air; and the entire skin surface is bombarded by new, often harsh, sensations. The skin elements with the largest representation in the sensory cortex of the brain are the hands and especially the thumbs, lips, tongue, pharynx, and feet—precisely those body parts that are involved when a baby crawls to the breast and latches on after childbirth (Montagu, 1986). Now the baby is in a condition of exterogestation—maturing outside the womb. The closer the external environment to the internal environment, the more the baby stabilizes and can turn his or her attention to growth and development. A normal baby placed in skin contact with the mother immediately after birth can crawl to the breast and begin breastfeeding in as little as 5 minutes, or at least within the first hour or so (Bullough, Msuku, & Karonde, 1989). Immediate and sustained skin-to-skin contact is so central to establishing breastfeeding that the Baby-Friendly Hospital Initiative (BFHI) includes close physical contact in step 4 and step 7 (WHO & UNICEF, 2009). A 2003 Cochrane review found statistically significant and positive effects of early skin-to-skin contact on the following factors: breastfeeding at 1 to 3 months postbirth (odds ratio 2.15); breastfeeding duration (mean weighted difference 41.99); maintenance of infant temperature in the neutral thermal range (odds ratio 12.18); infant blood glucose (mean weighted difference 11.07); (less) infant crying (odds ratio 21.89); and summary scores of maternal affectionate love touch during an observed breastfeeding within the first few days postbirth (standardized mean difference 0.73) (Moore, Anderson, & Bergman, 2007).

There is no research justifying the separation of a healthy mother and baby, yet this is a very common practice. Separating babies, even for procedures as allegedly benign as weighing and measuring, disrupts the infant's sucking response (Righard & Alade, 1990, 1992). Separating the mother and baby postbirth stresses both (Almeida et al., 2010; Bergman, Linley, & Fawcus, 2004; Meaney et al., 1995) and is actually painful for the infant (Jacobson & Bygdeman, 1998). Separation instantly and permanently raises stress hormones, including salivary cortisol. The separated baby experiences the trauma of hyperarousal and dissociation (protest–despair) simultaneously (Bergman et al., 2004). Thus, separated babies are more stressed and separated mothers are more stressed. Breastfeeding is comforting for both mother and baby.

In addition to alterations in oral motor functioning when separation occurs, separated babies cry more (Christensson, Cabrera, Christensson, Uvnas-Moberg, & Winberg, 1995). Crying increases risks of postbirth intracranial bleeds (Anderson, 1989). Symptoms of intracranial bleeds in term newborns include hypotonia or hypertonia, disturbed swallowing, disturbed sucking, transient apnea, and tremor or jerks (Avrahami, Amzel, Katz, Frishman, & Osviatzov, 1996).

Radiant electronic warmers separate the infant from the mother, have inconsistent temperature regulation, expose the infant to hospital-borne pathogens, destabilize the infant (Bergman et al., 2004), and are less effective in keeping the infant warm than direct skin-to-skin contact on the mother's body. Furthermore, when a baby is in an electronic warmer, he or she is not breastfeeding.

As harmful as separation is to mother and baby individually, separation impedes breastfeeding. Babies need to be physically close to their mother to breastfeed. Physical proximity, especially skin-to-skin contact, results in more episodes of breastfeeding, faster maternal response to baby's feeding cues, normal sucking patterns, thermal coregulation, immune protection for the infant, and more. Ball, Ward-Platt, Heslop, Leech, and Brown (2006) conducted a randomized trial of infant sleep locations on a postnatal ward and concluded that "suckling frequency in the early post-partum period is a well known predictor of successful breastfeeding initiation. Sleeping newborn babies in close proximity to their mothers (bedding-in) facilitates frequent feeding in comparison with rooming-in" (p. 1005). Safe bed sharing facilitates maternal rest (Quillin & Glenn, 2004), infant rest and recovery (Christensson et al., 1992), and breastfeeding (P. S. Blair, Heron, & Fleming, 2010;

McKenna, Ball, & Gettler, 2007). Conversely, separation stresses mothers and infants and compromises breastfeeding.

Recovery from and Resolution of Birth-Related Infant Problems

The three most important and effective strategies to help an infant recover from birth-related insults are (1) skin-to-skin contact, (2) skin-to-skin contact, and (3) more skin-to-skin contact. Skin-to-skin contact between baby and mother does not preclude or replace treatment of any injuries. "Healthy infants should be placed and remain in direct skin-to-skin contact with their mothers immediately after delivery until the first feeding is accomplished . . . Delay weighing, measuring, bathing, needle-sticks, and eye prophylaxis until after the first feeding is completed" (Gartner et al., 2005). Virtually all nonemergency procedures can be done with the baby resting on the mother's body or lying supine next to her in her bed. Let the mother and baby get to know one another without interruption (Morrison, Ludington-Hoe, & Anderson, 2006). Staff and family should fully support the mother's cues and requests for privacy or companionship, food and drink, warmth, and so on. Nursing staff should specifically discourage anyone other than the mother (including other hospital staff) from handling, holding, feeding, or otherwise removing the baby from the mother's arms or bed. Safety should be assured for mother and baby, of course, by unobtrusive and careful observation from a short distance. Nothing should be introduced into the baby's mouth other than the mother's breast until some time after the baby's first effective breastfeed. The BFHI steps 4, 6, 7, 8, and 9 address these strategies in detail.

Ten Steps to Successful Breastfeeding (WHO & UNICEF, 2009)

1. Have a written breastfeeding policy that is routinely communicated to all healthcare staff.
2. Train all healthcare staff in skills necessary to implement this policy.
3. Inform all pregnant women about the benefits and management of breastfeeding.
4. Help mothers initiate breastfeeding within half an hour of birth.
5. Show mothers how to breastfeed and how to maintain lactation even if they should be separated from their infants.
6. Give newborn infants no food or drink other than human milk, unless medically indicated.
7. Practice rooming-in; allow mothers and infants to remain together 24 hours a day.
8. Encourage breastfeeding on demand.
9. Give no artificial teats or dummies to breastfeeding infants.
10. Foster the establishment of breastfeeding support groups and refer mother to them on discharge from hospital.

Mother and baby should remain together throughout the recovery period, even after cesarean surgery or other operative procedures, with breastfeeding on cue 24 hours a day (BFHI steps 4, 7, 8, and 9). An undrugged baby kept with his or her mother may sleep deeply up to 3–4 hours after the first feed (Emde, Swedberg, & Suzuki, 1975) and then transition into and out of sleep for the next day or two with very frequent breastfeeding sessions. Before the moment of birth, the baby received nourishment continually through the umbilical cord and intermittently by sucking and swallowing amniotic fluid. Colostrum is thick, almost gel-like, and is released in relatively small quantities that are easier to manage during the first days of coordinating sucking, swallowing, and breathing. As the mother and baby adapt to external gestation with frequent unrestricted breastfeeding, the dyad's mutual breastfeeding dance continues to improve and mature.

However, some babies are too immature, injured, drugged, and/or otherwise compromised to feed effectively. In that case, follow three rules:

6. Feed the baby.
7. Support the mother's milk supply.
8. Keep the dyad together while the baby's problems are identified and resolved.

Smith's ABC protocol may be useful (**Figure 3-2**). The number 1 rule is always "feed the baby." The number 2 rule is "try the easy solutions that do not involve equipment first." The following is a sequential, three-step strategy. Stop when the mother and baby decide that successful breastfeeding has been achieved. The goal is staying at or returning to step 1, effective feeding directly at the breast. Many of the BFHI Ten Steps to Successful Breastfeeding are integrated into this protocol.

Step 1: Feed the Baby at the Breast (1–3 Days)

Goal: Rule out behavioral issues and minor mechanical issues. The first step is working with mother and baby together.

First, assure enough time is spent at the breast (BFHI steps 4, 7, 8). If the baby isn't near the food, she or he can't eat! To obtain enough calories, the baby should be at the breast at least 140 minutes per 24 hours, or an average of about 11 minutes per hour (De Carvalho, Robertson, Friedman, & Klaus, 1983; Kent et al., 2006). Many babies cluster feedings into 10- to 30-minute sessions, using one or both breasts, every 1 to 3 hours. After 6 weeks, babies may have one 4- to 5-hour sleep stretch per 24 hours. Other patterns are common; the total time at the breast matters.

Warning signs:

- There are consistently fewer than 8 feedings per 24 hours.
- The feedings are consistently less than 5–10 minutes per breast.
- Mother removes baby from the breast at a predetermined time.
- Any pacifier is used.
- Mother is worried that baby isn't getting enough milk.

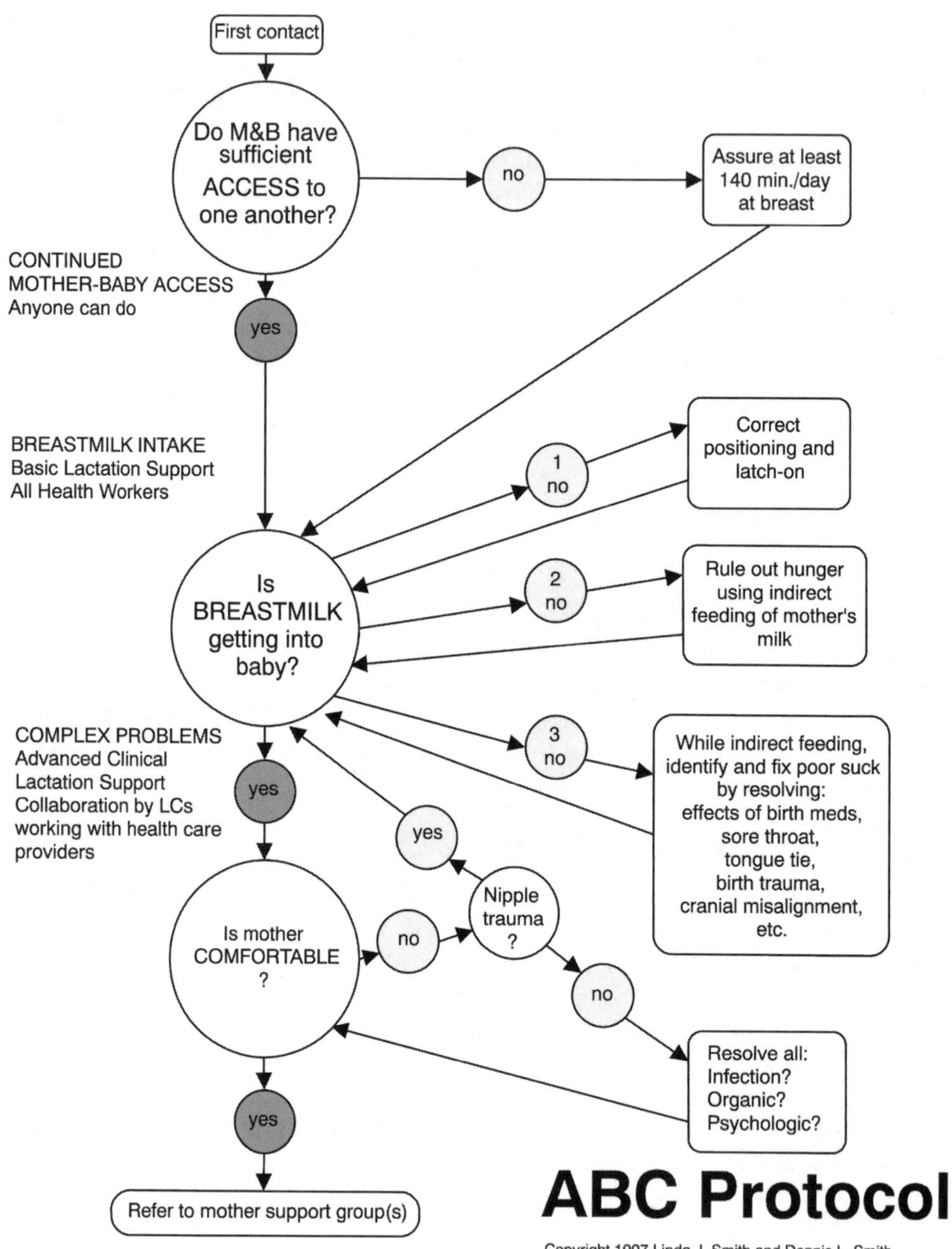

Figure 3-2 Smith's ABC protocol.

What to do: Get the baby to the breast!

- Keep mother and baby in nearly constant skin-to-skin contact for 24–48 hours.
- Maximize the amount of time the baby is at the breast, as continuously as possible.
- Stop all pacifier and bottle (artificial nipple) use. Pacifiers keep the baby away from the breast. All sucking should be at the breast.

Warning: If the mother will not or cannot bring the baby to the breast frequently for any reason, the baby is at immediate risk of inadequate caloric intake. Follow rule 1: feed the baby—with any reasonable source of nutrition, by any method—while addressing this issue. Breastfeeding is impossible without frequent breast contact. That's why it's called *breast*feeding.

Second, assure adequate milk transfer. The baby can be near food but not actually eating. Audible swallowing should be heard during most of the feed at a rate of about one swallow per second, with pauses between bursts of swallows (Riordan, Gill-Hopple, & Angeron, 2005).

Warning signs:

- There are consistently fewer than 8 or more than 16 feedings per 24 hours.
- Feedings are *consistently* shorter than 5 minutes or longer than 30 minutes (Kent et al., 2006).
- There is rapid sucking with little or no swallowing most of the time.
- Baby sucks 3–4 times, falls asleep, *stays at the breast*, and repeats this pattern.
- Mother's nipple is creased, cracked, flattened, or painful after feeding.
- Breast fullness does not change (soften) as a result of feeding.

What to do: Make sure milk is getting from the mother to the baby!

- Assure deep attachment (grasp) to the breast.
- Assure good alignment of the baby's body.
- Assure baby is sucking and swallowing properly.

When to go to step 2:

- Corrected positioning *does not* result in audible swallowing.
- Corrected positioning *does not* eliminate nipple compression or pain.
- Baby pulls away from breast, screams, or cannot stay at the breast.
- Baby does not come off the breast spontaneously with obvious satiety.

Step 2: Feed the Baby Expressed Milk Indirectly (Not at the Breast; 1–3 days) (BFHI Steps 5 and 6)

Goal: Continue to feed the baby while correcting short-term suck problems.

Because direct breastfeeding is not yet effective, indirect feeding of mother's own expressed milk while establishing lactogenesis is the next step. Poor sucking results in inadequate milk intake for the baby and causes milk retention, engorgement, and a subsequently lowered milk supply in the mother. Hunger may cause a poor or disorganized sucking response, resulting in a self-fulfilling vicious circle. Step 2 breaks this cycle by assuring adequate calories for the baby while maintaining or increasing the mother's milk production. The feeding method used in step 2 should correct early interferences and/or avoid compromising future direct breastfeeding. A disorganized suck caused by hunger may resolve in 2–5 days if artificial nipples are completely avoided and sufficient calories are consumed; feeding at the breast can then begin again.

First, get milk. To increase the milk supply, *remove milk from the breast more frequently and thoroughly*. Hand expression is the most effective method of milk expression in the first 48 hours; after that, using a hospital-grade electric breast pump with a double collection kit and manually expressing milk before and after pumping is recommended (Morton et al., 2009; Ohyama, Watabe, & Hayasaka, 2010). Collect milk in a pattern similar to how a normal baby would feed: at least 140 minutes per 24 hours, or about every 2 hours during waking hours and at least once or twice at night. When the breasts begin to feel full, express again. At each session, collect until the milk flow ceases, or at least past one let-down response (Meier et al., 2008). If the mother feels milk dripping or leaking at any time, *collect milk immediately*.

Warning signs:

- The milk volume does not increase in 2–5 days of determined pumping or expressing.
- Nipple or breast pain occurs or continues.
- The mother is taking hormonal contraceptives.
- The mother has ever had surgery on her breasts.

What does not matter:

- The mother's fluid intake, food quality, or food quantity.
- Telling the mother to rest and relax.

Second, feed the baby with anything other than an artificial teat (nipple). The goal is to provide calories while permitting or encouraging normal wavelike tongue movements. Feed the baby with a small open cup, spoon, or dropper (Collins et al., 2004; Howard et al., 2003). The use of a feeding tube device placed at the breast is not effective in step 2 because feeding tube devices placed at the breast do not remove milk from the breast. If a baby cannot get milk out of a breast filled with milk, it is unlikely she or he can get milk out of a tube placed at the breast.

Third, keep attempting to breastfeed the baby. After giving 1–2 ounces of milk (5–15 mL for babies younger than 3 days of age) by an alternate method, try breastfeeding. Placing the baby skin to skin on the mother's unclothed upper torso with the mother in a semireclining position often triggers breast-seeking behavior and self-attachment. Help the mother and baby achieve meticulous latch and positioning, preferably without touching the mother or baby (Colson, Meek, & Hawdon, 2008; Fletcher & Harris, 2000). Breastfeeding should be comforting and is desirable even if few calories are obtained. Monitor the baby's weight, stools, and urine with accurate equipment.

When to go to step 3:

- Breastfeeding causes nipple pain, compression, or damage.
- Baby continues to be unable to attach and feed from the breast.
- Baby's suck does not improve after 2–5 days of increased calories.
- Baby has a difficult time feeding from alternate devices.

Step 3: Find Out Why the Baby Cannot Obtain Milk at the Breast

Goal: Identify and fix the cause of the underlying suck problem.

Continue to feed the baby with mother's milk, using any feeding device that accomplishes effective, nonstressful feeding. Follow the number 1 rule: feed the baby. Consider *volume* of milk first, then *type* of milk, then feeding *method*. Denying a baby food to improve the suck is unjustified. Babies must receive adequate and appropriate caloric support while oral motor problems are solved. Help the mother maintain her milk supply in the most efficient manner. Because the baby's feeding problem has persisted despite previous strategies, further investigation is needed to identify whether this baby has a disorganized or dysfunctional suck. Disorganized and dysfunctional suck patterns are not corrected by using artificial nipples. An artificial nipple (teat) should be used only as a last resort for feeding. Many parents are at the last resort stage if step 3 becomes necessary.

Step 3 includes complete and careful medical evaluation and close follow-up by the baby's primary care provider. Breastfeeding does not cause sucking problems. However, sucking problems jeopardize the baby's nutritional status. Virtually all infant problems, including poor oral motor responses, are exacerbated by inadequate nutrition. Ineffective or inappropriate feeding practices may further compromise undernourished babies with feeding problems. In nearly all situations, human milk is best even if direct feeding at the breast is not possible or must be modified. Maintaining mother's milk supply is usually the easiest part of managing step 3 problems. The lactation consultant can continue to help the mother maintain a good milk supply and preserve and enhance whatever at-breast feeding is possible.

The reasons and remedies for suboptimal sucking responses in otherwise healthy babies are poorly studied. The underlying causes of poor sucking patterns may have long-term consequences to the baby that are unrelated to feeding. The following possibilities are areas to be explored in cooperation and collaboration with the entire healthcare team:

1. *Effects of labor medications:* Narcotic analgesia, epidural anesthesia, and general anesthesia can affect the baby's sucking and alertness for several hours to several weeks after birth.
   a. *To identify:* A history of maternal labor medication for pain relief is present (Smith, 2010).
   b. *Remedy:* Time is required. If the baby cannot suck well, hand express and use an effective breast pump to maintain the milk supply, starting within 6 hours after birth. Feed the milk to the baby using an alternate nonteat method until the effects of the medication have worn off. There should be noticeable improvement within 1 week, even if total resolution takes longer. If there is no improvement, seek further evaluation.
   c. *Cost:* Pump rental and patience are required.
2. *Sore throat from suctioning or intubation:* Vigorous suctioning or intubation may cause swelling or result in soreness in the mouth and/or throat. Some babies will react by biting, clenching their gums, and/or guarding their airway with strong tongue tip elevation.
   a. *To identify:* A history of suctioning or intubation is present.
   b. *Remedy:* Time and gentle, respectful oral experiences are required. A suctioned baby may not want anything in his or her mouth for a while, not even a breast. Cup feeding is usually the preferred strategy. Do not use pacifiers, fingerfeeding, or artificial nipples in this situation.
   c. *Cost:* Pump rental and patience are required.
3. *Head insult or injury during birth:* The use of forceps or vacuum extraction, prolonged pushing, excessive or persistent molding, or cephalohematoma may cause head pain and motor inhibition.
   a. *To identify:* A history of events during delivery and immediately postpartum is present.
   b. *Remedy:* Time, gentle patience, and posture changes are required. Treat the baby as if she or he has a severe headache. Keep the sore side or area up and higher than the baby's heart. Reduce sensory input by reducing noise and music, light, touch, and excessive motion. Maximize skin-to-skin contact upright against a parent's bare chest in a quiet, darkened place. If the baby can nurse effectively in one position, use it frequently without trying for variety! Cool cloths on the baby's head may help. Some clinicians suggest judicious use of infant pain relief

medications. Cup feeding of pumped milk may be more comfortable for the baby than feeding directly at the breast.

c. *Cost:* Pump rental and patience are required.

4. *Oral structural problems, especially tongue-tie (ankyloglossia):* See Chapter 8 for more information about ankyloglossia.

   a. *To identify:* Use a validated assessment tool. Visual clues include a heart-shaped or square-tipped tongue or a tongue that cannot extend past the lower lip without curling or denting. Functional clues include absent or reverse tongue peristalsis, the tongue tip cannot rise to the palate, the mother's nipples are creased and cracked across the tip or have unhealed wounds on the tip, or the baby cannot obtain milk at the breast.

   b. *Remedy:* Evaluation and treatment by a qualified healthcare professional is required. The professional will release the frenulum (perform a frenotomy, see Chapter 9) with sterile scissors and immediately have the baby put to the breast. Frenotomy can be done within hours of the baby's birth. Maternal comfort and infant sucking effectiveness are often improved immediately and continue to evolve over several days.

   c. *Cost:* Medical or dental outpatient surgical treatment is required, which may be covered by insurance.

5. *Misalignment of cranial bones during birth that does not spontaneously resolve in 1–2 weeks (Frymann, 1966):* A mechanically difficult birth may cause pressure on cranial sensory and motor nerves as they pass through the foramen between the infant's skull bones and sutures, which in turn can affect sucking, swallowing, and digestion. The vagus nerve can also be affected.

   a. *To identify:* Signs include gagging, weak suck, abnormal tongue movements, facial asymmetry (Wall & Glass, 2006), postural asymmetry, head molding persisting past 1 week, arching, plugged tear ducts, baby cannot turn head both ways easily, and palpable ridges along cranial suture lines.

   b. *Remedy:* Evaluation and treatment by a doctor of osteopathy, physical therapist, pediatric chiropractor, cranial-sacral therapist, or another qualified provider trained in manipulative techniques on infants is required. These therapeutic modalities are subtle, gentle, and have produced remarkable results (Fraval, 1998) (see Chapter 13).

   c. *Cost:* The cost varies and may be covered by insurance.

6. *Other medical or health problems in the baby:* Other medical or health problems may include cardiac abnormalities, neurological problems, severe allergies, fungal or other mouth infections, metabolic abnormalities, and other congenital issues. Some providers suggest that feeding behavior is the first thing to go wrong when a severe problem is developing in a baby. Always stay in close collaboration with the baby's primary care provider whenever step 3 becomes necessary.

The following is a summary of the protocol:

Step 1: Direct breastfeeding; keep mother and baby together (steps 4, 6, 7, 8, 9)

- Assure sufficient time at the breast (quantity issue).
- Assure effective feeding at the breast (quality issue).

Step 2: Indirect feeding of mother's own milk; keep mother and baby together (steps 5, 6)

- Maintain or increase mother's milk production.
- Feed the baby in a way that encourages proper tongue movements.
- Continue attempts to breastfeed directly.

Step 3: Find out why baby cannot feed at the breast; keep mother and baby together

- Continue indirect feeding with mother's milk while causes and remedies are investigated.
- Support the mother's milk supply, her efforts, and her motivation.
- Collaborate with other providers.

Summary

Obviously babies have to be born. The best way to prevent complications arising from birth practices is to minimize the use of interventions. A normal birth usually leads to normal breastfeeding. Complications during pregnancy, labor, and birth do occur, and properly used interventions can be life saving for the mother and/or baby. Even when they are necessary and properly used, interventions can have a profound negative effect on the infant, the mother, and the course of breastfeeding. The rate at which interventions are used is the chief concern, not the interventions themselves. The WHO and other health-policy bodies have published research-based data on the recommended rates of medically necessary interventions. In many places, local rates of induction, cesarean surgery, and epidural use far exceed medically necessary rates.

The 2009 WHO/UNICEF Baby-Friendly Hospital Initiative guidelines include Mother-Friendly Care (WHO & UNICEF, 2009). The Global Criteria for the BFHI Mother-Friendly Care Module contains these five principles:

- Encouraging women to have companions of their choice to provide continuous physical and/or emotional support during labor and birth, if desired
- Allowing women to drink and eat light foods during labor, if desired
- Encouraging women to consider the use of nondrug methods of pain relief unless analgesic or anaesthetic drugs are necessary because of complications, respecting the personal preferences of the women
- Encouraging women to walk and move about during labor, if desired, and assume positions of their choice while giving birth, unless a restriction is specifically required for a complication and the reason is explained to the mother

- Care that does not involve invasive procedures such as rupture of the membranes, episiotomies, acceleration or induction of labor, instrumental deliveries, or cesarean sections unless specifically required for a complication and the reason is explained to the mother (WHO & UNICEF, 2009, p. 36)

Lamaze International developed six Lamaze Healthy Birth Practices, each of which is fully supported by abundant research. The organization believes that the care practices, adapted from the WHO, promote, support, and protect nature's plan for birth:

1. Labor begins on its own
2. Freedom of movement throughout labor
3. Continuous labor support
4. No routine interventions
5. Nonsupine (e.g., upright or side-lying) positions for birth
6. No separation of mother and baby after birth with unlimited opportunity for breastfeeding (Lamaze International, 2010)

Regardless of what happens during childbirth, lactation consultants have a key role in helping mothers and babies establish breastfeeding. Lactation consultants are trained and skilled in observing, assisting, and monitoring the mother–baby dyad as they move along the continuum from internal gestation to exterogestation. Lactation consultants play an important role in documenting and bearing witness to the mother and baby outcomes that may be affected by birth interventions and in aiding the mother–baby dyad to overcome early and/or negative consequences of birth practices.

References

Almeida, N. D., Loucks, E. B., Kubzansky, L., Pruessner, J., Maselko, J., Meaney, M. J., & Buka, S. L. (2010). Quality of parental emotional care and calculated risk for coronary heart disease. *Psychosomatic Medicine, 72*(2), 148–155.

Amiel-Tison, C., Sureau, C., & Shnider, S. M. (1988). Cerebral handicap in full-term neonates related to the mechanical forces of labour. *Baillieres Clinical Obstetrics and Gynaecology, 2*(1), 145–165.

Anderson, G. C. (1989). Risk in mother–infant separation postbirth. *Image—The Journal of Nursing Scholarship, 21*(4), 196–199.

Apgar, V. (1953). A proposal for a new method of evaluation of the newborn infant. *Current Researches in Anesthesia and Analgesia, 32*(4), 260–267.

Avrahami, E., Amzel, S., Katz, R., Frishman, E., & Osviatzov, I. (1996). CT demonstration of intracranial bleeding in term newborns with mild clinical symptoms. *Clinical Radiology, 51*(1), 31–34.

Avrahami, E., Frishman, E., & Minz, M. (1993). CT demonstration of intracranial haemorrhage in term newborn following vacuum extractor delivery. *Neuroradiology, 35*(2), 107–108.

Ball, H. L., Ward-Platt, M. P., Heslop, E., Leech, S. J., & Brown, K. A. (2006). Randomised trial of infant sleep location on the postnatal ward. *Archives of Disease in Childhood, 91*(12), 1005–1010.

Baumgarder, D. J., Muehl, P., Fischer, M., & Pribbenow, B. (2003). Effect of labor epidural anesthesia on breast-feeding of healthy full-term newborns delivered vaginally. *Journal of the American Board of Family Practice, 16*(1), 7–13.

Beebe, L., Beaty, C., & Rayburn, W. (2007). Immediate neonatal outcomes after elective induction of labor. *Journal of Reproductive Medicine, 52*(3), 173–175.

Beilin, Y., Bodian, C. A., Weiser, J., Hossain, S., Arnold, I., Feierman, D. E., . . . Holzman, I. (2005). Effect of labor epidural analgesia with and without fentanyl on infant breast-feeding: A prospective, randomized, double-blind study. *Anesthesiology, 103*(6), 1211–1217.

Bergman, N. J., Linley, L. L., & Fawcus, S. R. (2004). Randomized controlled trial of skin-to-skin contact from birth versus conventional incubator for physiological stabilization in 1200- to 2199-gram newborns. *Acta Paediatrica, 93*(6), 779–785.

Bhutani, V. K., Donn, S. M., & Johnson, L. H. (2005). Risk management of severe neonatal hyperbilirubinemia to prevent kernicterus. *Clinics in Perinatology, 32*(1), 125–139, vii.

Blair, A. C., & Smith, L. J. (2007). *Birth injuries that affect breastfeeding*. Paper presented at the International Conference on the Theory and Practice of Human Lactation Research and Breastfeeding Management, Orlando, FL.

Blair, P. S., Heron, J., & Fleming, P. J. (2010). Relationship between bed sharing and breastfeeding: Longitudinal, population-based analysis. *Pediatrics, 126*(5) e1119–e1126. Advance online publication. doi:10.1542/peds.2010-1277

Boies, E., Chantry, C. J., Howard, C. R., & Vaucher, Y. (2004). *Clinical protocol # 10: Breastfeeding the near-term infant (35 to 37 weeks gestation)*. New Rochelle, NY: Academy of Breastfeeding Medicine.

Bullough, C. H., Msuku, R. S., & Karonde, L. (1989). Early suckling and postpartum haemorrhage: Controlled trial in deliveries by traditional birth attendants. *Lancet, 2*(8662), 522–525.

Caton, D., Frolich, M. A., & Euliano, T. Y. (2002). Anesthesia for childbirth: Controversy and change. *American Journal of Obstetrics and Gynecology, 186*(5 Suppl. Nature), S25–S30.

Chantry, C. J., Nommsen-Rivers, L. A., Peerson, J. M., Cohen, R. J., & Dewey, K. G. (2010). Excess weight loss in first-born breastfed newborns relates to maternal intrapartum fluid balance. *Pediatrics, 127*(1), e171-e179. Advance online publication. doi:10.1542/peds.2009-2663

Cheng, Y. W., Shaffer, B. L., & Caughey, A. B. (2006). The association between persistent occiput posterior position and neonatal outcomes. *Obstetrics and Gynecology, 107*(4), 837–844.

Christensson, K., Cabrera, T., Christensson, E., Uvnas-Moberg, K., & Winberg, J. (1995). Separation distress call in the human neonate in the absence of maternal body contact. *Acta Paediatrica, 84*(5), 468–473.

Christensson, K., Siles, C., Moreno, L., Belaustequi, A., De La Fuente, P., Lagercrantz, H., . . . Winberg, J. (1992). Temperature, metabolic adaptation and crying in healthy full-term newborns cared for skin-to-skin or in a cot. *Acta Paediatrica, 81*(6–7), 488–493.

Collins, C. T., Ryan, P., Crowther, C. A., McPhee, A. J., Paterson, S., & Hiller, J. E. (2004). Effect of bottles, cups, and dummies on breast feeding in preterm infants: A randomised controlled trial. *BMJ, 329*(7459), 193–198.

Colson, S. D., Meek, J. H., & Hawdon, J. M. (2008). Optimal positions for the release of primitive neonatal reflexes stimulating breastfeeding. *Early Human Development, 84*(7), 441–449.

Cotterman, K. J. (2004). Reverse pressure softening: A simple tool to prepare areola for easier latching during engorgement. *Journal of Human Lactation, 20*(2), 227–237.

De Carvalho, M., Robertson, S., Friedman, A., & Klaus, M. (1983). Effect of frequent breast-feeding on early milk production and infant weight gain. *Pediatrics, 72*(3), 307–311.

Emde, R. N., Swedberg, J., & Suzuki, B. (1975). Human wakefulness and biological rhythms after birth. *Archives of General Psychiatry, 32*(6), 780–783.

Evans, K. C., Evans, R. G., Royal, R., Esterman, A. J., & James, S. L. (2003). Effect of caesarean section on breast milk transfer to the normal term newborn over the first week of life. *Archives of Disease in Childhood. Fetal and Neonatal Edition, 88*(5), F380–F382.

Fletcher, D., & Harris, H. (2000). The implementation of the HOT program at the Royal Women's Hospital. *Breastfeeding Review, 8*(1), 19–23.

Fraval, M. M. (1998). A pilot study: Osteopathic treatment of infants with a sucking dysfunction. *Journal of the American Academy of Osteopathy, 8*(2), 25–33.

Frymann, V. (1966). Relation of disturbances of craniosacral mechanisms to symptomatology of the newborn: Study of 1,250 infants. *Journal of the American Osteopathic Association, 65*(10), 1059–1075.

Gartner, L. M., Morton, J., Lawrence, R. A., Naylor, A. J., O'Hare, D., Schanler, R. J., . . . American Academy of Pediatrics. (2005). Breastfeeding and the use of human milk. *Pediatrics, 115*, 496–506.

Glantz, J. C. (2005). Elective induction vs. spontaneous labor associations and outcomes. *Journal of Reproductive Medicine, 50*(4), 235–240.

Goland, R. S., Wardlaw, S. L., Stark, R. I., & Frantz, A. G. (1981). Human plasma beta-endorphin during pregnancy, labor, and delivery. *Journal of Clinical Endocrinology and Metabolism, 52*(1), 74–78.

Gray, L., Miller, L. W., Philipp, B. L., & Blass, E. M. (2002). Breastfeeding is analgesic in healthy newborns. *Pediatrics, 109*(4), 590–593.

Gray, L., Watt, L., & Blass, E. M. (2000). Skin-to-skin contact is analgesic in healthy newborns. *Pediatrics, 105*(1), e14.

Hall, R. T., Mercer, A. M., Teasley, S. L., McPherson, D. M., Simon, S. D., Santos, S. R., . . . Hipsh, N. E. (2002). A breast-feeding assessment score to evaluate the risk for cessation of breast-feeding by 7 to 10 days of age. *Journal of Pediatrics, 141*(5), 659–664.

Hofmeyr, G. J., Gulmezoglu, A. M., & Alfirevic, Z. (1999). Misoprostol for induction of labour: A systematic review. *British Journal of Obstetrics and Gynaecology, 106*(8), 798–803.

Hofmeyr, G. J., Gulmezoglu, A. M., & Pileggi, C. (2010). Vaginal misoprostol for cervical ripening and induction of labour. *Cochrane Database Syst Rev*(10), CD000941.

Howard, C. R., Howard, F. M., Lanphear, B., Eberly, S., deBlieck, E. A., Oakes, D., & Lawrence, R. A. (2003). Randomized clinical trial of pacifier use and bottle-feeding or cupfeeding and their effect on breastfeeding. *Pediatrics, 111*(3), 511–518.

Howard, C. R., Howard, F. M., & Weitzman, M. L. (1994). Acetaminophen analgesia in neonatal circumcision: The effect on pain. *Pediatrics, 93*(4), 641–646.

Jacobson, B., & Bygdeman, M. (1998). Obstetric care and proneness of offspring to suicide as adults: Case-control study. *BMJ, 317*(7169), 1346–1349.

Johnson, L., Bhutani, V. K., Karp, K., Sivieri, E. M., & Shapiro, S. M. (2009). Clinical report from the pilot USA Kernicterus Registry (1992 to 2004). *Journal of Perinatology, 29*(Suppl. 1), S25–S45.

Jonas, W., Johansson, L. M., Nissen, E., Ejdeback, M., Ransjo-Arvidson, A. B., & Uvnas-Moberg, K. (2009). Effects of intrapartum oxytocin administration and epidural analgesia on the concentration of plasma oxytocin and prolactin, in response to suckling during the second day postpartum. *Breastfeeding Medicine, 4*(2), 71–82.

Jonas, W., Nissen, E., Ransjo-Arvidson, A. B., Matthiesen, A. S., & Uvnas-Moberg, K. (2008). Influence of oxytocin or epidural analgesia on personality profile in breastfeeding women: A comparative study. *Archive of Women's Mental Health, 11*(5–6), 335–345.

Jordan, S., Emery, S., Bradshaw, C., Watkins, A., & Friswell, W. (2005). The impact of intrapartum analgesia on infant feeding. *BJOG, 112*(7), 927–934.

Kaul, B., Vallejo, M. C., Ramanathan, S., Mandell, G., Phelps, A. L., & Daftary, A. R. (2004). Induction of labor with oxytocin increases cesarean section rate as compared with oxytocin for augmentation of spontaneous labor in nulliparous parturients controlled for lumbar epidural analgesia. *Journal of Clinical Anesthesia, 16*(6), 411–414.

Kent, J. C., Mitoulas, L. R., Cregan, M. D., Ramsay, D. T., Doherty, D. A., & Hartmann, P. E. (2006). Volume and frequency of breastfeedings and fat content of breast milk throughout the day. *Pediatrics, 117*(3), e387–e395.

Kramer, M. S., Demissie, K., Yang, H., Platt, R. W., Sauve, R., & Liston, R. (2000). The contribution of mild and moderate preterm birth to infant mortality. Fetal and Infant Health Study Group of the Canadian Perinatal Surveillance System. *JAMA, 284*(7), 843–849.

Lamaze International. (2010). Lamaze healthy birth practices. Retrieved from http://www.lamaze.org/Default.aspx?tabid=90

Lapeer, R. J., & Prager, R. W. (2001). Fetal head moulding: Finite element analysis of a fetal skull subjected to uterine pressures during the first stage of labour. *Journal of Biomechanics, 34*(9), 1125–1133.

Lieberman, E., Davidson, K., Lee-Parritz, A., & Shearer, E. (2005). Changes in fetal position during labor and their association with epidural analgesia. *Obstetrics and Gynecology, 105*(5 Pt. 1), 974–982.

Lieberman, E., & O'Donoghue, C. (2002). Unintended effects of epidural analgesia during labor: A systematic review. *American Journal of Obstetrics and Gynecology, 186*(5 Suppl. Nature), S31–S68.

Loftus, J. R., Hill, H., & Cohen, S. E. (1995). Placental transfer and neonatal effects of epidural sufentanil and fentanyl administered with bupivacaine during labor. *Anesthesiology, 83*(2), 300–308.

Marshall, R. E., Porter, F. L., Rogers, A. G., Moore, J., Anderson, B., & Boxerman, S. B. (1982). Circumcision: II. effects upon mother–infant interaction. *Early Human Development, 7*(4), 367–374.

Marzalik, P. R. (2004). *Breastfeeding education in university nursing programs.* Chicago: University of Illinois.

McKenna, J. J., Ball, H. L., & Gettler, L. T. (2007). Mother–infant cosleeping, breastfeeding and sudden infant death syndrome: What biological anthropology has discovered about normal infant sleep and pediatric sleep medicine. *American Journal of Physical Anthropology, 134*(Suppl. 45), 133–161.

Meaney, M. J., O'Donnell, D., Rowe, W., Tannenbaum, B., Steverman, A., Walker, M., . . . Lupien, S. (1995). Individual differences in hypothalamic-pituitary-adrenal activity in later life and hippocampal aging. *Experimental Gerontology, 30*(3–4), 229–251.

Meier, P. P., Engstrom, J. L., Hurst, N. M., Ackerman, B., Allen, M., Motykowski, J. E., . . . Jegier, B. J. (2008). A comparison of the efficiency, efficacy, comfort, and convenience of two hospital-grade electric breast pumps for mothers of very low birthweight infants. *Breastfeeding Medicine, 3*(3), 141–150. doi:10.1089/bfm.2007.0021

Mollberg, M., Hagberg, H., Bager, B., Lilja, H., & Ladfors, L. (2005). Risk factors for obstetric brachial plexus palsy among neonates delivered by vacuum extraction. *Obstetrics and Gynecology, 106*(5 Pt. 1), 913–918.

Montagu, A. (1986). *Touching: The human significance of the skin* (3rd ed.). New York, NY: Harper and Row.

Moore, E., Anderson, G., & Bergman, N. (2007). Early skin-to-skin contact for mothers and their healthy newborn infants. Cochrane Database System Review, 3, (CD003519).

Morrison, B., Ludington-Hoe, S., & Anderson, G. C. (2006). Interruptions to breastfeeding dyads on postpartum day 1 in a university hospital. *Journal of Obstetric, Gynecologic, and Neonatal Nursing, 35*(6), 709–716.

Morton, J., Hall, J. Y., Wong, R. J., Thairu, L., Benitz, W. E., & Rhine, W. D. (2009). Combining hand techniques with electric pumping increases milk production in mothers of preterm infants. *Journal of Perinatology, 29*(11), 757–764. doi:10.1038/jp.2009.87

Netter, F. (1989). *Atlas of human anatomy*. Summit, NJ: CIBA-Geigy.

Nissen, E., Lilja, G., Matthiesen, A. S., Ransjo-Arvidsson, A. B., Uvnas-Moberg, K., & Widstrom, A. M. (1995). Effects of maternal pethidine on infants' developing breast feeding behaviour. *Acta Paediatrica, 84*(2), 140–145.

Ohyama, M., Watabe, H., & Hayasaka, Y. (2010). Manual expression and electric breast pumping in the first 48 h after delivery. *Pediatrics International, 52*(1), 39–43.

Peitsch, W. K., Keefer, C. H., LaBrie, R. A., & Mulliken, J. B. (2002). Incidence of cranial asymmetry in healthy newborns. *Pediatrics, 110*(6), e72.

Quillin, S. I., & Glenn, L. L. (2004). Interaction between feeding method and co-sleeping on maternal-newborn sleep. *Journal of Obstetric, Gynecologic, and Neonatal Nursing, 33*(5), 580–588.

Radzyminski, S. (2005). Neurobehavioral functioning and breastfeeding behavior in the newborn. *Journal of Obstetric, Gynecologic, and Neonatal Nursing, 34*(3), 335–341.

Ransjo-Arvidson, A., Matthiesen, A., Lilja, G., Nissen, E., Widstrom, A., & Uvnas-Moberg, K. (2001). Maternal analgesia during labor disturbs newborn behavior. *Birth, 28*, 5–12.

Righard, L., & Alade, M. O. (1990). Effect of delivery room routines on success of first breast-feed. *Lancet, 336*(8723), 1105–1107.

Righard, L., & Alade, M. O. (1992). Sucking technique and its effect on success of breastfeeding. *Birth, 19*(4), 185–189.

Riordan, J., Gill-Hopple, K., & Angeron, J. (2005). Indicators of effective breastfeeding and estimates of breast milk intake. *Journal of Human Lactation, 21*(4), 406–412.

Sepkoski, C. M., Lester, B. M., Ostheimer, G. W., & Brazelton, T. B. (1992). The effects of maternal epidural anesthesia on neonatal behavior during the first month. *Developmental Medicine and Child Neurology, 34*(12), 1072–1080.

Shah, P. S., Aliwalas, L. I., & Shah, V. (2006). Breastfeeding or breast milk for procedural pain in neonates. Cochrane Database System Review, 3, (CD004950).

Singhi, S. (1988). Effect of maternal intrapartum glucose therapy on neonatal blood glucose levels and neurobehavioral status of hypoglycemic term newborn infants. *Journal of Perinatal Medicine, 16*(3), 217–224.

Singhi, S., Chookang, E., Hall, J. S., & Kalghatgi, S. (1985). Iatrogenic neonatal and maternal hyponatraemia following oxytocin and aqueous glucose infusion during labour. *British Journal of Obstetrics and Gynaecology, 92*(4), 356–363.

Smith, L. J. (2010). *Impact of birthing practices on breastfeeding* (2nd ed.). Sudbury, MA: Jones and Bartlett.

Stellwagen, L., Hubbard, E., Chambers, C., & Jones, K. L. (2008). Torticollis, facial asymmetry and plagiocephaly in normal newborns. *Archives of Disease in Childhood, 93*(10), 827–831.

Tappero, E., & Honeyfield, M. (1993). *Physical assessment of the newborn*. Petaluma, CA: NICULink.

US Food and Drug Administration. (1998). Need for caution when using vacuum assisted delivery devices. Retrieved from http://www.fda.gov/MedicalDevices/Safety/AlertsandNotices/PublicHealthNotifications/ucm062295.htm

Vain, N. E., Szyld, E. G., Prudent, L. M., Wiswell, T. E., Aguilar, A. M., & Vivas, N. I. (2004). Oropharyngeal and nasopharyngeal suctioning of meconium-stained neonates before delivery of their shoulders: Multicentre, randomised controlled trial. *Lancet, 364*(9434), 597–602.

Vidaeff, A. C., & Ramin, S. M. (2008). Potential biochemical events associated with initiation of labor. *Current Medicinal Chemistry, 15*(6), 614–619.

Wall, V., & Glass, R. (2006). Mandibular asymmetry and breastfeeding problems: Experience from 11 cases. *Journal of Human Lactation, 22*(3), 328–334.

Wang, M. L., Dorer, D. J., Fleming, M. P., & Catlin, E. A. (2004). Clinical outcomes of near-term infants. *Pediatrics, 114*(2), 372–376.

Ward, R. C. (2003). *Foundations for osteopathic medicine* (2nd ed.). Philadelphia, PA: Lippincott Williams and Wilkins.

Wiklund, I., Norman, M., Uvnas-Moberg, K., Ransjo-Arvidson, A. B., & Andolf, E. (2009). Epidural analgesia: Breast-feeding success and related factors. *Midwifery, 25*(2), e31–e38.

World Health Organization & UNICEF. (2003). Global strategy for infant and young child feeding. Retrieved from http://www.who.int/nutrition/publications/infantfeeding/9241562218/en/index.html

World Health Organization & UNICEF. (2009). *Baby-Friendly Hospital Initiative: Revised, updated and expanded for integrated care*. Geneva, Switzerland: Author.

Zanardo, V., Nicolussi, S., Carlo, G., Marzari, F., Faggian, D., Favaro, F., & Plebani, M. (2001). Beta endorphin concentrations in human milk. *Journal of Pediatric Gastroenterology and Nutrition, 33*(2), 160–164.

CHAPTER 4

How Infants Learn to Feed: A Neurobehavioral Model

Christina M. Smillie

When a healthy, hungry human infant is with his mother, whether on her abdomen, in her arms, on her chest, or up on her shoulder, the infant will begin to make certain predictable movements, bobbing his head, pecking with his open mouth, moving his head and neck, flexing his arms and legs, and squirming and attempting to propel himself in one direction or another toward the breast.

This behavior has many variants, but it is a behavior we have all seen, as parents or professionals, in newborns only a half-hour old, in infants days and weeks and months old, and even in babies of a year or older. We see it in experienced breastfed infants, in newborns who have never been at breast, and even in those unfortunate infants who have had only trouble at the breast and who will cry and fret as soon as they reach the breast. We even see this pecking and twisting behavior in older artificially fed infants, completely inexperienced with the breast, when they are hungry and in their mother's or father's arms.

However, we do not see this breast-seeking behavior in deeply sleeping babies, nor in frantically crying babies. The full-blown behavioral sequence of bobbing and pecking and twisting is only seen in alert and hungry babies and occasionally in more muted form, in mildly sleepy but mildly hungry infants.

Such behaviors are often termed *rooting responses* or *feeding cues*. An inexperienced new mother, confused by her newborn's bobbing behavior, might ask, "What's my baby doing?" but most mothers appear to quickly learn to recognize this behavior at least as a sign of hunger. And some mothers, confident in their infant's competence, will even explain, "He's trying to get to the breast."

Those mothers are right, of course. These behaviors are not mere reflex responses or even simply signs of hunger, they are full-fledged and purposeful feeding behaviors, which, if recognized and not thwarted, can initiate a cascade of behaviors that not only take the baby to the breast, but also allow the baby to find the nipple and begin suckling. If his mother responds to his pecking and twisting, and supports rather than restrains his movement, even the naïve and inexperienced infant will then bob, bounce, gently fall, or throw his body down toward the breast. Once there, under a variety of specific facilitating circumstances that we will describe later in this chapter, the infant then has the opportunity to initiate a feed, reaching his wide-open mouth over the nipple to orally grasp the breast and begin to suckle.

However, Western culture has not prepared either mothers or professionals to expect such infant competence. On the contrary, the newborn is usually understood to be quite incompetent, his behavior restricted by unpredictable and intrusive reflex responses, insatiable drives, and neurological disorganization.

From this viewpoint, if the infant begins, apparently randomly, to peck and squirm, his mother will restrain her infant, protect the head and neck, and interfere with his movement. Without an expectation of competence, she will not see what her infant is trying to do.

It is the expectation of incompetence in the human infant that has kept us from seeing this ordinary mammalian behavior, a behavior consistent with what we know about other mammalian infants and the evolutionary roots of adaptive animal behavior.

Innate Mammalian Newborn Feeding Behaviors

Biologists have long recognized that mammalian behavior is both genetically scripted and environmentally adaptive. Human newborns, like all mammalian infants, are biological organisms uniquely adapted to the developmentally specific environmental habitat for which evolutionary forces have prepared them—the interactive environment of the mother's care.

This evolutionary preparation includes a rich repertoire of innate physiologic and neurobehavioral responses that allow the infant to adapt to, interact with, learn from, and even alter his environment to meet the infant's primary tasks of survival and growth. This is discussed in more detail in Chapter 2.

Innate Infant Feeding Behaviors in Nonhuman Mammals

From species to species, the immediate postnatal behaviors of all mammalian newborns are remarkably similar. After a short period of recovery, the newborn of each species, using a series of neurosensory cues to guide it, searches for and independently finds its mother's teat, grasps it with its mouth, and initiates feeding. The tiny kitten, eyes still sealed closed, nuzzles in, finds a teat, and begins to feed. The still-wet fawn struggles to its feet, reaches up to find a soft, hairless area, follows its nose, finds a teat, and begins feeding (D. Wiessinger, personal communication, 2003). The baby rat twists to turn itself over so it can crawl along its mother's underside, probes and scans to find the nipple, grasps it, attaches, and begins to suckle (Eilam & Smotherman, 1998). After just a month's gestation, the tammar wallaby (a tiny Australian marsupial) looks more embryonic than fetal, with its translucent and red epidermis, yet it crawls the long distance from its mother's perineum up her abdomen and into her pouch, then back down to attach to her teat, which looks almost as big as the neonate itself (Bergman, 2003).

All of this is done without maternal assistance. Nonprimate mammals do not have arms, and so most mammalian mothers could not easily assist their young with this first task even if they had the neuroendocrine priming to do so.

However, even in our primate cousin the monkey, the newborn apparently receives no help from its mother's arms as it seeks out its first meal. The mother macaque monkey, once she has manually pulled her infant from her birth canal, leaves it on her belly to rest. From there, the newborn monkey, independently and completely without its mother's assistance, climbs over her abdomen up to her chest, searches for and finds the nipple, and grasps it with its mouth to begin its first feeding (Rosenblum & Youngstein, 1974).

Innate Newborn Feeding Behavior in the Human Infant

It is only quite recently in Western medical literature that this same innate mammalian newborn behavioral sequence has been described in the human neonate. In 1977, the pioneering French obstetrician Michel Odent described the ability of the human newborn to use the rooting reflex in the first hour of life to search for and find the breast for an important "first, precocious suck" (Odent, 1977, p. 1118). The rooting reflex, Odent said, is more than a mere reflex. He called it "a very complex behavior pattern demonstrating a certain coordination between the mother–infant couple" (p. 1117). Analyzing the conditions necessary to facilitate this complex behavior, Odent explained that "one need only remember the rooting reflex involves all the special senses" (p. 1118), specifically, skin-to-skin touch "stimulated by caresses," the mother's scent, and the mother's voice. Interestingly, it was his impression that the latter was the primary stimulus, although he noted that this contradicted "what the scientists tell us." He did not include vision as an initiating stimulus toward the breast but observed that the infant opened his eyes while suckling. He cautioned against delivery room circumstances that interfered with the infant's use of these senses, and, noting that the mother's complementary behavior was also affected by her surroundings, he warned that "any oxytocic or analgesic drug can perturb the complex neuroendocrine reactions leading to the first suck" (p. 1118).

Ten years later, expanding on Odent's observations, Swedish researchers Ann-Marie Widström, Kerstin Uvnäs-Moberg, and their team at the Karolinska Institute in Stockholm described in a seminal study how routine gastric suction at birth could interfere with this innate neonatal behavior (Widström et al., 1987). A few years later, another Swedish research team, pediatrician Lennart Righard and midwife Margaret Alade, described how other hospital routines could also disrupt this neurobehavior (1990). The subsequent 1995 release of videotape from that study dramatically illustrated this previously unrecognized newborn behavior and broadened the audience for this message. That videotape showed two infants in the first hours of life, using first the stepping response to crawl up the mother's abdomen to find the breast and then the rooting response to locate the nipple, grasp it, attach, and begin suckling. This complex behavior they termed infant *self-attachment* (Righard & Frantz, 1995). Both Widström et al. and Righard and Alade initially emphasized the fragility of what was then felt to be a fleeting behavior, easily disrupted by common Western delivery room routines and best seen in the undisturbed first hour of life. In a later release of this material, Righard suggested that this behavior might be seen at least for a few weeks, or as long as the crawling or stepping reflex persists (Righard & Frantz, 2005).

Indeed, such behavior has since been documented in infants up to a month of age (Colson, Meek, & Hawdon, 2008). These authors videotaped a total of 93 breastfeeding episodes involving 40 breastfeeding dyads in the first postnatal month, demonstrating how maternal semireclined postures can facilitate this newborn behavior. Looking at the qualitatively defined "best" breastfeeding episode for each dyad, for nearly half the dyads the mothers were in a semireclined, flat, or side-lying posture, while for 21 of the 40 dyads, the mother was in a more traditional upright sitting posture when her infant's "best" breastfeeding episode was achieved. The authors found that more important than maternal posture was the infant's body position. In all the best recorded episodes, the infant's body was in close apposition to the mother's body.

Infant-Initiated Feeding Behaviors: Persistence Beyond the First Days of Life

A few years after the pioneering Swedish studies, Australian midwife and lactation consultant Heather Harris described several infants of a few weeks of age who had not yet learned to breastfeed and who had a history of significant prior trouble at the breast (1994). She found that when mother and baby were put together in a bathtub, with mother pouring warm water over the infant's back, these infants would move toward the breast and initiate breastfeeding on their own. Harris called this *cobathing*, a way to calm and relax both infant and mother in order to facilitate the infant's behavioral sequence. However, at the time, this technique became popularized as *rebirthing*. That term probably stemmed from the misconception that the infant's behavior was facilitated by the association of the bath water with the infant's earlier experience with amniotic fluid, suggesting perhaps a re-creation of those first 24 hours. Harris, however, does not see the water as requisite and has seen infants of various ages, in a variety of circumstances, who, when calmed, were able to take themselves to breast, grasp the nipple and a mouthful of breast, and feed (H. Harris, personal communication, 2003).

Kathryn Meyer, while a nursing student at Case Western under Gene Cranston Anderson, described in 1999 her accidental discovery of the value of kangaroo care to full-term infants who were experiencing difficulty learning to feed in the first days of life. During her rotation through the maternity floor, she discovered that if she simply left such a newborn infant alone, skin on skin on his mother's chest, the infant would find the breast on his own and be feeding comfortably when she returned a short time later (Meyer & Anderson, 1999).

In our breastfeeding medicine practice, both full-term and preterm infants have demonstrated that this instinct is not limited to the first weeks of life; indeed, our clinical experience suggests that this innate capability probably persists for at least a year or much longer (Smillie, 2001).

Karleen Gribble, an Australian researcher, has compiled 32 cases (Gribble, 2005) from adoptive mothers who reported that their postinstitutionalized adopted children spontaneously initiated breastfeeding-seeking behaviors without maternal invitation. This unsolicited behavior was described in children of various ages, ranging from 8 months to 12 years. In addition, many individual mothers, nurses, and lactation consultants have described anecdotal and seemingly chance experiences with this innate behavior in infants of various ages.

Despite these observations, we have found no literature describing this full infant-initiated sequence of behaviors occurring beyond the first month of life or suggesting a universality or persistence to this infant capability, nor have we found any well-articulated neurobehavioral explanation for these observations. What follows, then, are our best descriptions of what we have seen in our breastfeeding medicine practice over the past decade and a half and an attempt to look to the literature for an explanation of these observations.

That this remarkable innate competence has been so long unrecognized, at least in Western scientific literature, has allowed many to believe that it is an uncommon and unpredictable occurrence. But our observations (Smillie, 2001) and those of others (Bergman, 2003; Colson et al., 2008; Frantz, 2005; H. Harris, personal communication, 2003) demonstrate that, when understood and nurtured, these infant capabilities are quite robust, persistent, universal, and of important clinical significance. Nyqvist (2008) has shown that even very premature infants as young as 29 weeks gestational age have these capabilities. Indeed, our clinical experiences have demonstrated that this wonderful neonatal capability is not limited either to the first 24 hours of life or to the bathtub, and that, when recognized, this innate competence can help infants avoid or overcome a wide variety of difficulties encountered as they learn to breastfeed.

Baby-Led Learning

We describe this approach to initiating breastfeeding as *baby led* and prefer to use such terms as *baby-led learning* or *baby-led feeding*, rather than *infant self-attachment*, to acknowledge the interactive nature of the process, which involves the mother supporting the infant's state regulation (Schore, 2001), reading her infant's communications, and following her baby's cues.

Observations from Our Practice: The Neurobehavioral Cascade

When moved to the supine position, a baby will often flail and behave uncomfortably, like an upside-down turtle. In our clinical experience, the infant calms and relaxes when cuddled upright between his mother's breasts. The vertical position, like the prone position, stabilizes the infant's vestibular system, while the midline ventral position provides a stabilizing symmetric posture, minimizing intrusive postural reflexes (Morris & Klein, 2000; Wolf & Glass, 1992). With her baby snuggled on her chest, even a very insecure and unsure mother will usually begin stroking her infant, apparently instinctively, vocalizing and often attempting to make eye contact with her baby. Eye contact and the mother's voice help the infant remain calm and focused and enhances motor control. If the baby is in an upright position, neck support helps prevent intrusive reflex motor movements. A sequence of neurosensory cues will, in this context, direct the infant toward the breast. The smell of the milk helps orient the baby (Doucet, Soussignan, Sagot, & Schaal, 2009; Porter & Winberg, 1999; Varendi & Porter, 2001; Varendi, Porter, & Winberg, 2002), directing the baby to crawl in the direction of the breast, that is, from the mother's abdomen upward or from the mother's shoulder or upper chest downward. The sensation of the infant's upper chest against his mother, skin against skin, appears to promote a searching response in

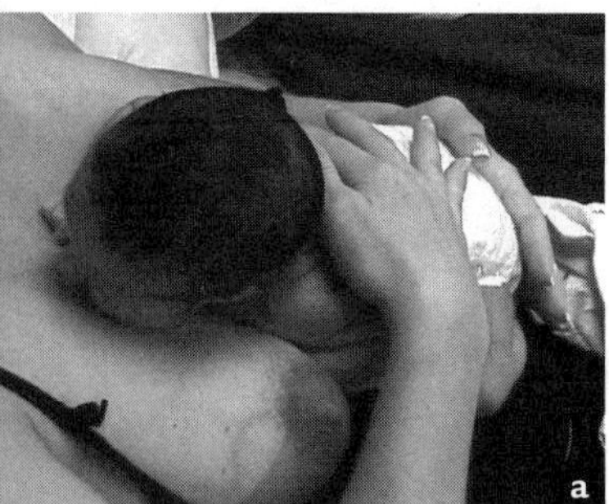

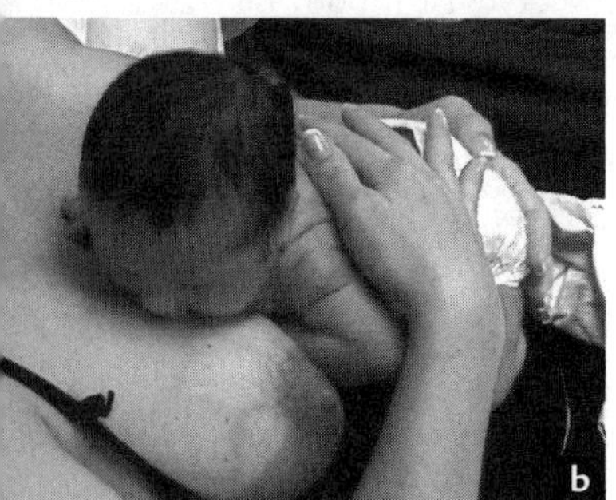

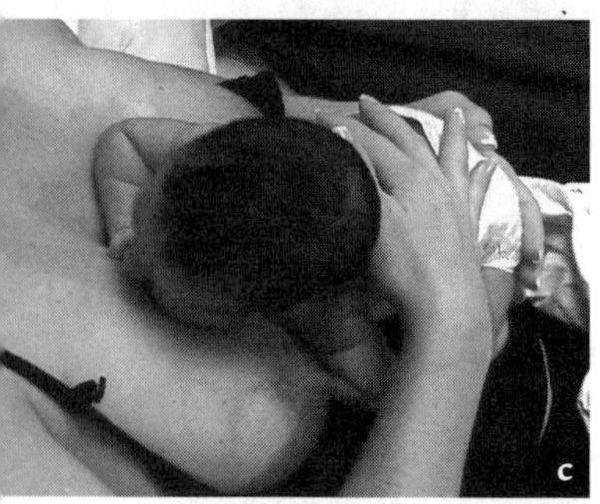

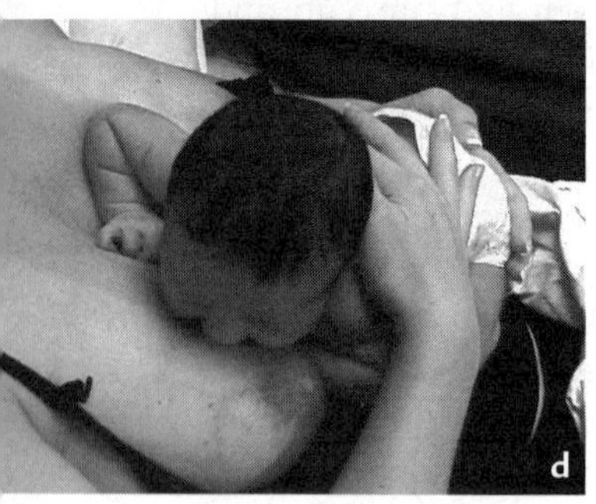

Figure 4-1 The searching response: This 8-second sequence (a, b, c, and d) shows a 10-day-old girl bouncing toward her destination. Using the rooting response, she feels her way with her cheeks, sweeping swiftly side to side.

the stable, hungry, quiet alert infant. The infant who is curled up, so that his chest is no longer in contact with the mother's skin, is less likely to initiate a move toward the breast, and yet as soon as his mother helps him straighten his torso, allowing him to feel his chest against her chest, the infant will begin or resume his searching.

The stepping or crawling reflex described by Righard and Alade (1990) is but one of many ways that infants can take themselves to the breast. We have observed that when mothers hold their infants in an upright position, their infants also find the breast, using arms and trunk to bob, bounce, throw themselves, or gently fall toward the breast. We differentiate all of these innate gross motor behaviors from the classic rooting behavior, which involves primarily the head and neck, by collectively terming such behaviors the *searching response* (**Figures 4-1 and 4-2**).

It appears that part of what stimulates the infant to begin the behaviors that will initiate feeding is the momentum begun by this searching behavior itself. If the searching baby is interrupted, shuts down, falls asleep, or becomes distressed, that momentum can be disturbed and attempts cease. However, if his mother brings him back to that neutral midline position, changing both his body position and his behavioral state, the baby may suddenly reinitiate his search, find the breast, and begin feeding.

What in the past was termed the *rooting reflex* is now called the *rooting response*, to acknowledge the complexity of this neurobehavior. Our observations reinforce the view that the rooting response and other associated feeding neurobehaviors are not simple stereotypical reflexes but are complex behaviors that vary with a choice of movements depending on the infant's state, body position, and sensory cues received.

Once the baby has moved closer to the nipple and into a feeding position, the mother's intuitive support of the infant's pelvis against her body allows the positional stability necessary for the neurobehavioral organization required

Figure 4-2 The searching response: The same infant depicted in **Figure 4-1**, a few seconds later. Once at the nipple, the sensation of the chin on the breast triggers another aspect of the rooting response, and the infant opens her mouth (a) to begin feeding (b).

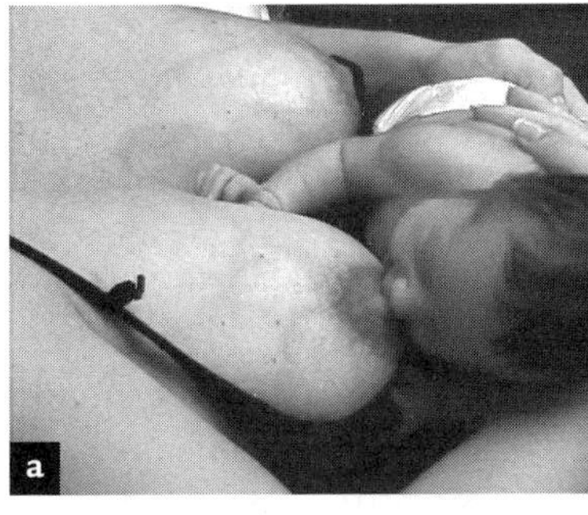

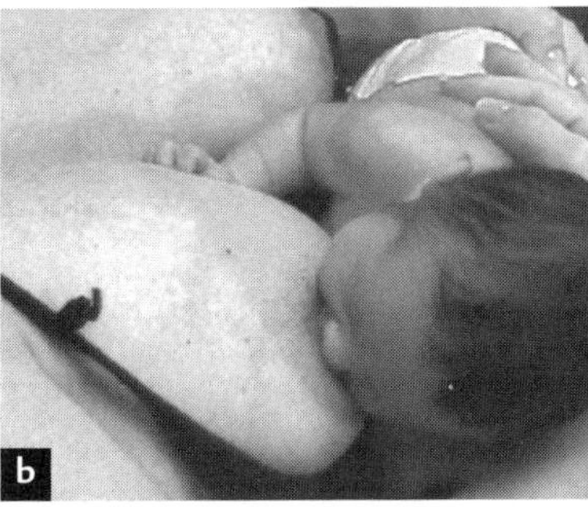

for feeding (Glover, 2004; Morris & Klein, 2000; Wolf & Glass, 1992). Comfortable and relaxed support to the infant's pelvis, trunk, and neck gives the infant the positional stability necessary for optimal motor control. A semireclined position promotes such stability (Colson et al., 2007).

With his neck slightly extended and head slightly back, the infant approaches the breast with his chin leading, rather than his mouth or nose, a position that allows the baby to open his mouth widely. In this way, the baby's nose is floating over the nipple in a sniffing position, and his chin, lower lip, and tongue are firmly on the breast, away from the nipple, when the pressure of the chin on the breast stimulates the baby to reach his upper lip up and over the nipple to grasp a mouthful of breast and begin to suckle.

However, if the infant's face loses contact with the mother's skin before the infant is able to finish this sequence, we've observed that the infant behaves as if he has been separated from his mother—he becomes anxious and distressed, his muscles tense, and he may arch his back, moving him even further away from his mother's body. His mouth may be only a half-centimeter away from the nipple, and his eyes may be closed or wide open, but if his face is not in contact with his mother's skin, the infant will behave as if the breast has been removed. Because such a very distressed infant often arches, the mother may misinterpret this disorganized behavior as the infant trying to get away from the breast. In actuality, however, the arching is not purposeful, but rather a reflexive sign of stress. The perceived separation has put the infant in the sympathetic or adrenergic state, disorganizing his behavior and making voluntary motor activity difficult. If his mother can calm him, as she helps his face or mouth resume contact with her breast (not shoving mouth to nipple, but permitting his face to touch the breast), the baby may relax and resume his rooting behavior. If his neurobehavioral state has been sufficiently disrupted, she may need to use specific comfort measures, for example, letting him suck on her finger or his own hand as she talks to him, or moving him away from the nipple and even back to a midline position before he can reorganize and resume the sequence.

Once at the breast, the infant's hand may brush the nipple, which in turn becomes erect. The infant's face, in contact with the mother's skin, turns toward the smell of her nipple and areola, and the classically described rooting behavior is seen. The work of Colson et al. (2008) confirms our observations: It is the firm pressure of the chin against the breast that then organizes the gape, stimulating the infant to open his mouth wide, reach down with his tongue, and grasp a mouthful of breast. It is then the infant's oral sensation of the breast filling the oral cavity—with the palate and buccal and lingual surfaces all in full contact with the breast—that stimulates the infant to begin suckling (Ardran, Kemp, & Lind 1958; K. Frantz, personal communication, 2006). Although some enthusiastic infants will begin suckling with only the smallest amount of breast in their mouths, or none at all, many infants will come off the breast if they do not get that big mouthful of breast that provides the significant intraoral contact that will initiate suckling. The nipple, firmed by contact with the infant's hand or mouth, when felt against the palate, provides the neurosensory stimulus to help sustain suckling (Weber, Woolridge, & Baum, 1986; Woolridge, 1986).

All of these are most likely instinctive, hardwired behavioral sequences that occur under specific circumstances. The association of sensorimotor feedback, the provision of milk, and the mother's relaxed demeanor probably provide the positive reinforcement for infant learning. The feeding process moves from an instinctively driven behavior to a learned behavior, from an innate situational response to the learned associations that make breastfeeding easy.

Why Haven't We Noticed This Before?

Most of the searching behaviors I've described here are probably quite familiar to the reader. Those of us who work with breastfeeding dyads often call many of these behaviors *feeding cues*. However, I contend that they are more than just a behavioral form of communication. If not obstructed, these movements initiate a cascade of behaviors that lead the baby to feed. When we view these behaviors as mere cues, we don't give the infant the opportunity to follow through and finish the full sequence.

As an infant tries to twist downward toward the breast, I've observed that parents and healthcare professionals who are unfamiliar with infant competence typically respond by restraining the infant. This cultural inclination to restrain and protect newborn head movements has kept many of us from noticing or utilizing this infant capability. That cultural ignorance of these infant capabilities has then upset this natural feeding paradigm; parental or professional interference with the innate maternal and infant behaviors that begin the feeding sequence, followed by an adult attempt to force the thus unprepared infant directly to the final step of the sequence (the oral grasp of the nipple that is often termed "latch"), can actually interfere with the infant's attempts to feed. The infant then appears incompetent, reinforcing the cultural misunderstanding, when in fact the infant's competence was being thwarted. If these contrary attempts to force the infant to feed are noxious or repetitive, the resulting stress and neurobehavioral disorganization can potentially result in learned association of feelings of distress with sensations at the breast, which are, in my view, the cause of apparent breast refusal.

Explaining Infant Competence: The Neurobehavioral Literature

To understand both the neurological basis for this infant competence and the many variations of this infant behavior, we need to look to infant and animal neurobehavioral literature.

Reflex Responses

Righard and Alade (1990) demonstrated that the *stepping* or *crawling* response is not merely a residual and useless primitive reflex; it is a vital behavior, just as the rooting response is. Although the pediatric neurology literature does not address how other infant reflexes might also help the infant feed, animal studies describe similar initial feeding behaviors, collectively termed the *mammalian feeding sequence*.

We know that the mother herself has reflexes that facilitate infant feeding. Nipple erection occurs in response to infant touch and to specific sensory and psychosocial signals (Widström et al., 1990). When an infant is held skin to skin, the maternal breast skin temperature changes quickly via vasodilation or constriction, rapidly responding to the infant's skin temperature, to maintain it within narrow euthermic limits (Ludington-Hoe et al., 2006; Ludington-Hoe, Nguyen, Swinth, & Satyshur, 2000). Somatosensory stimuli cause the release of pituitary oxytocin to initiate milk ejection and the release of a variety of gastrointestinal hormones in both mother and infant (Uvnäs-Moberg, Widström, Marchini, & Winberg, 1987; Widström et al., 1990). The reflex release of oxytocin elicits a variety of complex maternal physiologic, emotional, and behavioral responses (Matthiesen, Ransjö-Arvidson, Nissen, & Uvnäs-Moberg, 2001; Uvnäs-Moberg & Eriksson, 1996; Uvnäs-Moberg, Johansson, Lupoli, & Svennersten-Stjaunja, 2001).

Instinctive or Hardwired Neuroendocrine Programs for Behavior

Beyond simple reflex behaviors are far more complex patterns of instinctive behaviors for both mother and baby. Colson et al. (2008) term these innate behaviors *primitive neonatal reflexes*, using this term loosely to describe not only "inborn unconditioned reflex responses" (p. 442), but also more broadly "spontaneous behaviours and reactions to endogenous or environmental stimuli" (p. 442). Indeed, in the past several decades, rapid advances in the neurosciences (Guzzetta, 2009; Schore, 2005) are moving us away from seeing the infant as a passive automaton of mere reflex responses, but rather as a competent individual capable of using complex, highly differentiated motor and sensory abilities to interact with his social environment.

A slight drop in blood sugar may cause the infant to initiate a searching response (Marchini, Persson, & Uvnäs-Moberg, 1993), but a wide variety of different searching behaviors can occur in that context. These are far too complex to be merely reflexive, but they are, nevertheless, hardwired innate behaviors. Such instinctive patterns of behavior can be understood as neuroendocrine programs for behavior, which occur in specific environmental (autonomic, neurosensory, and social) circumstances (Marchini et al., 1993). If a hungry baby is in his calm mother's arms, the baby will be in a calm parasympathetic state, allowing him to look for the breast, facilitating both learning and feeding. If separated from his mother, the hungry baby will experience stress and enter a sympathetic or adrenergic state characterized by a rise in catecholamines and serum cortisol. This will make him squirm and cry, behaviors that help him get back to his mother (Bergman, 2003; Christensson, Cabrera, Christensson, Uvnäs-Moberg, & Winberg, 1995).

These instinctive behaviors can be disrupted. State regulation is important to permit organized feeding responses, even in the physical presence of the mother. Even when the infant is chest against chest in his mother's arms, if he is overly hungry and so distressed that his mother is unable to help him return to the calm quiet alert state, the infant may be unable to organize his behavior. The baby's own hunger, his instincts to feed, and insistent sensory cues from his mother's chest may overstimulate him, creating a clash between the distress of hunger and his own ability to achieve the state regulation necessary to relieve that distress. Once calmed, for example by sucking on his father's finger, the baby may now have the state regulation necessary to organize his motor behavior to search for the breast. Widström and Thingström-Paulsson (1993) demonstrated that when the newborn infant is permitted to initiate feeding on his own, he approaches the breast making licking movements, with his tongue down in a position that makes it easy to grasp the breast. However, when infants cry, they lift their tongues to their palates, making it impossible to grasp the breast. Infants forced to the breast likewise fail to drop their tongues.

The mother also has hardwired neuroendocrine patterns of behavior, her maternal instincts, which, like her baby's instincts, can be disrupted if she is unable to achieve her own state regulation. In the presence of her infant, the self-confident mother demonstrates a variety of predictable instinctive behaviors as she seeks to calm and communicate with her infant. Usually even the inexperienced mother will actively and spontaneously seek eye-to-eye contact with her infant, caress and stroke him in specific ways, vocalize, and demonstrate a predictable repertoire of responses to her infant's behaviors (Kjellmer & Winberg, 1994; Uvnäs-Moberg, 1994; Uvnäs-Moberg, Johansson, Lupoli, & Svennersten-Sjaunja, 2001). These oxytocin-mediated patterns of behavior can calm her infant, permitting the infant to follow his own instincts.

The Importance of Social Interaction to Infant State Regulation

More than five decades ago, British pediatrician and psychoanalyst Donald Winnicott observed that "There is no such thing as a baby, there is a baby and someone" (1958, p. 99). That is, he explained, it is only within the context of an adult's "good-enough care" (p. 100), typically the total mother–baby environment, that the baby can be understood. Since then, American pediatricians T. Berry Brazelton, John Kennell, and Marshall Klaus, psychotherapist Phyllis Klaus (Brazelton, 1979; Klaus, Kennell, & Klaus, 1995; Klaus & Klaus, 1998), and others have observed and chronicled the neurobehavioral competence of the infant, as facilitated by interaction with either the mother or an examiner.

Over the past several decades, research in a wide variety of disciplines has helped us better understand the neurophysiologic basis for these newborn behaviors. The American neuropsychoanalyst Allan Schore, in work integrating research from the neurosciences, psychology, behavioral pediatrics, and psychiatry, offers a compelling theoretical model that describes the right-brained communication between mother and infant as central both to the infant's psychophysiologic state regulation and to his ongoing psychoneurodevelopment (Schore, 2001). It is in episodes of "affective synchrony" (p. 23) with his mother, involving interactive resonance between the amygdalae, limbic systems, and right brains of both infant and mother, that the infant achieves the state regulation necessary for such important life-preserving functions as feeding.

This resonance between the nervous systems of mother and infant is achieved through direct sensory interaction—eye-to-eye contact, skin-on-skin contact, and vocal-auditory communication—and in this way permits what Schore describes as direct right-brain to right-brain communication. Thus connected, the mother-baby dyad exists as a single psychoneurobiological organism. In that context, connected to her infant via their right brains, the mother is able to help her infant with state regulation, first as her right brain resonates in tune with her infant's, and much later as this experience of attachment helps the infant to develop his own abilities for state regulation, autonomic regulation, and emotional regulation.

For the mother to communicate with her infant, she too must let her right brain lead. When the mother herself is in a calm and relaxed state, she is open to subtle communication with her newborn; she can connect and respond to her infant's behavior and with her response transfer that calm state regulation to her infant.

It has been said that in the postpartum period women tend to demonstrate a "cognitive deficit" (Eidelman, Hoffmann, & Kaitz, 1993). They can be quite daunted by such tasks as following verbal instructions, remembering dates or their baby's weights, paying attention to time, or counting diapers. This is not so much a total global cognitive deficit, but rather the effect of the mother's left brain taking a bit of a back seat to the right brain, making it easier for her to connect with her baby. Kaitz and Eidelman had earlier demonstrated with other colleagues that the postpartum mother can, without the sensory aid of vision, hearing or smell, identify her own infant from two other babies, merely by touch: by stroking the back of the infants' hands (Kaitz, Lapidot, Bronner, & Eidelman (1992). This shift in emphasis from left to right brain is likely mediated at least in part by high maternal postpartum endorphins and oxytocin levels and reinforced by recurrent neurosensory stimulation from her infant (Matthiesen et al., 2001; Uvnäs-Moberg & Eriksson, 1996; Widström et al., 1990). When a mother can allow her left brain to step back, she can make room for more of the right brain's holistic, intuitive, attentive, in-the-moment, emotionally based thinking. This permits the mother to think more like her baby does and to empathize with her baby, that is, to connect with him in both the colloquial sense and, as Schore would say, right brain to right brain, thus allowing the mother to better understand her baby's moment-to-moment needs and be attentive to his moment-to-moment communication.

I think the reason these newborn abilities have been so long overlooked in the Western world is that mothers and newborns are so rarely left together, just to relax and connect, without a left-brained agenda for what mother or infant was supposed to do. Only in that first hour of life, or later, sitting together in a warm bathtub, could mothers and babies just relax and enjoy each other while not feeding. When the mother leaves her left brain's agenda behind and follows her right-brained instincts to simply calm and relax her infant, only then can her feelings coincide with the baby's, and the two right brains begin to resonate as one. Thus I believe that the key to what we are seeing, when an infant can search and find the breast to feed, is the state regulation made possible by this right-brain to right-brain maternal–infant communication, which Schore has so elegantly explained.

Nearly two decades before Schore proposed this model, French pediatric neurologist Claudine Amiel-Tison and her colleague, pediatrician Albert Grenier (1983), described an alert newborn state that they distinguished from Prechtl's simple "quiet alert" state, a state they termed the *communicative state*. These physicians noted that, when examining a baby in the first months of life, they were able to elicit more advanced and organized infant neurobehavior than might otherwise be seen at that age, if the infant was already in this more socially interactive alert state. Recognizing that this observation could be very useful to the neurologic examination of the very young infant, they developed a technique for facilitating this alert behavioral state by transiently "liberating" the newborn from the intrusive reflex motor activity that usually inhibits the infant's voluntary movement. They hypothesized that neck instability was the primary trigger for most of these intrusive neonatal primitive motor reflexes. They noted that when the examiner supported the infant's neck and shoulders, rocking the infant while making eye contact and socializing verbally with the infant, after a few minutes the infant would "appear charmed," fixing on the examiner's eyes, making social facial expressions, and attempting to vocalize responsively. In this "communicative" state, a 2- or 3-week-old infant could be transiently "liberated" from intrusive obligatory reflex motor movements and could even support his own head and neck with minimal examiner intervention (Amiel-Tison & Grenier, 1983, *passim*).

Although Amiel-Tison and Grenier focused their attention on the stabilized neck, their monograph describes the adjunct use of eye-to-eye contact, rocking, and social vocalization. These interactions with the infant create precisely the right-brained interactions that Schore (2001) later conceptualized as key to infant state regulation.

The two French physicians devised this technique specifically to aid their neurologic exam of the newborn, with no discussion of any broader implications for their findings. Nevertheless, their method demonstrates how new parents get to know their newborns—"charming" the infant with eye contact and social verbalization, thus stabilizing the infant's autonomic regulation and permitting better motor control. No wonder so many mothers tell us their babies held their heads up all by themselves at only a few days of age, when our developmental texts tell us it should not happen for another couple of months! And, of course, it is that same liberated motor control that I believe permits the infant to follow his sense of smell, search for the breast, find the nipple, grasp the breast, and suckle.

Neuroendocrine Correlates of Behavior

Over the past few decades a large literature has developed demonstrating how skin-to-skin care facilitates both newborn autonomic stability and breastfeeding behaviors (Bergman, Linley, & Fawcus, 2004; Moore, Anderson, & Bergman, 2007). At the same time, much research throughout the world has further helped us understand the neuroendocrine correlates of both maternal (Matthiesen et al., 2001; Pedersen, 1997; Rosenblatt, 1994; Uvnäs-Moberg, 1994; Uvnäs-Moberg & Eriksson, 1996; Uvnäs-Moberg, Johansson, Lupoli,

& Svennersten-Sjaunja, 2001) and infant (Christensson et al., 1995; Christensson et al., 1992; Luddington-Hoe, Cong, & Hashemi, 2002; Marchini et al., 1993) behavior and their interaction (Kjellmer & Winberg, 1994; Nelson & Panksepp 1998; Rosenblatt 1994; Swain, Lorberbaum, Kose, & Strathearn, 2007). A physiologic drop in blood sugar can trigger hunger (Marchini et al., 1993), or a minute rise in serum osmolality will trigger vasopressin release (Marchini & Stock, 1997), and either can then cause the initiation of infant feeding behaviors. A variety of tactile, visual, olfactory, and auditory sensory cues will, in the context of hunger, direct the infant's feeding behaviors toward the breast.

Infant Learning

Many studies have shown us that infants learn quite quickly by making associations between certain somatosensory experiences (for a summary of these studies, see Klaus & Klaus, 1998). Milk transfer can quickly reinforce and teach a baby how to suckle as the infant makes an association between milk flow and a particular oral motor sensory pattern and a particular autonomic state.

Maternal–Infant Interactions

The interactive behavior between mother and baby constitutes a continuous neuropsychological and neurobehavioral dance. A variety of neurosensory mediators are involved in these mutually reinforcing maternal and infant neuroendocrine responses, which affect the state regulation of both mother and baby, as well as physiologic and social processes necessary for infant survival.

These interactions may be positive or negative, and mutual reinforcement may promote or disturb homeostasis. The infant's calm, responsive behavior may aid maternal learning just as much as maternal state regulation aids infant learning. Conversely, infant distress provokes maternal distress, evoking physical tension, which in turn can interfere with her ability to calm her baby, listen to her instincts, or make use of verbal instructions she may have been given.

On the other hand, when mothers are able to see their babies searching for the breast, they are usually quite impressed by their infant's spontaneous movements. The mother's positive response to seeing her infant's competent behavior helps calm both mother and baby further, so that the mother's arms, if tensed, often begin to relax, and her body language encourages her infant on his mission, allowing the infant to maintain the neurobehavioral organization needed to follow through with the complex cascade of behaviors necessary to initiate feeding.

To do this, the infant needs not only his mother's emotional support, but also her physical support. There is no one right way to achieve this; any open, nonjudgmental, supportive environment can facilitate both physical and state stability. A relaxed, semireclined maternal posture (Colson et al., 2008) offers one way to provide both infant positional stability and a relaxed maternal emotional state, both of which allow the mother to support her infant's state regulation. If the mother is unable to comfortably offer the physical support her infant needs, she may not have the opportunity to see what her infant can do (Nyqvist, 2008.)

Baby-Led Learning: From Theory to Practice

The infant's feeding behaviors we describe here are not rare or idiosyncratic. Since we started using this approach in 1996, we have witnessed no exceptions to the healthy hungry infant's primary inclination to search for the breast. Predictable factors affect the infant's ability to maintain the organized neurobehavioral state that enables the cascade of innate behaviors to trigger the final moves that end in feeding. The infant's ability to remain organized, his mother's ability to facilitate her infant's neurobehavioral organization, past experiences at the breast—all of these affect whether or not the searching behavior will conclude in an actual feed. However, whether or not the infant is able to complete the behavior, the search itself appears to be quite universal, and it appears far more complex and varied than the simple rooting reflex that begins with a brush to the cheek.

How Babies Can Learn to Feed: An Alternative Approach

Breastfeeding, for both mother and baby, is a motor-sensory procedural task mediated by right-brained processes. Just as one cannot learn to ride a bicycle by reading a manual, step-by-step instructions can confuse the mother, making her feel awkward and making the process more difficult. Colson et al. (2008) have suggested that skills-based methods for teaching breastfeeding may interfere with maternal intuitive learning.

1. First, We Start with a Calm Baby

The key to seeing these infant-initiated seeking and feeding behaviors is to permit both mother and baby to be calm and relaxed while interacting with each other, with no other agenda. The process of learning to feed can be facilitated by protecting mother and infant from stress and by allowing the infant to lead the process. Instructions, if any, should be minimal and reassuring in their simplicity. Because oxytocin makes a mother intuitively responsive to her infant (Uvnäs-Moberg, 1994; Uvnäs-Moberg & Eriksson, 1996; Uvnäs-Moberg et al., 2001), we need only to encourage the mother to follow her baby's lead and let her own instincts, intuition, and impulses (i.e., her right brain) guide her.

2. Skin on Skin (or Not!) in Any Comfortable Position

The mother starts by simply holding her baby, skin on skin if the baby is within the first week or so of life, more likely with a light shirt after the baby has become habituated to clothing, so the baby's body and the mother's body are in continuous contact along the length of the baby's torso. The mother might begin by placing her baby's chest against her chest in any position they both find cuddly and comfortable. The mother might be sitting, semireclined, or even standing, and the infant's face will not necessarily be near the breast at all. Colson's group noted that in the semireclined position, the mother's lap opens up, allowing the infant better access to the breast, while gravity holds the baby securely and snugly in the continuous and stable body contact that facilitates the infant's searching behaviors. The mother might instinctively begin caressing or stroking her infant or perhaps begin talking to her baby or trying to make eye contact if possible, so that they are just relaxing and enjoying each other's company, with no other agenda, on baby time (**Figure 4-3**).

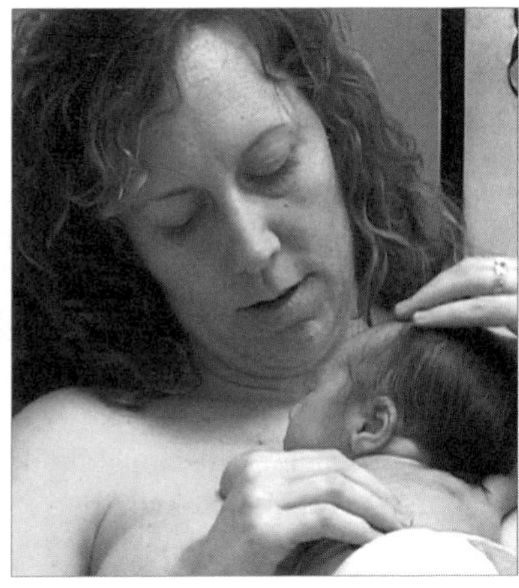

Figure 4-3 The mother begins by simply holding her baby in any comfortable position. Note this mother's hands: Without instruction, as she enjoys her baby's company, she is intuitively stroking and caressing her infant, calming and relaxing the baby.

3. Mother Keeps Infant Calm and Follows Baby's Lead

As her baby begins to move toward one breast (as in **Figure 4-1**), the mother follows her baby's lead, intuitively helping if needed as her baby moves in the direction of one breast or the other. If she is sitting, she might stabilize her baby's hips at her waist. If he takes a position across her lap, his body will likely take something close to a 45-degree angle, with his hips snugly below her opposite breast. If she holds her baby under her arm, his body may end up wrapped around her waist, hips near her back. If she is standing, her lap will be gone, so her natural instinct to give support to her baby's hips and shoulders will be reinforced. If she is semi-reclined, her hands will be free to respond as needed to her baby's moves.

The mother helps her infant along as she instinctively speaks in a calming and encouraging way, strokes the infant, and perhaps makes eye contact. It is important that she follow her instincts to keep her baby calm and happy. If her baby shows any tension, she may want to move the baby away from the breast or nipple if necessary to calm the baby. As the baby moves toward one breast, she can follow his lead, helping him maintain physical contact with the breast, allowing his face and cheek to touch the breast. If she is sitting or standing, her support to her baby's hips gives his body the stability to allow his search, and her support of his shoulders allows the baby to tilt his head back, with his chin firmly against her breast.

When the baby approaches the breast from underneath, it allows chin contact with the full underside of the breast, which encourages the baby to open his mouth wide.

Although many parents and professionals often lament that the baby's hands get in the way, the infant's hand movements are innate, predictable, and an important and purposeful part of the newborn's feeding script (Genna & Barak, 2010; Klaus & Klaus, 1998; Matthiesen et al., 2001). The infant's hands massage and press on the breast, adding to maternal oxytocin release. Allowing the infant to suck on his hands will usually be calming so the baby can resume his search, particularly if his mother reassures him with her voice and body language. Indeed, it is often the adult's hand that gets in the infant's way; the mother's hand, cupped under her breast, can interfere with the infant's movements, particularly if cupping her breast is an instructed method rather than a thoughtless, momentary, and transient instinctive movement. When left to their instincts, mothers often, without instruction, raise the breast if needed by placing their flat hands palm side down on the upper breast, briefly raising the breast by pressing or sliding the skin upwards from above (in a manner similar to that illustrated later in **Figure 4-5**), as needed, so the breast still hangs comfortably and undistorted by her hands, allowing the infant's chin to make full and firm contact with the full curved underside of the breast. The feel of that breast fullness on her baby's chin will stimulate the baby to open his mouth widely, and then, reaching his upper lip upwards over the top of the nipple, the baby can then grasp a mouthful of breast and begin suckling (**Figure 4-4**).

No One Correct Way

There will be many variations on how this is done (see, for example, **Figure 4-2**), because babies and mothers come in many sizes, shapes, and personalities. Women can have short or long torsos, large or small breasts, and babies can be small or large, long or short. So, mothers and babies will not all fit together in the same way. A large-breasted woman whose nipple points down may find that her baby moves down low below where her breasts naturally fall and may end up nearly on his back, his eyes and face looking up at her, chin under the breast. Or, she might instinctively lift the breast from above, raising the nipple just enough for her infant to feed easily (**Figure 4-5**). If she prefers, she may find that reclining helps open up her lap and makes her baby's journey easier. On the other hand, a

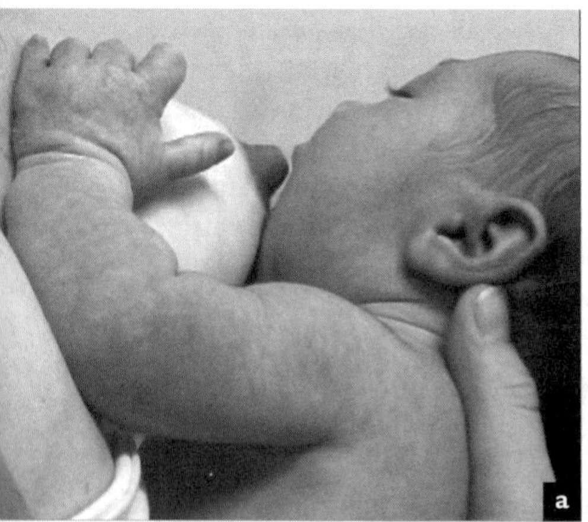

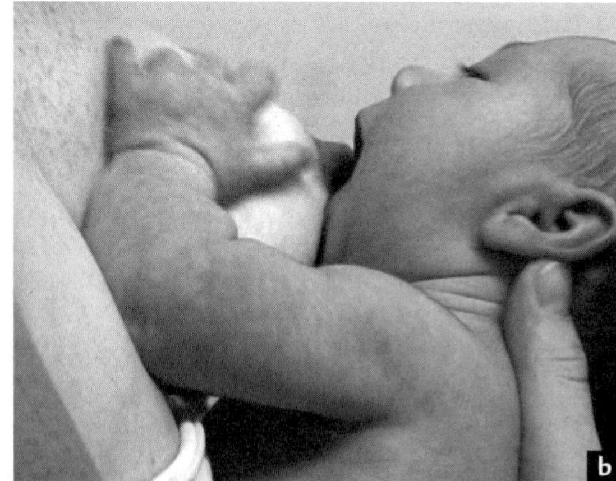

Figure 4-4 With his chin firmly on the breast (a), this infant instinctively reaches his upper lip up, as he is about to take the breast (b). Note that his mother's hand supports his back, because they are in a relatively upright position, but she is not guiding him. In another situation, she might instinctively briefly use her hands to help, in subtle response to something in her infant's behavior.

small-breasted woman whose nipples point straight out may well find her baby in a more tummy-to-tummy position and may or may not find it more comfortable for her baby to nurse in a somewhat more vertical position, his hips down by her waist, as her baby looks up at her.

When we cease giving the mother specific rules as to what she should do, she is free to follow her own hardwired maternal instincts, facilitated by the confidence she gets from watching her infant's competent behavior.

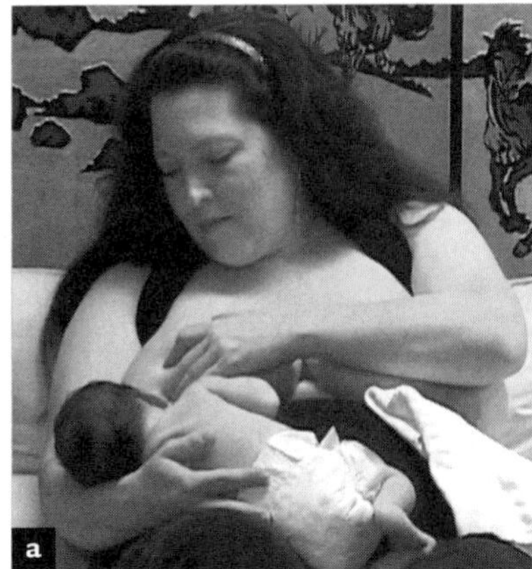

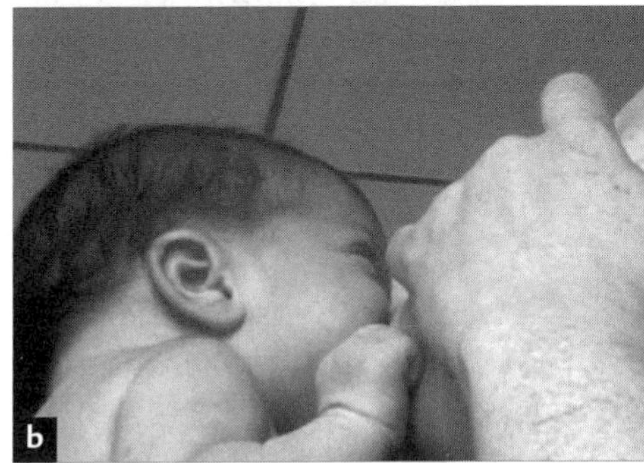

Figure 4-5 This mother uses her hand to raise her breast from above (a), making it easy for her infant to feed low in her lap (b). In another situation, with a baby just about to feed, a mother might instinctively use the palm of her hand in a similar way, but perhaps only briefly—just long enough to assist her infant as he takes the breast. This is an easy move that many mothers choose instinctively, without instruction. It is also easily taught, usually with a single, nearly wordless demonstration.

How Babies Can Relearn to Feed: An Approach to Distressed Behavior at the Breast

In our practice, we use this baby-led approach not only for initial mother–infant learning, but also for the wide variety of feeding problems that can be seen when these innate processes have been impeded. Premature or ill infants who have been long separated from their mothers' arms may need a long period of skin-on-skin reacquaintance before they are ready to learn.

Babies who have been repeatedly pushed forcefully to the breast, bypassing their instincts, may learn to associate distress with the breast. Thus, when placed skin on skin, these babies will usually still search for the breast and move toward the nipple, but when they get close to the breast they can suddenly become disorganized, their tongues rise to their palates, and they become so tense and distressed that they are unable to follow through to grasp the breast. They may even arch, cry, or pull away from the breast. Although many term this *breast refusal*, it is not clear whether the infant is actually refusing the breast or simply distressed at being too disorganized to feed. Fortunately, an understanding of infant neurobehavior and basic principles of conditional learning allows this problem to be easily addressed.

Such babies simply need the opportunity to regain trust and a positive association with the breast. This can be done by stopping all attempts to make the baby breastfeed. The baby will need to be fed expressed breastmilk via an alternative means, usually for a day or two, but occasionally for as long as a week or more, depending on such variables as how noxious the initial experience was, the level of the baby's and the mother's distress, how long this negative experience had been reinforced, the baby's and mother's personalities, and their home and family circumstances.

During this time of exclusively alternative feeds, the mother and baby can reestablish trust via repeated periods of safe, quiet, skin-on-skin time after alternative feedings when the infant is not hungry so the baby has no impulse to search for the breast.

After trust has been reestablished, the baby forgets the negative associations and will be able to again follow his natural instincts that lead to the breast. We usually advise a mother that the first several times she permits the baby to go to breast should not be by plan, calendar, or clock. Instead, these first (usually nonconsecutive) times will be initiated only on her maternal instinctive (right-brained) impulse so that she gives the baby the opportunity to search for the breast only when the baby is displaying one of those particularly alert and social moments and appears more grown-up than usual, that is, when the baby is in what Amiel-Tison and Grenier called the "communicative state."

Even older babies who have never been to breast can learn to feed in this manner. Although we know of anecdotal instances of infants as old as 10 and even 20 months (D. Wiessinger, personal communication, 2011) who have surprised their mothers by independently initiating feeding for the first time in this manner, such instances are rare; it is much easier for infants in the first 3 months of life. After infants reach 4 or 5 months of age, when developmentally they are more and more distractible, their curiosity and high activity can interfere with the calm and focused behavioral state that allows them to follow through on their instincts for the breast.

Our Role in Helping Mothers and Babies as They Learn to Breastfeed

Our role, as healthcare professionals, is to convey this information in a calm, relaxed way, allowing each mother to feel comfortable and confident so that she can help her baby be comfortable and competent. That often means we offer this information with more visual and physical demonstration than verbal instruction so that we show her what we mean by speaking to her right brain, without using the kind of left-brained language that can often sound more complicated and technical than the mother's postpartum brain is prepared to handle. We certainly need not use the language of this chapter; a woman need not become a lactation consultant herself to feed her baby.

What we want to convey with our demeanor, and our emotional connection with the mother, is our confidence in her and her baby. We let her know that we believe in her, we convey the confidence that of course she will be able to do this, and we reassure her that any negative experiences up to this point were not her fault. In this way, she can, as she begins to trust the process, convey those same right-brained messages to help her infant feel relaxed, calm, and competent.

When a mother intuitively speaks to her infant, the infant's responsive behavior can reassure her. Without instructing the mother to speak to her baby, the clinician can encourage the mother by modeling the behavior, talking to the infant in thoughtful and perhaps amusing ways about his emotions. And when the mother spontaneously speaks to her infant, and she usually does, the clinician can comment on how the infant calms to her speech or remark on how the infant paused to listen or sped up suckling in response.

We want to encourage the mother to enjoy the process of learning, to recognize that this can take time, just like learning to walk or dance or ride a bike. She may need reassurance about her ability to mother. We want to emphasize that this is all a normal part of mothering—that the problems that brought her to seek help do not mean that she's incompetent.

It is helpful also to interpret her baby's behavior, to show her how competent her infant is. If her baby gets on the breast and immediately comes off, only to try again, she may be confused and think her baby is doing something wrong. The clinician can tell her how smart her infant is, that he knows he didn't get on quite far enough or didn't get the flow just right and wants to try again. Or if the baby comes off the breast and quits, that's fine, too; the clinician can say that the infant knows his limits and needs to chill a bit.

Whatever is going on, it is instinct at work, so the clinician can always reinterpret the behavior for the mother as normal and as positive. As the clinician interprets and reassures the mother, she will be better able to relax over time. The clinician can then point out how her being more relaxed is also helping her baby.

It helps to tell the mother that her job is not to learn to breastfeed, nor to make her baby learn. Her job is simply to keep her infant calm and relaxed and comfortable so her baby can learn. As Nils Bergman repeatedly says in his lectures, "mothers don't breastfeed; babies breastfeed" (2001). Letting her know that it is her baby who is doing the learning can take considerable self-imposed pressure off her and encourage her own self-confidence.

There is no one right way to do this. The key is to use right-brain techniques to give mothers the confidence they need to keep their babies calm, which in turn promotes feeding-directed infant behavior, which then reinforces the mother's confidence. By modeling patience and calmness, the healthcare professional can elicit in the mother the autonomic and emotional state that she needs to help her baby. It is through helping her baby be relaxed, alert, and calm, and in the parasympathetic state, that the mother can allow her infant to follow his instincts to search, root, grasp the breast, and learn to feed. And then, as she watches her baby's innate behavior, her own confidence increases, and in this way the two help each other as they begin their journey.

References

Amiel-Tison, C., & Grenier, A. (1983). Expression of liberated motor activity (LMA) following manual immobilization of the head (J. Steichen, P. Steichen-Asch, & C. P. Braun, Trans.). In C. Amiel-Tison & A. Grenier (Eds.), *Neurologic evaluation of the newborn and the infant* (pp. 87–109). New York, NY: Masson.

Ardran, G. M., Kemp, F. H., & Lind, J. A. (1958). Cineradiographic study of breast feeding. *British Journal of Radiology, 31*, 156.

Bergman, N. J. (2003). Humans and kangaroos—a biological perspective. *Conference Syllabus*, International Lactation Consultants Association, Sydney, Australia.

Bergman, N. (2001). Kangaroo mother care: Restoring the original paradigm for infant care and breastfeeding. Presentation at La Leche League International Physician's Seminar, July 7, 2001, Chicago, IL.

Bergman, N. J., Linley, L. L., & Fawcus, S. R. (2004). Randomized controlled trial of skin-to-skin contact from birth versus conventional incubator for physiological stabilization in 1200- to 2199-gram newborns. *Acta Paediatrica, 93*(6), 779–785.

Brazelton, T. (1979). Behavioral competence of the newborn infant. *Seminars in Perinatology, 3*(1), 35–44.

Christensson, K., Cabrera, T., Christensson, E., Uvnäs-Moberg, K., & Winberg, J. (1995). Separation distress call in the human neonate in the absence of maternal body contact. *Acta Paediatrica, 84*, 468–473.

Christensson, K., Siles, C., Moreno, L., Belaustequi, A., De La Fuente, P., Lagercrantz, H., . . . Winberg J. (1992). Temperature, metabolic adaptation and crying in healthy full-term newborns cared for skin-to-skin or in a cot. *Acta Paediatrica, 81*, 488–493.

Colson, S. D., Meek, J. H., & Hawdon, J. M. (2008). Optimal position for the release of primitive neonatal reflexes stimulation breastfeeding. *Early Human Development, 84*(7), 441–447.

Doucet, S., Soussignan, R., Sagot, P., & Schaal, B. (2009). The secretion of areolar (Montgomery's) glands from lactating women elicits selective, unconditional responses in neonates. *PLoS One, 4*(10), e7579. doi:10.1371/journal.pone.0007579

Eidelman, A. I., Hoffmann, N. W., & Kaitz, M. (1993). Cognitive deficits in women after childbirth. *Obstetrics and Gynecology, 81*(5 Pt. 1), 764–767.

Eilam, D., & Smotherman, W. P. (1998). How the neonatal rat gets to the nipple: Common motor modules and their involvement in the expression of early motor behavior. *Developmental Psychobiology, 32*, 57–66.

Genna, C. W., & Barak, D. (2010). Facilitating autonomous infant hand use during breastfeeding. *Clinical Lactation, 1*(1), 15–20.

Glover, R. (2004). Lessons from innate feeding abilities transforms breastfeeding outcomes. *Conference Syllabus*, International Lactation Consultants Association, Scottsdale, AZ.

Gribble, K. D. (2005). Post-institutionalized adopted children who see breastfeeding from their new mothers. *Journal of Prenatal and Perinatal Psychology and Health, 19*(3), 217–234.

Guzzetta, F. (2009). Psychomotor development: The beginning of cognition. In F. Guzzetta (Ed.), *Neurology of the infant* (pp. 37–54). Montrouge, France: John Libbey Eurotext.

Harris, H. (1994). Remedial co-bathing for breastfeeding difficulties. *Breastfeeding Review, 11*(10), 465–468.

Kaitz, M., Lapidot, P., Bronner, M., & Eidelman, A. I. (1992) Parturient women can recognize their infants by touch. *Developmental Psychology, 28*(1), 35–39.

Kjellmer, I., & Winberg, J. (1994). The neurobiology of infant–parent interaction in the newborn: An introduction. *Acta Paediatrica, 397*(Suppl.), 1–2.

Klaus, M. H., Kennell, J. H., & Klaus, P. H. (1995). *Bonding: Building the foundations of secure attachment and independence*. New York, NY: Addison-Wesley.

Klaus, M., & Klaus, P. (1998). *Your amazing newborn*. Reading, MA: Perseus Books.

Ludington-Hoe, S. M., Cong, X., & Hashemi, F. (2002). Infant crying: Nature, physiologic consequences, and select interventions. *Neonatal Network, 21*(2), 29–36.

Ludington-Hoe, S. M., Lewis, T., Morgan, K., Cong, X., Anderson, L., & Reese, S. (2006). Breast and infant temperatures with twins during shared kangaroo care. *Journal of Obstetrics and Gynecology Neonatal Nursing, 35*(2), 223-231.

Ludington-Hoe, S. M., Nguyen, N., Swinth, J. Y., & Satyshur, R. D. (2000). Kangaroo care compared to incubators in maintaining body warmth in preterm infants. *Biological Research for Nursing, 2*(1), 60–73.

Marchini, G., Persson, B., & Uvnäs-Moberg, K. (1993). Metabolic correlates of behaviour in the newborn infant. *Physiology and Behavior, 54*, 1021–1023.

Marchini, G., & Stock, S. (1997). Thirst and vasopressin secretion counteract dehydration in newborn infants. *Journal of Pediatrics, 130*(5), 736–739.

Matthiesen, A. S., Ransjo-Arvidson, A. B., Nissen, E., & Uvnäs-Moberg, K. (2001). Postpartum maternal oxytocin release by newborns: Effects of infant hand massage and sucking. *Birth, 28*(1), 13–19.

Meyer, K., & Anderson, G. C. (1999). Using kangaroo care in a clinical setting with fullterm infants having breastfeeding difficulties. *MCN. The American Journal of Maternal Child Nursing, 24*(4), 190–192.

Moore, E. R., Anderson, G. C., & Bergman, N. (2007). Early skin-to-skin contact for mothers and their healthy newborn infants. *Cochrane Database of Systematic Reviews, 18*(3), CD003519.

Morris, S. E., & Klein, M. D. (2000). *Pre-feeding skills: A comprehensive resource for mealtime development* (2nd ed.). Tucson, AZ: Therapy Skill Builders.

Nelson, E., & Panksepp, J. (1998). Brain substrates of infant–mother attachment: Contributions of opioids, oxytocin, and norepinephrine. *Neuroscience and Biobehavioral Reviews, 22*, 437–452.

Nyqvist, K. H. (2008). Early attainment of breastfeeding competence in very preterm infants. *Acta Paediatrica, 97*(6), 776–781.

Odent, M. (1977). The early expression of the rooting reflex. In: *Proceedings of the 5th International Congress of Psychosomatic Obstetrics and Gynaecology, Rome, Italy*. London: Academic Press, 1117–1119.

Pedersen, C. (1997). Oxytocin control of maternal behavior: Regulation by sex steroids and offspring stimuli. *Annals of the New York Academy of Sciences, 807*, 126–145.

Porter, R. H., & Winberg, J. (1999). Unique salience of maternal breast odors for newborn infants. *Neuroscience and Biobehavioral Reviews, 23*, 439–449.

Righard, L., & Alade, M. (1990). Effect of delivery room routines on success of first breast-feed. *Lancet, 336*, 1105–1107.

Righard L., Frantz, K. (Director). (1995). *Delivery self-attachment* [VHS tape]. Los Angeles, CA: Geddes Productions [out of print].

Righard L., Frantz, K. (2005). *Delivery self-attachment* [DVD]. Los Angeles, CA: Geddes Productions. Available from http://www.geddesproduction.com/breast-feeding-delivery-selfattachment.php

Rosenblatt, J. S. (1994). Psychobiology of maternal-behavior: Contribution to the clinical understanding of maternal behavior among humans. *Acta Paediatrica, 3*(Suppl. 397), 3–8.

Rosenblum, L. A., & Youngstein, K. P. (1974). Developmental changes in compensatory dyadic response in mother and infant monkeys. In M. Lewis & L. A. Rosenblum (Eds.), *The effect of the infant on its caregiver* (pp. 141–161). New York, NY: John Wiley.

Schore, A. N. (2001). The effects of a secure attachment relationship on right brain development, affect regulation, and infant mental health. *Infant Mental Health Journal, 22*, 7–66.

Schore, A. N. (2005). Back to basics: Attachment, affect regulation, and the developing right brain: Linking developmental neuroscience to pediatrics. *Pediatric Review, 26*, 204–217.

Smillie, C. M. (2001). How newborns learn to latch: A neurobehavioral model for self-attachment in infancy [Abstract PL9]. *Academy of Breastfeeding Medicine News and Views, 7*, 23.

Smillie, C. M. (Writer). (2010). *Baby-led breastfeeding: The mother–baby dance* [DVD]. Available from http://www.geddesproduction.com/breast-feeding-baby-led.php

Swain, J. E., Lorberbaum, J. P., Kose, S., & Strathearn, L. (2007). Brain basis of early parent–infant interactions: Psychology, physiology, and in vivo functional neuroimaging studies. *Journal of Child Psychology and Psychiatry, 48*(3–4), 262–287.

Uvnäs-Moberg, K. (1994). Oxytocin and behaviour. *Annals of Medicine, 26*(5), 315–317.

Uvnäs-Moberg, K., & Eriksson, M. (1996). Breastfeeding: Physiological, endocrine and behavioural adaptations caused by oxytocin and local neurogenic activity in the nipple and mammary gland. *Acta Paediatrica, 85*, 525–530.

Uvnäs-Moberg, K., Johansson, B., Lupoli, B., & Svennersten-Sjaunja, K. (2001). Oxytocin facilitates behavioural, metabolic and physiological adaptations during lactation. *Applied Animal Behaviour Science, 72*(3), 225–234.

Uvnäs-Moberg, K., Widström, A.-M., Marchini, G., & Winberg, J. (1987). Release of GI hormones in mother and infant by sensory stimulation. *Acta Paediatrica Scandinavica, 76*, 851–860.

Varendi, H., & Porter, R. H. (2001). Breast odour as the only maternal stimulus elicits crawling towards the odour source. *Acta Paediatrica, 90*, 372–375.

Varendi, H., Porter, R. H., & Winberg, J. (2002). The effect of labor on olfactory exposure learning within the first postnatal hour. *Behavioral Neuroscience, 116*(2), 206–211.

Weber, F., Woolridge, M. W., & Baum, J. D. (1986). An ultrasonographic analysis of sucking and swallowing in newborn infants. *Developmental Medicine and Child Neurology, 28*, 19–24.

Widström, A.-M., Ransjö-Arvidson, A. B., Christensson, K., Matthiesen, A.-S., Winberg, J., & Uvnäs-Moberg, K. (1987). Gastric suction in healthy newborn infants: Effects on circulation and developing feeding behaviour. *Acta Paediatrica Scandinavica, 76*, 566–572.

Widström, A.-M., & Thingström-Paulsson, J. (1993). The position of the tongue during rooting reflexes elicited in newborn infants before the first suckle. *Acta Paediatrica, 82*, 281–283.

Widström, A.-M., Wahlberg, V., Matthiesen, A.-S., Eneroth, P., Uvnäs-Moberg, K., Werner, S., & Winberg, J. (1990). Short-term effects of early suckling and touch of the nipple on maternal behavior. *Early Human Development, 21*, 153–163.

Winnicott, D. W. (1952/1958). Anxiety associated with insecurity. In *Collected papers: Through paediatrics to psycho-analysis* (pp. 97–100). Oxford, England: Basic Books.

Wolf, L. S., & Glass, R. P. (1992). *Feeding and swallowing disorders in infancy: Assessment and management.* Tucson, AZ: Therapy Skill Builders.

Woolridge, M. W. (1986). The anatomy of infant sucking. *Midwifery, 2*(4), 164–171.

CHAPTER

5

They Can Do It, You Can Help: Building Breastfeeding Skill and Confidence in Mother and Helper

Rebecca Glover and Diane Wiessinger

In cultures past, we breastfed during our own first few years of life, then observed it frequently and at very close range as we grew. By the time we were mothers, we had a rock-solid confidence in our own and our babies' abilities. But personal memory and observation had largely vanished by the second half of the 20th century. By the beginning of the 21st century, our culture had lost its belief that birth and breastfeeding work. Mothers and babies who might have managed by following the instinctive flow of behaviors from birth to breastfeeding found that flow destroyed by birth interventions and inappropriate breastfeeding help. Today, mothers and helpers alike tend to *hope* that breastfeeding will work, and *know* that bottle feeding will work.

This chapter is a work in progress, an ongoing attempt to relearn breastfeeding and to regain confidence in the normal interactions of mother and baby that have made lactation so successful through all of human—indeed, all of *mammalian*—history.

Because all mothers are female, and with apologies to all of us mothers of girls, we will be referring to all of the babies as male for the sake of an easy distinction between mothers and babies.

Self-Efficacy Theory and Breastfeeding

Throughout life, the healthy human brain grows new connections in response to the environment, the task at hand, and our thoughts and imaginings (Doidge, 2010). Repetition of those experiences and thoughts—like the repetition of piano scales—builds stronger and more lasting neural pathways, making future successes more likely. We too often overlook the fact that the expectation of success provides neural reinforcement through a process called self-efficacy.

Self-efficacy is a person's belief in his or her ability to accomplish a task or deal with a challenge. It is quite different from self-esteem, which relates to our sense of self-worth. The higher a person's sense of self-efficacy—his or her expectation that success will follow effort and perseverance—the more likely that person is to make the effort and persevere to success (Noel-Weiss, Bassett, & Cragg, 2006; Noel-Weiss, Ruppe, Craig, Bassett, & Woodend, 2006).

Since Bandura first published his theory of self-efficacy in 1977, a large body of academic papers and studies has shown that an individual's expectation of success has a powerful influence on his or her accomplishments in fields as diverse as education, health, athletics, business, and international affairs (Stajkovic & Luthans, 1998). People with a strong sense of self-efficacy

- see problems as challenges to be mastered;
- develop increased interest in and commitment to the activities in which they are involved;
- recover readily from setbacks and disappointments.

People with a weak sense of self-efficacy

- avoid challenging situations, believing that they will fall short;
- focus on their shortcomings and negative outcomes;
- quickly lose confidence in the face of problems (Bandura, 1994).

It is no surprise that a strong sense of breastfeeding self-efficacy can be a great help to the breastfeeding mother who experiences early problems. Dunn et al. (2006, p. 93) found that maternal confidence was a stronger predictor of breastfeeding outcome than supplementation or perception of support. The importance of maternal self-efficacy has been demonstrated or discussed by Blyth et al. (2002); Buxton et al. (1991); Creedy, Dennis, Blyth, Moyle, Pratt, & De Vries (2003); Dennis (1999, 2006); O'Campo, Faden, Gielen, & Wang (1992); Papinczak & Turner (2000); Kingston, Dennis, & Sword (2007); and many others. Dennis has been instrumental in promoting breastfeeding self-efficacy in numerous ethnic and social groups (2010), yet it remains an often-neglected part of breastfeeding support.

Pathways to Breastfeeding Self-Efficacy

There are four main routes by which we build self-efficacy:

7. Performance accomplishment or task mastery
8. Vicarious experience
9. Verbal persuasion
10. Emotional and physiological state

Performance accomplishment, as it pertains to breastfeeding, means that every successful experience increases a mother's belief in her ability to breastfeed. Success breeds success, highlighting where we should focus our efforts initially. *Supporting birth practices that minimize interventions and mother–baby separation; facilitating extended postbirth skin-to-skin contact; and encouraging the biological nurturing approach described in this chapter together form a package that can help convince a mother of her own and her baby's competence and ability to succeed.* However, because "successful experiences increase self-efficacy, [and] repeated failures diminish it" (Dennis, 1999, p. 196), the second half of this chapter will discuss how the remaining sources of self-efficacy information can culminate in breastfeeding success *if* the previously described experiences do not.

Vicarious experience is what mothers would have gained by seeing other women breastfeed. "Much human behavior is developed through modelling: observing others" (Bandura, 1977, p. 192). Modelling is especially important for people who have limited prior experience or are uncertain of their own abilities (Pajares, 2002). Having successful behaviors modeled for them helps mothers avoid excess trial and error; the repetition of errors can diminish self-efficacy.

Vicarious experience is the concept underlying step 10 of the Baby-Friendly Hospital Initiative: "Foster the establishment of breastfeeding support groups and refer mothers to them on discharge from the hospital or clinic" (World Health Organization & UNICEF, 1989, p. iv). Its placement (last) among the steps is unfortunate, for mothers need to have successful breastfeeding modelled repeatedly *before* their babies are born. *Prenatal and postnatal attendance at mother-to-mother groups deserves our strong, early, enthusiastic, repeated support.* We need to understand that unless mothers observe successful breastfeeding behaviors, they will turn automatically to what our culture perceives as successful infant feeding, for bottle feeding models abound (**Figure 5-1**).

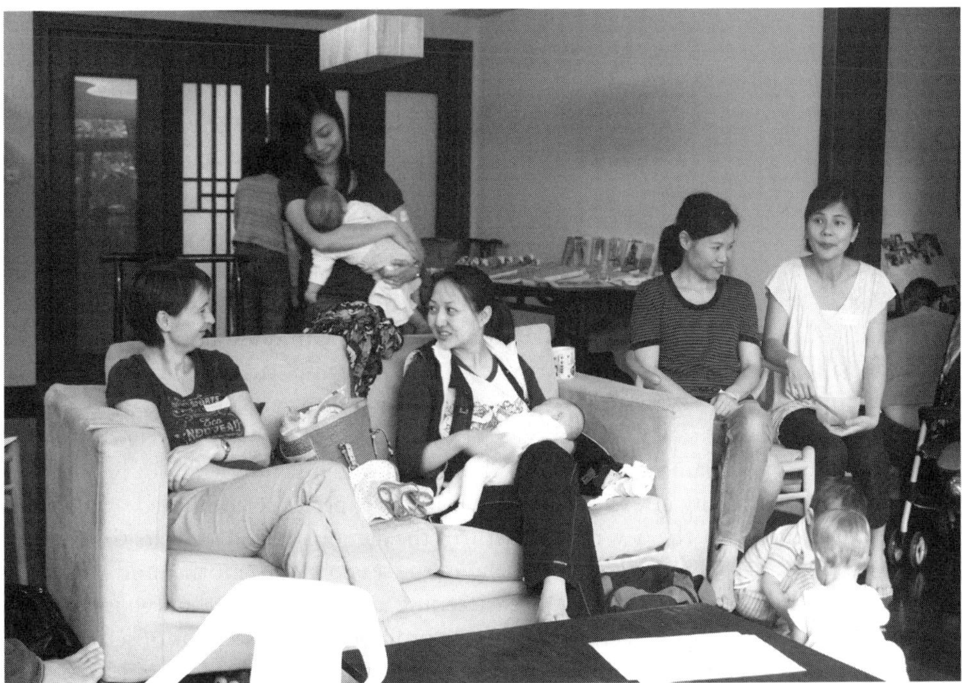

Figure 5-1 Mother-to-mother groups enhance breastfeeding self-efficacy.

Repeated modelling of successful outcomes and breaking a complex behavior into easy steps have been shown to improve self-efficacy (Bandura, 1977). Given the many stumbling blocks 21st-century mothers face, breastfeeding success will not always be immediate, but when we can accurately demonstrate innate breastfeeding behaviors to a mother, it can be achieved one step at a time. The use of visual media, such as videos and DVDs, pictures, graphics, and demonstrations with a doll, can provide mothers with effective vicarious learning experiences. Participatory modeling, discussed in more detail later in this chapter, is an especially effective form of vicarious experience.

Verbal persuasion includes encouragement and additional verbal information that is relevant, comes from a source the mother finds credible, and clearly contributes to improved success. It can be a valuable tool for us, but it is easier to undermine verbally than to build self-efficacy verbally. Raising expectations without providing the conditions for success "will most likely lead to failures that discredit the persuaders and further undermine the recipients' perceived self-efficacy" (Bandura, 1977, p. 198). The helper who says breezily, "You're looking great; just keep trying," builds no self-confidence in a woman who is breastfeeding in pain, and too many such comments may prompt her to look elsewhere for help or leave her feeling that breastfeeding simply doesn't work. Inappropriate verbal persuasion is perhaps our least effective way to help. Appropriate verbal persuasion combined with participatory modelling can be one of our best ways to help.

Of course, pain, stress, fatigue, anxiety, and fear affect a new mother's **emotional and physiological state**, reducing her self-efficacy. Simply alleviating a new mother's pain or stress and making her comfortable physically and emotionally can improve her belief in her breastfeeding abilities; when we help a mother with breastfeeding, her own emotional and physical comfort should always come first.

Participatory Modelling to Enhance Self-Efficacy

Your most helpful colleague, assuming you don't always have a group of successfully breastfeeding mothers at your elbow, may be a floppy newborn-sized doll. Too often, the breastfeeding helper tries to use verbal persuasion techniques alone. "You need to close the gap between you and your baby." ("Close the gap?" the tired, frustrated new mother thinks. "I don't even know what that means!") But the helper with a doll in tow can demonstrate, step by step, how to ensure that the baby is closely applied to the mother's body, explaining what she is doing and why it is important. A helper with a doll represents a highly effective form of vicarious experience combined with verbal persuasion. At each step, the new mother returns the demonstration (repeats the helper's actions with her own baby) so that, by the end of the session, both mother and helper are confident that at least this stage of the breastfeeding experience has been well integrated. This participatory modelling has been shown to promote strong feelings of self-efficacy, whether it involves a breastfeeding mother and her helper or an athlete and his coach. Demonstration, repetition, and repeated small successes are a powerfully effective route to success. Even before breastfeeding itself is successful, participatory modelling that leads to or enables a series of smaller successes can strengthen a mother's self-efficacy so that she remains eager to reach her breastfeeding goals. Imagine the pleasure the mother of a nonlatching baby can derive simply from knowing how to make herself and her baby fit comfortably together.

Self-Efficacy and the Breastfeeding Helper

In helping a mother learn to breastfeed her baby, you are actually helping her lay down neural pathways for success! Just as a baby's early stress level may have lifelong implications for his or her ability to handle stress (Teicher, Andersen, Polcari, Anderson, & Navalta, 2002), the kind of support a mother receives from you can influence whether her breastfeeding efforts are made from a position of confidence or defeat. But to help her gain that confidence, you need to exude confidence yourself. Reread the characteristics of high and low self-efficacy, substituting an image of a breastfeeding helper for your image of a new mother, and it will ring just as true.

This book is all about strengthening your own sense of self-efficacy by giving you a capacious tool kit with which to approach breastfeeding problems. Mothers and babies have innate abilities that you will learn how to recognize and encourage, contributing greatly to the likelihood of breastfeeding success when there are problems. In realizing that you can build a mother's self-confidence, we hope you will build your own as well.

Use (Your Expertise) Only as Needed

With today's highly medicalized, disempowering births and counterproductive cultural learning, you will often find yourself needing your expertise with normal breastfeeding pairs, in addition to helping mothers and babies with abnormal issues. In either situation, remember that unnecessary and excessive interference, insistence on a specific approach, and a rigid adherence to guidelines force a mother out of her normal peripartum right-brained learning mode and have caused a great deal of breastfeeding failure in recent decades. Explanations (which are inevitably somewhat left brained) should be kept to a minimum. They should be simply stated and be rich in analogies, playfulness, demonstrations, and confidence in breastfeeding success. Examples of analogies and playful demonstrations appear in boxes throughout the text, phrased as you might talk to the mother. The concept that each supports is in parentheses.

Think of yourself as an interpreter. You need to know as much of the breastfeeding language as possible. And from that vast vocabulary you need to select only those words that *this* mother and baby need in *their* situation, for their next step. You have many options to choose from. Use them sparingly.

Biological Nurturing®, or Laid-Back Breastfeeding

A first-time mother, postcesarean, with damaged nipples and a hard-to-latch baby about a month old, slumped back against the pillows on her couch one afternoon. She had just struggled through another feeding, and she knew her baby enjoyed napping prone between her breasts, his cheek against her skin. After a bit he stirred, lifted his head, and began to search drowsily for her breast. Too tired to sit up again, she shifted her breast and supported his head with her upper arm. He latched easily and comfortably. Throughout his half-asleep feeding, she found herself giggling at the ridiculous position they had invented. But because it broke all the rules and because she lacked further reinforcement, at their next feeding she returned to the rigid, ineffective, "correct" approach she had been taught. Her nipple pain did not resolve for another 2 months.

This mother's experience as she leaned back encapsulates all that is good about what Colson has termed *biological nurturing*® (2008) (www.biologicalnurturing.com) or *laid-back breastfeeding*. The mother was relaxed and comfortable, neither completely upright nor completely supine, her baby had plenty of room to maneuver, he was able to use his powerful rooting reflex along with many other reflexes, gravity was a help to both of them, she found the experience to be extremely pleasant, and they were both entirely free of rules. Let's take those one at a time (**Figures 5-2a through 5-2c**).

Mothers Need to Be Comfortable

The mother described above was fully supported—head, neck, shoulders, back, arms, legs—in a relaxed and sustainable position. It was an ideal—indeed, a necessary—starting point for their success.

Babies Belong to an Upright Species

Gorillas, chimpanzees, and other upright apes hold their infants upright against their chests to feed. Modern humans might do the same, but sitting creates a lap, the lap shortens our torso, and there is no room on that sitting-shortened torso for a nearly upright infant. Paintings from centuries past may show the mother with one foot on a low stool, baby sloping downward across her lap. Experienced mothers often cross one leg over another to create that slope, dropping the baby's hip onto their thigh to angle the baby's body further.

Current instruction and modern nursing stools and nursing pillows, in contrast, encourage a completely horizontal baby lying completely on his side with his legs unsupported, while his mother is completely vertical—an arrangement not usually seen among other primates and probably not selected instinctively by mothers. Indeed, mothers who are told to position their babies at right angles to their own torsos may complain that they can't see the baby's face or can see only one eye; the urge to be *en face* with our babies (our eyes in alignment with theirs) is a powerful one (Kashiwagi & Shirataki, 1995). In recent years, mothers have also been instructed to lie supine and let their baby do it all. No mother would do this without instruction, of course; we are not only a vertical species, we are interactive. Breastfeeding is something mothers and babies engage in together.

It is worth noting that babies in biological nurturing positions may "ground" themselves by planting the sole or ball of at least one foot on a maternal body part, often her thigh.

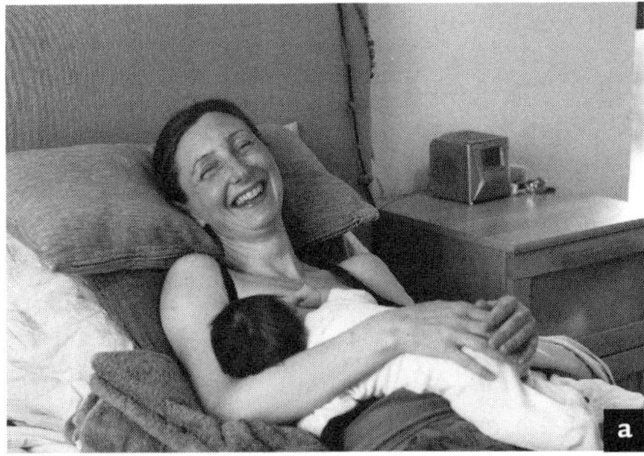

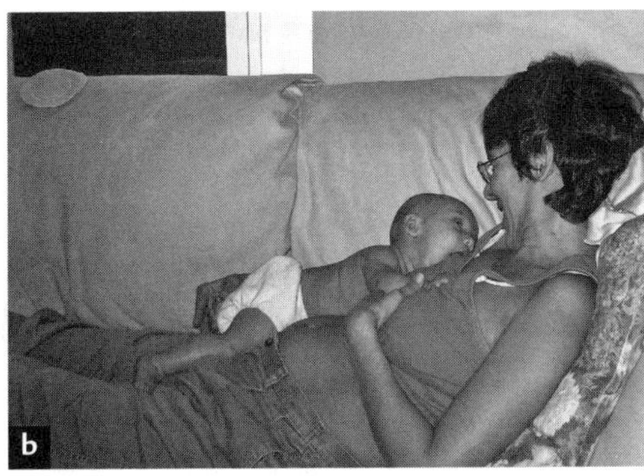

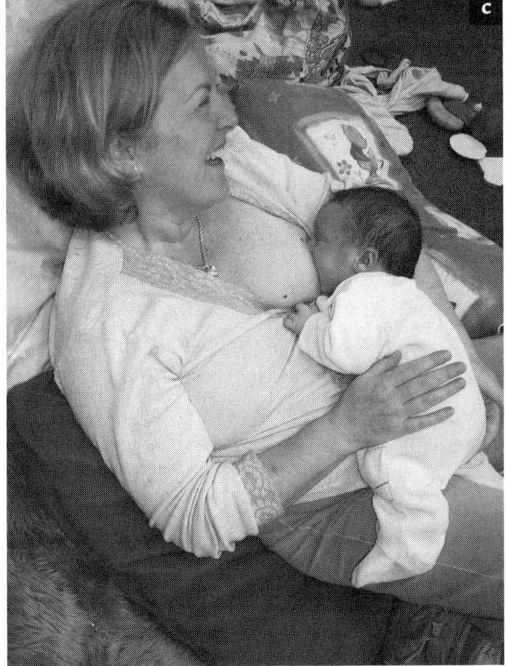

Figure 5-2 Biological nurturing, or laid-back breastfeeding. Note the smiles!

Alternatively, mothers may instinctively play with their baby's feet, as if supporting the bottoms of the feet. These are behaviors that may take on greater meaning as we add to our knowledge of maternal and infant feeding interactions in more upright postures. Colson (2008) lists "plantar grasp" as one of the primitive neonatal reflexes (PNRs) that facilitates feeding (see **Figure 5-2b**).

Leaning Back Opens the Torso

Because she leans back, the laid-back mother's lap disappears, in effect creating a longer torso that allows her baby considerable freedom of movement and a whole range of possible positions. Indeed, her baby can lie anywhere on her body like the hour hand on a clock face centered on her nipple. alongside hers, making the range of possible baby positions truly 360 degrees and allowing for a baby placement that, for instance, completely avoids a cesarean incision (Colson, Meek, & Hawdon, 2008; Colson, 2010).

When a mother leans back, the location of the nipple itself changes. Babies need good access to the part of the breast below the nipple (from the baby's perspective); an open torso tends to lift the underside of the breast away from the abdomen, allowing the baby access from any direction that mother and baby choose. When a mother lies back comfortably, a new world of positioning possibilities presents itself.

Babies Who Are with Their Mothers Feed on Their Own Timetable

A newborn's feedings are driven by more than hunger. Shifting hormones and levels of alertness, no doubt along with undiscovered triggers, can result in numerous feedings, which are important to the establishment of good milk production. These opportunities are missed when mother and baby are not together. Indeed, a baby at breast may feed without waking at all. Where this culture can usually count early-day feedings on one or two hands, mothers who begin motherhood with biological nurturing may have difficulty counting them at all.

The Rooting Reflex Is Not a Mistake of Nature

In the early 1980s, lactation consultants in our fledgling profession realized that a common cause of nipple pain was the baby who fed supine in his seated mother's arms. When a supine baby's cheek brushed his mother's nipple, his powerful rooting reflex caused him to turn in that direction with a gaping, seeking mouth, but the tugging and shallow mouthful that often resulted tended to cause pain. Starting with the baby already facing the breast, reasoned the lactation consultants, eliminated the head turn, along with any torque on the nipple. Next, they reasoned that a baby already facing the breast should be held away from the nipple until his mouth was fully open, so that he took a full mouthful of breast. However, newborns normally attach to the breast by feel and smell rather than by sight, anchoring their chin deeply in the breast first, and attaching at a moment of their, not their mother's, choosing.

Backing the baby away from the breast, which was often done to avoid a premature latch, also prevented the baby from understanding his location or anchoring his lower jaw on the breast, contributing to his difficulties and perhaps making clamping and tugging more likely. The precise moment of latch was determined, no doubt to the baby's complete surprise, by someone other than the baby. The phenomenon of healthy babies who wouldn't latch began.

In contrast, when a baby lies on his mother's sloping chest, he lies fully supported *with his face turned to the side*. His cheek now touches her skin, stimulating him to lift his head and right it—a move that both aligns his head and body and triggers a wide, searching mouth. Rooting to the side, a powerful reflex avoided for decades, comes so readily into play in biological nurturing that babies can feed without fully waking, as the woman described earlier found when she broke the rules and lay back

Hard-to-Get Ice Cream (Seeking)

Imagine yourself blindfolded. Now imagine the frustration of having an ice cream spoon being touched to your lips by someone else and then having it retreat into the darkness. If you finally figure out "ice cream spoon!" you're likely to make a grab for it with your mouth when you think it will work. Babies find the breast by feel, and they land their chins before they start to suck. The lip tickling that was recommended in the past tended to end in forward-reaching lips, a barely-open mouth as the baby tried to understand what was happening and why, and a tight grip to try to hang on if he was able to attach.

with her baby. Indeed, many babies who have difficulty attaching and feeding in more alert states can do so with much greater ease and maternal comfort if they are offered the breast from a biological nurturing position during light sleep.

A biological nurturing position tends to trigger many more reflexes that just the rooting reflex. Some have not previously been associated with feeding, and some have been assumed (because babies were oddly held or poorly stabilized) to interfere with feeding. But as Colson points out (2010), why would a baby have readily-released reflexes that run counter to his own best interests? Gravity holds at least part of the answer.

Gravity as an Ally

The mother who sits bolt upright, flat lapped, fights gravity at every step. To keep herself upright and maintain a hold on her baby, she must stay fully awake. ("Breastfeeding is exhausting me," she may complain.) She may need to apply additional pressure to keep him truly stable against her. ("My arm gets so tired.") If the baby senses any instability, he may begin flailing in an attempt to stabilize himself, to which she may respond with swaddling or arm holding. ("This takes three hands!") If he begins the normal behavior of head bobbing to find her nipple, gravity pulls his head away from her instead of toward her. ("I don't think he likes breastfeeding.") While most of these vertical-mother difficulties can be overcome with instruction, the very need for instruction is a problem. Gravity is her enemy.

If, however, she leans back comfortably against pillows or bedding that support her head, neck, shoulders, back, and body, with her baby prone on top of her, gravity maintains her position for her. It maintains her baby's position. It keeps the baby solidly and stably against her with their bodies closely applied. It draws the baby's head toward the mother with every head bob and helps him maintain his attachment once he latches. Its consistent, persistent whole-body support facilitates the release of at least 20 infant reflexes, some of which had not previously been associated with feeding (Colson, 2008). For example, the arm cycling and fighting behavior that a baby often displays when loosely held by an upright mother reverts to a series of instinctive behaviors that support effective feeding when she lies back somewhat. Gravity becomes her friend.

Hormonal Complexion

The mother who giggled through her experiment in laid-back breastfeeding may well have been responding to the high level of oxytocin that the casual, instinct-based positions of biological nurturing seem to encourage. Colson (2008, 2010) sometimes sees a "hormonal complexion"—flushed cheeks, drooping eyelids, gentle smile or half smile, even an apparent disconnection from the world associated with high oxytocic pulsatility—when mothers have a relaxed, gravity-as-friend feeding. The mothers in Figures 5-2A through 5-2C certainly express a degree of pleasure not often seen when mothers follow a checklist.

Rules? What Rules?

Colson (2010) describes, rather than prescribes, the biological nurturing positions that mothers and babies assume: a longitudinal lie when mother's and baby's long axes are parallel, a transverse lie when they are roughly at right angles. The most commonly chosen lie is an oblique one, with the baby angling somewhat across the mother's body, for example, from her left breast toward her right hip. When one lie isn't effective, or for other reasons of their own, mother or baby may spontaneously shift. Some mothers hold or manipulate their breast, others do not. Some wait for the baby to self-attach, others may plop the baby's mouth directly over the nipple. Most opt for light clothing on both themselves and their babies. Before the helper intervenes, it would be beneficial to observe patiently for a while! Biological nurturing is not about rules, it's about a mother and baby creating their own success.

The Importance of Fumbling

Mothers who are not following instructions tend to make numerous small movements as they help their baby attach. While the first edition of this book described a baby's innate ability to find the breast and attach, it is important to remember that a baby *does not normally manage this alone*. Baby-led shouldn't mean mother-dead. Left alone, a mother will stroke the baby from head to foot, shift his position or head or limbs, shift her own position and breast, play with his hands or feet, perhaps do it all again. An onlooker may see her actions as delaying the attachment. A closer look will probably reveal that they help. New-mother fumbling offers the baby a rapid-fire smorgasbord of arrangements, often made in response to his own movements. Because the baby is geared to seize the moment, the mother's arrangements and rearrangements tend to shorten the time it takes him to find what works best and increase the likelihood of success. Over time, the mother's motions subside to those few moves that she has learned work.

A Summary of Biological Nurturing (Laid-Back Breastfeeding)

Whatever feeding position a mother uses should offer physical and mental ease, appropriate breast availability, flexibility, and close application of the baby's body to the mother's body. Biological nurturing, although not the only arrangement that meets these criteria, is a very easy, flexible approach for most new mothers, and it is one that can be encouraged for all mother–baby pairs between feedings, regardless of how they choose to feed, because of the pleasure it offers mother and baby. *The mother chooses her angle of recline, her baby's position, whether and how they are clothed, and whether and how to hold or move her breast and her baby. She is the organizer and brain that arranges and rearranges conditions to which the baby responds reflexively.* Gravity helps the mother and baby fit together in a manner of their choosing and rechoosing, without gaps or strain. Biological nurturing is relaxing and hormonally advantageous to both mothers and babies and allows them a freedom similar to what they no doubt enjoyed in eons past, when mothers came to the breastfeeding experience with a powerful sense of self-efficacy and were able to transition without interference through birth to feeding.

Some mothers continue to use some variation of biological nurturing for many months. Others quickly begin to use a more upright posture for breastfeeding after a few days or weeks of lying back, but an opened torso while seated in an ordinary chair continues to be useful to many. Colson (2010, p. 46) uses the term "sacral sitting" for this use of the sacrum rather than ischial tuberosities for primary chair contact, usually with her shoulder blades against the back of a chair (**Figure 5-3**). In any case, biological nurturing can be thought of as one form of training wheels for breastfeeding—an approach that gives new mothers extra rest and gives babies a stable base and a rich source of feeding stimuli while they both learn their roles.

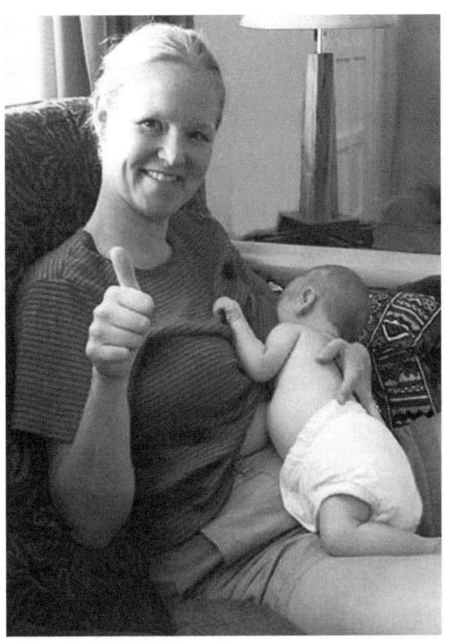

Figure 5-3 Sacral sitting.

Leaving a mother and baby to find their own path, with a bit of help in finding a comfortable laid-back position, is proving to be a highly effective starting point for successful breastfeeding. One hospital (I. Taubman, personal communication, 2009) now posts in every maternity room a photograph of a mother semireclining in her hospital bed, one arm loosely cradling her breastfeeding newborn, while she gently holds her baby's hand. "This is so easy," the poster says, quoting the mother. And most of the time, it is!

Undoing the Recent Past

What about those times when a mother and baby can't just do it? Self-efficacy studies tell us that breaking a new skill into small steps is helpful. However, the steps that many mothers learn today are counterproductive. Mothers learn these steps—sideways baby, lift the breast, tickle the lips, pull the baby on—from websites, books, and "experts." They try their best to follow a left-brained checklist at a time when they should be happily settled in their right brains. As one mother explained, "I didn't breastfeed because the nurse never came to show me how." And the checklist approach, so foreign to the normal start of breastfeeding, has resulted in this comment from another mother: "Women of my generation are convinced that breastfeeding doesn't work." Do we hear you whispering "poor self-efficacy"?

A bonus of biological nurturing is simply that it's different. A mother can't apply the rules that she learned from her books and websites and "experts," because the topography has changed. And with that change, she becomes open to a new set of ideas explained in a new way.

Presucking Behaviors: A Closer Look

Babies need first to be *stabilized* so they can concentrate on feeding and have a position of security and strength from which to move. Once they are stable, they begin *seeking* behaviors that bring them to the breast, using an instinctive, forward-reaching head position and head bobbing, both of which require that their heads be free to move. When they sense the nipple nearby, they find a place where they can anchor the lower jaw and perform a *scooping* motion that brings adequate breast and nipple into the mouth. The *sucking* that results is the focus of other chapters in this book.

Stabilizing: Bodies Facing Each Other, Open, and Closely Applied

All newborn mammals are uneasy if they are placed on their backs. They struggle to right themselves—to feel the ground or nest or mother's body against their chest and belly. Human infants are calmer when their chest and belly are against a firm support—preferably against an adult body. The Moro reflex (startle response) does not occur when the baby's entire front is held securely, without gaps, against an adult body. The human baby who rides on the mother's hip, the gorilla baby who clings to the mother's back, the premature infant in kangaroo care, even the baby in a colic hold—facing away from the adult but with firm pressure from the adult's forearm along the baby's chest and belly—are all stabilized by the position in which they are held. This externally-generated stability is called *positional stability* (Morris & Klein, 1987). For smooth, calm execution of the complex sequence of movements required for attachment and feeding, babies work best from a stable base, just as the position of a golfer's feet on solid ground affects the strength and accuracy of the swing. But unlike the golfer, a baby younger than 3 to 4 months cannot provide that stability independently. Gravity or adult hands must help. Gravity provides stability for a baby in biological nurturing positions. A seated mother provides stability for her infant when she holds her prone baby's back across the shoulder blades against her body (**Figure 5-4**).

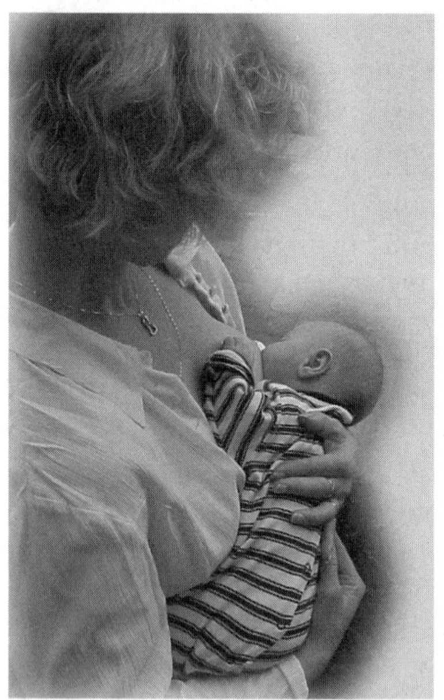

Figure 5-4 Open torso, positionally stable baby.

Adult mammals—and older babies—are capable of internally-generated *postural stability*; their more mature nervous systems allow them to feel stable in a variety of positions. However, "in the newborn stability is dependent on the development of neck and shoulder girdle stability *which are in turn* dependent upon trunk and pelvic stability" (Morris & Klein, 1987; italics added); for true stability, the baby's whole body must be turned toward and supported against the mother's body.

Creating a stable base for a breastfeeding infant also involves ensuring both midline and proximal stability. *Midline stability*—the stabilization of an imaginary line down the center of the infant's body—provides a stable base from which the infant can move the muscles on each side of the midline more effectively. Symmetrical movement of the muscles in the infant's neck, head, jaw, tongue, pharynx, and larynx allow for easier feeding. If the infant's midline is compromised, those muscles will be compromised to an equal degree; babies who have any form of physical asymmetry usually exhibit difficulty with effective feeding. Midline stability also gives babies a "sense of center," helping them focus their attention on their mouth and the breast in front of them (Morris & Klein, 1987, p. 18).

Once a baby is at or near the mother's breast and nipple, midline stability is not quite enough. The baby now needs to be able to lift his head and neck to refine his search. Physical and occupational therapists point out that proximal stability promotes distal mobility: stabilizing a body part closer to our core lets us move more skillfully a related body part that is farther away. When our forearm rests on a firm surface, our hand moves a computer mouse more accurately. With our wrist braced on the desktop, we have a steadier hand for the finer motion of placing the cursor. In the same way, stabilizing a baby's shoulders gives *proximal stability* to his head, neck, and oral area, allowing him much better mobility and control (Morris & Klein, 1987, p. 14).

A baby in a biological nurturing position achieves midline and proximal stability almost automatically; the seated mother must help her baby maintain stability by holding her baby firmly against her open torso, with as wide an angle as possible between her torso and lap. Supporting the baby behind his back and shoulders helps to open *his* body as well and ensures close, gap-free contact. Allowing the baby's lower hip to drop toward or onto the mother's thigh means that gravity helps her maintain whole-body stability for him.

Seeking: Lower Face Contacts Breast, Baby Free to Move

In order to bob about in search of and finally to reach for his mother's nearby nipple, an infant needs considerable strength in the neck's extensor muscles. Parents may say, proudly, "He could lift his head up when he was only a week old." In fact, that

What Do Baby Mammals Do? (Stabilizing)

Picture a mammal, any mammal, as a newborn. Imagine it on its back. What does it do? It thrashes and tries to get on its stomach where it feels stable and in control. Human newborns are no different. Your baby needs to hug your body, front to front, in order to feel truly secure.

Yes, You Have Instincts! (Self-Efficacy)

When you pick up your crying baby and hold him against your shoulder, swaying and patting his back, you have instinctively made him positionally stable and vertical, both of which are calming to him, and you've "put the baby in the kitchen"; from your shoulder, a hungry baby can move surprisingly quickly to your breast. No instincts for breastfeeding? Assuming your breast is uncovered, you have just done all you really need to do to help your baby nurse. Your baby can make the trip from your shoulder to your nipple all by himself!

First Stability, Then Supper (Stabilizing)

Imagine being offered a sandwich while you're walking on a narrow beam. "Not now," you say, "wait until I'm more stable." It's hard to think about a meal when you're feeling wobbly. No wonder babies who feel a gap between themselves and their support surface may flail their arms or pedal with their feet; they don't feel secure. One thing at a time, please! Stability first! Lean back with your baby, even very slightly, stabilize the baby's whole front in a prone position on your own front, with no gaps between you, and watch the flailing stop.

ability exists in all healthy babies from birth, provided they have a stable shoulder girdle from which to lift (Morris & Klein, 1987). The baby will use those extensor muscles to adopt a distinctive posture—head lifted and tilted back, so that the baby approaches the breast with the chin and mouth leading. This is the infant's "instinctive feeding position" (Glover, 2004, p. 87) (**Figure 5-5**).

Lifting the head into the instinctive feeding position is not entirely the work of the neck's extensor muscles. The hyoid bone and the muscles that attach to it have a key role (Wolf & Glass, 1992). The hyoid, a U-shaped bone in the neck located between the mandible and the larynx, is the only bone in the body that does not articulate with another bone. It is the attachment site for a number of muscles involved in large and small motor skills for breastfeeding. Some of these muscles connect to the clavicle, scapula, and cervical vertebrae (the shoulder girdle). Others connect to the skull, mandible, pharynx, and larynx; still more control and support the tongue. Collectively, the muscles attached to the hyoid bone are responsible for most of a baby's seeking, scooping, and suckling behaviors, and their ability to function is directly affected by the position of the infant's head and neck (**Figure 5-6**). Positional stability of the baby's body allows for proximal stability of the shoulder girdle, which allows for the strong and controlled movements of the head and neck that are part of the rooting reflex.

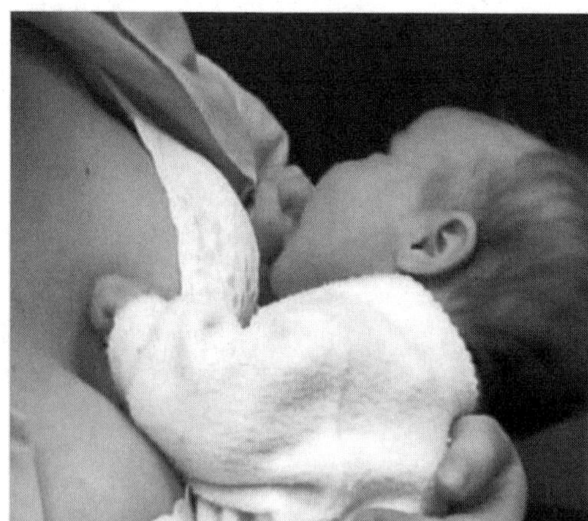

Figure 5-5 The instinctive position.

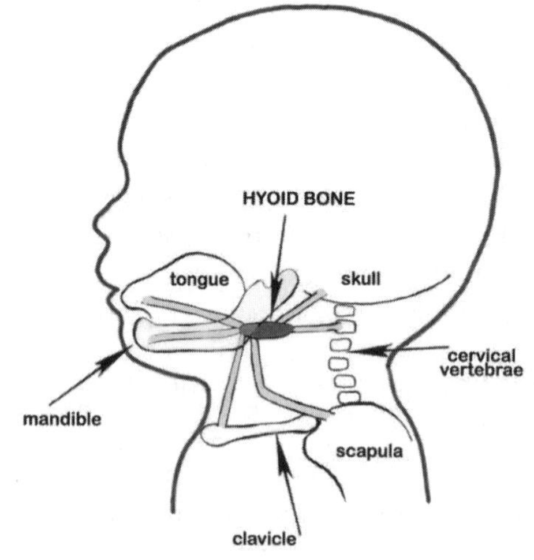

Figure 5-6 Schematic of hyoid bone and its muscle attachments to other bones.

As the previous chapter noted, a whole constellation of stimuli and responses can be considered part of the rooting reflex. Cheek or lower-face contact is especially helpful to the infant who is trying to locate lunch. A baby in a biological nurturing position automatically lies with this cheek on his mother's skin. The seated mother can begin by bringing any part of the baby's cheeks or lower face into contact with her breast; if the baby gets lost, the mother can quickly reorient the baby by resting his cheek on the skin near her nipple. This maneuver can also "unstick" a baby who is caught in a reflex loop, repeatedly sucking his hands at breast, pushing away, and coming back to his hands rather than to the breast. In either maternal position, placing the baby so that he will ultimately need to lift his chin and mouth to reach for the nipple will probably elicit the instinctive feeding position.

When gravity is his ally, the baby will lift and drop, lift and drop, bobbing his head about to find exactly where he wants to be. This normal woodpecker-like behavior is problematic for a baby in a seated mother's arms, unless she leans back enough to allow gravity to pull his head toward her body. A mother who sits with her torso completely vertical may report that the baby doesn't want to feed because she sees him swinging his head away from her breast. In fact, the baby is performing a normal behavior in an abnormal position; when gravity becomes her ally, she can see the behavior for what it is: competently performed breast seeking.

In the instinctive feeding position, an infant's head is neither fully flexed nor fully extended. The baby maintains it in a comfortable midrange, optimizing both his strength and his control as he gapes. In essence, the baby is about to take a very large bite from a very large sandwich.

Have a Sandwich (Scooping)

Consider keeping a fat toy sandwich among your tools—more fun for helper and mother alike!

When we eat a fat sandwich, we don't hold it vertically. Our jaws run horizontally; the upper one is fixed, the lower one is moveable. (See what happens when a finger rests on your upper lip when you chew, and when it rests on your chin. Only the chin finger moves.) To take the biggest mouthful, we plant our moveable jaw—our working jaw—well underneath the sandwich. We don't worry about the fingers on top of the sandwich; we may even use them to help tuck some of the bread under our upper lip.

The more deeply we plant our lower jaw under the sandwich, the bigger the bite we can take as we rock the top of the sandwich into our mouth. We don't focus on our upper jaw; it's the lower one that needs a big hunk of sandwich on it, so we keep the fingers under the sandwich (in this case our thumbs) well out of the way.

If the sandwich were suspended hands free, as a breast is, we wouldn't approach it straight on if we wanted a big bite. We certainly wouldn't approach it from above, which would require that we swing our working jaw—our chin—away from the food as we dip our head toward it. Instead, we would approach from slightly below, head tipped back, with our lower jaw lifting toward the underside of the sandwich. Babies like that same head-back arrangement.

Scooping: Clear Access Below the Breast Allows the Chin to Anchor

We aren't finished with stability yet! Once a baby finds the right spot near the nipple, his lower jaw swings open and he anchors his chin and bottom lip on the breast. Anchoring is just another word for stabilizing. The baby's head, well controlled as it is, is still a newborn head; without a solid breast attachment, he may grip or tug with his lips or jaws to maintain his position—ouch! That solid anchoring of chin and lower lip on breast benefits both baby and mother.

Ultrasound studies (Woolridge, 1986) indicate that, when attachment is good, a baby takes in enough breast to fill his mouth. The nipple comes to rest close to the junction of the hard and soft palate, and the infant's bottom lip, tongue, jaw, and chin lie deeply and securely under the breast tissue. With this essential mouthful in place (**Figure 5-7**), the baby can feed comfortably and effectively. The "critical area for attachment" is described as the "region below the nipple [from the baby's perspective], apposed to the baby's lower jaw and tongue" (Woolridge, 1986, p. 175). The mouthful is asymmetrical, with as much breast as possible on the lower jaw; the upper jaw may be placed just past the nipple base.

As a baby prepares to attach to the breast, his lower lip tends to be 3–4 cm from the nipple base and is usually folded back against his chin. Babies tend not to anchor their chins in the breast until the nipple is near their nose or upper lip—within reach but a head tilt away.

If the mother chooses to hold her breast, she needs to remember that any fingers on the lower jaw side need to be far away from her nipple to ensure that her baby has a clear runway and landing place for his chin and bottom lip on the breast below her nipple.

A baby who is positioned so that he must tuck his chin to reach the nipple will find his all-important lower jaw actually swinging away from the breast, destabilizing his jaw and making it all but impossible to attach to a short-shafted nipple. While he may be able to attach to a longer nipple with his chin tucked, the nipple must stretch, the latch is likely to be painful, and the lack of breast tissue over the tongue may compromise milk intake.

One of the most valuable forms of help a mother can give her baby as he attaches to the breast is to bring him back below her nipple if he moves past it. Babies simply cannot attach easily with a tucked chin, and although they are quite good at creeping forward or dropping sideways, they are not skilled at going backward.

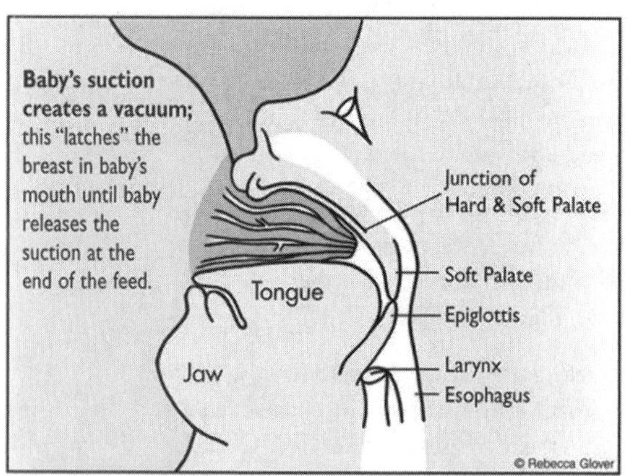

Figure 5-7 The essential mouthful.

The Helping Continuum

The previously described basics apply to almost every baby, from birth to 3 or 4 months old, who is learning to breastfeed. Simply being aware of babies' needs and sequences and making them available through the mother–baby interactions of biological nurturing is often all that is needed. Help the mother recognize and respond to her baby's presucking behaviors, reminding her of their normalcy, and *make sure she has access to a local mother-support group.* Mother and baby will learn from each other and will shorten their latching process and alter their positioning considerably as they go. The mother will skip over steps that her baby no longer requires, and the baby will correctly read signals that are sloppily, absent-mindedly, or only partially given in the shorthand style of every comfortable nursing couple. Attend a mother-to-mother breastfeeding group and you will see a wide range of normal latching behaviors among experienced mothers and babies. Any technique—*any* technique—that allows for mutual comfort and an efficient transfer of milk at breast is correct breastfeeding.

Other babies may need a more hands-off approach, and still others may need extra guidance or specialized equipment. All these babies form a continuum of helping situations.

Baby-Led Self-Attachment

Some babies have been overhelped or have had interventions that distressed them; these babies may need to feel completely free to do it all themselves at first. It may be helpful for the mother to find a biological nurturing position in which she can see her baby comfortably when he lies between her breasts, low enough that he needn't twist to reach them. In truly baby-led self-attachment, the mother keeps her role almost entirely passive, limiting her help to ensuring the following:

Chin Lifted Means Wide Mouth (Seeking, Scooping)

Press on the back of your head, tuck your chin toward your chest, and open your mouth wide. You'll find the size of your gape restricted. Notice where the back of your tongue is during this exercise: probably humped up against the soft palate, where the nipple would normally go! Now cradle your neck and let your head fall back. You can open your mouth in a cavernous gape, and your tongue lies on the floor of your mouth, out of the way of where the nipple would be and almost unable to retract or hump. Pressing on a baby's head makes latching much more difficult for him.

The gag reflex is also less sensitive with your head in the instinctive feeding position. Try touching your soft palate with your finger, first with your mouth wide open and your chin down, then with your mouth wide open and your head in the instinctive feeding position.

Try taking several large, quick swallows from a full glass of water, first with your chin down, then with your chin slightly—not dramatically—raised. The mouth is bigger and swallowing is more comfortable, for both adults and babies, when the head is in the instinctive feeding position.

- Stabilizing: If the baby draws his knees up, creating an ongoing gap, the mother can gently, with soothing and stroking, restore full frontal contact. If you or she senses that even light clothing is a hindrance, discuss the value of skin-to-skin contact with her.
- Seeking: If the baby fusses, the mother can return him to her midline, gently arranging for his cheek or lower face to contact her breast, or she can use other calming measures, including sitting or standing to settle him.
- Scooping: If the baby overshoots the target by sliding his mouth past the mother's nipple, she can place the baby's cheek near her nipple or reposition the baby on her body so he must move forward to reach her breast.

A mother whose baby needs a truly baby-led approach at first will find that he accepts and appreciates her input more and more as they both gain confidence in breastfeeding. As they both relax, they will also begin to rely on techniques of their own devising.

Infant Feeding Sequence (Seeking)

Every mammal is born with the ability to move instinctively to its mother's nipple. This *infant feeding sequence*, or series of predictable and standardized moves that end with suckling, often involves a little bit of help from mom. A horse stands up and may nudge her newborn in the general direction, a dog lies down and may do the same, but finding the nipple and latching on is basically the baby's role for each mammal species. For some, the infant feeding sequence is so preset that they can't latch on if they are placed directly in front of a nipple. The human infant feeding sequence is much less rigid, but a baby who seems confused or angry at the breast may do fine if he is allowed to go through his sequence from the start, especially if his mother is in a laid-back position.

When Technique Is Necessary: Mother-Sped and Mother-Led Breastfeeding

Sometimes a mother must take a more active role from the start. The helping situations along this part of the continuum all involve the same general stabilizing, seeking, scooping, and sucking components as biological nurturing. But they also require that mother and helper pay attention to these components in finer detail (**Table 5-1**).

Mother-Sped Breastfeeding

Mother-sped attachments range from simply speeding up the process by bringing the baby directly to the breast (common to almost all mothers once they and their babies gain some experience) to mothers being required to step in and help. Birth medications, separations, or minor anatomical variations, such as tongue-tie or a very receding chin, can leave a baby confused about his mother's landscape or how to make use of it. Prematurity, neurological issues, and other more substantial anomalies may require an even more active role on the mother's part; some gentle maternal guidance can help any normal, hungry baby who does not latch spontaneously.

When a mother needs to take the lead, either nudging the process along or actually taking over, we can be the most useful by helping her to help herself through

Table 5-1 The Helping Continuum: A Summary of Presucking Behaviors and Approaches

These seven fundamental behaviors apply to all holds and positions.

Fundamental Behaviors		Approach: Biological Nurturing	Approach: Baby-Led	Approach: Mother-Sped	Approach: Mother-Led
		Biological Nurturing *Mother's behaviors stimulate but don't direct (normal baby); mother is active partner.*	**Baby-Led** *Mother almost entirely passive; fundamental behaviors are nonetheless triggered (useful for reluctant baby).*	**Mother-Sped** *Mother provides proactive guidance to trigger fundamental behaviors (useful for reluctant baby, anatomical variations).*	**Mother-Led** *Mother may provide total guidance at every step (useful for prematurity, neurological issues).*
Stabilizing Triggers the release of innate responses in both mother and baby and leads to . . .	1. Mother and baby face each other *Allows midline stability*	Mother chooses angle of recline, places baby prone on her chest/abdomen, close to her breast		Mother makes herself comfortable, turns baby's whole body to face her own body	
	2. Mother and baby's bodies are **open** against each other *Eliminates gaps*	Mother's semi-reclining posture and baby's prone position open their bodies		Mother sits with a straight back, upright or slightly reclined, holding baby's back and shoulders; mother places baby in prone position on her open body	
	3. Baby is **closely applied** to mother's body *Calms, triggers reflexes, provides a stable base*	Gravity keeps baby closely applied to mother's body; mother repositions baby when and as she sees fit		Baby's chest is closely applied to the base or side of the breast with baby's body completely supported on his mother	
		Prevents random reflex responses (arm cycling, hand to mouth, head shaking, and back arching)			
Seeking Stimulates rooting, gaping, and tongue extrusion reflexes, and leads to . . .	4. Baby's lower face is **in contact** with the chest/breast *Stimulates seeking behaviors*	Gravity keeps baby's lower face, cheeks, chin, and lips against mother's body/breast		Baby's lower face makes good contact with breast (provided baby is stabilized as above)	
	5. Baby can **move to the breast/nipple** *Especially his head*	Baby moves freely on mother's abdomen; mother shifts breast, body, and baby as she sees fit, holds breast as she sees fit	Baby moves freely on mother's abdomen; mother prevents excessive motion, moves baby if he "overshoots"	Holding baby across the shoulders, ensures baby's head is free to life and orient to the nipple	Mother may gently support her baby's head in the instinctive position as she aligns mouth and breast

(continues)

Table 5-1 The Helping Continuum: A Summary of Presucking Behaviors and Approaches *(continued)*

Fundamental Behaviors		Approach			
		Biological Nurturing *Mother's behaviors stimulate but don't direct (normal baby); mother is active partner.*	**Baby-Led** *Mother almost entirely passive; fundamental behaviors are nonetheless triggered (useful for reluctant baby).*	**Mother-Sped** *Mother provides proactive guidance to trigger fundamental behaviors (useful for reluctant baby, anatomical variations).*	**Mother-Led** *Mother may provide total guidance at every step (useful for prematurity, neurological issues).*
Scooping Results in large mouthful of breast and leads to . . .	6. Baby has clear **access to the breast below the nipple** *Allows adequate mouthful*	Baby moves his mouth up the breast "mountain" to find the nipple, before swinging his jaw down to anchor on the breast		Mother may tilt her nipple up, centering it above baby's top lip, offering baby more breast below the nipple	
	7. Baby **anchors** chin and bottom lip on breast *Allows fine motor control of mouth without tugging on breast or nipple*	Gravity keeps baby's chin and lips "in touch" with the breast as he opens wide, anchors his chin and lower lip, and scoops in a good mouthful of breast		Mother keeps baby's chin and lips "in touch" with the breast below the nipple and, as he opens wide, hugs him extra close, helping to anchor the chin and lower lip at the moment of latching	
Sucking	See Chapters 1 and 8 for a detailed discussion of infant suck				

Source: Courtesy of Rebecca Glover.

the processes described in the self-efficacy section of this chapter: modelling, participatory modelling, visual images (vicarious learning), and relevant information broken into simple steps that show the mother how to support and work with her baby's innate reflex behaviors (verbal persuasion).

If possible, share video footage of babies seeking, finding, and attaching by feel. DVDs are wonderful because they allow you to pause on a frame and talk to the mother about the image. If you do not have video at hand, use your doll and demonstrate what the baby can do, *describing each fundamental behavior*, what stimulates it, and the action the baby is likely to take in response to the stimulus (**Table 5-1**). Mothers are built to follow their baby's lead; knowing what their baby can do is the first step toward their knowing how to help.

Sitting Up . . . Almost

When a laid-back posture isn't working, many mothers will want to sit more upright. But even though the mother's arms and hands must now take over gravity's role to some extent, an *open posture* remains the foundation for all of the other fundamental behaviors. What she sits on can help a great deal. Chairs with arms can restrict mother and baby's freedom of movement; couches that are too low, saggy, or deep can produce a curled posture. The addition of a cushion or some extra foam under the couch seat and extra cushions behind the mother's back can help open her posture. A small cushion or rolled-up towel can provide lumbar support, improving the mother's comfort and maintaining an open upper body.

In this seated-but-open posture, the mother sits on her sacrum rather than her ischia, her back is comfortably straight (though angled backward slightly), her shoulders are wide, and her arms drop to her sides. Her straight, slightly reclined back lifts her breasts and flattens her abdomen, creating a more open space for the baby to be positioned prone on her body, with arms and hands resting against the mother's body, one on each side of the breast. Much of the baby's weight falls onto her body, while the weight of her hands and forearms falls on the baby's body, and gravity is once again their ally (**Figure 5-8**).

A mother who needs or wishes to be fully vertical when helping her baby to attach can relax back against good support once her baby is attached and feeding well. A forward-leaning position (common in this culture with a nursing pillow holding the baby) is rarely helpful, in part because of the gaps it creates. *But remember that* rarely *is not* never; *no position should be rejected out of hand.*

Think Flat to Flat (Stabilizing)

You, the helper, can curl your body forward, displaying how this tilts your breasts and nipples down toward your abdomen (postpartum breasts often rest on a postbirth tummy, especially in larger women). Then, with a bit of dramatic flourish, uncurl. As you lift your shoulders up and back, the mother can see that this lifts the breasts and flattens the abdomen. Immediately position a doll on your body (as in **Figure 5-4**), modeling how a straight, uncurled upper body opens the mother's posture, creating space for her baby's body. Mother and baby can "fit together like two pieces of a jigsaw puzzle" (Colson, 2008).

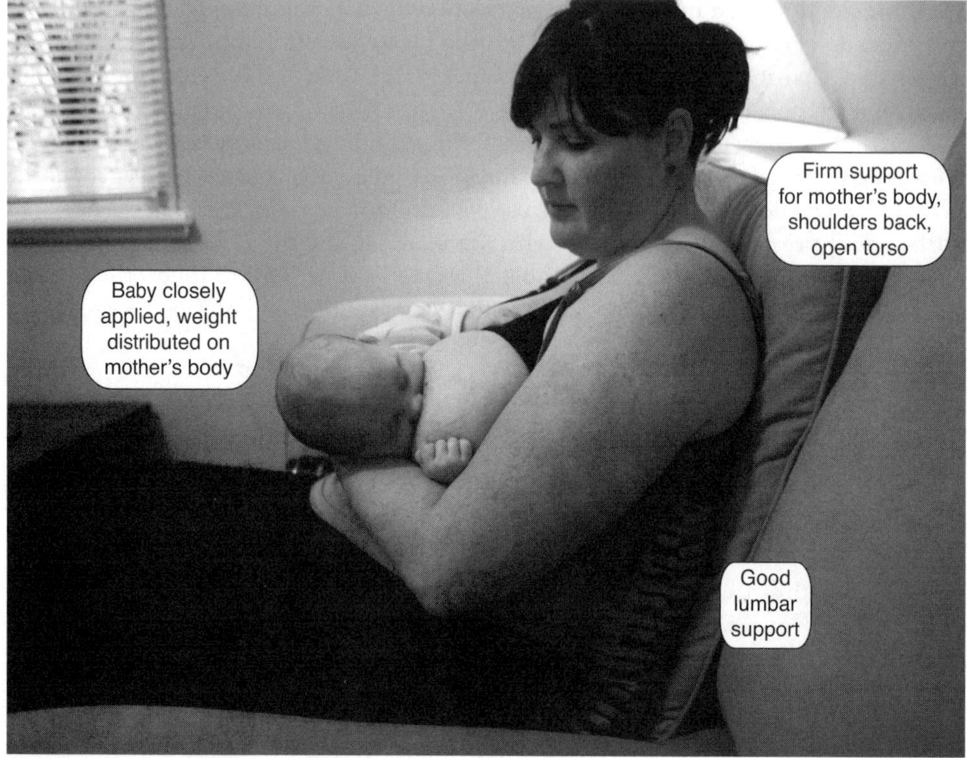

Figure 5-8 The seated-but-open posture: seated, straight back, angled back slightly, shoulder blades against chair, good lumbar support.

As well as optimizing infant-maternal contact, the baby's stability, and the strength and effectiveness of reflex movements, a prone posture on the mother's body prevents some reflex responses that appear to hinder or distract the baby from attaching well. It is common to see a mother struggling with a baby who is reflexively responding to random stimuli with arm cycling, hand to mouth movements, head shaking, and back arching *simply because he is not positioned closely enough against his mother's body.*

A Cradle Hold That Makes Sense

Mothers in modern cultures have often learned vicariously to cuddle the baby in the crook of the arm with a hand on the baby's bottom, a practice that curls the baby into a comma; pulls the baby's torso away from the mother's body; restricts the baby's head movement; tucks his chin; and puts the mother, not the baby, in control of his approach to the nipple. Combine all that with cultural practices of swaddling and bottle feeding and the cultural norm of supporting a baby's head, and the accumulated images tell the mother to cradle her cueless, clueless baby supine in her arms, being sure to support the head while trying to point a nipple into his mouth.

With participatory modelling, and using your own body or a model breast and a doll, you can quickly help a mother understand that the way she holds her baby affects his posture and access to her breast. Using demonstrations and clear descriptions, calmly walk her through a more effective approach, ensuring that she succeeds at each step, breaking it into smaller steps as needed.

Participatory Modelling Steps: Cradle Hold

1. Hold the baby's back with one hand across his shoulder blades (same hand and breast). With your wrist in a neutral position, fitting snugly into the nape of the baby's neck, drop your shoulder and arm into a normal posture.
2. Use your hand to uncurl the baby, turn the flat, open body to face you, and place the baby in a prone position underneath your breasts, closely applied to your open body. The baby's chest will be snuggled against the base or side of the breast, and his arms may encircle it like an underwire bra (see the box titled Hands Up!) (**Figures 5-9 and 5-10**).
3. Position the baby's chest and upper shoulder against the lower inner quadrant of the breast (just below the cleavage). When he reaches up for the breast, his chin and mouth can find the sweet spot just below the nipple.

Hands Up! (Stabilizing)

Imagine lying prone and lifting your head, first with one hand across your chest and then with a hand on each side of your body near your shoulders. Which position gives you the most strength and stability?

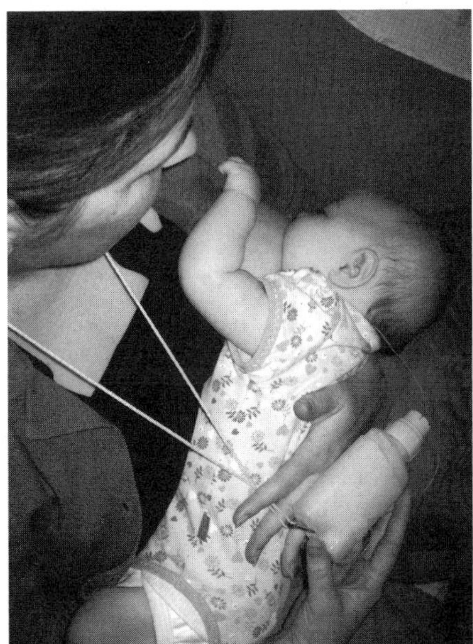

Figure 5-9 (Left) Baby uncurled, prone-like, closely applied, chest to breast, arms encircling breast, instinctive head position.

Figure 5-10 (Below) Chest against side of larger breast. Note open body, head tilted back slightly, chin into breast, nose clear of breast.

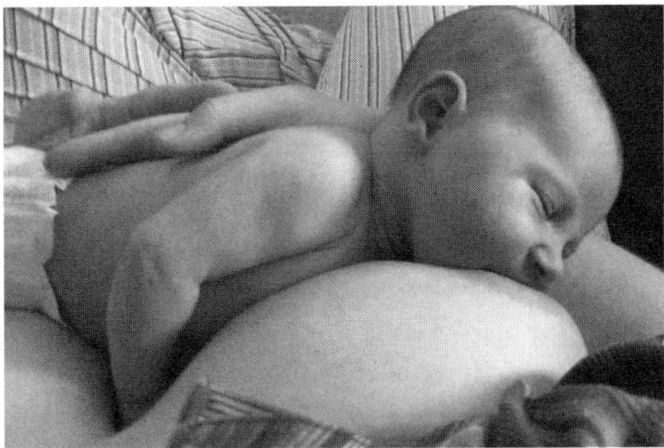

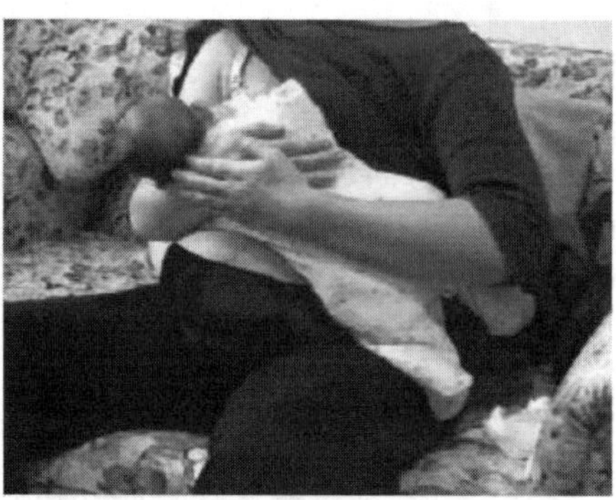

Figure 5-11 Cradle hold, with baby's leg resting on mother's thigh.

How Close Is Close Enough? (Stabilizing)

If your baby lies in your arms without you leaning back a bit, there may be a gap between the baby's body and yours. The baby's body may be against yours in a nice, straight line, but he may not be as well supported as you think. Try standing up while you hold the baby's front against yours and notice how you hug him more closely. Now your two bodies fit together like two pieces of a jigsaw puzzle, with the baby's flat, open body against your flat, open body. That's what gravity can do for you if you lean back a bit while you nurse. Now, have a seat, but keep that closeness.

4. Use an appropriate angle for the baby's body. Sitting up—even sacral sitting—can reduce the area in which the baby's body can fit; the mother's breast size and length will determine the extent to which the baby must be swung sideways. For very long-breasted women and very large women, see the variations discussed later. In general, however, the baby will be angled downward, his feet clearly lower than his head.
5. After you have modelled the necessary step or steps for a mother, coach her to accomplish them successfully with her own baby (**Figure 5-11**).

Cross-Cradle Hold: Another Training Wheels Option

The cross-cradle hold (left breast, right hand) can be helpful in specific circumstances, but its use has many more potential problems than the alternatives of laid-back breastfeeding and the cradle hold. Once the baby understands his role, it is important for mother and baby to experiment with more relaxed, interactive approaches. For many mother–baby combinations, the mother's hands will eventually rest on the baby's back, one hand over the other, at her midline. For these couples, cradle hold and cross-cradle hold become irrelevant. Rest your hands on your own stomach, one over the other. Now change which one is on top. Does it really matter?

Participatory Modelling Steps: Cross-Cradle Hold

1. Hold your baby's lower shoulder in the palm and heel of your hand (opposite breast and hand), with your fingers extending well past the lower shoulder and your pointer finger and thumb *lightly* positioned just behind the baby's ears, forming a passive cradle at the nape of the baby's neck.
2. Allow your baby's body to drape downward at an oblique angle, from your breast to your opposite thigh. This not only improves the baby's position, but also moves your wrist, forearm, and elbow closer to your body, increasing the strength and comfort of the hold. You will instantly feel the difference.

3. Keep your wrist straight and flattened out against your baby's back. Remember, muscles work best in the midrange, neither flexed nor extended. A flat, straight wrist keeps your baby's body uncurled (chest to breast) and optimizes the strength, function, and comfort of your hand and wrist.
4. Turn your baby's open body to face you, and place him in a prone position on your open body. As described for the cradle hold, the baby's chest will be snuggled against the base or side of the inner lower quadrant of your breast, with his lower shoulder tucked under your breast and his upper shoulder just below your cleavage.
5. Keep your body and your shoulders in a normal posture at all times (**Figure 5-12**).

Cross-Cradle Training Wheels (Stabilizing)

Who wants to ride a bicycle, as an adult, with training wheels still attached? Just as those training wheels can slow you down or catch in potholes, the mother-controlled, baby-restricting cross-cradle hold is more tiring and can even cause a resentful baby in later months. If you use cross-cradle training wheels at the start, experiment with ways that allow you just to hold your baby, start to finish, once you both know your roles. You'll both be glad you did!

Coaching: Hitches and Hints

It is common to see a mother who uses this hold twisting her body, moving her shoulder, and therefore *moving her breast away from her baby*. What follows is a chain reaction as she tries to chase the breast with the baby. A blanched thumbnail indicates that the mother is *gripping* the baby's head with her thumb and fingers, rather than holding the baby's shoulder with the heel of her hand and flattened wrist. It usually teams with a cocked wrist that curls the baby's body forward, and the mother uses her grip to push her baby's head onto or over the nipple. This overriding of all the baby's innate reflexes is usually unsuccessful. Keeping her hand and wrist in a more neutral—not cocked—position helps prevent wrist strain, keeps the baby's chest to the breast, and provides the baby with solid positional stability and all that flows from it.

Mothers may have been told to hitch the baby's bottom up under the arm, but this shifts her attention to holding the baby's bottom against her body instead of holding his chest and shoulders against the base or side of her breast. Consider it an unhelpful hitch.

As a final check for all mothers, observe that the mother's shoulders and arms are relaxed and dropped into a neutral position, the baby is closely applied to her body with no gaps, and she is relaxed against good back and lumbar support.

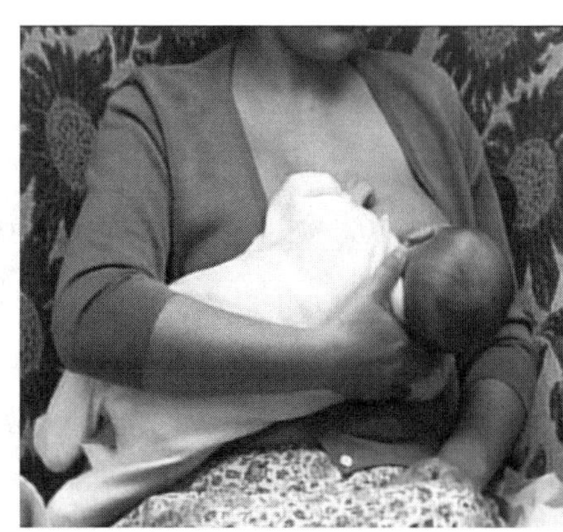

Figure 5-12 Cross-cradle hold.

When there are latching problems, human babies, like other primates, often attach more easily in oblique or vertical (long axis to long axis) positions. *There is one common exception.* A postbirth tummy, nature's pillow, can be an impediment to a gap-free position. Try positioning the baby horizontally, closely applied to the mother's body *immediately* under the breasts, and supported on her postbirth tummy (**Figures 5-13a and 5-13b**).

Seeking Behavior with a Seated Mother

Whether the mother lies back or sits, her baby needs the sensory stimuli of the breast on his lower face to seek the nipple and attach well. The introduction in Smillie's DVD (2007) provides some excellent seeking footage of a baby working her way cheek-by-cheek to the nipple. However, nothing will top the personal experience of a mother seeing her own baby respond to the touch of his face on her breast. This is easy to arrange; healthy, hungry babies free of birth medications can be relied on to do it every time!

Breast and Mouth Alignment

If a baby is positioned well, as previously described, good breast and mouth alignment can be almost automatic for many mother–baby pairs. However, if a mother has large breasts or there are other anatomical variations, she may need some additional modeling or relevant information.

Participatory Modelling Steps: Breast and Mouth Alignment

1. Keep your baby's chest snug against the base or side of your breast, with no gaps. Remember that the baby moves best from a stable base and must be uncurled, with hands near his head, to lift his head into the instinctive feeding position.
2. Keep some part of your baby's lower face in good contact with the breast. Keep it uppermost in your mind that your baby *feels* his or her way on your breast. The

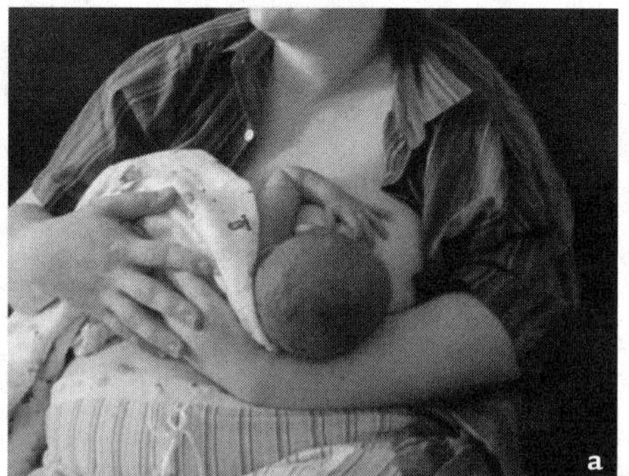

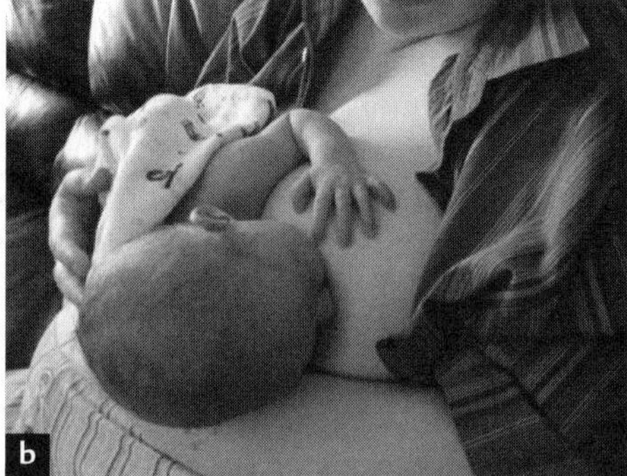

Figure 5-13 Horizontal baby in space (a) between breasts and (b) postpartum tummy.

unbroken touch of face on breast stimulates the baby to look up the mountain and find the nipple.

3. Keep your nipple at or above your baby's top lip and watch his chin and lips center on the breast just *below* the nipple—the starting block from which his jaw swings open to anchor his chin and *lower* lip and scoop up a good mouthful of breast. This may occur automatically or it may be helpful to use a finger or thumb to position your nipple for your baby.
4. To use a finger or thumb to tilt your nipple up, place the pad of your finger (if using the cradle hold) or thumb (if using the cross-cradle hold) just *above* your nipple and *parallel* to your baby's top lip. Press gently to tilt your nipple up and shape the top of your breast like an appropriately-angled sandwich. (See the box titled Have a Sandwich.) Use your finger or thumb to move and center your nipple above your baby's top lip, so that your nail, nipple, and baby's nose are aligned. Your finger may even be under your baby's top lip briefly at the moment of attachment (**Figures 5-14 and 5-15**).

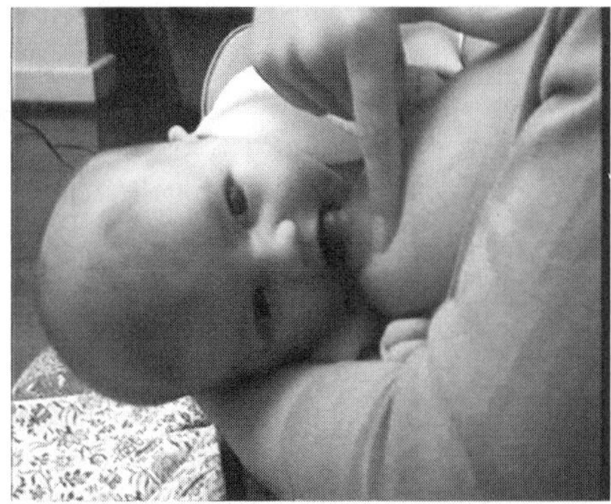

Figure 5-14 A well-placed finger or thumb.

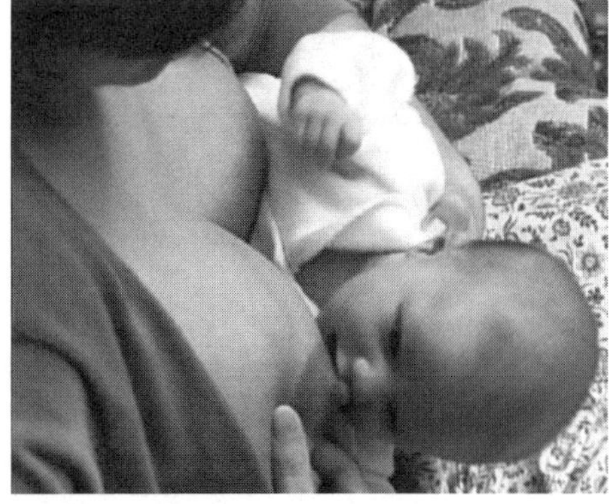

Figure 5-15 Keeping the nipple above top lip allows bottom lip to "anchor" lower on breast.

Coaching: Hitches and Hints

If a baby must tuck his chin toward his chest while trying to reach a nipple directly in front of or below his mouth, he may, in frustration, end up *lifting* his chin into the instinctive position, only to find his mouth in open space, well past the breast and nipple, rooting near his mother's elbow! Show the mother how her baby is seeking the breast but needs his whole body moved toward her midline to position his chest against the inner lower quadrant of her breast, with his chest and upper shoulder effectivly in her cleavage. Now when the baby reaches up for the nipple it will be right in front of his nose!

Some babies may have learned to reach down rather than up for the nipple. If the mother keeps her nipple above her baby's top lip, rather than chasing his mouth with it, he will begin to look up for it. Rushing the baby or trying to bring the nipple to his mouth during this brief period of relearning will likely confuse him.

The mother may feel that her nipple should be in front of her baby's mouth. ("I can't see how the nipple is going to fit in his mouth," she may exclaim.) However, if her nipple is presented directly to her baby's mouth, he will probably respond with forward-reaching lips and fall short of a deep mouthful. The exercises described in the box titled Chin Lifted Means Wide Mouth can give the mother firsthand insight into the value of good breast and mouth alignment.

If a mother complains of strained, painful wrists, you may find that she flexes her wrist and holds her elbow away from her body as she uses her thumb to position her nipple for the baby. Physical pain and discomfort will lower her sense of self-efficacy. Show her how to flatten the heel of her hand and wrist against the side of her body. This improves her comfort and turns the pad of her thumb toward her baby's mouth instead of away from it. When using a finger to tilt her nipple in the cradle hold, the mother's wrist and arm should be relaxed across the top of her breasts.

A mother who is using the cross-cradle hold may be frustrated because her baby attaches for only a few seconds and then comes off the breast. She may have been removing her thumb and hand from the breast immediately after the baby attaches, causing the breast to drop out of the baby's mouth. Show her how to position her baby's body to stabilize her breast in its normal position and provide reciprical support for the baby. Relaxing her hold on her breast gradually, after swallowing starts, will help her maintain baby and breast as a single unit.

Holding the baby's head or pushing it forward will inhibit or prevent the rooting, gape, and tongue extrusion reflexes, making seeking and latching difficult or even impossible. Therefore, no part of a mother's hand or arm should support the *back* of the baby's head.

Keeping the nipple above the baby's top lip can help him scoop in a bigger mouthful of breast below the nipple. Because actions speak louder than words, mothers might find the exercise in the Staying in Touch box useful to reinforce the importance of the instinctive feeding position and the value of keeping the nipple above the baby's top lip (**Figure 5-16**).

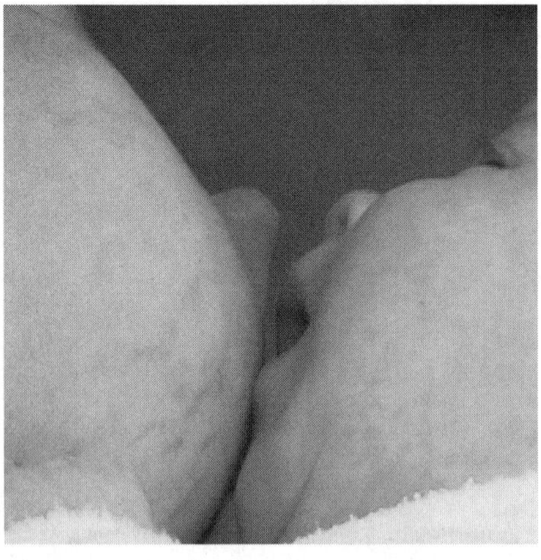

Figure 5-16 Good breast and mouth alignment.

A Good Mouthful

An effective and fun way to help a mother understand how her baby takes the best possible mouthful of breast is to use the analogy of a very fat sandwich or hamburger (described in the box titled Have a Sandwich). This analogy models the relevance of shaping the breast parallel to the baby's lips; offering him the breast "below" the nipple (from his perspective); and allowing the baby's head to tilt back as he brings his chin and bottom lip forward to anchor them well away from the nipple, allowing for the biggest possible mouthful of breast.

Everything is covered in one playful analogy that the mother can experience firsthand.

Participatory Modelling Steps: A Good Mouthful

1. With your baby's lips and chin positioned at the starting block, focus on having the part of your breast nearest his lower lip the nipple become the mouthful. The nipple is attached; it will follow! *If you present your breast, not your nipple, to the baby*, your nipple will be the last part of the breast to enter his mouth, and it will unfold deep inside (**Figures 5-17a through 5-17d**). Glover's DVD (2005) has demonstrations and animated illustrations of this approach.
2. Keeping unbroken mouth-breast contact, *wait* for your baby to open his lower jaw *wide.*
3. *Wait* for your baby's chin to anchor on the breast with his bottom lip, 3–4 cm from the base of your nipple. (The farther his bottom lip is from the nipple, the bigger the mouthful your baby will take.)

Staying in Touch (Scooping)

Position your thumb vertically at your lips, with your thumbnail resting on your upper lip. Keeping your thumb in that position, open your mouth as wide as possible while keeping your bottom lip in constant contact with your thumb.

Your head needs to tilt back to keep your bottom lip and jaw touching your thumb. In the same way, your baby has to tilt his head back to keep his chin touching your breast while he latches on.

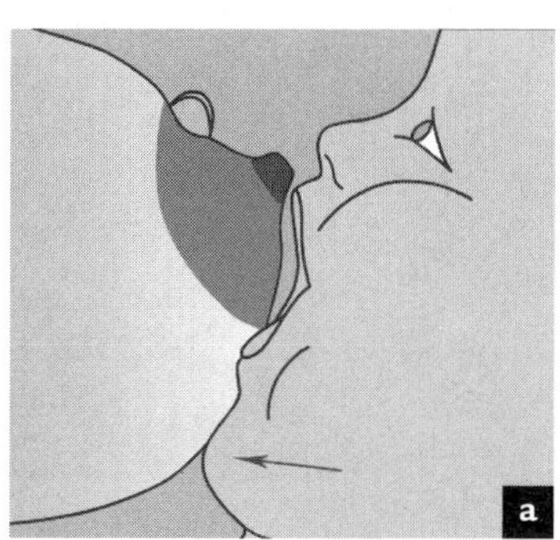

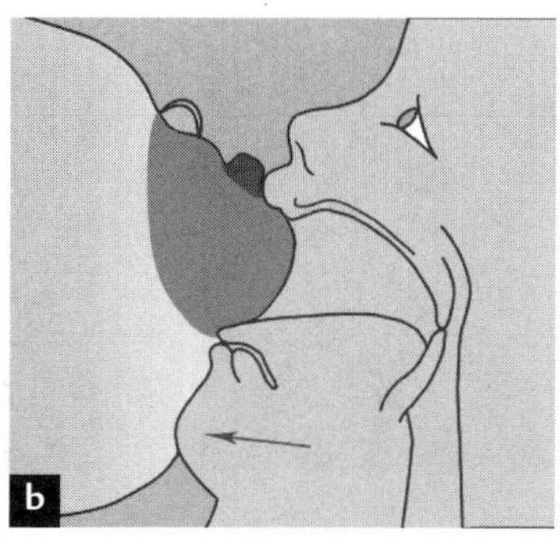

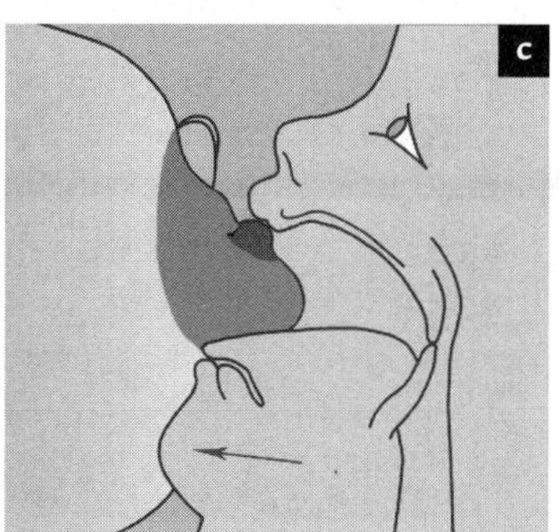

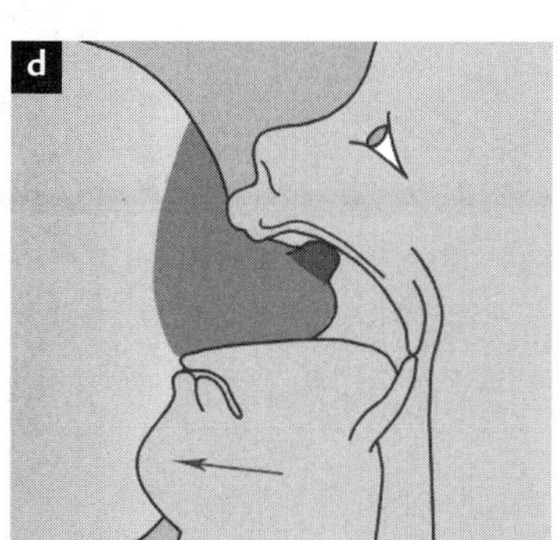

Figure 5-17 The nipple is attached; it will follow! Note: Baby moves to breast, not breast to baby.

4. Then, hug your baby's body closer, using the *heel of your hand and wrist* only.
5. Watch your baby's chin and bottom lip sink into your breast.
6. Watch *all* the breast above the bottom lip roll down into your baby's mouth and your nipple brush or fold under the baby's top lip (**Figures 5-18a through 5-18c**).

Coaching: Hitches and Hints

How big a mouthful the baby takes also depends on how wide the baby's mouth is when his lips close on the breast. Wherever the lips touch the breast, *all* the breast and nipple tissue between the lips goes into baby's mouth. If a mother holds her baby too far from the breast or hesitates at baby's crucial moment of readiness, the baby will have begun to close his mouth before his lips reach the breast, and he will take a smaller portion of breast into the mouth. A too-small mouthful is not only likely to be painful, it also may not stimulate the baby to begin sucking. It is worth waiting for that wide mouth. After a few successful experiences, a mother can usually anticipate and recognize the moment when her baby's searching mouth suddenly opens wide and he is ready to attach.

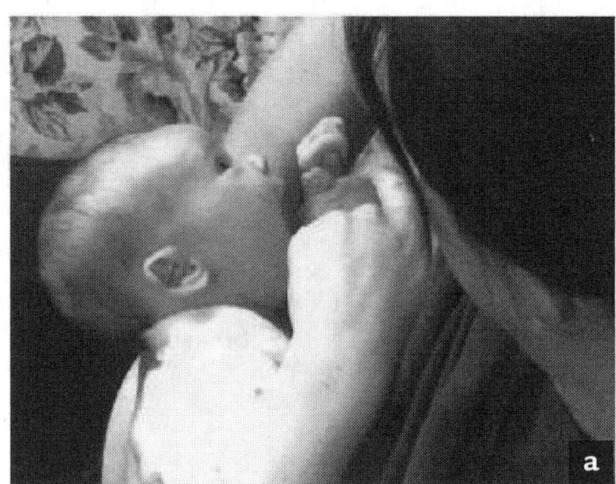
a

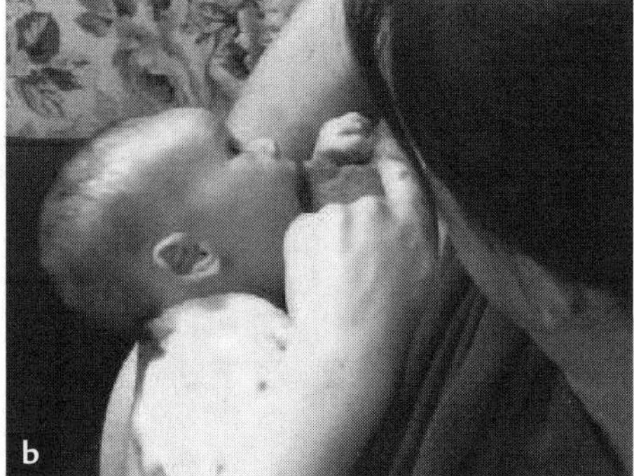
b

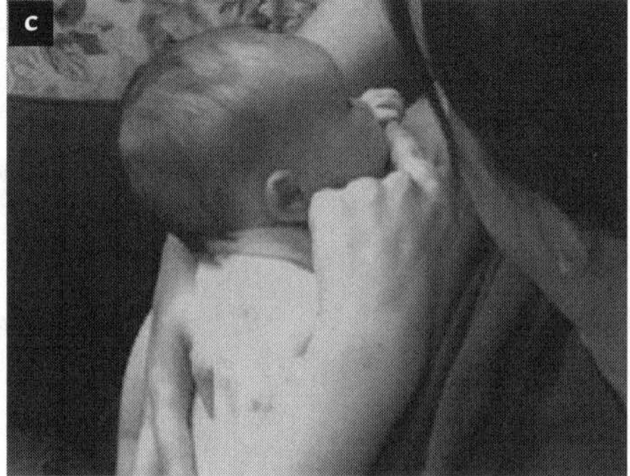
c

Figure 5-18 Wide mouth–nipple at or above top lip.

Shallow attachment appears to be the principal cause of painful, ineffective feeding. Anatomical variations in mother or baby cause attachment difficulties because they interfere with the infant's ability to scoop in a sufficient mouthful of breast. In these circumstances, a mother can help her baby attach more deeply by hugging him extra close at the moment of attachment.

Mothers should avoid moving the breast toward the baby's mouth. You may see a mother pushing her breast toward her cleavage and her baby in the opposite direction, with frustrating results for both. Even when a baby needs help to attach well, any movement of the breast into the mouth must occur *after* the chin and bottom lip anchor firmly on the breast. Much of the finesse of mother-led latching comes from our right brains, but here are a few thoughts that may help:

- Catch the lower lip if needed: Occasionally, it may be helpful not only to shape the sandwich and tilt the nipple, but also to catch the lower lip and jaw of the open mouth with the breast. The idea is *not* to put the breast into the baby's mouth, but to catch the lower lip and jaw of the baby's open mouth with that portion of breast below the nipple, holding the baby's mouth open fractionally longer and wider as he is brought onto the breast.
- Help the baby take a good mouthful of breast: A mother can help her baby to latch deeply by catching a good amount of breast below the nipple and then using her finger or thumb (positioned as previously described) to press the breast into her baby's mouth as she hugs his shoulders closer, bringing his chin, bottom lip, and mouth onto the breast. Remember the sandwich analogy. In this variation, the mother not only lands the lower jaw on the sandwich, she also uses the finger nearest the baby's upper jaw to stuff some extra bread into his mouth! The aim is to fill the baby's mouth with breast to maximize oral sensory input, which is the "least invasive means of applying appropriate orofacial stimuli" for infants with suck problems (Bovey, Noble, & Noble, 1999, p. 26).
- Exaggerate breast shaping: This may be useful for a baby who does not respond normally to the previously described assistance, increasing sensory input by firming and shaping the breast. Instead of using just one finger or thumb to shape the breast, the mother uses one hand to narrow the sandwich, tilting the nipple as previously described and also using her hand to shape the entire breast between her fingers and thumb. One digit presses near the base of the nipple where the baby's upper lip will land, while the rest of her fingers scoop under the breast to create a sandwich shape that runs parallel to the baby's lips. To ensure that ample breast below the nipple is available to the baby, the lower fingers must be far from the nipple—usually well off the areola and perhaps even kept as far away as the breastbone. Her fingers may be very close to the upper lip, but *not* to the lower lip. The mother may find this works best if she shapes her left breast with her left hand, or her right breast with her right hand. Her hand can come from either below the breast, as in **Figure 5-19**, or above the breast.

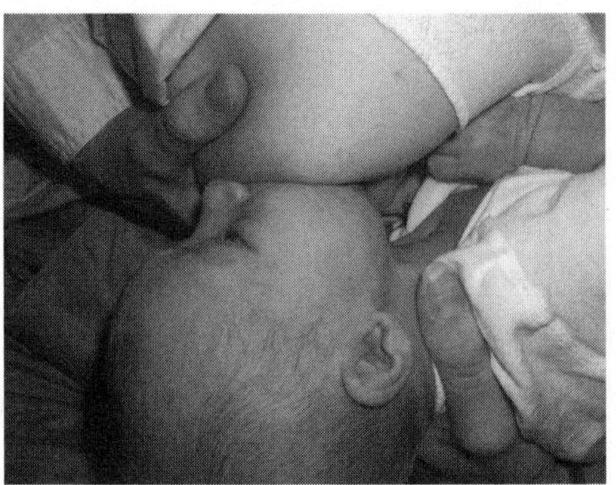

Figure 5-19 Exaggerated breast shaping, hand below the breast.

- Shape the breast rather than supporting it: For most mother–baby pairs, the mother need only shape the breast where it rests naturally, relaxing and removing the shaping hand after the baby begins active sucking. Lifting it from its normal position usually means she must continue to hold it throughout the feed; releasing it will cause it to drop out of the baby's mouth. Some babies do require that the breast be held throughout the feed in order for them to maintain an adequate mouthful, and a long-breasted woman with downward-pointing nipples may need to lift her breast for effective positioning.

Other Holds and Approaches

The new and only rule for helping mothers is that there are no unbreakable rules. Mothers have found it easiest to nurse cross-legged with the baby's bottom dropped into the "hole" in their lap, standing, lying, with baby wrapped around their side or kneeling at their side, or simply putting their nipple straight into the baby's mouth. Here are several common variations.

Side-Lying

A baby who is struggling to breastfeed when his mother is upright may be more willing to attach when she lies on her side on a firm, flat surface. In one side-lying approach (**Figure 5-20a**), the mother makes herself comfortable and balanced on her side. She lifts her lower breast, which may have tucked beneath her somewhat, and sets it back down on the bed so that her nipple is its natural baby's cheek height above the mattress. She rolls the baby onto his side, facing her, with his lower shoulder below her breast, probably with her nipple near his eye. In this position, if the baby rocks his head back, his mouth will usually cover her nipple nicely. As it does so, she may press the *middle* of his back in slightly more to help him finish the latch. The baby's body will usually arch slightly backward, and he will be looking up at his mother's face. Pressing the baby's shoulders toward her may cause his face to burrow into the breast instead of encouraging the instinctive feeding position. Tilting the nipple and shaping the breast may be helpful, but the breast sandwich, if it is used, should run floor to ceiling in order to run parallel to the baby's lips.

Unless the baby latches fairly quickly, the mother may find that he has wriggled up past her nipple. Since a baby cannot move down the bed independently, she can pull him back down for another try. She may need to do this several times; even newborns creep remarkably well! **Figures 5-20b and 5-20c** demonstrate other common side-lying positions.

Figure 5-20 Mother-sped attachment, side-lying.

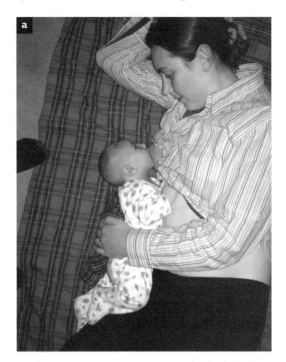

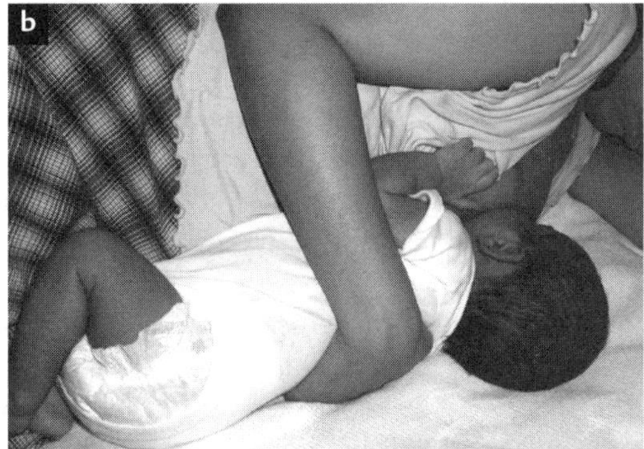

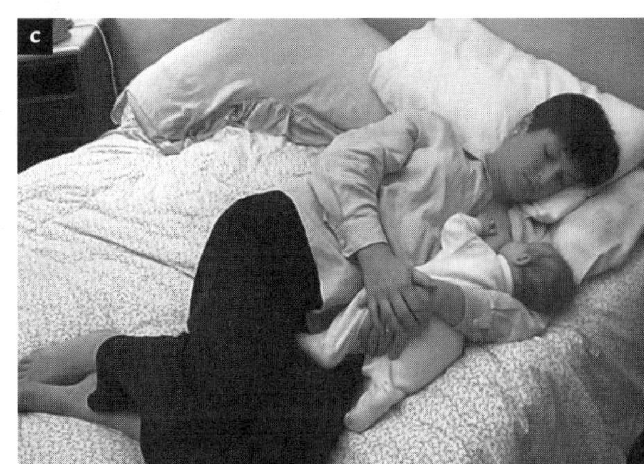

A slightly extended head is simple to achieve by lying down, and it can help a baby cope with a fast flow or receding chin.

The gap that may exist between mother and baby in some side-lying positions can be problematic for some pairs; she can bring his legs and lower torso toward her, which may help. The gap can also be an asset for the infant who has been traumatized at the breast and who prefers some freedom from touch at first.

Some form of side-lying is, of course, what most comfortable breastfeeding pairs will adopt for nighttime nursing, and it is well worth learning.

Long-Breasted Mothers and Mothers with Downward-Pointing Nipples

Some breasts are so long that there is little room for the baby beneath them. The nipple may point down, which means that stabilizing the baby's chest against the mother's body puts the baby in the wrong place.

When a mother's breast is long or large, the baby's stability can come not from her torso but from the breast itself. Remember, babies can feel secure in any position, provided they have firm pressure on their chest and belly and are positionally stable. A long- or large-breasted mother can hold her baby slightly higher than her breast's resting position, so that a gentle portion of the breast's weight rests on the baby's chest. In the cradle hold, with her baby held sunny-side up below her breast, rather than against her torso, the mother's forearm helps to stabilize her breast from the side, the breast and baby become a unit, and the breast is less likely to slip from the baby's mouth.

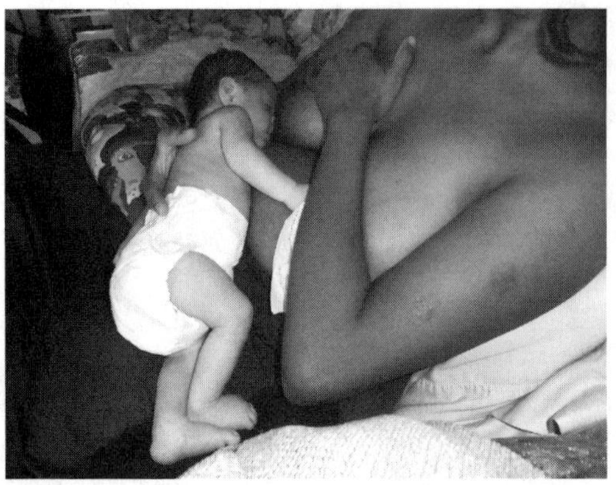

Figure 5-21 Mother slides thoracic skin to roll nipple upward.

A variation of this cradle hold can help the baby with torticollis or other neck or shoulder problems. If the baby's painful side is held against the mother, with his arm across his middle, his body more supine than usual, and the breast lying partially on the baby's chest, the mother's breast, baby's arm, and baby's body can support one another.

If the mother's breast is especially long or if she cannot see her nipple, she can use the palm of one hand on the thoracic skin above her breast, or on the breast itself, to lift and hold the entire breast and angle the nipple slightly more forward (**Figure 5-21**). Others may prefer to lift the breast by holding it in the palms of their hands (left breast, left hand) or by using a scissor hold with nipple and adequate lower-jaw breast tissue protruding between the index and middle fingers (left breast, right hand). Some very long-breasted mothers may spread their legs and drop the baby's bottom into the space created.

Larger Women

A larger mother may need help finding a position in which her baby can approach her breast with a straight and open body, mouth lifted and head tilted back into the instinctive position. Laid-back positions are often effective, perhaps with the baby angled more completely across the mother's body. This can help prevent the baby's nose from becoming buried in breast tissue. A very large woman may sometimes find it easier to sit fairly upright and hold her baby nearly horizontally on the shelf below her breasts as described earlier in this chapter. The cross-cradle hold may not be helpful; it can be difficult for this mother to reach an arm across her body. One mother did well cradling her supine baby's head in her hand, extending that arm straight in front of her and lightly resting her breast on the baby's body. Experimentation can result in surprising and effective approaches (**Figures 5-22 and 5-23**).

Mother-Led Breastfeeding

Prematurity and neurological or physical difficulties are well covered elsewhere in this book; this is simply a reminder that the same fundamentals are important, whether the baby sees to them himself or his mother sees to them for him. When the mother is providing extensive assistance, she will likely be helped by sacral sitting. It's no accident that kangaroo care for premature infants involves having the mother neither vertical nor supine.

The details will vary with the baby's needs, but keeping in mind the steps from **Table 5-1** will help the mother and her assistant make appropriate choices. Sucking *always* requires a baby with some sucking ability. However, the mother can perform the prefeeding steps

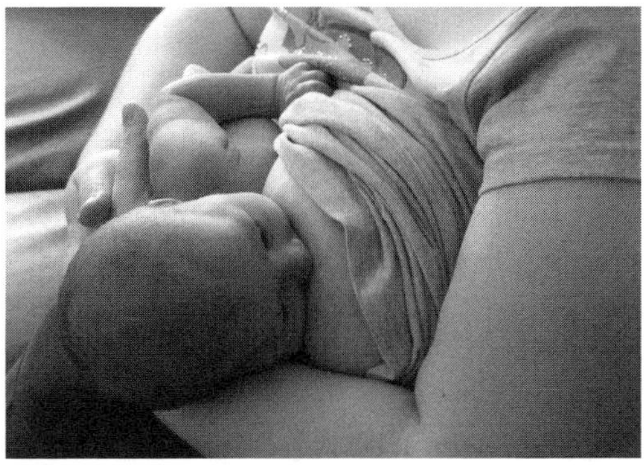

Figure 5-22 Larger mother stabilizes baby against breast, breast against arm.

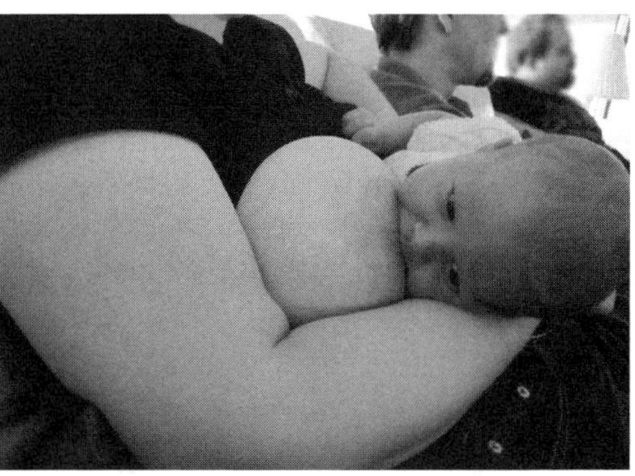

Figure 5-23 Sacral sitting with a larger breast. Note lumbar support and how arm and baby stabilize the breast where it falls.

for even a very low-muscle-tone baby (this is one time when holding a baby's head—respectfully and in appropriate alignment—may be helpful). Specialized approaches for these special situations are what the rest of this book is about.

However a baby feeds, spending all or much of each day in biological nurturing positions and baby wearing (**Figure 5-24**) is one of the fastest, most pleasurable routes toward competent, pleasurable breastfeeding.

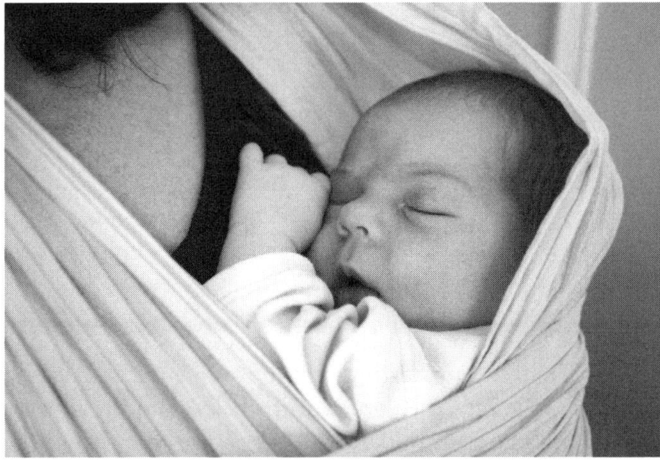

Figure 5-24 Baby-wearing–where babies belong.

Road to Health (Self-Efficacy)

Taking over most of the breastfeeding work for the baby who needs it is very much like your mother propping you up in bed when you were sick, placing a bed tray across your legs, and even spoon feeding you, blotting the dribbles from your chin for you. Sucking in the soup and swallowing it were up to you; your mother took care of everything that made sucking and swallowing possible—encouraging you to eat, your position, and bringing the food to your mouth in a form you could manage. The extra help you're giving your baby right now is almost always—like your mother's help—temporary. It is just part of helping your baby eat appropriately and get healthy.

Choosing an Approach

There is no immutable order to the approaches along the helping continuum. Not every approach makes sense for every mother and baby, and aspects of one approach can certainly be combined with another approach. Some vigorous babies are nonetheless helped by exaggerated breast shaping. A baby who has had numerous bad experiences at the breast might do best moving straight to lying down to give him a completely new experience from the start. If you know that the baby has developed an aversion to the breast, you might want to encourage at least a few days of near-continuous holding, using an alternate feeding method, before going further. If you know that others have tried without success to help a mother and baby, you might move more quickly to an artificial aid—perhaps one described in the next section.

Sometimes an office visit is simply ill timed. The overly hungry baby may need at least part of his meal first, by some familiar means, before he can begin to learn. If the baby isn't hungry at first, you and the mother have some time for discussion and modelling. If he is in a deep sleep, you can use the session to describe and demonstrate techniques she can use at home (see the section on self-efficacy), offer encouragement, and share your confidence in the baby's and her innate abilities. (Remember that lighter sleep states can be an optimal time for bringing a baby to breast in biological nurturing positions!) Above all, stay in touch with the mother and help her find additional sources of encouragement! One mother simply wasn't willing to hear about biological nurturing with her twins during the first two visits; she needed to give up on the old-style rules in her own time. Another reported that there came a day when "my baby just looked different to me," and breastfeeding proceeded uneventfully from that point. We can provide insights and enthusiasm, we can even provide tools like those in the next section, but it is the mother and baby who ultimately make breastfeeding happen.

When Technique Is Not Enough

Jumping through a fiery hoop is an unnatural act for a tiger, but it can learn to do so through a combination of patience, mutual trust, technique . . . and tools. Breastfeeding is an entirely natural act for a baby. When patience, trust, and technique are insufficient to help a normal baby feed at a normal nipple and breast, there are some tools that may be helpful. For a more complete discussion of these and other tools, see Genna (2009).

Dripped Enticement

Dribbling a bit of expressed colostrum or milk on the nipple with an eyedropper or syringe can sometimes encourage a baby to begin licking, tasting, and showing interest. Tucking a dropper, syringe, or periodontal syringe into the corner of the baby's mouth after an unenthusiastic latch, and adding a few drops of milk as the baby sucks, may cause the baby to swallow, draw in a bit more breast, and perhaps begin sucking. If the baby is truly hungry, however, he may need to take in significant calories before he is able to breastfeed effectively.

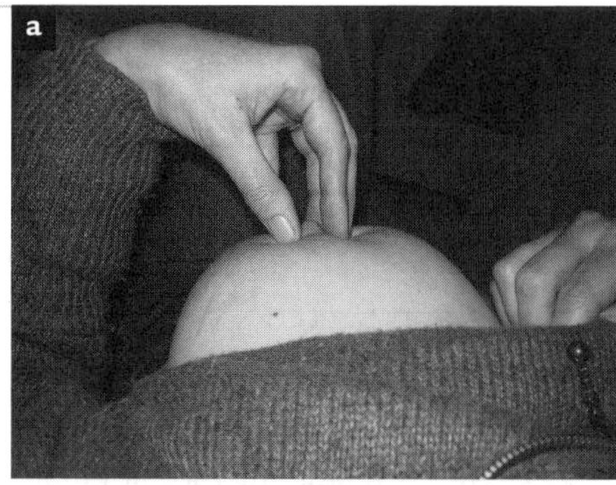

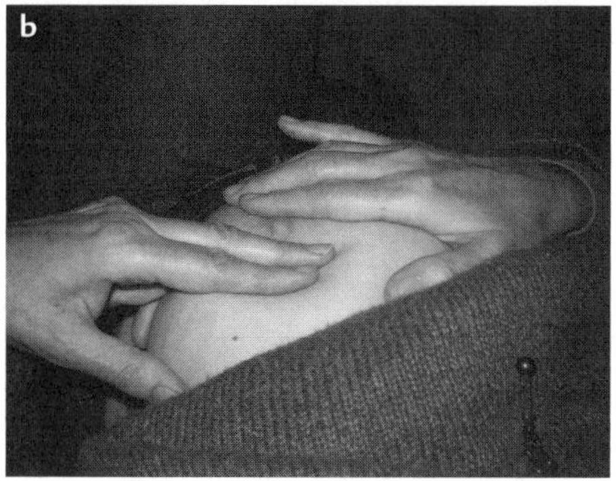

Figure 5-25 Reverse pressure softening.

Reverse Pressure Softening

Initial engorgement can make it difficult for a baby to attach. One of the best tools in this situation is the mother's own fingers. All five fingertips of one hand can be pressed around the base of her nipple for approximately a minute, or about as long as it takes her to hum a lullaby. The pressure moves fluids deeper into the breast, softening and indenting the area that the baby needs for attachment just as a fingertip pressed into any pitting edema creates a soft, temporary dent. The mother can also press with the sides of two or more fingers, perhaps laying an index finger at the nipple base where the baby's upper lip will be and two fingers from the opposite hand where the baby's lower jaw will land, with the fingers running parallel to where the baby's lips will be (Cotterman, 2004) (**Figures 5-25a and 5-25b**).

Suction Device

Necessity is the mother of invention. For a quick, inexpensive aid for babies who were unable to attach to inverted nipples, try a syringe whose diameter is slightly larger than the mother's nipple diameter. Remove the piston and cut off the needle end. Slide the piston into the cut end, creating a small suction device with a smooth open end. The mother places the smooth end over her nipple and draws back the piston until her nipple everts, but not so far that it causes discomfort (**Figure 5-26**). If the syringe fills with milk and loses suction, she pulls the piston out farther. After about a minute, she releases the suction by depressing the piston and offers her breast to the baby before the nipple inverts. Most babies who require this temporary aid learn quickly to attach to their mothers' less-than-prominent nipples without preliminaries (Kesaree, Banapurmath, Banapurmath, & Shamanur, 1993). Commercial suction devices, including Supple Cups, are available that can help evert nipples prenatally, or they can be used between feedings.

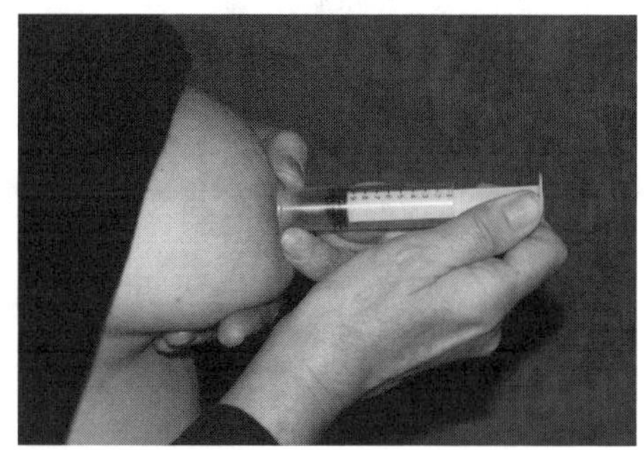

Figure 5-26 Suction device for inverted nipple.

Bottle Feeding as a Prelude to Offering the Breast

A baby may be more receptive to breastfeeding if he has taken at least part of a meal first. If the mother likes, the bottle can be tucked under her arm when she is seated, so that her baby can be held against her as if for breastfeeding, with the bottle teat close to her nipple.

Bait and Switch

The mother holds the baby as if for breastfeeding, but in such a way that she can also offer a bottle. Sitting upright and holding the bottle under her arm is one such position. Upright and holding the baby along her side, with the baby looking up at her, is another. She offers several swallows from the bottle, then quickly removes the bottle and offers her breast. The baby will probably refuse. She immediately offers several more swallows from the bottle, then offers the breast again. After several such back-and-forth offerings, the baby may have gained enough energy and interest to attach to the breast and begin feeding. The shorter the time between removing the bottle and offering the breast, the more likely

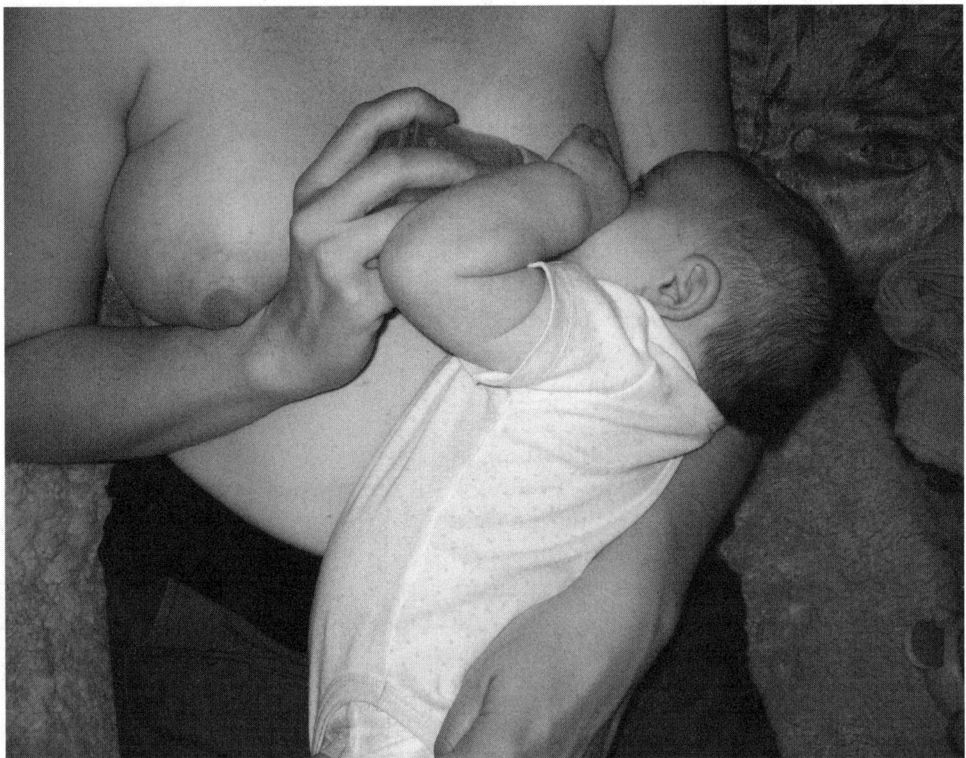

Figure 5-27 Bait and switch.

the baby is to shift his suckling behavior to the breast (**Figure 5-27**). In the end, even if he does not attach to the breast, the baby will have been fed. For a full discussion of paced bottle-feeding technique, see Chapter 11.

Nipple Shield

The human nipple is soft and tends to retreat from a baby if he mouths it before latching. In contrast, a nipple shield stays very assertively *there*, allowing the baby to feel it, play with it, grasp it correctly or incorrectly, even push it away with his tongue. Its unchanging shape can make it a very helpful bridging tool for a baby who is suspicious of the breast, who is accustomed to a bottle teat, or who has decided that there is no reason to try. Premature infants may actually increase their milk intake with the help of a shield; it keeps the mother's nipple from sliding away from a weaker baby with thinner buccal fat pads during the pauses between suckling bursts (Meier et al., 2000).

Modern silicone nipple shields have a stiff nipple section and a very soft rim. They come in several nipple diameters and nipple lengths. While the nipple shield chosen needs to accommodate the mother's nipple comfortably, it must also match the infant's palate length. Wilson-Clay and Hoover (2008, p. 58) suggest selecting the shield "with the shortest available teat and smallest base diameter" given the mother's anatomy. When a baby latches deeply on a well-fitted shield, the thin and flexible rim usually allows him to milk the breast with near-normal efficiency. This level of efficiency was not possible with the old latex shields.

To attach the shield, the mother can grasp the shield's rim between her thumb and fingers, with the nipple section facing away from her. She stretches the base of the teat open as if she is trying to turn the teat inside out, and brings the lower edge of the nipple section onto the breast, beginning well below her own nipple and stretching the shield over the nipple, centering the shield's nipple over her own. This brings a good portion of her breast and nipple into the shield, with slightly more tissue below her nipple, helping to ensure that her baby will take more breast into the mouth with the shield. Because the base of the nipple section has been stretched onto the breast, it grips the breast and is less readily dislodged. The mother brings the baby onto the breast and shield, with his head tilted back and mouth open wide. As the baby's bottom lip and chin sink into the rim of the shield, well below the nipple, his top lip will glide over the upper surface of the shield's nipple section, facilitating a deep and asymmetrical latch. A baby who is able to attach well can take a truly effective mouthful of breast and suckle almost as if the nipple shield does not exist (**Figures 5-28a through 5-28d**).

Some nipple shields have a portion of the rim cut away to remove any barrier between the baby's nose and the mother's skin. They can be difficult to apply to the breast using the method previously described. An alternate approach is for the mother to hold the shield on opposite sides at the outside edge using the thumb and index finger of each hand, with the nipple section facing away from her. With her middle fingers, she gently applies pressure to the tip of the shield's nipple portion until it begins to collapse, pushing until the nipple

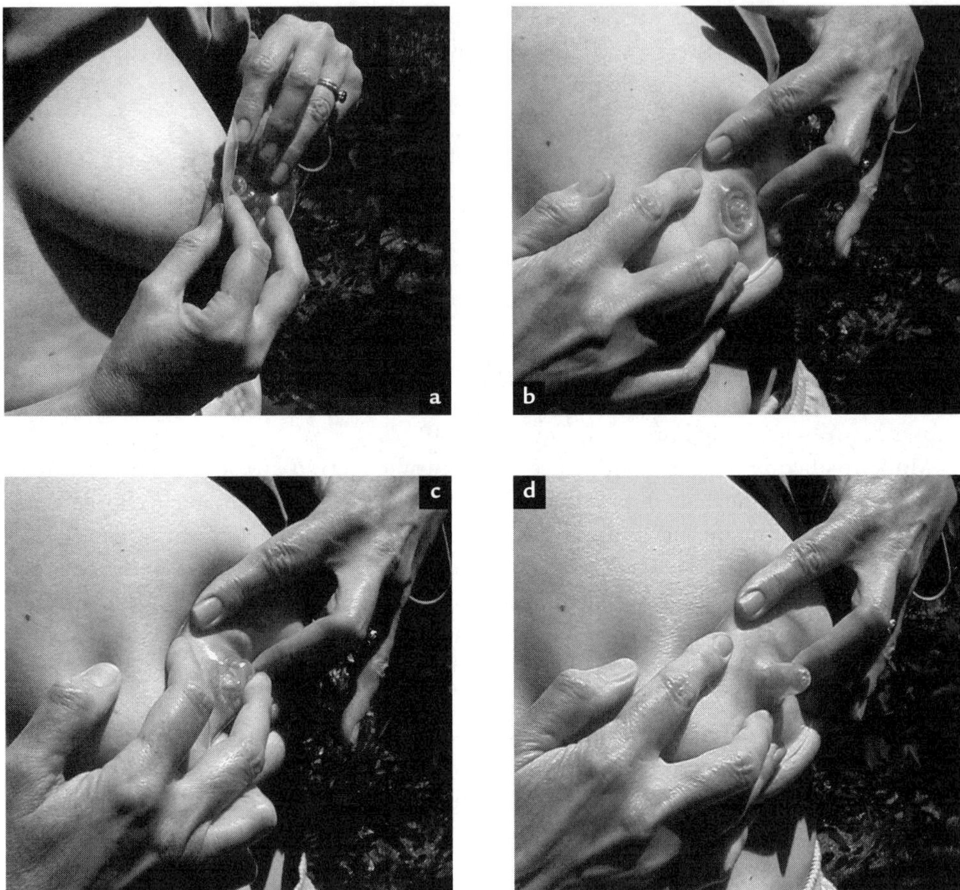

Figure 5-28 Applying a nipple shield.

section is just a little longer than her own nipple. She places the partially inverted shield over her nipple, the rim curling away from her breast. Using the first two fingers from each hand, she slides the backs of her fingernails down the slope of the shield's nipple. When her fingertips touch the bottom of the moat around it and the pads of her fingers touch the outer edge of the moat, she stops sliding her fingernails and uses the pads of her fingers to stretch the moat out onto the areola. Her nipple tip is drawn into the shield as the moat disappears (L. Pohl, personal communication, 2006).

The rim of a shield may curl over the baby's nose while he feeds; however, the nipple section stays in the baby's mouth, and the rim will not interfere with his breathing. If the baby repeatedly dislodges the shield, a piece of tape along the upper edge can help to hold it in place. Moistening the underside may also help.

At times, a baby's inability to breastfeed effectively with a shield simply reflects his inability to breastfeed effectively without it; these mother–baby pairs will need additional support in the form of milk expression and an alternate feeding method. However, nipple shields have helped many babies learn to latch and to associate the breast with food, and they often give the mother of a nonlatching baby a way to enjoy her baby at breast while they learn to breastfeed.

Until a baby using a shield has demonstrated a normal feeding pattern and normal pattern of weight gain, his growth should be followed closely. Babies can use a nipple shield ineffectively, spending long periods of time at breast without significant intake.

Most babies relinquish the shield without difficulty after they gain some competence and confidence; an occasional baby continues to rely on a nipple shield for months or, rarely, for the duration of the breastfeeding relationship. Breastfeeding with a shield is still breastfeeding.

Pillow

Pillows probably cause more breastfeeding problems than they solve. Pillows are usually not helpful if they raise the baby above the natural level of the mother's nipple, create a crevice into which the baby can roll, cause his body to lie across the other breast instead of below it, or prevent the close application of his body to his mother's. Pillows encourage a horizontally positioned baby, rather than the angled-down position of earlier generations. In addition, mothers can become pillow dependent, unable to nurse with the spontaneity and adaptability that easy breastfeeding requires. Although an ordinary pillow can support a mother's arm or back, a specialized breastfeeding pillow is rarely useful. Biological nurturing positions are usually much more useful than pillow-supported positions. However, a firm, flat pillow can allow some distance for a baby who resists close contact. It can serve as a bait-and-switch platform, perhaps even with a nipple shield in place so the baby can approach the breast with only the lightest maternal touch, allowing him to explore the shield at will. Pillows for nursing twins together were considered all but essential until our rediscovery of laid-back positions; the mother of twins who leans back comfortably may find that she can simply cradle a baby in a near-longitudinal lie on each side, resting a baby's cheek on each breast. A one-sided wriggle can move one baby's cheek against her breast, bringing the nipple toward his mouth as he turns to grasp it; a wriggle on her other side repeats the process for the second twin.

Supplemental Feeding Device

Normally used to supplement a baby who can attach to the breast, a supplemental feeding device can occasionally help a baby who is having difficulty attaching to a very flat-nippled breast by providing a focal point for his efforts. Held or taped so the tubing runs along the underside of the breast (on top of the baby's tongue when suckling) and extends slightly beyond the nipple tip, the added stimulus can make a nearly featureless breast less confusing.

Conclusion

When any fluid act is broken into discrete components—when a right-brained, body-sense activity like dancing, tennis, walking, bicycling, or breastfeeding is taught or performed in left-brained steps—fluidity disappears and instinct bows to instruction. But many of the lessons we have learned from our decades of disruptive, left-brained breastfeeding analysis can help certain mothers and babies. If we can facilitate smooth, instinctive, right-brained breastfeeding with little more than a nudge or suggestion, most of the time we can drop into the background of an interaction in which we do not rightly belong. When aids *are* used with a normal mother and baby, be sure that they will help to move the mother and infant toward a normal relationship, ideally with breastfeeding as the cornerstone.

Learning to breastfeed can take time. Simply encouraging the mother to enjoy ample, preferably gravity-as-friend, time with her baby and to follow her baby's lead are often the most important suggestions of all. With time, with repeated positive experiences, and with a mother and (if necessary) a helper who respect and work with the baby's innate abilities, the great majority of normal babies will eventually begin to feed normally.

Helping a mother and baby breastfeed requires more than an understanding of positioning, tools, and techniques. It requires an understanding of one's own limitations and of the mother's and baby's limits today and in the future. It requires access to other helping resources, including mother-support groups. And it requires full confidence in the basic breastfeeding process. This is, after all, how all mammal babies eat.

It is easy to exhaust a mother and baby with attempts and experiments, so that breastfeeding fails before it begins. Be ready to find more experienced help *before* the mother's emotional wells run dry. The goal is not to have the baby breastfeed today, or to be the one who made it work, but to help ensure that mother and baby will be a happy breastfeeding pair in the future. Is there someone else who might help her more efficiently? Then refer the mother, go with her, and add to your skills by observing.

The future may see better and simpler bridging tools that help a baby make the transition from bottle to shield, or shield to breast. But interventions can harm as easily as they can heal, and far too many mothers today find themselves pumping for months simply because they were not encouraged to attend local mother-support groups or were not told about the simplicity of lying back with their babies. Start with the basics; they will take you far.

In addition to improving your tool kit and confidence with the ideas in this book, be sure to take a little time to support the mother-to-mother groups and birth activists in your area. We will truly be doing our job when we're able to help the majority of mothers and babies *avoid* breastfeeding problems, rather than helping to solve them.

References

Bandura, A. (1977). Self-efficacy: Toward a unifying theory of behavioural change. *Psychology Review, 84*(2), 191–215.

Bandura, A. (1994). Self-efficacy. In V. S. Ramachandran (Ed.), *Encyclopedia of human behavior* (Vol. 4). New York, NY: Academic Press.

Blyth, R., Creedy, D., Dennis, C.-L., Moyle, W., Pratt, J., & De Vries, S. (2002). Effect of maternal confidence on breastfeeding duration: An application of breastfeeding self-efficacy theory. *Birth, 29*, 278–284.

Bovey A. R., Noble R., & Noble, M. (1999). Orofacial exercises for babies with breastfeeding problems. *Breastfeeding Review, 7*(1), 23–28.

Buxton, K. E., Gielen, A. C., Faden, R. R., Brown, C. H., Paige, D. M., & Chwalow, A. J. (1991). Women intending to breastfeed: Predictors of early infant feeding experiences. *American Journal of Preventive Medicine, 7*(2), 101–106.

Colson, S. (2008). *Biological Nurturing: Laid-back breastfeeding* [DVD]. Available from http://www.biologicalnurturing.com

Colson, S. D., Meek, J. H., & Hawdon, J. M. (2008). Optimal positions for the release of primitive neonatal reflexes stimulating breastfeeding. *Early Human Development, 84*(7), 441–449.

Colson, S. (2010). *An introduction to Biological Nurturing.* Amarillo, TX: Hale.

Cotterman, K. J. (2004). Reverse pressure softening: A simple tool to prepare areolae for easier latching during engorgement. *Journal of Human Lactation, 20*(2), 227–223.

Creedy, D., Dennis, C.-L., Blyth, R., Moyle, W., Pratt, J., & De Vries, S. (2003). Psychometric characteristics of the Breastfeeding Self-Efficacy Scale: Data from an Australian sample. *Research in Nursing and Health, 26*, 143–152.

Dennis, C.-L. (1999). Theoretical underpinnings of breastfeeding confidence: A self-efficacy framework. *Journal of Human Lactation, 15*, 195–201.

Dennis, C.-L. (2006). Identifying predictors of breastfeeding self-efficacy in the immediate postpartum period. *Research in Nursing & Health, 29*, 256–268.

Dennis, C.-L. (2010). Mothering transitions research. Retrieved from http://www.cindyleedennis.ca/research/1-breastfeeding/specific-publications

Doidge, N. (2010). *The brain that changes itself.* New York, NY: Penguin.

Dunn, S., Davies, B., McCleary, L., Edwards, N., & Gaboury, I. (2006). The Relationship between Vulnerability Factors and Breastfeeding Outcome. *JOGNN, 35(1), 87-96.*

Genna, C. W. (2009). *Selecting and using breastfeeding tools.* Amarillo, TX: Hale.

Glover, R. (2004). Lessons from innate feeding abilities transform breastfeeding outcomes. *ILCA Conference Syllabus*, Scottsdale, AZ. 87-94.

Glover, R. (2005). *Follow me mum* [DVD]. Available from http://rebeccaglover.com.au/video.html

Kashiwagi, H., & Shirataki, S. (1995). Development in mother–infant en face interaction of high-risk newborn infants: A longitudinal follow-up from 0 to 7 months. *Early Human Development, 43*(3), 245–270.

Kesaree, N., Banapurmath, C. R., Banapurmath, S., & Shamanur, K. (1993). Treatment of inverted nipples using a disposable syringe. *Journal of Human Lactation, 9*(1), 27–29.

Kingston, D., Dennis, C.-L., & Sword, W. (2007). Exploring breastfeeding self-efficacy. *Journal of Perinatal and Neonatal Nursing, 21*(3), 207–215

Meier, P. P., Brown, L. P., Hust, N. M., Spatz, D. L., Engstrom, J. L., Borucki, L. C., & Krouse, A. M. (2000). Nipple shields for preterm infants: Effects on milk transfer and duration of breastfeeding. *Journal of Human Lactation, 16*(2), 106–114.

Morris, E. S., & Klein, M. D. (1987). *Pre-feeding skills.* San Antonio, TX: Therapy Skills Builders.

Noel-Weiss, J., Bassett, V., & Cragg, B. (2006). Developing a prenatal breastfeeding workshop to support maternal breastfeeding self-efficacy. *Journal of Obstetric, Gynecologic, and Neonatal Nursing, 35*(3), 349–357.

Noel-Weiss, J., Ruppe, A., Craig, B., Bassett, V., & Woodend, K. A. (2006). Randomized controlled trial to determine effects of prenatal breastfeeding workshop on maternal breastfeeding self-efficacy and breastfeeding duration. *Journal of Obstetric, Gynecologic, and Neonatal Nursing, 35*(5), 616–624.

O'Campo, P., Faden, R. R., Gielen, A. C., & Wang, M. C. (1992). Prenatal factors associated with breastfeeding duration: Recommendations for prenatal interventions. *Birth, 19*(4), 195–201.

Pajares, F. (2002). Overview of social cognitive theory and of self-efficacy. Retrieved from http://www.emory.edu/EDUCATION/mfp/eff.html

Papinczak, T. A., & Turner, C. T. (2000). An analysis of personal and social factors influencing initiation and duration of breastfeeding in a large Queensland maternity hospital. *Breastfeeding Review, 8*, 25–33.

Smillie, C. M. (2007). *Baby-led breastfeeding: The mother–baby dance* [DVD]. Available from http://www.geddesproduction.com

Stajkovic, A. D., & Luthans, F. (1998). Self-efficacy and work-related performances: A meta-analysis. *Psychological Bulletin, 124*, 240–261.

Teicher, M. H., Andersen, S. L., Polcari, A., Anderson, C. M., & Navalta, C. P. (2002). Developmental neurobiology of childhood stress and trauma. *Psychiatric Clinics of North America, 25*, 397–426.

Wilson-Clay, B., & Hoover, K. (2008). *The breastfeeding atlas* (4th ed.). Manchaca, TX: Lactnews Press.

Wolf, L. S., & Glass, R. P. (1992). *Feeding and swallowing disorders in infancy: Assessment and management.* San Antonio, TX: Therapy Skills Builders.

Woolridge, M. W. (1986). The "anatomy" of infant sucking and aetiology of sore nipples. *Midwifery, 2*, 164–176.

World Health Organization & UNICEF. (1989). *Protecting, promoting, and supporting breastfeeding: The special role of maternity services. A joint WHO/UNICEF statement.* Geneva, Switzerland: Author.

CHAPTER 6

The Goldilocks Problem: Milk Flow That Is Not Too Fast, Not Too Slow, but *Just* Right

Or, Why Milk Flow Matters and What to Do About It

Lynn S. Wolf and Robin P. Glass

Introduction

Successful breastfeeding is one of the first achievements of the newborn infant. Immediately after birth the baby is able to root, grasp the breast, and begin to suckle. The ease with which this generally occurs leads many to think of newborn feeding as a simple skill. Infant feeding, however, is a very complex activity that requires exquisite coordination of three foundation processes: sucking, swallowing, and breathing. The coordination of these processes, and thus the success of the baby's feeding, is easily influenced by the flow rate of the liquid the baby is ingesting. A high flow rate can lead to significant incoordination, aspiration, and/or feeding refusal. A slow flow rate might help a baby with respiratory illness return to feeding, but for another baby it may lead to poor weight gain. This chapter will provide an overview of sucking, swallowing, and breathing; their coordination; and how flow rate impacts the success or difficulty of breastfeeding. The assessment of flow rate during breastfeeding will be discussed, along with management of feeding problems related to flow rate.

Foundations of Infant Feeding: A Triad of Skills

Thoroughly understanding the skills that form the foundation for infant feeding provides the framework to identify feeding problems. This triad of skills includes sucking, swallowing, and breathing. It is important to have a working knowledge of each skill and an appreciation of their coordination during infant feeding.

Sucking

During breastfeeding, the infant's sucking leads to latch at the breast and milk transfer. As described throughout this book, successful latch is necessary for successful breastfeeding. After latching, ongoing sucking is key to establishing the flow rate and determining how sucking, swallowing, and breathing are coordinated. Infant sucking is organized into bursts of sucks interspersed with pauses (**Figure 6-1**). At the beginning of a feeding, the bursts are long with infrequent and short pauses. Over the course of the feeding, the sucking bursts gradually become shorter, and pauses are longer, until at the end of the feeding the young baby is sucking occasionally with long pauses between sucks (Chetwynd, Diggle, Drewett, & Young, 1998; Mathew, Clark, Pronske, Luna-Solarzano, & Peterson, 1985). If the infant is fed on both breasts (paired feeding), this pattern is typically repeated on each breast, though the duration of active sucking and milk intake is typically less on the second breast (Drewett & Woolridge, 1979, 1981). The flow rate during sucking bursts will vary depending on the availability of milk in the breast, the competence and strength of the baby's suck, and the quality of the latch.

During nutritive sucking bursts (when there is active fluid flow), infants suck at a rate of approximately one suck per second. This is in contrast to nonnutritive sucking (such as on a finger or pacifier), when the baby sucks more rapidly at about two sucks per second (Wolff, 1968). Fluid flow is the reason for this difference. During nutritive sucking, the baby's sucking rate is slower to accommodate swallowing.

The strength of the suck is also a factor influencing flow rate. Sucking strength is developed as the baby creates two types of pressure: positive pressure (or compression) and negative pressure (or suction). A healthy term baby has some control over the type and amount of pressure that is generated (Sameroff, 1968). At the breast, the interaction of pressure components is complex. Suction is necessary for the baby to latch to the breast, to draw the breast deeply into the mouth, and to maintain latch appropriately. If the baby does not create adequate suction, the baby will chomp at the breast and the latch will not be effective. If latched appropriately, the baby will suckle with both compression and suction pressure. We know that milk can be released from the breast using suction alone (as occurs when using a breast pump) or by compression alone (as with manual expression), and we now understand how milk release relates to these pressure components during breastfeeding. Geddes and colleagues (Geddes, Kent, Mitoulas, & Hartmann, 2008; Ramsay & Hartmann, 2005) performed ultrasound studies, done with intraoral pressure monitoring, to demonstrate that milk flows from the breast into the baby's mouth at peak negative pressure, or during the point of strongest suction, indicating that suction plays a major role in milk removal from the breast. Although milk may not flow during compression, or typically be expressed into the baby's mouth during breastfeeding, the sensory components of this pressure to the breast and nipple may play a role in hormonal regulation of the milk ejection

NUTRITIVE SUCKING (NS)

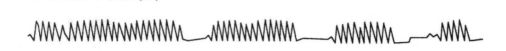

Figure 6-1 Nutritive sucking burst pause pattern.

reflex. It appears likely that each baby develops a unique balance of sucking pressures, over time, determining the relative amount of compression versus suction to use with his or her own mother to create optimal milk flow. It is also likely that the mother's breast learns to respond to the particular characteristics of a baby's sucking pattern, modifying the milk release pattern over time. Thus, milk flow at the breast is related to both mother and baby factors. Developing synchrony between mother and baby to establish functional milk flow is often one of the challenges of early breastfeeding. If abnormal oral structures or movements, or maternal factors, interfere with this process, the baby may have trouble latching or appear to be latched yet not create adequate milk flow.

Sucking movements are seen in utero starting at 14–16 weeks, and they progressively mature in terms of pressure components and coordination. Thus sucking is immature in premature infants, especially those babies born at less than 36 weeks gestation. Lau and colleagues (Lau, Alagugurusamy, Schanler, Smith, & Shulman, 2000) have used pressure monitoring during early bottle feeding to demonstrate that in premature infants compression develops first, though it initially lacks organization into clear sucking bursts. This compressive force begins to form rhythmic bursts around 34 weeks gestation. Suction begins to emerge at this point but is not coordinated with compression until 36–38 weeks gestation. Additionally, premature infants feeding on a bottle show an immature pattern of bursts and pauses, with shorter bursts, longer pauses, and less rhythmicity (**Figure 6-2**). Each of these factors impacts the rate of milk flow the baby is able to create, with more mature infants showing sucking patterns that are more effective in creating milk flow. The developmental progression of these skills has important implications for a premature infant who is trying to latch and maintain latch during breastfeeding. Although maturation of feeding skills usually follows a typical sequence, each infant will mature at his or her own rate.

Swallowing

Swallowing is a complex task involving precise timing and coordination of the many muscles within the mouth, pharynx, larynx, and esophagus and is controlled by the activity of cranial nerves. A swallow occurs when enough milk is present in the mouth to stimulate the numerous sensory receptors in the posterior oral cavity. The swallow carries milk through the pharynx into the esophagus and stomach while protecting the airway. In young infants, once mother's milk supply has been established, one nutritive suck usually produces a quantity of milk (bolus) that fills the oral cavity and initiates a swallow. This creates a suck to swallow ratio of 1:1 (Bu'Lock, Woolridge, & Baum, 1990; Weber, Woolridge, & Baum, 1986). If the flow rate is very low, more sucks will be needed to fill the oral cavity and trigger a swallow. The suck to swallow ratio might be three or more sucks to one swallow. Older infants have larger oral cavities, so two or three normal volume sucks may be taken before a swallow is required. Fluid flow is the key to determining the ratio of sucks to swallows (Mathew & Bhatia, 1989).

An important function of the swallowing process is airway protection. During initiation of swallow, the soft palate elevates to close the nasal passages, and fluid flows into

Stage	Sample Tracings	Suction/Expression Amplitude Range of Tracings (mm Hg)	Description
1A and 1B	Suction	Absent	No suction
	Expression	+0.5 to +1.0	Arrhythmic expression
	Time (sec)		and
	Suction	−2.5 to −12.5	arrhythmic alteration of suction/expression
	Expression	+0.5 to +1.0	
2A and 2B	Suction	Absent	No suction
	Expression	+0.2 to +0.4	Arrhythmic expression
	Time (sec)		and
	Suction	−7.5 to −15.0	arrhythmic alteration of suction/expression
	Expression	±0.2	Presence of sucking bursts
3A and 3B	Suction	Absent	No suction
	Expression	+0.8 to +1.0	Rhythmic expression and rhythmic suction/expression: · Suction amplitude increases · Wide amplitude range · Prolonged sucking bursts
	Time (sec)		
	Suction	−15 to −75	
	Expression	+0.5 to +0.7	
4	Suction	−50 to −75	Rhythmic suction/expression: · Suction well defined · Decreased amplitude range
	Time (sec)		
	Expression	+0.5 to +0.7	
5	Suction	−110 to −160	Rhythmic/well defined suction/expression: · Suction amplitude increased · Sucking pattern similar to that of full-term infant
	Time (sec)		
	Expression	+0.6 to +0.75	

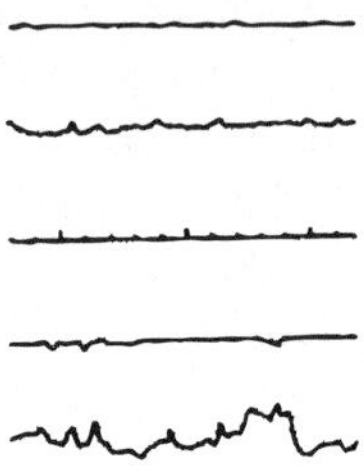

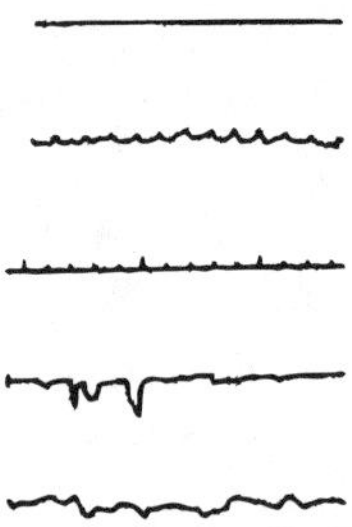

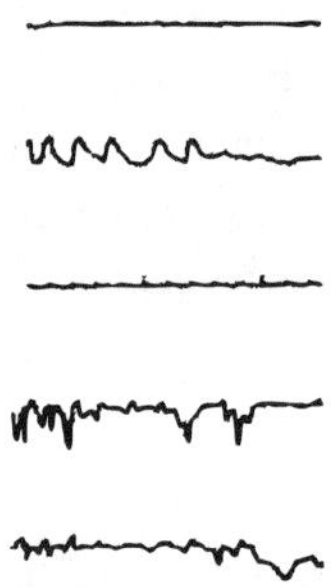

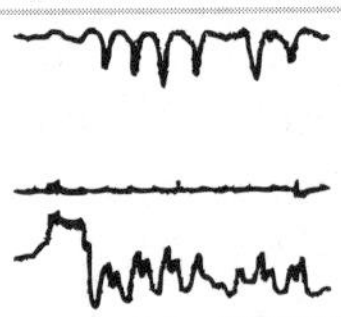

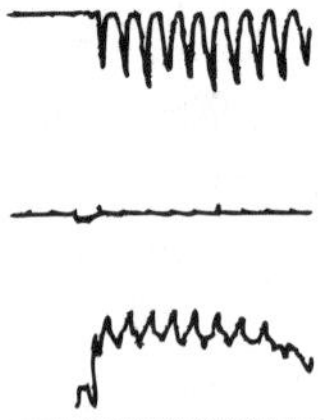

Figure 6-2 Maturation of expression and suction in premature infants.

the pharynx by movement of the tongue. To protect the airway, the larynx then elevates, the epiglottis moves downward to cover the laryngeal opening tightly, and the vocal cords adduct (pull together). Next, the upper esophageal sphincter relaxes, and the bolus moves into the esophagus. Finally, the structures return to their resting positions—the soft palate sits on the base of the tongue with the nasal passages open, the epiglottis has uncovered the larynx, and the upper esophageal sphincter is closed. All of this occurs in about 0.1 seconds (Tuchman, 1993).

If the airway is not fully protected during swallowing, milk can be aspirated into the lungs. This can happen before, during, or after the swallow. If timing of the initiation of swallow is delayed, milk moves into the pharynx before the airway is protected and can then enter the airway *before* the swallow has been initiated. When the swallow sequence has been initiated, if the airway is not fully sealed, fluid can be aspirated *during* the swallow. If a safe swallow occurs but food is not fully cleared from the pharynx, it can be aspirated into the airway during breathing, leading to aspiration *after* the swallow (Wolf & Glass, 1992). The amount of material aspirated can vary from occasional microaspiration to consistent frank aspiration. Some infants may cough or choke with aspiration; however, many do not. An immature infant may stop breathing and become apneic to prevent more food from coming into the lungs (Mortola & Fischer, 1988). In infants of all ages, aspiration can also be silent, with no apparent external response or evidence.

The flow rate has an important relationship to swallowing function. If the flow is very low, multiple sucks may occur before a swallow is necessary. This slower rate of swallowing allows the baby more time to organize the initiation of each swallow. If the bolus is very large or moving at a very fast speed (high flow), timing of the initiation of swallow may be compromised. This can lead to inadequate protection of the airway as the bolus passes through the pharynx and can result in aspiration.

Breathing

Breathing is a critical process for the success of infant feeding and has a strong relationship to flow rate. For the baby, feeding is work, not unlike exercise for adults. This requires adaptability of the respiratory system. During sucking and swallowing, opportunities to breathe are reduced, so the baby must have respiratory reserve to compensate for these ventilatory reductions. The baby needs to be able to adjust the rate and depth of breathing in order to integrate breathing into the sucking-swallowing sequence. During nutritive sucking bursts, breaths are short and less frequent. During pauses, they may be more rapid and deeper (**Figure 6-3**).

Medical conditions that impact breathing affect the baby's respiratory adaptability (**Table 6-1**). Feeding problems are frequently associated with these conditions, and it is often the respiratory portion of the feeding process that underlies the problem. Flow rate plays a significant role in determining how much time the baby has available to breathe during feeding. In general, the higher the flow rate, the less time available for breathing, so the greater the respiratory challenges for the baby (Wolf & Glass, 1992). Altering the flow rate can sometimes improve feeding in babies with respiratory compromise.

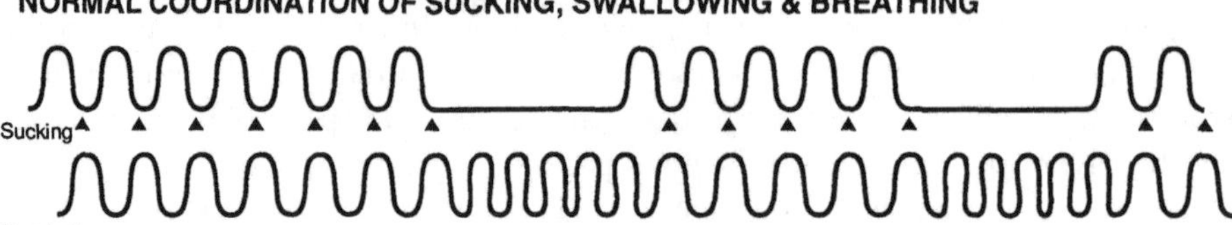

Figure 6-3 Breathing coordinated with sucking and swallowing.

Coordination of Sucking, Swallowing, and Breathing

In infants, as in adults, breathing ceases during swallowing. The pharynx is the centerpiece of this activity, serving as a conduit to move air from the nose and mouth to the lungs and to move food from the mouth to the stomach (**Figure 6-4**). At rest the structures are aligned for breathing, and alterations are made during swallow. It is this dual role that creates the need for coordination of sucking, swallowing, and breathing, and it leads to many of the challenges of infant feeding. If air moves into the stomach, the baby may be gassy. More significantly, if milk moves into the lungs, aspiration occurs, which can lead to a variety of secondary symptoms such as respiratory illness or feeding refusal.

Multiple studies confirm that during infant feeding, breathing stops during each swallow. This presents a unique challenge for the infant who swallows after each suck and must rapidly switch between swallowing and breathing. Selley and associates (Selley, Ellis, Flack, & Brooks, 1990) have depicted this clearly, showing exquisite rhythmic coordination of these processes for the mature newborn. While feeding, the baby sucks, stops breathing to swallow, then starts breathing again. This cycle repeats approximately once each second during the sucking burst. The need to frequently stop breathing causes the infant

Table 6-1 Medical Conditions Affecting Respiratory Function

Central Nervous System	Upper Airway	Lower Airway	Lung Parenchyma	Thoracic
Central apnea Periodic breathing Tumors Hypoxic ischemic encephalopathy (HIE)	Micrognathia Choanal atresia Tracheo-laryngo-malacia Paralyzed vocal cords Hemangiomas	Respiratory distress syndrome Respiratory syncytial virus (RSV) Meconium aspiration Primary alveolar collapse	Collapsed lung Pulmonary hemorrhage Pulmonary hypertension	Diaphragmatic hernia Paralyzed diaphragm Rib anomalies Cardiac anomalies

to draw on respiratory reserves during sucking bursts. During a sucking pause, breaths are rapid and deep, allowing some catch up in breathing (**Figure 6-3**). Like other aspects of feeding, the coordination of sucking, swallowing, and breathing shows a maturational sequence. Although term infants can have incoordination of sucking, swallowing, and breathing, it is more common in premature babies. Flow rate can have a significant affect on this process, with premature infants particularly vulnerable; this will be discussed in detail in the following section.

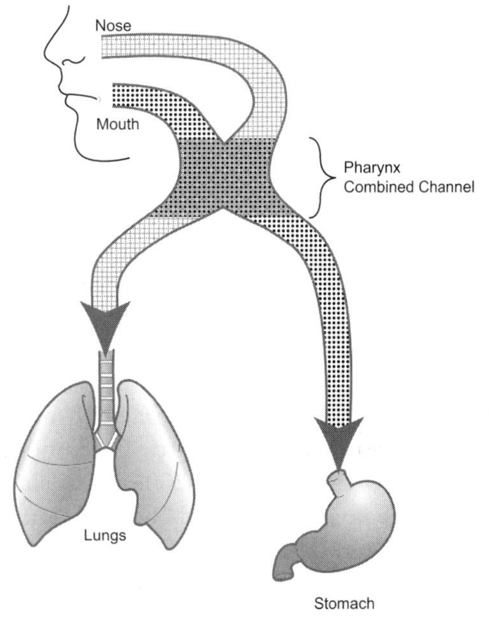

Figure 6-4 Dual role of the pharynx.

The Relationship Between Flow Rate and Coordination of Sucking, Swallowing, and Breathing

In addition to the sequential organization of sucking, swallowing, and breathing during infant feeding, there is also an interrelationship among these components. Each can affect the others and thus further impact the baby's feeding performance. Flow plays an important role in these relationships. High flow, whether it is actually high or just perceived by the baby as high, can upset the delicate balance of sucking, swallowing, and breathing coordination.

Flow and the Relationship Between Swallowing and Breathing

Whether at the breast or simply managing saliva, every time the baby swallows, breathing must pause momentarily. The higher the swallowing rate, the more often breathing will be interrupted. During a vigorous nutritive sucking burst, the young baby swallows after each suck, thus pausing breathing enough to lower the respiratory rate, tidal volume (size of each breath), and minute ventilation (amount of air inhaled per minute). This lowers the amount of available oxygen and leads to a slight, but measurable, decrease in oxygen saturation, even if it remains in the normal range (Mathew et al., 1985). The longer the nutritive sucking burst lasts, the greater the reductions in ventilation. Many babies with an elevated respiratory rate are most comfortable with lower flow, so they need to swallow less often and thus have more time for breathing.

High flow leads to a higher swallowing rate and even less time for breathing. In some cases when the flow is too high for the baby, sucking and swallowing will continue, but breathing will stop. This results in feeding-induced apnea, which is characterized by a vigorous and rhythmic sucking burst, with swallows to clear the food but no breathing interspersed with suck and swallow. These apneic pauses, of even 2–3 seconds, can lead to falling oxygen saturations, bradycardia, coughing or choking, and/or lethargy (Gewolb, Vice, Schwietzer-Kenny, Taciak, & Bosma, 2001). This pattern is more prevalent in premature infants but can be seen occasionally in term infants (Hanlon et al., 1997).

In other cases, high flow can affect the integrity of the swallow. If the baby is swallowing rapidly there may not be time to adequately protect the airway before the bolus moves through the pharynx. This can lead to aspiration. Typically, each swallow will be followed by exhalation, possibly affording the baby some airway protection (Gewolb & Vice, 2006). High flow may affect timing of the swallow–breathe relationship such that the baby is more likely to inhale after swallowing.

Flow at the breast is variable throughout the feeding. When the baby first latches to the breast there is very little flow, until the mother's milk ejection reflex (MER) is initiated (Mizuno & Ueda, 2006). This slow ramping up of milk flow may allow the baby to prepare for the rapid coordination of swallowing and breathing required with full milk flow. During the MER, the flow will be steady and then taper as the MER subsides. The length and volume of the MER will vary for each mother, but this periodic natural reduction in flow during breastfeeding allows the baby the opportunity to continue sucking with less frequent swallowing, thus having more time to breathe until the next MER is stimulated. This variability in flow pattern during breastfeeding provides more opportunity for breathing than during bottle feeding, unless the mother's flow is excessive. Similarly, for the neonate, the small volumes of colostrum available in the first few days of life will not overpower the baby's swallow–breathe abilities as they begin the adjustment to extrauterine life. Newborns who are given bottles immediately are known to cough and choke frequently because they are not fully prepared for the task of coordinating swallow and breathe in this high flow situation (Bamford, Taciak, & Gewolb, 1992).

Flow and the Relationship Between Sucking and Breathing

Milk flow is typically high during sucking bursts and when sucking is strong. Milk flow is typically low or absent when sucking strength is poor and during sucking pauses. When there is little or no flow, the baby does not need to swallow, allowing for an increase in respiratory rate, tidal volume, and minute ventilation. During times of low flow or during a sucking pause, an actively feeding baby may actually seem to pant as he or she catches up on breathing.

If high flow overwhelms breathing, the baby may alter the sucking pattern. One strategy is to use to a pattern of short sucking bursts. This allows more pause time, where catchup breathing can occur. If mother's milk is flowing very rapidly, moving to short sucking bursts may not be possible, and the baby may use prolonged compression to try to stop the flow and allow breathing. Another strategy is that the baby simply pulls away from the breast in order to stop sucking and move to a breathing pause.

In some cases, babies may refuse to suck if they perceive the breathing adjustments as too stressful. Other babies learn to suck with very little pressure as a way to reduce the flow rate. These same babies may love nonnutritive sucking on a finger or a pacifier because it gives them the comfort of sucking without the stress of handling flow and making breathing adjustments. Although we may be tempted to look for ways to increase flow for these inefficient feeders, if respiratory difficulties underlie their sucking patterns, this strategy can make the situation worse (Wolf & Glass, 1992).

Flow and the Relationship Between Sucking and Swallowing

Sucking sets up the initiation and timing of swallowing, so it has a very direct impact on swallowing performance. If the baby is sucking at a fast rate and each bolus requires a swallow, the swallowing rate will be high. During fast flow, the swallowing structures need to move and recover quickly, with little time for breathing or for timing errors. Regardless of the sucking rate, milk flow can be high and bolus size can be large if the baby's sucking is strong or mother's milk flow is very abundant. This may lead to premature spillage of the bolus into the pharynx, poor timing of the swallow, and possibly aspiration.

When a baby has a primary swallowing dysfunction, he or she may be reluctant to create any fluid flow in an effort to avoid swallowing. The baby may refuse to suck nutritively, though he or she may be eager to suck nonnutritively and/or may show significant stress cues during nutritive sucking (Wolf & Glass, 1992).

Factors to Consider in Assessing Flow Rate

When the flow rate is optimal for a baby, breastfeeding performance and nutrition are supported. The baby can take the amount of food needed in a reasonable amount of time, without distress. When the flow is too fast, the baby can show physiologic compromise and behavioral stress and may become a reluctant feeder or even refuse to feed. If the flow rate is too slow, the baby will spend excessive time and energy feeding and/or have inadequate intake. The appropriate flow rate for any baby is individual and based on that baby's physical skills, temperament, and medical condition. Before the flow is adjusted, the clinician must consider a variety of factors. The questions in each of the following sections can be used to guide the assessment of flow rate and its impact on the infant.

Sucking

Evaluating various characteristics of sucking can help determine the reasons that the flow rate may be too high or too low:

- Is the baby able to create suction? Compression?
- Can the baby alternate between suction and compression?
- What is the strength of the baby's suction?
- How long is the sucking burst?

- What is the rate of nonnutritive and nutritive sucking?
- Is the baby able to latch effectively to the breast?
- Are the baby's sucking mechanics and abilities similar in all situations, or do they vary among breast sucking, nonnutritive sucking, and bottle sucking or other alternate feeding method?
- Could the strength or rate of suck be creating flow that is too high?
- Could the strength of suck or quality of latch be leading to poor milk transfer and low flow?

When milk flow at the breast is low, we must determine whether the underlying issue is poor milk supply or the baby's inability to transfer milk. If milk is present but the baby is not able to obtain it, irregularities in latching and/or sucking are often present. We must then determine whether these are primary problems for the baby or if the latch-suck problems are the baby's attempt to keep the flow low to compensate for another problem.

Swallowing

There is a strong relationship between flow rate and swallowing function. Understanding the signs of swallowing dysfunction helps the clinician evaluate the infant's performance in this area:

- Does the baby have signs or symptoms of swallowing dysfunction?
  - History of pneumonia or frequent respiratory illness
  - Coughing or choking frequently during feeding
  - Apnea during feeding
  - Rattly, wet-sounding breathing during or after feeding
  - Preference for nonnutritive sucking
  - Pulling away at the start of the MER

Although swallowing dysfunction (dysphagia) is not common, it may be seen in former premature infants, babies post heart surgery, those with neurologic or anatomic problems, severe gastroesophageal reflux, and even occasionally in healthy infants (L. A. Newman, Keckley, Petersen, & Hammer, 2001; Sheihk et al., 2001; Suskind et al., 2006). Breastfeeding does not protect a baby from swallowing dysfunction or aspiration. Aspiration of human milk, however, is more likely to be silent and may be less likely to lead to respiratory infections. In the breastfeeding baby, coughing and choking and reluctance to nurse are frequently attributed to overactive MER or hyperlactation. In this situation the baby should be carefully evaluated for swallowing dysfunction, including a trial with controlled flow at a lower rate (partially emptied breast, or bottle if necessary). Babies with a true swallowing dysfunction will usually also have problems in a normal flow situation.

If it appears the baby may have a primary swallowing problem, a more detailed evaluation by an experienced healthcare professional is indicated. This may include clinical evaluation of swallowing and/or a videofluoroscopic swallowing study (also known as a modified barium swallow). This test can assess swallowing function and safety and explore treatment options. Based on the results of this test, interventions that may be considered include providing a controlled, low flow rate or using thickened liquid. These treatments may require feeding away from the breast, and in some cases oral feeding of any kind may not be safe. Human milk can still be supplied, and pacification at the freshly pumped breast may be possible, depending on the severity of the infant's dysphagia. See Chapter 11 for more information.

Breathing

Although it is often overlooked during a feeding assessment, careful evaluation of breathing status during feeding can help to uncover the reason for many infant feeding problems:

- What is the baby's respiratory rate before, during, and after feeding?
- Is the baby showing increased work of breathing?
- Does the baby have stridor?
- How is the baby's energy and endurance?
- How often and how long are the breathing pauses?
- Does the baby have any diagnosis that would affect breathing?

Breathing issues are often overlooked in evaluating feeding problems, but in infants they can be a key component of a feeding problem. It is important to appreciate the baby's baseline respiratory status, and how it changes during feeding, in order to gauge the impact of respiratory issues. If a baby with breathing problems is also having feeding problems, reducing flow is often helpful. Although some babies will modify sucking patterns to reduce flow on their own, others eagerly generate high flow, only to become stressed or overwhelmed by the flow.

Listening to the quality of breathing helps identify the location of the difficulty. The presence of stridorous, high-pitched, noisy respiration suggests some type of airway obstruction (**Table 6-1**), which will make it hard for the baby to breathe adequately during feeding. Hearing wet or rattly breathing suggests swallowing problems.

Coordination of Sucking, Swallowing, and Breathing

Rhythmicity is a hallmark of infant feeding that results from normal coordination of sucking, swallowing, and breathing. Clinicians should have an understanding of normal, as well as atypical, patterns of coordination:

- What is the baby's pattern of coordination?
    - *Normal:* In the early part of feeding, swallowing and breathing are smoothly integrated into bursts of at least 20–30 sucks.

- *Short sucking bursts:* Sucking bursts early in the feeding last only 3–5 sucks, with frequent and perhaps lengthy breathing pauses.
- *Feeding-induced apnea:* During sucking bursts, the baby swallows but does not breathe. This may lead to oxygen desaturation, coughing or choking, or pulling away from the milk flow.

When poor coordination of sucking, swallowing, and breathing is noted, it is important to investigate the underlying reasons for the pattern that is observed. Short sucking bursts may be seen in a baby who is premature or weak and lacks stamina to sustain sucking. A baby who has respiratory or swallowing problems may use short sucking bursts to limit the milk flow. This pattern may also be seen if the mother has little milk or if the baby is not able to transfer the milk. If feeding-induced apnea is observed, it may be a primary problem of coordination for the baby due to maturational or neurologic issues, or it could be related to high milk flow.

Assessing Flow Rate During Breastfeeding

Determining flow rate during breastfeeding is done by direct and indirect methods of observation.

Sucking Rate

Observing the sucking rate is a quick and simple method to screen for rate of flow during breastfeeding:

- How fast is the baby sucking?
  - Two or more sucks per second: Nonnutritive sucking
  - One suck per second: Nutritive sucking
- Does the rate change throughout the feeding?
- When do changes occur?

If the baby is sucking at two sucks per second or faster, the sucking is probably nonnutritive and the flow is low. This faster sucking rate is typical of the first 10–60 seconds at the breast, before the MER. When the milk flow begins, the baby's sucking rate should slow down to about one suck per second. This is characterized by a brief pause in jaw movement when the jaw is at its lowest point during the sucking cycle. Much of the feeding should be characterized by sustained active sucking at this nutritive sucking rate. If only small portions of the baby's feeding exhibit this type of nutritive sucking activity, the overall flow is probably low. The total length of time at each breast does not correlate with the amount of milk transferred.

Swallowing Rate

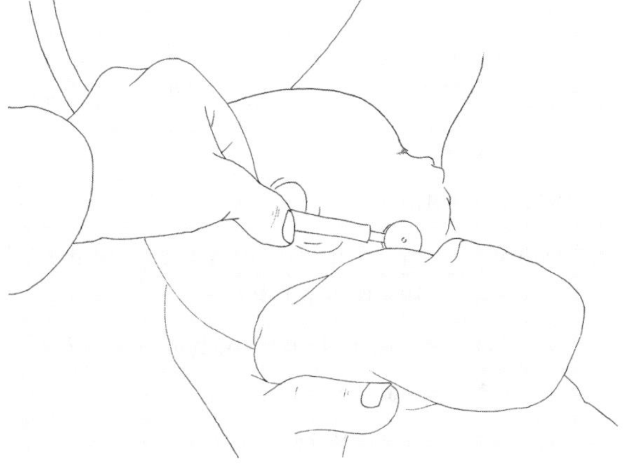

Figure 6-5 Cervical auscultation.

The swallowing rate reflects the flow rate and is an excellent method of estimating flow. The assessment of the swallowing rate is enhanced by using a stethoscope to amplify the swallow sounds:

- How many sucks occur before each swallow?

A ratio of one to three sucks per swallow should indicate normal flow as long as this rate is sustained over the majority of the feeding. If clear swallows are heard less frequently, the flow may be low. Typically, swallowing has been determined by listening for soft swallow sounds. This method may miss the more subtle swallows that are not always evident to the naked ear. A more precise method is cervical auscultation. This method uses a neonatal-size stethoscope placed laterally on the baby's throat to distinctly hear swallowing and breathing sounds (Vice, Heinz, Giuriati, Hood, & Bosma, 1990) (**Figure 6-5**). (See also the section on cervical auscultation in Chapter 1.)

Behavioral Cues

Although it is decidedly low tech, a baby's behavior, in conjunction with other observations, can provide the clinician with information about the flow rate:

- How wakeful is the baby before and during feeding?
- Does the baby quickly fall asleep at the breast?
- Is the baby content at the breast but cries when taken off?
- Does the baby look distressed during feeding?
- Does the baby pull away from the breast?
- Is the baby fussy while feeding?
- Does the baby resist going to the breast?
- Is the baby very fidgety or wiggly during feeding?

The baby's behavior can give important information about the flow rate and how the baby copes with it. Babies who get milk at a rate they can handle generally have open eyes and an intent look. Babies who get inadequate flow often become sleepy early in the feeding, seem to fall asleep, or seem uninterested. A content baby who cries when taken off the breast also may not be getting adequate milk transfer. Babies who receive a very high flow rate will often show stress cues. One baby might generate high flow and momentarily show stress but then settle into a pattern of rapid but comfortable feeding. Other babies in the same situation may show stress in their eyes, turn their head away, or stop sucking.

Test Weights

Test weights are a definitive measure of intake. When compared to feeding time, it provides information on the flow rate:

- How much milk has the baby taken?
  - On each breast?
  - Cumulatively?
- How long has it taken?

By weighing the baby before and after breastfeeding with a digital scale accurate to 1–2 grams, the overall flow rate can be objectively determined (Meier, Lysakowski, & Engstrom, 1990). This method is accurate and often gives surprising results. A mother who is worried that her baby stays at the breast for only 5 minutes and will not nurse often may learn that her baby gets 3 ounces in 5 minutes—a very high flow rate. Another mother with a good milk supply and a baby who nurses constantly may learn that her baby is eliciting a very low flow rate, getting only 0.5 ounces in 15 minutes.

Milk Production

The amount of milk mother has available, and the ease with which it is transferred to the baby during the MER, can be highly correlated with the flow rate. The clinician should consider the following information about milk production when assessing flow:

- Is it adequate, low, or abundant?
- How has milk production been determined?
- Are there signs of overactive let-down?
- Is the mother exclusively breastfeeding?
- Is the mother expressing milk?

When there are problems related to flow, it should be determined if they are related to the mother's milk supply or if they are baby-sided issues. Assessing the baby's performance without accurate information on the mother's supply may lead to an inaccurate understanding of the problem:

- A mother can have a normal flow, but the baby perceives it as too high and may have inadequate intake or other feeding problems.
- A mother can have abundant milk production, yet believe that she has little milk when her baby feeds quickly and is unsettled.

- A mother can have an oversupply and/or robust MER, which causes the baby to pull away, cough or choke, or become resistant to eating.
- The mother can have an adequate supply, yet the baby generates little flow, indicating a baby-sided feeding problem. Milk production will decrease rapidly if milk is not removed from the breast.
- The mother can have low production, thus the baby generates low flow.

Simply observing the baby at the breast may give an inaccurate indication of the mother's milk supply. Objective measurements, such as doing test weights and then having the mother pump any residual milk, are more accurate. The total that the baby transferred plus the pumped milk would be the mother's potential supply for that feeding. If the baby is not feeding at the breast, pumping with a high-quality breast pump will determine the mother's milk supply. Keep in mind that when using a pump, the mother may not transfer milk in the same way that she does for her baby.

Common Diagnoses Related to Flow Issues

Prematurity

Many premature babies struggle with breastfeeding, and flow issues may contribute to these difficulties. The following information can help focus the assessment of feeding problems:

- At what gestational age was the baby born, and what is the current corrected age?
- What is the baby's respiratory status, including respiratory rate, need for oxygen, work of breathing, and endurance?
- Can the premature baby sustain suck adequately (length of burst and suction pressure) at the breast to create the necessary flow?
- What is the pattern of suck-swallow-breath control?
- Is there any evidence of feeding-induced apnea?
- If the baby is struggling with feeding, has there been a trial with controlled low flow?

Premature infants often have medical and/or maturational issues that lead to sensitivity to high flow during feeding. Respiratory distress syndrome and chronic lung disease are often seen in premature infants and are associated with a high resting respiratory rate, increased work of breathing, poor respiratory reserve, and low endurance. High flow, or even normal flow, may not be tolerated by these babies who often prefer nonnutritive sucking or very low flow. Maturational issues also impact feeding, with younger preemies typically having more feeding problems. One maturational issue preterm babies are prone to is feeding-induced apnea, which is exacerbated by high flow. Immaturity may also lead to trouble maintaining latch and creating adequate milk flow at the breast. How preterm infants are cared for, how early they initiate breastfeeding, and their individual medical conditions help determine their feeding competence. See Chapter 7 for more information on breastfeeding preterm infants.

Oral-Facial Anomalies

Feeding problems are common among babies with oral-facial anomalies such as cleft lip and/or palate, Pierre Robin sequence, hemifacial microsomia, and macroglossia. When assessing babies with these diagnoses, the clinician should consider the following:

- Can the baby create suction during sucking?
- What is the suction strength?
- Are there associated breathing issues?
- Is there airway obstruction (stenosis, malacia, glossoptosis, etc.)?
- Is there evidence of swallowing dysfunction?

A baby with oral anomalies, including any oral cleft, is often unable to create suction. The research of Geddes and colleagues (Geddes et al., 2008) has underscored the important role of suction in breastfeeding, so if suction cannot be created, typical breastfeeding generally is not successful. For an isolated cleft lip, the soft breast tissue may fill the gap and allow the baby to create suction and latch effectively to the breast. For a cleft palate, it is not possible to create suction, so latch is inadequate, milk flow is limited, and supplementation is required. Partial breastfeeding during the MER, or the use of a pressure-assisted supplemental device at the breast, may be strategies to allow a baby with cleft palate to come to the breast.

When an oral-facial anomaly, such as micrognathia (small lower jaw) with glossoptosis (a posteriorly placed tongue that intermittently occludes the airway), causes intermittent airway obstruction, feeding will be limited by difficulty breathing and coordinating breathing with sucking and swallowing. Reducing the flow may be helpful, but the intake may still be inadequate. Babies with oral-facial anomalies are also at increased risk for swallowing disorders, so it is important to observe for signs of swallowing dysfunction. See Chapter 8 for more on this issue.

Respiratory Compromise

Because respiration plays such an important role in infant feeding, the clinician should pay particular attention to respiratory issues when assessing feeding problems:

- Does the baby have a medical diagnosis that could impact respiratory function (**Table 6-1**)?
- What is the baby's respiratory status prior to feeding?
  - Respiratory rate
  - Need for additional oxygen

    - Need for breathing treatments or medications
    - Work of breathing
    - Energy level
    - Signs of obstruction (stuffy nose, snorty breathing, wheezing, stridor, breathing pauses)
- How do the baby's respiratory parameters change with feeding?
- If the baby is struggling to breathe during feeding, has there been a trial in a controlled low-flow situation?
- Are the oral feeding expectations appropriate for the baby's respiratory status?

A baby with compromised respiratory status will often require ongoing intervention, such as oxygen or breathing treatments, or have a high respiratory rate and/or work of breathing. All of these issues make handling the ventilatory reductions associated with feeding and coordinating sucking, swallowing, and breathing much more challenging. High flow exacerbates this and further reduces opportunities for breathing. The baby may use a pattern of short sucking bursts, or suck with less pressure to try to limit the flow. Even when the baby uses normal feeding patterns, energy and endurance may be limited due to the increased work required during feeding. Because the baby often takes in less than expected and feeds slowly, the temptation is to increase the flow rate. This group of babies, however, may do better with a lower flow rate to assist them with respiratory stability, and reduced expectations for total oral intake.

Intervention Strategies to Alter Flow

When it has been determined that high or low flow rate is a factor in an infant's feeding problems, there are a variety of methods to change flow rate in order to improve feeding performance.

Increasing Flow

There are several reasons to increase flow during breastfeeding. The most frequent reason is to improve the nutrition of a baby who is not achieving adequate milk transfer. This baby may be failing to gain weight or growing at an inappropriately slow rate. It is important to determine if this is due to baby-sided factors, such as inability to latch or suck effectively, or inadequate milk supply from the breast.

Another reason to increase flow is to improve the sucking pattern. A chomping and biting sucking pattern may be observed when the baby has difficulty generating flow at the breast, resulting in painful nursing and/or inadequate milk transfer. Increasing flow may help the baby use a more functional and appropriate sucking pattern with greater suction. Some caution is necessary when increasing flow. If the baby is intentionally limiting the flow due to breathing or swallowing problems, increasing the flow may be detrimental to the baby.

Increasing Flow Without a Feeding Tube Device

Optimizing the latch frequently improves flow. The baby must be wakeful to latch well and actively participate in breastfeeding. Parents should be taught how to fully wake their baby for feeding, and they will benefit from instruction in identifying feeding cues so they are able to respond to their baby at opportune times. Specific techniques to improve the baby's latch might include activities to increase the baby's mouth opening, strengthen the baby's suck (see Chapter 11), and find the best position (see Chapters 5 and 12).

If the baby appears to have a good latch and suck, but the milk flow still seems inadequate, techniques to stimulate milk flow can be added. If there appears to be a delayed MER, with the baby frustrated and unwilling to suck long enough to stimulate milk flow, it may be helpful for mother to prepump so milk is available more quickly. While the baby is sucking, it can be effective for the mother to use deep compression with moderate to strong squeezing of the breast to increase flow, and then release the compression when the baby pauses (Newman & Pitman, 2000).

For premature infants, it is common for the mother to have a good milk supply but for the baby to transfer very little milk. The strength and coordination of suction is not fully developed in premature infants and may lead to inability to sustain latch and transfer milk. The use of a nipple shield has been found to aid milk transfer significantly for those premature infants who cannot breastfeed well without one, because more of their energy goes into removing milk and less goes into staying latched to the breast (Clum & Primomo, 1996; Meier et al., 2000). For a nipple shield to be effective in augmenting flow for a premature infant, it should be sized to the infant's mouth. Nipple shields may also aid milk transfer in term infants who have trouble sustaining suction at the breast.

If the mother has a marginal or poor milk supply, increasing her supply should increase the flow. Milk supply can be increased by frequent milk expression with a hospital-grade electric breast pump, the use of galactogogues (such as domperidone, metoclopramide, or fenugreek and other herbs), and by spending time with the baby at the breast or in skin-to-skin contact.

Feeding Tube Devices

When the methods described in the previous section do not result in a sufficient increase in flow, or if it is clear that the mother has a low milk supply, a feeding tube device can be considered. These devices add milk flow from an external source. When recommending these devices to a mother, the lactation specialist should be sensitive to the mother's verbal and nonverbal communication to determine her acceptance of the device. Providing adequate, hands-on instruction in the use of the device is crucial to ensuring success. Commonly used devices are the Supplemental Nursing System (SNS; Medela), the Lact-Aid Nursing Trainer, and a feeding tube (such as a 5 French gavage tube) attached to a syringe or placed in a bottle of milk.

Adding flow at the breast using a feeding tube device can be a strategy to improve the sucking pattern and efficiency. Some babies suck using an excessive amount of compression and limited suction, resulting in inefficient milk transfer and/or breast pain for mother. These babies may show a normal sucking pattern during each MER but may revert to a pattern of excessive compression and limited suction as the flow of milk abates. In this situation, the lactation specialist should identify the point during nursing when the baby needs increased flow to improve the sucking pattern. Although some babies will need increased flow throughout the entire feeding, others may need it only when milk flow from the MER slows. The supplemental device is set up at the beginning of the feed but is not used or opened until the baby requires additional flow. With training, most mothers are able to start the flow of the tube feeding device to correspond with their baby's needs. For a healthy infant, this should increase the flow rate so the baby swallows after most sucks. Each suck should be a long draw rather than a short chomp.

Feeding tube devices can be helpful for any baby with diminished endurance and/or weak suck, including babies with prematurity or congenital heart disease. To augment milk flow, the tube feeding device may be used throughout the entire feeding or started as the baby tires. For a baby with low endurance, the lactation specialist must take care not to overwhelm the baby's suck, swallow, and breathe abilities with a flow rate that is too high. A slower flow rate with a ratio of three or four sucks per swallow may be needed to support the baby's abilities.

The rate of milk flow can be adjusted when using any of these devices. For the SNS, the tube size can be selected to give the appropriate flow rate. The Lact-Aid Nursing Trainer and feeding tube and syringe can be squeezed to change the flow. For tube-in-bottle devices, the container can be elevated to increase the flow. As the flow rate is increased with any of these devices, the lactation specialist needs to be attentive to signs of excessive flow. An appropriate flow rate occurs when the baby is able to breathe regularly while sucking, and breathing is inhibited only in the moment of swallowing. If the baby is holding its breath, looking distressed, or coughing and sputtering, the baby's suck–swallow–breathe capacities have been overwhelmed, and flow from the device should be slowed.

Decreasing Flow

The unique flow characteristics at the breast usually support excellent control and coordination of sucking, swallowing, and breathing. There can be times, however, when flow at the breast leads to lack of coordination regardless of the mother's actual flow rate. Feeding-induced apnea, although more prevalent during bottle feeding, can also be observed during breastfeeding, even in healthy infants. Medical diagnoses such as respiratory distress can result in an elevated respiratory rate, making it difficult to coordinate swallowing and breathing even when the flow rate is typical. In these cases, methods to decrease the milk flow may be considered.

At times, the quantity of the mother's milk production, or the vigor of her MER, can overwhelm even a baby who has normal skills to coordinate sucking, swallowing, and breathing. Too often, however, difficulty with coordinating sucking, swallowing, and breathing is immediately diagnosed as an overactive letdown. The problem is attributed to the mother, when the difficulty may actually lie with the baby. This results in treatment strategies that do not improve the problem, because they do not deal with the root cause. The lactation specialist should carefully evaluate the baby's respiration at baseline and during feeding, how well breathing is coordinated with sucking and swallowing, and if there are any concerns about the safety of swallowing. If problems are noted, the flow may need to be reduced. In identifying methods to slow the flow, the lactation specialist needs to identify which changes might be needed on the mother's part and which might be needed on the baby's part.

Mother-Sided Methods

As the mother feels her MER approaching, she can momentarily take her baby off the breast and allow the strong flow to fall on a cloth. Prepumping to reduce the initial milk flow may offer a short-term solution, but in the long term it can result in more milk, which compounds the problem. Feeding the baby on only one breast at each feeding may gradually lower the mother's milk supply so her MER is not as brisk. A similar strategy is block feeding, where mother uses only one breast for gradually increasing periods of 2 to 6 hours of feeding before moving to the other side for a similar period. Some mothers have one breast that makes more milk or has a more brisk MER, so she can start each feeding on the slower breast, and the baby is not as hungry and vigorous when switching to the faster breast.

An additional method for slowing milk flow during breastfeeding was suggested by Carol Chamblin, IBCLC (personal communication, March 30, 2007). Chamblin teaches mothers to press on the breast with a flat hand to temporarily collapse some ducts when the infant shows signs of struggling with flow.

Baby-Sided Methods

Changing the baby's position during nursing can decrease the flow. Positions where the baby is below the breast (such as the standard cradle or football hold) should be avoided because gravity assists the flow of milk. Alternate positions that eliminate gravity include mother and baby lying side by side in bed or having the mother recline with the baby lying prone on her chest. In the latter position, the milk will travel slightly uphill, so it potentially does the most to slow the flow.

If feeding-induced apnea is present during breastfeeding, external pacing can be used to help the baby coordinate breathing with sucking and swallowing. This is a technique that systematically imposes breathing breaks for a baby who is not spontaneously breathing at appropriate intervals. During active milk flow, if the baby has not taken a breath after 3–5 suck or swallows, the mother needs to help the baby take a breathing break. For some babies, simply touching their cheek, talking to them, and/or moving them may encourage them to stop sucking and take a few breaths. Other babies need to be unlatched while they take two to four breaths. The baby's mouth should continue to touch the mother's breast, so the baby knows that the feeding will resume quickly. This technique sets the pace of breathing for a baby who does not have appropriate internal control of breathing coordination. In many cases, pacing is needed only for the first few minutes of feeding when the baby is sucking eagerly, when the mother is having her first and strongest MER, and when the flow is very high. Although this technique may sound disruptive to nursing, it may actually make a baby who latches easily more comfortable. Feeding-induced apnea is not only exhausting for the baby, but it also can lead to oxygen desaturation, microaspiration, and general stress. External pacing allows the baby to continue breastfeeding while remaining physiologically stable.

Conclusion

The rate of milk flow is an important aspect of infant feeding, and within breastfeeding there is a dynamic relationship around flow—mother and baby both contribute to the rate of milk flow. If the flow is too low, because the mother has inadequate milk supply or the baby is not able to access it, the baby will not thrive at the breast. If the milk flow is too high, because of abundant supply or because the normal flow is too high for a particular baby, the baby will be uncomfortable at the breast. Our job is to help mothers and babies adjust flow so it is not too high, and not too low, but just right.

References

Bamford, O., Taciak, V., & Gewolb, I. H. (1992). The relationship between rhythmic swallowing and breathing during suckle feeding in term neonates. *Pediatric Research, 31*(6), 619–624.

Bu'Lock, F., Woolridge, M. W., & Baum, J. D. (1990). Development of coordination of sucking, swallowing and breathing: Ultrasound study of term and preterm infants. *Developmental Medicine and Child Neurology, 32*(8), 669–678.

Chetwynd, A. G., Diggle, P. J., Drewett, R. F., & Young, B. (1998). A mixture model for sucking patterns of breastfed infants. *Statistics in Medicine, 17,* 395–405.

Clum, D., & Primomo, J. (1996). Use of a silicone nipple shield with premature infants. *Journal of Human Lactation, 12*, 287–290.

Drewett, R. F., & Woolridge, M. W. (1979). Sucking patterns of human babies on the breast. *Early Human Development, 3*(4), 315–320.

Drewett, R. F., & Woolridge, M. W. (1981). Milk taken by human babies from the first and second breast. *Physiology and Behavior, 26*, 327–329.

Geddes, D. T., Kent, J. C., Mitoulas, L. R., & Hartman, P. E. (2008). Tongue movements and intra-oral vacuum in breastfeeding infants. *Early Human Development, 4*, 471–477.

Gewolb, I. H., & Vice, F. L. (2006). Maturational changes in the rhythms, patterning, and coordination of respiration and swallow during feeding in preterm and term infants. *Developmental Medicine and Child Neurology, 48*, 589–594.

Gewolb, I. H., Vice, F. L., SchwietzerKenny, E. L., Taciak, V. L., & Bosma, J. F. (2001). Developmental patterns of rhythmic suck and swallow in preterm infants. *Developmental Medicine Child Neurology, 43,* 22–27.

Hanlon, M. B., Tripp, J. H., Ellis, R. E., Flack, F. C., Selley, W. G., & Shoesmith, H. J. (1997). Deglutition apnoea as indicator of maturation of suckle feeding in bottlefed preterm infants. *Developmental Medicine and Child Neurology, 39*(8), 534–542.

Lau, C., Alagugurusamy, R., Schanler, R. J., Smith, E. O., & Shulman, R. J. (2000). Characterization of the developmental stages of sucking in preterm infants during bottle feeding. *Acta Paediatrica, 89*(7), 846–852.

Mathew, O. P., & Bhatia, J. (1989). Sucking and breathing patterns during breast- and bottlefeeding in term neonates. *American Journal of Disease in Children, 143,* 588–592.

Mathew, O. P., Clark, M. L., Pronske, M. L., LunaSolarzano, H. G., & Peterson, M. D. (1985). Breathing pattern and ventilation during oral feeding in term newborn infants. *Journal of Pediatrics, 106,* 810–813.

Meier, P. P., Brown, L. P., Hurst, N. M., Spatz, D. L., Engstrom, J. L., Borucki, L. C., & Krouse, A. M. (2000). Nipple shields for preterm infants: Effect on milk transfer and duration of breastfeeding. *Journal of Human Lactation, 16*(2), 106–114; quiz 129–131.

Meier, P. P., Lysakowski, T. Y., & Engstrom, J. L. (1990). The accuracy of test-weighing for preterm infants. *Journal of Pediatric Gastroenterology and Nutrition, 10,* 62–65.

Mizuno, K., & Ueda, A. (2006). Changes in sucking performance from non-nutritive sucking to nutritive sucking during breast- and bottle-feeding. *Pediatric Research, 59*(5), 728–731.

Mortola, J. P., & Fischer, J. T. (1988). Upper airway reflexes in newborns. In O. P. Mathew & G. Sant'Ambrogio (Eds.), *Respiratory function of the upper airway* (Vol. 35, pp. 303–357). New York, NY: Marcel Dekker.

Newman, J., & Pitman, T. (2000). *The ultimate breastfeeding book of answers.* Roseville, CA: Prima.

Newman, L. A., Keckley, C., Petersen, M., & Hammer, A. (2001). Swallowing function and medical diagnoses in infants suspected of dysphagia. *Pediatrics, 108*(6), e106.

Ramsay, D. T., & Hartmann, P. (2005). Milk removal from the breast. *Breastfeeding Review, 13*(1), 5–7.

Sameroff, A. J. (1968). The components of sucking in the human newborn. *Journal of Experimental Child Psychology, 6*(4), 607–623.

Selley, W. G., Ellis, R. E., Flack, F. C., & Brooks, W. A. (1990). Coordination of sucking, swallowing and breathing in the newborn: Its relationship to infant feeding and normal development. *British Journal of Disorders of Communication, 25*(3), 311–327.

Sheikh, S., Allen, E., Shell, R., Hruschak, J., Iram, D., Castile, R., & McCoy, K. (2001). Chronic aspiration without gastroesophageal reflux as a cause of chronic respiratory symptoms in neurologically normal infants. *Chest, 120,* 1190–1195.

Suskind, D. L., Thompson, D. M., Gulati, M., Huddleston, P., Liu, D. C., & Baroody, F. M. (2006). Improved infant swallow after gastroesophageal reflux disease treatment: A function of improved laryngeal sensation? *The Laryngoscope, 116,* 1397–1403.

Tuchman, D. N. (1993). Physiology of the swallowing apparatus. In D. N. Tuchman & R. S. Walter (Eds.), *Disorders of feeding and swallowing in infants and children* (pp. 1–26). San Diego, CA: Singular Publishing Group.

Vice, F. L., Heinz, J. M., Giuriati, G., Hood, M., & Bosma, J. (1990). Cervical auscultation of suckle feeding in newborn infants. *Developmental Medicine and Child Neurology, 32,* 760–768.

Weber, R., Woolridge, M. W., & Baum, J. D. (1986). An ultrasonographic study of the organisation of sucking and swallowing by newborn infants. *Developmental Medicine and Child Neurology, 28,* 19–24.

Wolf, L. S., & Glass, R. P. (1992). *Feeding and swallowing disorders in infancy: Assessment and management.* Austin, TX: ProEd.

Wolff, P. H. (1968). The serial organization of sucking in the young infant. *Pediatrics, 42*(6), 943–955.

CHAPTER 7

Breastfeeding Preterm Infants

Kerstin Hedberg Nyqvist

Breastfeeding Rates in Preterm Infants

In spite of the particular importance of human milk feeding for children born preterm (a gestation of less than 37 weeks) or with low birth weight (LBW, less than 2500 g) (Feldman & Eidelman 2003; Schanler 2001; Smith, Durkin, Hinton, Bellinger, & Kuhn, 2003), breastfeeding rates in industrialized countries are lower than rates observed in term infants and show considerable variation. Differences in rates can be attributed to several factors. One major explanation is probably the general attitude to breastfeeding in society at large. Other contributing factors are mothers' right to maternity leave from work and maternal allowance during the infant's hospitalization and after discharge.

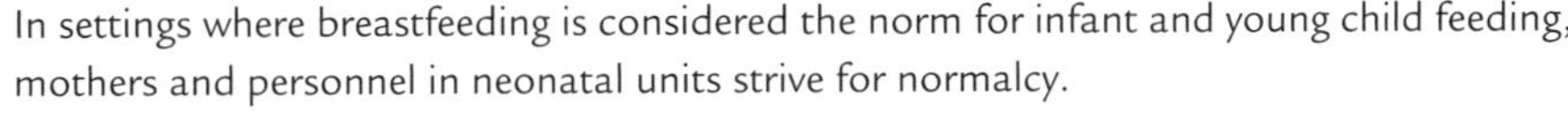

In settings where breastfeeding is considered the norm for infant and young child feeding, mothers and personnel in neonatal units strive for normalcy.

When breastfeeding is regarded as a matter of personal choice and bottle feeding is considered normal, this attitude is reflected in lower breastfeeding incidence.

Special Characteristics and Needs of Preterm Infants

Preterm infants have special characteristics and needs, including the following:

- *External characteristics:* Typical features of a preterm infant are thin arms and legs and low muscle tone when the infant is resting. The mouth is small, and the infant lacks fat pads in the cheeks, which help to stabilize movements of the tongue and jaws during oral feeding. Preterm infants' immature appearance may impart the false impression that they lack the prerequisites for oral feeding.
- *Physiological immaturity:* The cardiorespiratory system of a preterm infant is immature, with bradycardia, irregular respiration, and apnea (pause in respiration of more than 20 seconds). Difficulty maintaining adequate oxygen saturation is the main concern during feeding. Decisions about choice of feeding method are primarily based on protection of the infant's physiological stability.

- *Metabolic immaturity:* A lack of sufficient subcutaneous fat, brown fat, and glycogen contribute to increased risk of hypothermia and hypoglycemia in a preterm infant. This necessitates protection from cold stress during breastfeeding by skin-to-skin contact or adequate clothing, and frequent feeding.
- *Neurologic immaturity:* An immature motor system and low muscle tone make it difficult for a preterm infant to attain and maintain head control and a position with flexed hips, knees, and feet, as well as flexed arms with the hands joined in the midline near the face. Without adequate support, the infant is unable to stay fixed at the breast, with a straight trunk and neck; instead, the tendency is to curl into a slumped posture. Low muscle tone results in poor latch, less efficient sucking, and difficulties in staying fixed at the breast.

A preterm infant spends more time in a diffuse, drowsy state and has frequent shifts in states (e.g., between diffuse sleep and active awake). Signs of waking up are subtle (slightly more irregular respiration, gasps, grimaces, movements in lips and tongue, raised eyebrows, diffuse movements). Direct light is an obstacle to eye opening. Periods of focused alertness are short. Instead, a glassy-eyed look and a surprised look with wide-open eyes are common, indicating limited ability to handle visual stimuli.

The infant is easily overloaded by stimuli (touch, sounds, visual input, light), especially when they occur simultaneously. Habituation, the capacity to shut out common environmental stimuli, does not mature until term age. Voices in a normal conversational tone and activity in the visual field cause stress, displayed as irregular respiration and movements, and reduce the time available for activities directed at the breast.

Considering all these differences, the common assumption that breastfeeding is inappropriate until a certain maturational level is not surprising. However, research has shown that this is not the case.

Assessment of Readiness or Facilitation of Competence

Criteria for Initiation of Oral Feeding

Decisions about the initiation of breastfeeding in preterm infants are often based on an assessment of readiness. A certain maturational level has been the most common criterion, such as a postmenstrual age (PMA, gestational weeks from the first day of the last menstrual period) of 34 weeks (Comrie & Helm, 1997) or 32 weeks (Cousins, 1999; Lemons, 2001; Wheeler, Johnson, Collie, Sutherland, & Chapman, 1999). It has been suggested that infants at a gestational age (GA) of less than 32 weeks should be allowed to suck only at their mother's emptied breast, whereas mothers of infants at 32–33 weeks can be allowed to breastfeed without restriction (Meier, 2001). A minimum weight is also a common criterion. Another approach for testing readiness to feed is evaluation of sucking vigor during pacifier or finger sucking (Comrie & Helm, 1997). Several screening methods and guidelines have been elaborated for assessment of feeding skills and for introduction of oral feedings (McCain, 2003; Thoyre, Shaker, & Pridham, 2005; White-Traut, Berbaum,

Lessen, McFarlin, & Cardenas, 2005). But these methods were based on bottle feeding. As explained in the following discussion, the initiation of breastfeeding should be based on facilitation of competence instead of assessment of readiness.

Physiological Stability During Breastfeeding

Coordination of sucking, swallowing, and breathing is considered a requirement for commencing oral feeding. Because of fear of physiological compromise, preterm infants' physiological response to oral feeding has been explored extensively. However, in the absence of breastfeeding research, conclusions drawn from infants' reactions to nipple (bottle) feeding have been incorrectly applied to breastfeeding. A study of bottle feeding, which noted apnea, bradycardia, and oxygen desaturation during sucking, described the respiratory control in preterm infants as immature at 35–36 weeks (Mathew, 1988).

Comparisons of preterm infants' physiological responses to breast- and bottle feeding have clearly demonstrated differences in favor of breastfeeding.

Common observations during bottle feeding were uncoordinated sucking and swallowing, reduced breathing, higher incidence of bradycardia, apnea and desaturation, lower levels of oxygen saturation, progressive postfeed decline of transcutaneous oxygen saturation, and lower temperature, whereas the same infants—also very preterm infants—remained stable during breastfeeding (Blaymore Bier et al., 1997; Chen, Wang, Chang, & Chi, 2000; Dowling, 1999). Apnea during swallowing (deglutition apnea) is more frequent in bottle-fed preterm infants than in term infants (Hanlon et al., 1997).

These differences are easily explained: at the breast, the infant is in control of sucking, swallowing, and breathing in a pattern that permits physiological stability. A breastfed infant with an immature sucking pattern holds the breath during suckling and breathes during pauses, reflected in brief desaturations that resolve shortly after the termination of a sucking burst. After a period of rapid breathing, the respiration slows down and the infant spontaneously begins to suck again. This is no cause for concern, provided that the infant is allowed to decide the pace. Higher body temperature during breastfeeding is explained by the skin-to-skin contact and higher chest temperature in breastfeeding women, due to the effects of oxytocin (Uvnas-Moberg & Eriksson, 1996).

Obstacles to infant self-regulation during bottle feeding are the size of the hole in the nipple, the force of gravity that makes milk flow, and manipulation by the caregiver who tries to coax the infant to continue sucking, leading to oxygen desaturation and a postfeed period with low saturation or, if the percentage of supplemental oxygen was increased during the feed, before it can be decreased to the prefeed level.

Risk of aspiration has also been considered a possible hazard. However, even very preterm infants respond to fluid in the larynx via an upper airway chemoreflex (Davies, Koenig, & Thatch, 1989). In addition, observational studies of breastfeeding in preterm infants have not found aspiration to occur in an immature sucking pattern.

Preterm infants maintain physiologic stability during breastfeeding, provided that the mother is sensitive to the infant's behavioral and physiological cues.

Facilitation of Breastfeeding by Developmentally Supportive Care

Infant motor development is enhanced by modification of care and the caregiving environment according to the infant's current maturational stage of central nervous system development, which is accomplished by supporting the infant's own activities for self-regulation (Nyqvist, Ewald, & Sjödén, 1996). During the intense process of brain development during the second half of pregnancy, the organization of the cortex is influenced by the infant's exposure to touch, hearing, vision, taste, odor, and proprioceptive and vestibular experience.

The Newborn Individualized Developmental Care and Assessment Program (NIDCAP) is a clinical model for structured infant assessment and provision of care in harmony with infants' current developmental stage and medical status (Als, Lawhon, Duffy, McAnulty, Gibes-Grossman, & Blickman, 1994). The infant is perceived as an active individual who responds to sensory input by signs of strength or sensitivity and activities for self-regulation. The infant's responses are observed in autonomic signs, motor behavior, behavioral states, and activities related to interaction with the social and physical environment (**Table 7-1**). Decisions on the timing and progression of oral feeding are based on the infant's current threshold of tolerance (Ross & Browne, 2002). Younger age at the first oral feeding and last tube feeding were observed in preterm infants after modification of the physical environment in the nursery to make it less stressful (Becker, Grunwald, Moorman, & Stuhr, 1991). Very preterm infants who received care structured according to regular NIDCAP observations attained full bottle or breastfeeding earlier than infants with conventional care (Als et al., 1994).

The interaction between the infant and a parent or other caregiver is a dialogue in which both participants exert a mutual influence on each other. A sensitive caregiver modifies his or her behavior and the environment according to the infant's ongoing responses. When the caregiver acts according to his or her own agenda, the infant responds by increasing the incidence and severity of signs of sensitivity (**Table 7-2**). The NIDCAP program emphasizes parents' unique role in their infant's life. All steps are taken to enable parents to be present in the unit, participate in decisions regarding infant feeding on equal terms with professionals, and take over the responsibility for their infant's feeding and care as soon as they are willing to do so.

Protecting the Milk Supply

Initiation and Frequency of Breastmilk Expression

A variation in markers of the onset of copious milk secretion after birth (milk citrate, lactose, sodium, and total protein) indicates that some mothers of preterm infants may take longer to establish their milk production (Cregan, De Mello, Kershaw, McDougall, & Hartmann, 2002). This finding underscores the importance of initiation of regular, frequent milk expression as soon as possible, for example, beginning before 6 hours postdelivery (Furman, Minich, & Hack, 2002). Manual expression during the first 3 days after birth may contribute to success in lactation (Ohyama, Watabe, & Hayasaka, 2010). Combining manual expression and electric breast pumping may also be beneficial (Morton et al., 2009). Expressing milk at least 6–7 times per 24 hours has been associated with subsequent sufficient milk production (Hill, Brown, & Harker, 1995). Simultaneous pumping increases the chances of a higher milk yield; gentle breast massage may further increase milk production

Table 7-1 Infant Cues of Approach and Avoidance During Breastfeeding According to NIDCAP

Cues of Approach	Cues of Avoidance
Autonomic System	
Regular heart rate and respiration	Fast or slow heart rate Irregular fast or slow respiration
Adequate oxygen saturation	Respiratory pauses, apnea, hypoxia
Stable skin color: pink or red	Pale, mottled, dusky, cyanotic, flushed, color shifts
Stable digestive functions	Spits up, gags Bowel movement grunting Sighs, gasps
Occasional startles and twitches	Hiccough Startles, twitches, tremor
Motor System	
Maintains muscle tone Achieves and maintains flexed arms, legs, trunk, and gaping mouth	Low muscle tone in hands, arms, legs, trunk, and face Shows tongue
Tucks him- or herself closer to the breast Braces hands/feet against mother's body Brings/holds hands to face or mouth Smiles Mouthing, licking Laps milk	High muscle tone: extended posture, tense Active extension of arms/legs Arches head and/or trunk backwards, turns away Fans or splays (spreads out) fingers
Rooting, sucking Grasping Holds onto finger, breast, etc. Molds to mother's trunk	Clenches fists Grimaces Stretches out tense tongue Exaggerated flexion Does not mold to mother's trunk
Smooth, coordinated movements	Diffuse squirming Jerky, uncoordinated movements

(continues)

Table 7-1 Infant Cues of Approach and Avoidance During Breastfeeding According to NIDCAP *(continued)*

Cues of Approach	Cues of Avoidance
Behavioral States	
Stable periods of sleep or alertness Deep sleep States are easy to distinguish	Light/diffuse sleep Low/diffuse states (drowsy, diffuse movements with closed eyes) Short periods of alertness
Looks at mother, orients, with focused look	Swift state transitions Open eyes with glassy-eyed look or stares with a tense, surprised, frightened look
Smooth state transitions: calm waking up, falls asleep easily	Difficult to calm down Irritable Frenetic activity
Shuts out stimuli easily	Crying Limited ability to shut out disturbing stimuli
Attention, Interaction	
Orients towards mother's face, voice, other objects or events Raises eyebrows Frowns	Looks away Stares in another direction Eyes "float" from side to side or roll around
Purses lips as if saying "oh"	Fusses, cries, turns drowsy, closes eyes
Speech movements, imitates facial expression	Yawns, sneezes
Cooing sounds	Cues of avoidance in autonomic/motor/ behavioral system

(Jones, Dimmock, & Spencer, 2001). Mothers who prefer sequential pumping can be advised to repeatedly alternate breasts because this may result in higher volumes.

In industrialized countries, manual expression is mainly used as a complement to breast pumps. Because it is easier to collect colostrum by manual expression directly into a small cup, mothers should be offered instruction soon after delivery to stimulate their milk production. This practice also gives mothers proof of their ability to produce milk in spite of preterm birth. Ideally, these mothers who provide their infants' nutrition can borrow an electric breast pump, free of charge, for use at home during their infant's hospitalization. A

Milk Volumes in Order of Magnitude Depending on Pumping Strategy

Simultaneous pumping + breast massage > simultaneous pumping without breast massage > sequential pumping + breast massage > sequential pumping without breast massage.

hand pump may work for some mothers, but these are best for casual use, when the mother is outside the home or the hospital.

Early attainment of milk production that exceeds the infants' current needs should be encouraged (Hill, Aldag, & Chatterton, 1999). All of the mothers who attained a weekly

Table 7-2 Maternal Behavior During Breastfeeding Preterm Infants

Sensitivity	Lack of Sensitivity
Positions the infant at the breast at signs of waking, when the infant is awake, and at subtle signs of interest in sucking.	Positions the infant at the breast when asleep and shows no signs of interest in sucking.
Selects a quiet place where the infant is shielded from direct light, noise, activity, and visual input.	Selects a place with direct light, noise, a high level of activity, and visual input for the infant.
Sits in an upright or semireclined position (or lies down). Places the infant on a cushion or the like for positioning.	Blocks the infant's access to the breast.
Supports an infant position with straight trunk, head directed forwards, mouth in front of nipple.	Holds the infant with inadequate support for head and trunk, the infant's trunk is not straight, the head is turned sideways, the mouth is not in front of the nipple.
Places the infant with arms and legs flexed, using her clothes or KMC binder or the like for support and protection from cold stress. Gives consistent support for a correct position with still hands.	Holds the infant in a position with extended arms/legs. No clothes/other support for the infant's position. Does not cover the infant.
If the infant shows extension movements: Gently helps the infant to regain a flexed position. Offers the infant the breast by gently touching his lips with nipple/finger to elicit rooting.	Moves her hands often. Does not respond to extension movements. Changes the infant's position often. Does not adjust the position when needed.
When the infant does not respond: Lets him rest, waits for signs of interest in sucking/waking up. At signs of rooting, pulls the infant closer to her body, with the nose touching the breast and the chin pressed into the breast.	Opens the infant's mouth. Inserts the nipple into the infant's mouth. Continues her efforts to make the infant latch on in spite of no response. Holds the infant loosely, at some distance from her body. Nose and chin do not touch the breast, or the nose is "pressed into" the breast.
Is attentive to the infant's position at the breast.	Does not notice incorrect position.
Makes appropriate adjustments when needed.	Does not make any adjustments.

(continues)

Table 7-2 Maternal Behavior During Breastfeeding Preterm Infants *(continued)*

Sensitivity	Lack of Sensitivity
Focuses her attention mainly at the infant; does not pay much interest in the environment.	Focuses her attention at the environment; looks at the infant occasionally.
Has a relaxed face.	Looks worried, stressed, uncomfortable, or bored.
When the infant makes long pauses during sucking: Encourages sucking by talking or gently depressing breast tissue in front of the infant's nose to elicit the sucking reflex by tactile stimulation of the hard palate. Is mainly quiet, may talk sometimes in a soft voice with the infant's father, staff, or other parents.	Does not stimulate sucking, or stimulates the infant repeatedly by tickling face and body, patting, rocking, talking, moving the breast, or repositioning. Does not notice lack of response. Talks in a loud voice with infant's father, staff, or other parents.
Lets the infant suck until he stops and lets go of the breast.	Interrupts or terminates breastfeeding while the infant is still sucking.

production of more than 3500 ml at the end of the second week were able to maintain sufficient milk production at weeks four and five, whereas this was achieved by only 54% of mothers who produced 1700 ml and none of the mothers with a weekly production of less than 1700 ml.

Facilitation of Breastmilk Production

The mother can express her milk in a special pumping room. Some mothers like to express their milk at the infant's bedside, where they can look at or touch the infant during pumping—provided there are adequate arrangements for privacy. At home, the mother can arrange a cozy place for pumping where she has everything she needs within reach. Because stress is an obstacle to the milk ejection reflex (MER), the mother should be informed about what women in her situation have found helpful: sit in a comfortable chair, have something to drink and something to read, listen to music or the radio, or watch TV. The MER can be triggered by gentle massage of the nipples before pumping, looking at the baby's photo, imagining the baby, and holding or smelling clothes worn by the baby.

After some time, mothers may experience reduced milk production in spite of frequent and regular pumping. Counselling about the impact of stress, pain, anxiety, exhaustion, grief, etc. on the MER and milk production is important so the mother does not believe that her milk will disappear completely. Telling her about relactation may inspire her belief in her own capacity and help her to persevere in pumping or increasing pumping frequency.

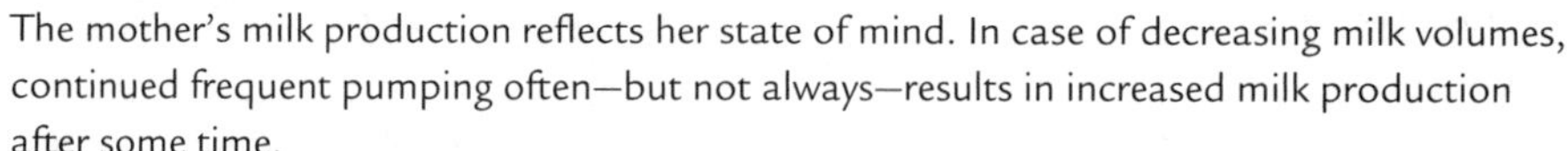

The mother's milk production reflects her state of mind. In case of decreasing milk volumes, continued frequent pumping often—but not always—results in increased milk production after some time.

Observing Breastfeeding in Preterm Infants

Breastfeeding policies for preterm infants are based on healthcare professionals' perception of what can be expected from these infants. Meier and Anderson (1987) described a burst-pause pattern in infants at 32–36 weeks, initially with sucking bursts of 3–7 sucks or isolated sucks. A few days later, some infants managed bursts of 10–15 consecutive sucks. The author developed the Preterm Infant Breastfeeding Behavior Scale (PIBBS) and performed the first prospective descriptive study ever of the development of preterm infants' breastfeeding behavior (**Table 7-3**) (Nyqvist, Rubertsson, Ewald, & Sjödén, 1996). This is a method for direct observation by professionals and mothers of levels of oral motor competence (see **Figures 7-1 and 7-2**). The aim is to obtain a basis for practical suggestions to the mother about enhancement of the infant's breastfeeding competence. The method can also be applied to term infants (Radzyminski, 2003).

Table 7-3 Breastfeeding Observation According to the PIBBS

Mark/record data in the box for the description that agrees with the infant's best performance.

Date										
Time										
Rooting (lip movements, mouth opening, tongue extension, hand to mouth/face movements, head turning, squirming)										
No rooting										
Some rooting										
Obvious rooting (simultaneous mouth opening + head turning)										
How much of the breast was inside the infant's mouth?										
None, the mouth merely touched the nipple										
Part of the nipple										
Whole nipple										
Nipple and part of the areola										
Latched on and stayed fixed										
Did not stay fixed										
Stayed fixed for less than 1 minute										
For how many minutes did the infant stay fixed before she/he let go of the breast (including pauses for resting or sleep, with part of the breast inside the mouth)? *Minutes 1–≥10*										

(continues)

Table 7-3 Breastfeeding Observation According to the PIBBS *(continued)*

Sucking (sucking burst = number of consecutive sucks)										
No activity directed at the breast										
Did not suck, only licked/tasted milk										
Single sucks, occasional short sucking bursts (2–9 sucks)										
2 or more short sucking bursts, occasional long bursts (> 10 sucks)										
2 or more consecutive long sucking bursts										
Longest sucking burst										
Maximum number of consecutive sucks before a pause										
Swallowing										
No swallowing was noticed										
Occasional swallowing										
Repeated swallowing										

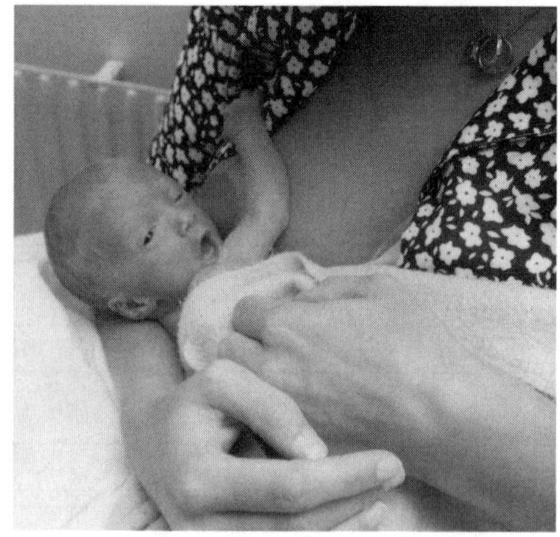

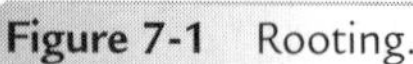

Figure 7-1 Rooting.

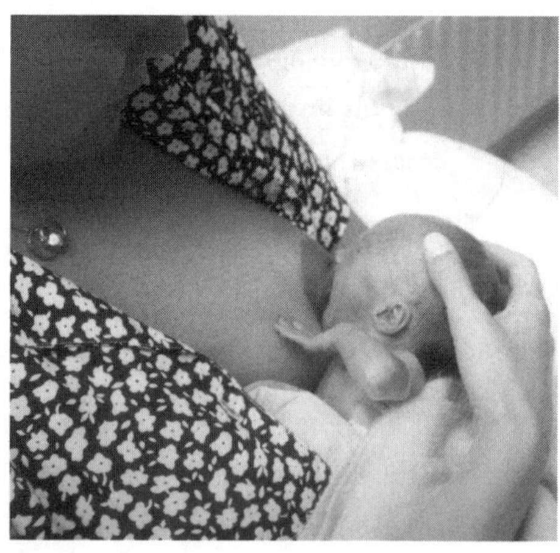

Figure 7-2 Latch.

Early Breastfeeding Competence in Preterm Infants

All 71 mothers of 71 singletons, born at a GA between 26 and 35 weeks, without serious illness, used the PIBBS as a breastfeeding diary, providing more than 4000 PIBBS records (Nyqvist, Ewald, & Sjödén, 1999). Breastfeeding was initiated as soon as the infant was able to breathe without a ventilator or continuous positive airway pressure (CPAP), irrespective of current PMA, age, or weight. The mother received weekly breastfeeding counselling based on the PIBBS (**Table 7-4**). As soon as there were signs of milk intake, test weighing before and after each breastfeed was introduced.

The first breastfeed occurred at 27 weeks PMA. Breastfeeding milestones are presented in **Table 7-5**. Irrespective of PMA on the first day with breastfeeding, all infants rooted (the majority showed obvious rooting) and latched on, half of them efficiently. Most infants stayed fixed for short periods, 5 minutes or less. Nearly all infants engaged in single sucks or short sucking bursts. Obvious rooting, efficient areolar grasp, and staying fixed at the breast for long periods were observed as early as 28 weeks. Some infants sucked in long sucking bursts, even bursts of 30 or more sucks, at 32 weeks. The longest sucking burst data showed large variation. Mothers perceived repeated audible swallowing at 31 weeks at the earliest.

Ninety-four percent of the infants were breastfed at discharge from hospital, 80% fully and 14% partly. Some infants reached full breastfeeding with an immature sucking pattern (mainly short sucking bursts and respiration occurring during pauses). On the day of attainment of full breastfeeding, several infants were able to ingest large volumes, whereas others mainly took small volumes, with a maximum of 40 ml (Nyqvist, 2001). Infants with apnea treatment and a longer period of separation from their mothers (number of days when the mother was not living in a parent room in the unit) established breastfeeding at a higher PMA and postnatal age (Nyqvist & Ewald, 1999). Low GA at birth was associated with early efficient breastfeeding behavior and a high incidence of full breastfeeding. This supports the theory that infant motor development occurs with experience (Thelen & Vogel, 1989). Oral motor competence is triggered when the nipple touches the infant's lips, the nipple touches the hard palate, and milk flows into the infant's mouth.

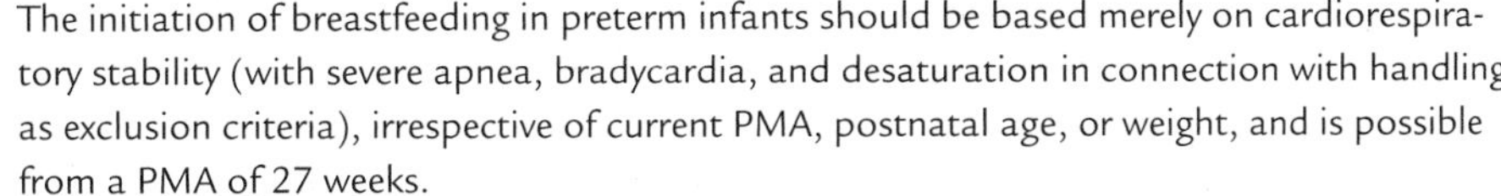
The initiation of breastfeeding in preterm infants should be based merely on cardiorespiratory stability (with severe apnea, bradycardia, and desaturation in connection with handling as exclusion criteria), irrespective of current PMA, postnatal age, or weight, and is possible from a PMA of 27 weeks.

Individual Sucking Patterns

Considerable variability in sucking patterns, sucking intensity and frequency, and duration of pauses were found in a study of 26 infants at 32–37 weeks PMA, using surface electromyography (**Figure 7-1**) (Nyqvist, Farnstrand, Edebol Eeg-Olofsson, & Ewald, 2001). The

Table 7-4 Practical Advice Based on Breastfeeding Observation According to the Preterm Infant Breastfeeding Behavior Scale (PIBBS)

Rooting: The infant does not root.
Support and advice: Give the mother suggestions about touching the infant's lips with the nipple or a finger to elicit rooting. Inform her that (a) touching the infant's cheek or corner of the mouth may cause restless movements, but elicits the rooting reflex in a term infant, and (b) that crying is a late hunger cue.

How much of the breast is inside the infant's mouth: Nothing, part of the nipple, or the whole nipple but no areola.
Support and advice: Give the mother suggestions for how she can stimulate rooting, and pull the infant closer when she or he has a wide open mouth and the tongue down. Touching the infant's palm may stimulate mouth opening (the palmomental reflex) when she or he approaches term age. Inform her that signs of a good latch are: the tip of the infant's nose touches the breast, the chin is burrowed into the breast, and infant is able to stay fixed.

Latching on and staying fixed: The infant does not stay fixed at all or only for short periods.
Support and advice: Suggest to the mother that she pull the infant closer. If the infant's nose is pressed into the breast, she should pull the buttocks closer. Ask her to avoid pressing down breast tissue and avoid using the "scissors hold."

Sucking: The infant does not commence sucking, or takes very long pauses with calm breathing while being awake, without sucking.
Support and advice: Suggest to the mother that she talk to the infant, and depress breast tissue gently in front of the infant's nose (makes the nipple touch the hard palate, which elicits the sucking reflex). She could also touch the infant's palm.

Swallowing: No sound of swallowing is perceived (a silent sound when the airways close, or the sound of gulping in case of a rapid milk flow).
Support and advice: Inform the mother that it is difficult to hear this sound. Also tell her that it is impossible to estimate milk intake from an observation of sucking pattern, sucking duration, and sounds of swallowing.

Lack of improvement in spite of application of suggested advice.
Support and advice: If no improvement occurs in spite of application of the above-mentioned advice repeated times (the infant does not latch on, lets go of the breast repeatedly, sucks minimally in spite of being awake, ingests minimal volumes of milk or the milk consumption does not increase, in spite of sucking), suggest the use of a nipple shield and assess the effects.

Table 7-5 Developmental Milestones in Preterm Infants' Progress in Breastfeeding

Events	*n*	Postmenstrual Age Median (range)	Postnatal Age Median (range)
Initiation of breastfeeding	71	33.7 (27.9–35.9)	1 (0–20)
First nutritive sucking (> 5 ml)*	71	34.3 (30.6–37.7)	8 (1–46)
Exclusive breastfeeding	57	36.0 (33.4–40.0)	19 (2–68)

*Verified by test-weighing (the electronic scales in the level II nursery gave infants' weight to the nearest 5 g).

proportion of time spent sucking ranged between 10% and 60% of a breastfeeding episode. Corresponding data for mouthing (movements in lips, tongue, and jaw other than sucking) and pauses was 2% to 35% and 12% to 67%, respectively. The longest sucking burst ranged from 5 to 96 sucks; this long sucking burst was noted at 34 weeks.

Common restrictions in the duration of breastfeeds, for example giving a mother–infant pair a maximum time of 15 or 30 minutes, are unwarranted. The infant is not exhausted by a long time at the breast because the infant is in control of his or her pattern of sucking, swallowing, breathing, and resting.

Mental Checklist for Practical Breastfeeding Support

Information Before the Delivery

When there is enough time, a mother admitted for impending preterm delivery (and the father) should be informed about how the infant will be fed, the lactation process, the benefits of breastmilk, and the value of initiating breastmilk expression as early as possible. She should also be told about skin-to-skin care (SSC)—the Kangaroo Mother Care method—and when she can commence breastfeeding.

Skin-to-Skin Care

Encouragement of early, prolonged mother–infant SSC, without unfounded restrictions, is a fundamental strategy for support of lactation and breastfeeding. The mother immediately notices when the infant is waking up; she feels movements and changes in the respiratory pattern, hears subtle sounds, and can see eye opening and early signs of interest in sucking. This helps her to utilize her baby's short periods of alertness in an optimal way.

Prevention of Stressful Events

Plan the infant's care in order to avoid stressful events before breastfeeding . For preterm infants, diaper changes, washing, and bathing constitute stressful experiences and deplete the infant's reserve of energy, and they should not be performed immediately before breastfeeding (Mörelius, Hellström-Westas, Carlén, Norman, & Nelson, 2006). On the other hand, a moderately preterm infant may wake up more easily during diaper changes.

Physiological Monitoring

For infants with tendencies for apnea, bradycardia, and desaturation, physiological monitoring of heart rate, respiration, and oxygen saturation at the mother's breast is advisable. When the infant has shown adequate stability during breastfeeding, monitoring can be discontinued and replaced by the mother's assessment of her baby's breathing pattern and skin color.

Armchair, Footstool, Pillow

Provide the mother with an armchair of the correct height. Assist her in finding a comfortable position, with adequate support for her back and arms. Offer her a pillow, if needed, as a positioning aid and a footstool to rest her feet and to facilitate the infant's position close to her body, with the head at the same height as the breast.

Breastfeeding Positions

Encourage the mother to hold her preterm baby skin-to-skin under her clothes, covered by a blanket and–if the infant is very small–wearing a cap in order to prevent heat loss. Suggest that she try different breastfeeding positions. The overhand (transitional) hold is the most practical position for small infants (**Figure 7-3**), followed by the football hold (**Figure 7-4**), but there are alternative ways of achieving a functional position. Describe how to hold the infant close to her trunk, with the infant's head extended, the neck and trunk aligned, and the arms and legs flexed (with the lower arm tucked around the mother's body, under the breast). Explain why a preterm infant needs adequate head support in order to stay at the breast.

A Supportive Physical Environment

If possible, breastfeeding should take place in privacy in a parent room or a separate breastfeeding room. In the nursery, the mother can be offered privacy by a curtain, screen, or partitioning wall, or by placing the armchair with her back turned against the room. It is essential that the environment is as calm as possible, with conversations taking place in a low voice and no disturbing sounds. The infant's eyes should be protected from direct light and activity in the visual field.

A Professional's Presence

Offer your presence in connection with the first few breastfeeding sessions. Sit down by the mother to guide her interaction with the infant and to answer questions.

No Unfounded Restrictions

The infant's time at the breast should not be restricted unless there are definite reasons, such as a medical procedure that must take place at a certain time. Instead, the mother should be encouraged to allow the infant plenty of time to suck and rest between periods of activity.

Realistic Expectations

GA at birth, past and present medical problems, normal variations in development, and individuality contribute to infants' progress. Maturational level alone cannot be applied as a criterion for an expectation of incidence and duration of periods of alertness, feeding frequency, sucking behavior, or milk intake.

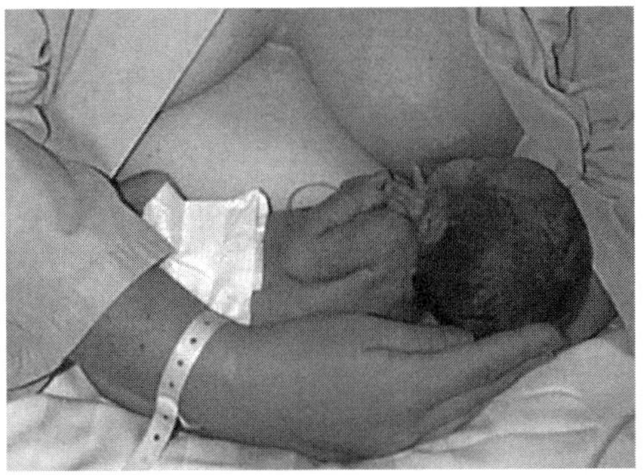

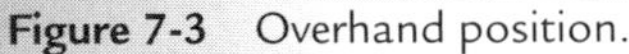

Figure 7-3 Overhand position.

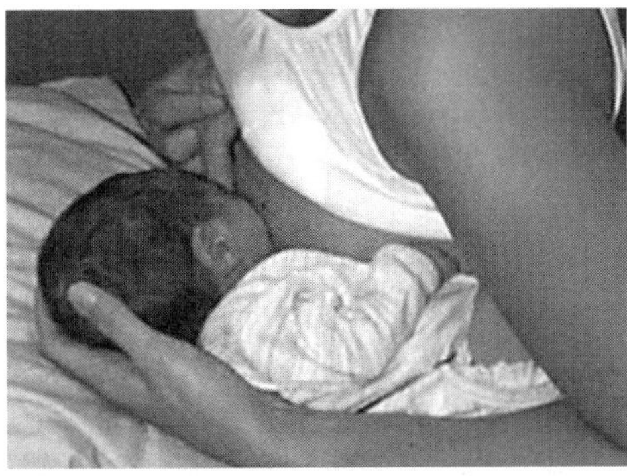

Figure 7-4 Football hold.

Guidance of Mother–Infant Interaction

By interpretation of infant behavior according to the NIDCAP model, optimal opportunities are created for the infant's activities directed at the breast. Point out the infant's signs of alertness and robustness, such as availability for stimulation at the breast and signs that the infant is tired and needs to rest, which indicate that stimulation should be withheld.

Tell the mother about preterm infants' response to touch; advise her to hold the infant with still hands after a comfortable position has been achieved. Caressing, patting, tickling, and rocking usually result in movements that obstruct successful breastfeeding (squirming, extension of arms and legs, arching head and trunk, pulling away from the breast, and irregular respiration with pauses).

Aims of a Breastfeeding-Supportive Feeding Policy

To support optimal infant growth, satisfy infants' need for sucking, achieve a feeding situation that is as normal as possible with respect to parent–infant contact and physical environment, entrust parents with the normal parental task of feeding as soon as possible, enable mothers to breastfeed, terminate a regulated feeding schedule with fixed times and volumes as soon as possible, and support breastfeeding (ideally exclusive breastfeeding).

Use of Alternative Feeding Methods Related to Breastfeeding

Cup Feeding

Cup-fed infants soon learn how to take milk from a cup, and the method is not time consuming if it is performed correctly (Gupta, Khanna, & Chattree, 1999; Malhotra, Vishwambaran, Sundaram, & Narayanan, 1999). Before a parent cup feeds the first time, a nurse should demonstrate how to hold the baby in an upright position and how to hold the cup; spillage is measured to ensure the prescribed milk intake (Dowling, Meier, DiFiore, Blatz, & Martin, 2002; Nyqvist & Strandell, 1999). Compared to bottle feeding, preterm infants are more stable during cup feedings, with lower heart rates, higher oxygen saturations, and lower incidence of oxygen desaturations (Marinelli, Burke,

& Dodd, 2001; Rocha, Martinez, & Jorge, 2002) because the infant controls the pace and volume of milk intake (Lang, 1994).

> Cup feeding is the first choice as alternative oral feeding method, when full oral feeding cannot be achieved wholly by breastfeeding, and it can be introduced from a PMA of 29 weeks. A cup is used (1) when the infant is awake for a feed in the mother's absence, and (2) after a breastfeed when the infant has not taken enough milk, does not want to suck, and is awake.

Tube Feeding

Compared to bottle supplements, preterm infants who received supplementation by tube were more likely to be breastfeeding at discharge (Kliethermes, Cross, Lanese, Johnson, & Simon, 1999). The use of a permanent indwelling naso- or orogastric feeding tube is common during the period of transition from full enteral to full oral feeding, but it may negatively influence sucking. Shiao et al. (1995) observed lower minute ventilation and tidal volume, lower pulse rate, and lower oxygen saturation when the infant sucked with a nasogastric tube than without the tube. Infants sucked more forcefully and took more milk without the tube. Pacifier sucking during tube feeding has been associated with decreased intestinal transit time and more rapid weight gain (Bernbaum, Pereira, Watkins, & Peckham, 1983) and a decrease in restless states (DiPietro, Cusson, Caughy, & Fox, 1994).

One approach is to regard tube feeding as an invasive practice and limit tube feeding to situations when an infant cannot be fed by cup because of prematurity, medical problems, or exhaustion. This policy is supported by evidence of risks for poor sucking ability and feeding problems in infants with prolonged exposure to tube feeding (Bier, Ferguson, Cho, & Vohr, 1993; Hawdon, Beauregard, Slattery, & Kennedy, 2000). On the other hand, the use of an indwelling tube is justified when the infant cannot be fed orally because of serious illness or when frequent tube feeding is needed. An infant with an occasional tube feeding requirement can have a new tube inserted and removed in connection with each feed. Staff can offer to teach parents how to tube feed as soon as the infant shows sufficient physiologic stability during feeding. Parents can also be offered the opportunity to perform tube insertion, especially in case of early discharge for home care.

> A breastfeeding-friendly tube feeding policy should include the following components:
>
> - Preferably, the infant is held (ideally skin to skin) by a parent while being fed.
> - An infant who has commenced breastfeeding is tube-fed at the mother's breast.
> - An infant who cannot be positioned at the mother's breast during tube feeding, including infants with ventilator or CPAP treatment, is offered
>   - the opportunity to suck a pacifier during each tube feed
>   - a small portion of breastmilk (0.5–1.0 ml) in the beginning of each tube feed by gentle administration via a syringe on one side of the tongue, combined with pacifier sucking

Bottle Feeding: An Exception When the Mother Intends to Breastfeed

In addition to the negative physiological effects, bottle feeding constitutes an obstacle to breastfeeding because facial muscles are activated in a way that differs from the oral motor pattern used during breastfeeding. Bottle feeding promotes the view of feeding as the provision of fixed volumes at fixed intervals by anybody—it does not require the mother's presence. Furthermore, it is mainly a feeding method, in contrast with breastfeeding, which is also the newborn infant's main strategy for self-regulation during the process of adaptation to the extrauterine environment.

In a feeding policy based on prioritizing breastfeeding, bottle feeding is considered appropriate when the mother

- is unable to breastfeed for medical reasons
- is unable to attain a milk production that satisfies her infant's needs in spite of her efforts
- does not intend to breastfeed, which ought to be a result of an informed decision and can have psychological explanations
- explicitly demands to use a bottle after information about advantages of cup feeding and reasons for a restrictive attitude toward bottle feeding

Nipple Shield

For term infants, caution is recommended by some authors regarding the use of nipple shields because of a possible risk of reduced milk transfer. In contrast, mothers' use of a nipple shield while breastfeeding their preterm babies was associated with higher milk consumption (Meier et al., 2000). Indications for nipple shield use, mentioned by these authors, were when the infant had difficulties in latching onto or staying fixed at the breast. The shield also helped to remind infants about sucking when they kept falling asleep at the breast; it resulted in longer sucking bursts and longer periods of wakefulness.

Transition from Full or Partial Enteral Feeding to Full Breastfeeding

The following guidelines are based on evidence and clinical experience in the unit where the author is working. Since their introduction, the PMA when infants reach full breastfeeding has decreased gradually. Healthy preterm infants are often discharged with full breastfeeding around 1 month before the expected date of birth, many at 34 weeks, and several at 33 weeks. A few infants reach full breastfeeding at 32 weeks (**Table 7-6**).

Initiation of Breastfeeding

Breastfeeding is initiated as soon as the infant has been weaned off the ventilator and CPAP and does not show severe physiologic instability, irrespective of current PMA, age, or weight. (Exceptions can be made for moderately preterm infants with CPAP who are

Table 7-6 Breastfeeding Progress in a Very Preterm Girl

Infant: GA at birth: 30 weeks + 5 days, birth weight 1,525 g, length 41 cm, ventilator treatment 8 hours, CPAP 12 hours.

Mother: Multipara, age 39 years, nonsmoker

Day	PMA	Weight, g	Events Related to Feeding/Breastfeeding
0	30 + 5	1,525	Tube feeding, every 3 hours donor milk and colostrum.
1	30 + 6	1,525	Tube feeding, donor milk, and mother's own milk.
2	31 + 0	1,495	Commenced breastfeeding. Nurses' report: "Sucks very well, hungry." Cup fed in mother's absence.
3	31 + 0	1,425	Lowest weight (-7%)
4	31 + 2		Mother transfers to parent room in the NICU.
5	31 + 3	1,445	Milk intake 9 times: 1–25 ml. Tube fed 4 times.
9	32 + 0	1,530	Regained birth weight.
10	32 + 1	1,555	Semi-demand feeding introduced. Tube fed once. Transferred from incubator to water bed in open crib.
11	32 + 2	1,555	Reached exclusive breastfeeding: 20–50 ml. "Spent the night in the mother's bed."
12	32 + 3	1,595	Test-weighing is terminated.
14	32 + 5	1,645	Water bed removed from open crib.
15	32 + 6	1,650	Home care by parents.
18	33 + 2	1,749	Discharged from hospital. Follow-up at neonatal follow-up clinic in hospital and local child health center.

sufficiently stable and dissatisfied with just pacifier sucking.) Additional oxygen via nasal prongs (nasal cannula) is no obstacle. The first time a mother positions her infant at the breast, suggestions are given about alternative breastfeeding positions, and a breastfeeding observation is made. Breastfeeding sessions are not restricted in frequency or duration. The timing and volume of supplementary feeds are planned on an individual basis to ensure attainment of a sufficient daily milk volume. The assessment of the infant's need of supplementation, timing, volume, and feeding method is made jointly by the mother and nurse in charge.

Breastfeeding mothers in the maternity unit are encouraged to come for breastfeeding during the night, and—upon agreement—the nurse telephones the mother when her infant wakes. When a mother leaves the neonatal unit, she informs the nurse how long she will be absent and how she can be reached (telephone, cell phone).

Transition from Scheduled Interval Feeding, to Semidemand Feeding, to Demand Feeding

Internationally, feeding regimens based on intervals of 2-, 3-, and 4-hour feeds are common in infants who are not breastfed fully. However, small infants tolerate frequent feeding intervals of 2 hours, with small volumes, more easily. The advantage of an initial 2-hourly feeding schedule is the message conveyed to the mother that a frequent feeding pattern, resembling breastfeeding, is natural. For very small preterm infants, hourly feeds may be even more appropriate.

Test weighing is introduced at signs of milk intake at the breast—audible swallowing or appearance of fresh milk when the feeding tube location is assessed by aspiration of gastric contents with a syringe. The goal is to reduce the number of tube feeds and the duration of the infant's exposure to a tube and to facilitate early attainment of exclusive breastfeeding. Mothers who find test weighing stressful are offered alternative strategies for reduction of supplementation (discussed later).

As soon as the infant ingests about half the volume of milk prescribed for a feed (once is enough), the scheduled interval feeding regimen is terminated and a total daily milk volume is prescribed. The mother is reminded that a variable intake pattern is normal in breastfed children. The mother is encouraged to offer the breast to the infant (1) whenever the infant shows any sign of interest, and (2) when a maximum of about 3 hours have passed since the last breastfeed, in order to encourage state transition; the sensation of the nipple touching the mouth and the taste of milk may elicit awakening.

The volumes of milk taken at the breast are recorded and added. The mother and the nurse decide jointly when the infant needs supplementation by tube or cup in order to reach the daily volume. The nurse responsible for each shift has the ultimate responsibility for ensuring consumption of the target daily volume. When the infant reaches full breastfeeding (or partial breastfeeding, when mixed feeding is required), test weighing is discontinued. The infant is weighed once a day or every 2–3 days initially to ensure adequate weight gain.

> Definitions used here:
>
> Semidemand feeding (or ad libitum feeding): Constant assessment of the infant's feeding cues for facilitation of frequent breastfeeding, combined with active encouragement of breastfeeding after long periods of rest, with supplemental feeds given whenever needed in order to reach the daily prescribed milk volume.
>
> Demand feeding: The neurological development has reached a stage when the brain is able to coregulate behavioral states with hunger and satiety, and feeding can be based entirely on the infant's hunger cues.

When the infant reaches term age, the immature sucking pattern is replaced by a mature sucking pattern with long bursts of rhythmical sucking interspersed with breathing, and the infant can safely be fed on demand. Many infants are discharged home from the hospital fully breastfeeding when they are still premature. Their mothers usually need to keep up the semidemand regimen for some time; they may have to awaken the infant, day and night, to avoid overly long interfeed intervals and reach a sufficient number of feeds per day. This is crucial for avoiding breastfeeding malnutrition; an infant who does not consume enough milk does not grow or may even lose weight, may present with late hyperbilirubinemia, and may become dehydrated with high levels of sodium and chloride (hypernatremic dehydration), a serious condition that is prevented by adequate breastfeeding and/or supplemental feeding by cup or tube when indicated (Cooper, Atherton, Kahana, & Kotagal, 1995).

The infant's feeding plan is established jointly by the mother or parents and the nursing staff. A graph can be used to identify the infant's current phase in the establishment of breastfeeding together with the mother and to prepare her for the following phases (**Figure 7-5**).

Strategies for the Transition from Enteral Feeding to Breastfeeding

Test Weighing

When the infant shows progress in milk intake, test weighing boosts mothers' confidence. It proves their infant's actual intake, is helpful for planning supplementation, and may reduce the time required to reach full breastfeeding. No difference in breastfeeding confidence was found between mothers of preterm infants who used test weighing during

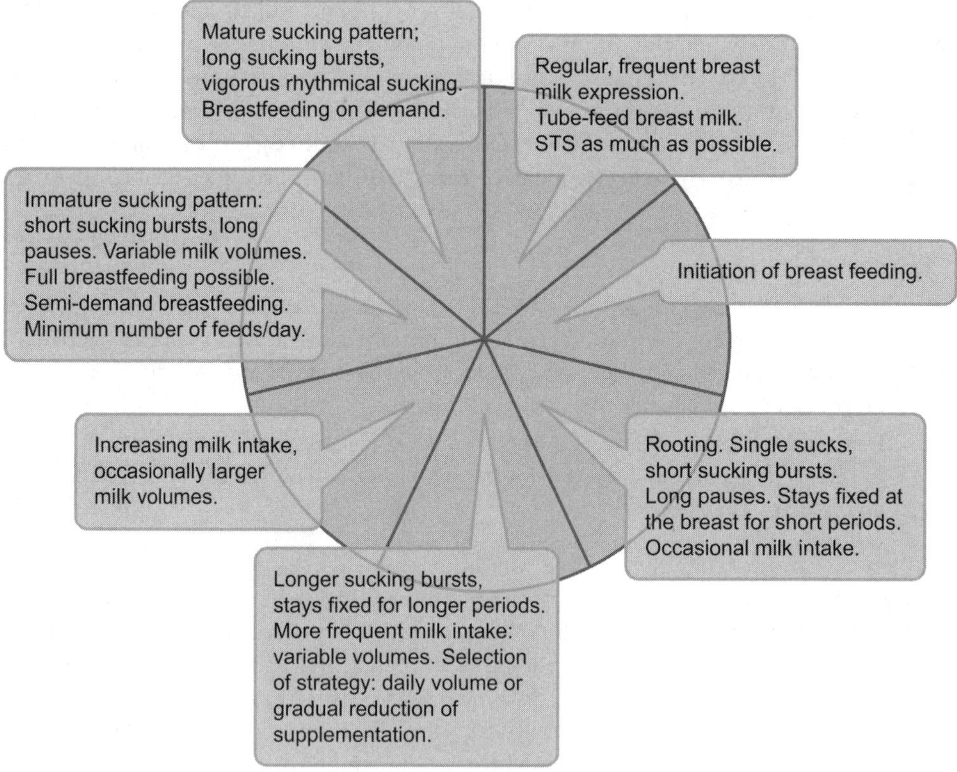

Figure 7-5 Phases in the mother and infant's progress in breast milk feeding and breastfeeding.

hospitalization and those who did not (Hall, Shearer, Mogan, & Berkowitz, 2002). Mothers of preterm infants who are discharged early in the process of establishing breastfeeding may find test weighing particularly valuable (Kavanaugh, Mead, Meier & Mangurten, 1995) because the primary concerns of these mothers are adequacy of their milk production and milk transfer to their infants (Hill, Hanson, & Mefford, 1994).

Gradual Reduction of Supplementation or According to Clinical Indices

Another alternative is to reduce supplementation gradually according to a schedule. A third approach is to base decisions on the assessment of the infant's sucking vigor and pattern and sounds of audible swallowing, so-called clinical indices of milk intake. However, this method is not reliable for evaluation of milk intake when used by mothers and nurses, not even in healthy children born at term (Meier, Engstrom, Fleming, Streeter, & Lawrence, 1996).

No differences in rates of any or exclusive breastfeeding at discharge were found between two Swedish neonatal intensive care units (NICUs); one applied test weighing and the other applied gradual reduction and clinical indices (Funkquist, Tuvemo, Jonsson, Serenius, & Nyqvist, 2010). However, the infants in the test-weighing NICU attained exclusive breastfeeding and were discharged at a lower PMA than the other NICU: median (range) 36 (33–38) versus 37 (34–39) weeks. Nevertheless, test weighing may constitute a risk of making breastfeeding seem like fulfillment of a duty and cause feelings of guilt if the mother is unable to produce or transfer enough milk (Flacking, Ewald, Nyqvist, & Starrin, 2006).

Individual Strategies

A middle course between these strategies is to ask mothers what they perceive as helpful. When the infant's progress is slow, the test-weighing procedure may become an additional source of stress and disappointment for the mother. Instead of opportunities for enjoyable interaction, breastfeeding may be perceived as merely a way of providing nutrition, a duty to be fulfilled. In that case, gradual reduction of milk volumes is preferred. If the mother wishes, test weighing can be performed for a 24-hour period once or twice a week for assessment of the pace of supplement reduction.

Early Discharge and Home Care

The usual criteria for transfer of the infant to home care are medical stability, absence of apneic episodes, ability to maintain normal body temperature in an open crib (with clothes, cap, and adequate bedding or by SSC), and some oral intake at the breast. Parental criteria are readiness to take their infant home, ability to feed by tube and/or cup, and reported confidence in taking over the infant's care. Basic requirements are a safe home environment, access to a telephone, and means of transportation to the hospital. Scales should provided free of charge as long as the infant is test weighed. A minimum period of 1 or a couple of days at home before the infant's formal discharge from the hospital, with telephone support, is required as a trial period. Daily rounds and communication about the infant's growth and planning of the infant's feeding occurs over the telephone. The parents have access to telephone counselling by a nurse and neonatologist around the clock and can return to the hospital whenever they wish. Before formal discharge from the neonatal unit, relevant information about the infant, including breastfeeding status, is communicated to the local child health center (child health services are provided free of charge in Sweden). The infant's health and growth is monitored carefully at the neonatal follow-up clinic and the child health center.

The Kangaroo Mother Care Method

At the same time as practices evolved in industrialized countries stipulating assessment of preterm infants' readiness to feed and advocating caution in introduction of oral feeding, the Kangaroo Mother Care (KMC) method was launched in Colombia (Gomez, Sanabria, & Marquette, 1992). KMC is based on kangaroo position, kangaroo feeding policy, and early discharge in kangaroo position. Alternative articles of clothing used for holding an infant in the kangaroo position are shown in **Figures 7-6 and 7-7**. Cup or spoon feeding is used to supplement breastfeeding. Outcomes in terms of improved lactation and breastfeeding have been noted (Hurst, Valentine, Renfro, Burns, & Ferlic, 1997). In a multicenter study of KMC, the breastfeeding and breastmilk feeding rates at discharge were 83%, 98%, and 80% (Cattaneo, Davanzo, Worku, et al., 1998).

In the Western world, SSC periods of about 1 hour per day are common, not necessarily occurring every day. But as evidence of benefits of the method kept appearing, the International Network on Kangaroo Mother Care recommended that in settings with ample healthcare and medical resources, "KMC can be applied to LBW infants of any postconceptional age from 28 weeks and onward, of any gestational age, of any weight (as low as 600 g), . . . as tolerated by the mother–infant dyad, by the family and by the health care system"

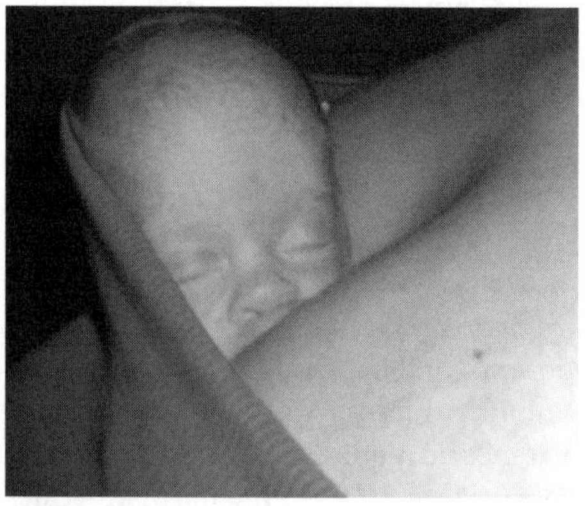

Figure 7-6 Kangaroo care blouse.

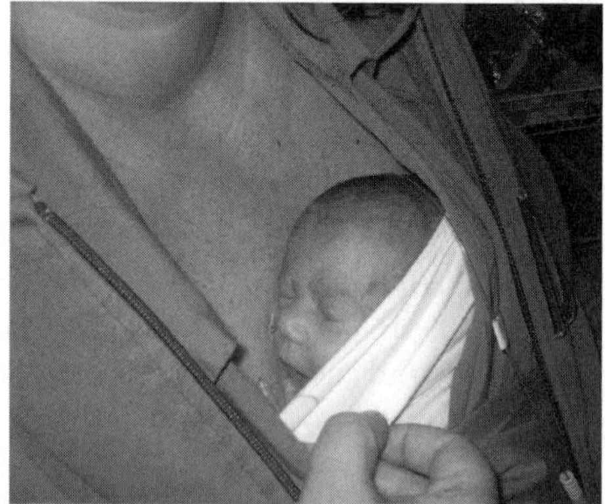

Figure 7-7 Kangaroo care top.

(Cattaneo, Davanzo, Uxa, & Tamburlini, 1998). In 2003, the World Health Organization included KMC among the methods recommended for high-quality neonatal care and published guidelines for practical implementation (World Health Organization, 2003).

Table 7-7 describes a moderately preterm infant who had nearly uninterrupted SSC contact with his mother (father acting as substitute) during his hospital stay. He was placed on his mother's chest immediately after birth and transported in this position to the NICU, where his parents roomed in with him in a parent room. The mother breastfed at any subtle cue of interest from her baby, initially twice per hour. During nights the mother coslept with him in the kangaroo position. Because his mother breastfed him frequently and he sucked well, no supplementation was introduced. Regular blood glucose tests were made, and his weight was followed closely. The reader is reminded that most preterm infants require variable periods of supplementation by tube and/or cup before they are breastfed fully. The case report is presented to highlight the need for reevaluation of current common feeding policies and practices with a view to modifying them so they agree with infants' actual abilities. In an industrialized country such as Sweden, continuous KMC—including uninterrupted KMC from birth, when possible—may be accepted by most parents, may have a favorable impact on breastfeeding, and may reduce the duration of the infants' hospital stay.

Conclusion

By learning from evidence and experience from different parts of the world, lactation consultants can improve policies and practices, which will help mothers of preterm infants to attain their personal goals for breastfeeding in the best possible way.

Table 7-7 Continuous Kangaroo Mother Care from Birth

Infant: GA 34 weeks + 4 days, birth weight 2,835 g, vaginal birth, Apgar 9-9-10
Mother: multipara, age 30 years, nonsmoker

Day	PMA	Weight, g	Events Related to Feeding/Breastfeeding
0	34 + 4	2,835	Uninterrupted skin-to-skin contact with mother from birth. Very frequent breastfeeding (initially twice/hour). No supplementation. Regular B-Glucose tests.
3	35 + 0	2,578	Lowest weight (-9%).
4	35 + 1	2,635	STS interrupted for phototherapy on water bed in an open crib 1 day because of hyperbilirubinemia.
5	35 + 2	2,670	Bilirubin levels do not require treatment. B-Glucose tests never showed any hypoglycemia. Home care program.
8	35 + 5	2,734	Discharge from hospital with exclusive breastfeeding. Never required any supplementation. Follow-up at neonatal follow-up program in hospital and local child health center.

References

Als, H., Lawhon, G., Duffy, F. H., McAnulty, G. B., Gibes-Grossman, R., & Blickman, J. G. (1994). Individualized developmental care for the very low-birth-weight preterm infant. *JAMA, 272,* 853-858.

Becker, P. T., Grunwald, P. C., Moorman, J., & Stuhr, S. (1991). Outcomes of developmentally supportive nursing care for very-low-birth-weight infants. *Nursing Research, 0,* 150-155.

Bernbaum, J. C., Pereira, G. R., Watkins, J. B., & Peckham, G. J. (1983). Nonnutritive sucking during gavage feeding enhances growth and maturation in premature infants. *Pediatrics, 71*(1), 41-45.

Bier, J. A., Ferguson, A., Cho, C., Oh, W., & Vohr, B. (1993). The oral motor development of low-birth weight infants who underwent orotracheal intubation during the neonatal period. *American Journal of Diseases in Children, 147,* 858-862.

Blaymore Bier, J. A., Ferguson, A. E., Morales, Y., Liebling, J. A., Oh, W., & Vohr, B. R. (1997). Breastfeeding infants who were extremely low birth weight. *Pediatrics, 100,* e3.

Cattaneo, A., Davanzo, R., Uxa, F., & Tamburlini, F. (for International Network on Kangaroo Mother Care). (1998). Recommendations for the implementation of kangaroo mother care for low birth-weight infants. *Acta Paediatrica, II*(87), 440-445.

Cattaneo, A., Davanzo, R., Worku, B., Surjono, A., Echeverria, M., Bedri, A., & Tamburlini, G. (1998). Kangaroo mother care for low birthweight infants. A randomized controlled trial in different settings. *Acta Paediatrica, I*(87), 976-985.

Chen, C. H., Wang, T. M., Chang, H. M., & Chi, C. S. (2000). The effect of breast- and bottle-feeding on oxygen saturation and body temperature in preterm infants. *Journal of Human Lactation, 16,* 21-27.

Comrie, J. D., & Helm, J. M. (1997). Common feeding problems in the intensive care nursery: Maturation, organization, evaluation and management strategies. *Seminars of Speech and Language, 18,* 239-261.

Cooper, W. O., Atherton, H. D., Kahana, M., & Kotagal, U. R. (1995). Increased incidence of severe breastfeeding malnutrition and hypernatremia in a metropolitan area. *Pediatrics, 96*(5 Pt. 1), 957-960.

Cousins, R. (1999). Breast feeding the preterm infant in the special care baby unit: The first feed. *Journal of Neonatal Nursing, 5,* 10-14.

Cregan, M. D., De Mello, T. R., Kershaw, D., McDougall, K., & Hartmann, P. E. (2002). Initiation of lactation in women after preterm delivery. *Acta Obstetrica Gynecologica Scandinavica, 81,* 870-877.

Davies, A. M., Koenig, J. S., & Thatch, B. T. (1988). Upper airway chemoreflex responses to saline and water in preterm infants. *Journal of Applied Physiology, 64*(4), 1412-1420.

DiPietro, J. A., Cusson, R. M., Caughy, M. O., & Fox, N. A. (1994). Behavioral and physiologic effects of nonnutritive sucking during gavage feeding in preterm infants. *Pediatric Research, 36*(2), 207-214.

Dowling, D. A. (1999). Physiological responses of preterm infants to breast-feeding and bottle-feeding with the orthodontic nipple. *Nursing Research, 48,* 78-85.

Dowling, D. A., Meier, P. P., DiFiore, J. M., Blatz, M., & Martin R. J. (2002). Cup-feeding for preterm infants: Mechanics and safety. *Journal of Human Lactation, 18,* 13-20.

Feldman, R., & Eidelman, A. I. (2003). Direct and indirect effects of breast milk on the neurobehavioral and cognitive development of premature infants. *Developmental Psychobiology, 43,* 109-119.

Flacking, R., Ewald, U., Nyqvist, K. H., & Starrin, B. (2006). Trustful bonds: A key to "becoming a mother" and reciprocal breastfeeding. Stories of mothers of very preterm infants at a neonatal unit. *Social Science and Medicine, 62*(1), 70-80.

Funkquist, E. L., Tuvemo, T., Jonsson, B., Serenius, F., & Nyqvist, K. H. (2010). Influence of test weighing before/after nursing on breastfeeding in preterm infants. *Advances in Neonatal Care, 10,* 33-39.

Furman, L., Minich, N., & Hack, M. (2002). Correlates of lactation in mothers of very low birth weight infants. *Pediatrics, 109*(4), e57(e57).

Gomez, H. M., Sanabria, E. R., & Marquette, C. M. (1992). The mother kangaroo programme. *International Journal of Child Health, 3*(1), 55-67.

Gupta, A., Khanna, K., & Chattree, S. (1999). Cup feeding: An alternative to bottle feeding in a neonatal intensive care unit. *Journal of Tropical Pediatrics, 45*, 108–110.

Hall, W. A., Shearer, K., Mogan, J., & Berkowitz, J. (2002). Weighing preterm infants before and after breastfeeding: Does it increase maternal confidence and competence? *American Journal of Maternal and Child Nursing, 27*(6), 318–326.

Hanlon, M. B., Tripp, J. H., Ellis, R. E., Flack, F. C., Selley, W. G., & Shoesmith, H. J. (1997). Deglution apnea as indicator of maturation of suckle feeding in bottle-fed preterm infants. *Developmental Medicine and Child Neurology, 39*, 534–542.

Hawdon, J. M., Beauregard, M., Slattery, J., & Kennedy, G. (2000). Identification of neonates at risk of developing feeding problems in infancy. *Developmental Medicine and Child Neurology, 42*(4), 235–239.

Hill, P. D., Aldag, J. C., & Chatterton, R. T. (1999). Effects of pumping style on milk production in mothers of non-nursing preterm infants. *Journal of Human Lactation, 15*, 209–215.

Hill, P. D., Brown, L. P., & Harker, T. L. (1995). Initiation and frequency of breast expression in breastfeeding mothers of LBW and VLBW infants. *Nursing Research, 44*, 352–355.

Hill, P. D., Hanson, K. S., & Mefford, A. L. (1994). Mothers of low birthweight infants: Breastfeeding patterns and problems. *Journal of Human Lactation, 10*, 169–176.

Hurst, N., Valentine, C. J., Renfro, L., Burns, P., & Ferlic, L. (1997). Skin-to-skin holding in the neonatal intensive care unit influences maternal milk volume. *Journal of Perinatology, 17*(3), 213–217.

Jones, E., Dimmock, P. W., & Spencer, S. A. (2001). A randomised controlled trial to compare methods of milk expression after preterm delivery. *Archives of Disease in Childhood, Fetal and Neonatal Edition, 85*, F91–F95.

Kavanaugh, K., Mead, L., Meier P., & Mangurten, H. H. (1995). Getting enough: Mothers' concern about breastfeeding a preterm infant after discharge. *Journal of Obstetric, Gynecologic and Neonatal Nursing, 24*, 23–32.

Kliethermes, P. A., Cross, M. L., Lanese, M. G., Johnson, K. M., & Simon, S. D. (1999). Transitioning preterm infants with nasogastric tube supplementation: Increased likelihood of breastfeeding. *Journal of Obstetric, Gynaecologic and Neonatal Nursing, 28*, 264–273.

Lang, S. (1994). Cup-feeding. An alternative method. *Midwives Chronicle and Nursing Notes, 107*, 171–176.

Lemons, P. K. (2001). Breast milk and the hospitalized infant: Guidelines for practice. *Neonatal Network, 2087*, 47–52.

Malhotra, N., Vishwambaran, L., Sundaram, K. R., & Narayanan, I. (1999). A controlled trial of alternative methods of oral feeding in neonates. *Early Human Development, 54*, 29–38.

Marinelli, K. A., Burke, G. S., & Dodd, V. L. (2001). A comparison of the safety of cupfeedings and bottlefeedings in premature infants whose mothers intend to breastfeed. *Journal of Perinatology, 21*, 350–355.Mathew, O. P. (1988). Respiratory control during nipple feeding in preterm infants. *Pediatric Pulmonology, 5*, 220–224.

McCain, G. C. (2003). Evidence-based guidelines for introducing oral feeding to healthy preterm infants. *Neonatal Network, 22*(5), 45–50.

Meier, P. P. (2001). Breastfeeding in the special care nursery. Prematures and infants with medical problems. *Pediatric Clinics of North America, 48*, 425–442.

Meier, P., & Anderson, G. C. (1987). Responses of small preterm infants to bottle- and breastfeeding. *American Journal of Maternal and Child Nursing, 12*, 97–105.

Meier, P. M., Brown, L. P., Hurst, N. M., Spatz, D. L., Engstrom, J. L., Borucki, L. C., & Krause, A. M. (2000). Nipple shields for preterm infants: Effect on milk transfer and duration of breastfeeding. *Journal of Human Lactation, 16*(2), 106–114.

Meier, P. P., Engstrom, J. L., Fleming, B. A., Streeter, P. L., & Lawrence, P. B. (1996). Estimating milk intake of hospitalized preterm infants who breastfeed. *Journal of Human Lactation, 12*, 21–26.

Mörelius, E., Hellström-Westas, L., Carlén, C., Norman, E., & Nelson, N. (2006). Is a nappy change stressful to neonates? *Early Human Development, 82*(10), 669–676.

Morton, J., Hall, J. Y., Wong, R. J., Thairu, I., Benitz, W. E., & Rhine, W. D. (2009). Combining hand techniques with electric pumping increases milk production in mothers of preterm infants. *Journal of Perinatology, 29*, 757–764.

Nyqvist, K. H. (2001). The development of preterm infants' milk intake during breast feeding. *Journal of Neonatal Nursing,* (7), 48–52.

Nyqvist, K. H., & Ewald, U. (1999). Infant and maternal factors in the development of breastfeeding behavior and breastfeeding outcome in preterm infants. *Acta Paediatrica, 88*, 1194–1203.

Nyqvist, K. H., Ewald, U., & Sjödén, P.-O. (1996). Supporting a preterm infant's behaviour during breastfeeding: A case report. *Journal of Human Lactation, 12*(3), 221–228.

Nyqvist, K. H., Ewald, U., & Sjödén, P.-O. (1999). Development of preterm infants' breastfeeding behavior. *Early Human Development, 55*, 247–264.

Nyqvist, K. H., Farnstrand, C., Edebol Eeg-Olofsson, K., & Ewald, U. (2001). Early oral behaviour in preterm infants during breastfeeding: An EMG study. *Acta Pediatrica, 90*, 658–663.

Nyqvist, K. H., Rubertsson, C., Ewald, U., & Sjödén, P. O. (1996). Development of the preterm infant breastfeeding behavior scale (PIBBS), a study of nurse-mother agreement. *Journal of Human Lactation, 12*, 207–219.

Nyqvist, K. H., & Strandell, E. (1999). Evaluation of a cup feeding protocol in a neonatal intensive care unit. *Journal of Neonatal Nursing, 2*. 31–36.

Ohyama, M., Watabe, H., & Hayasaka, Y. (2010). Manual expression and electric breast pumping in the first 48 h after delivery. *Pediatrics International, 52*, 39–43.

Radzyminski, S. (2003). The effect of ultra low dose epidural analgesia on newborn breastfeeding behaviors. *Journal of Obstetric Gynecologic and Neonatal Nursing, 32*(3), 322–331.

Rocha, N. M. N., Martinez, M. E., & Jorge, S. M. (2002). Cup or bottle for preterm infants: Effects on oxygen saturation, weight gain, and breastfeeding. *Journal of Human Lactation, 18*, 132–138.

Ross, E. S., & Browne, J. V. (2002). Developmental progression of feeding skills: An approach to supporting feeding in preterm infants. *Seminars in Neonatology, 7*, 469–475.

Schanler, R. (2001). The use of human milk for premature infants. *Pediatric Clinics of North America, 48*, 207–219.

Shiao, S. Y. P. K., Youngblut, J. A. M., Anderson, G. C., DiFiore, J. M., & Martin, R. J. (1995). Nasogastric tube placement: Effects on breathing and sucking in very-low-birth-weight infants. *Nursing Research, 44*(2), 82–88.

Smith, M. M., Durkin, M., Hinton, V. J., Bellinger, D., & Kuhn, L.. (2003). Influence of breastfeeding on cognitive outcomes and age 6–8 years: Follow-up of very low birth weight infants. *American Journal of Epidemiology, 158*, 1075–1082.

Thelen, E., & Vogel, A. (1989). Toward an action-based theory of infant development. In J. Lockman & N. Hazen (Eds.), *Action in social context*. New York, NY: Plenum.

Thoyre, S. M., Shaker, C. S., & Pridham, K. F. (2005). The early feeding skills assessment for preterm infants. *Neonatal Network, 24*(3), 7–16.

Uvnas-Moberg, K., & Eriksson, M. (1996). Breastfeeding: Physiological, endocrine, and behavioural adaptations caused by oxytocin and local neurogenic activity in the nipple and mammary gland. *Acta Paediatrica, 85*, 525–530.

Wheeler, J. L., Johnson, M., Collie, L., Sutherland, D., & Chapman, C. (1999). Promoting breastfeeding in the neonatal intensive care unit. *Breastfeeding Review, 7*, 15–18.

White-Traut, R. C., Berbaum, M. L., Lessen, B., McFarlin, B., & Cardenas, L. (2005). Feeding readiness in preterm infants. *American Journal of Maternal and Child Nursing, 30*(1), 52–59.

World Health Organization. (2003). *Kangaroo mother care: A practical guide*. Geneva, Switzerland: Author.

CHAPTER 8

The Influence of Anatomic and Structural Issues on Sucking Skills

Catherine Watson Genna

Ankyloglossia (Tongue-Tie)

Ankyloglossia, or tongue-tie, is considered a minor anomaly. It may be isolated or may occur with other midline defects. Ankyloglossia is caused by insufficient apoptosis during prenatal differentiation of the tongue from the floor of the mouth. The cells that attach the tongue to the floor of the mouth normally regress from anterior to posterior, leaving a small remnant of attachment called the lingual frenulum. The lingual frenulum is an extension of the oral mucosa to the tongue and is poorly vascularized and poorly innervated at birth. If the lingual frenulum is too inelastic or too short, if it failed to regress and extends along the underside of the tongue, or if it is placed too close to the gum ridge, tongue function will be restricted. Many combinations of length, placement, and elasticity are possible, affording a wide range of potential effects on feeding skills.

Tongue Mobility

Tongue mobility is often assessed by the infant's ability to extend the tongue tip over the gum ridge. Tongue extension in a tongue-tied infant generally decreases as the infant opens the mouth wider (tongue retraction increases with gape). Because a wide gape is vital to a deep latch, and the tongue contacting the breast is the stimulus for latch, tongue retraction interferes with attachment. Retraction (pulling back) with gape may cause the infant who can keep the tongue over the gum ridge while sucking an adult finger to be unable to do so during breastfeeding, where a wider gape is required (**Figure 8-1**). The presence of the tongue tip over the lower gum during sucking is important to prevent the bite reflex from being stimulated. Normally, the tongue tip extends over the lower lip with the mouth wide open. Tongue extension can be elicited by a touch to the front (not the tooth-bearing surface) of the lower gum in infants (**Figure 8-2**). Infants with slightly more posterior tongue attachments may be able to extend the tongue over the gum ridge, but traction from the restrictive frenulum will cause the tongue tip to be pulled under and the posterior tongue to elevate (**Figure 8-3**).

Tongue elevation is more vital in suckling because elevation of the anterior tongue stabilizes the breast in the mouth while the posterior tongue depresses to draw milk out.

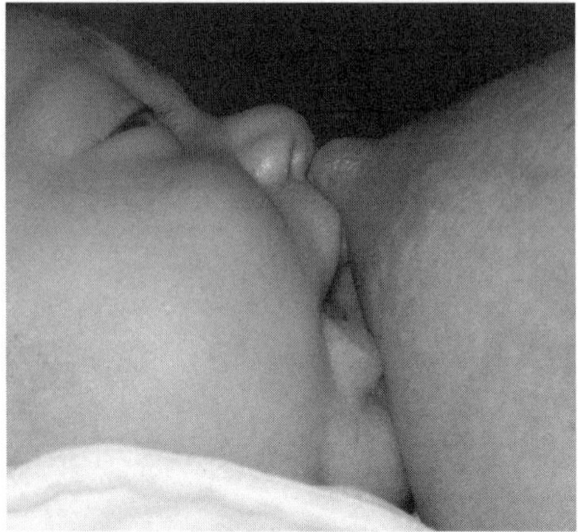

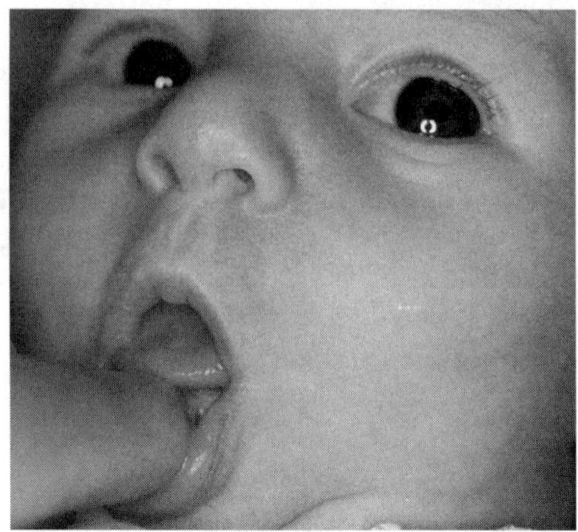

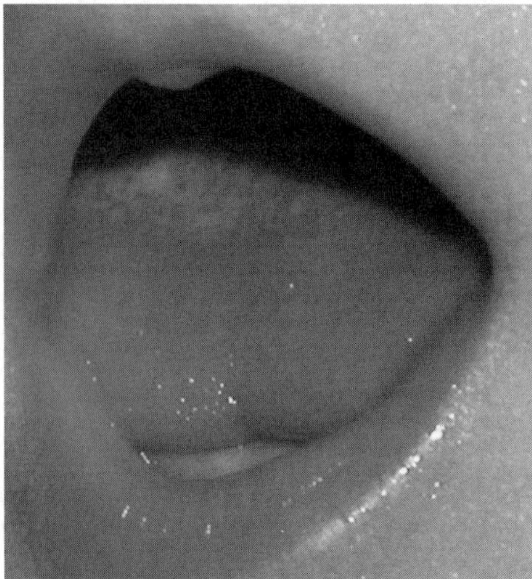

Figure 8-1 (top left) Tongue retraction with gape prevents the infant from grasping the breast.

Figure 8-2 (top right) Stimulating tongue extension by touch to the front surface of the lower gum. Note that in normal tongue extension, the tongue tip remains flat and extends well out over the lower lip.

Figure 8-3 (left) Restricted extension due to tongue tie.

The sequential front-to-back wavelike movements of the anterior tongue may also move milk toward the pharynx during swallowing and are probably important in initiating a coordinated swallow. Tongue elevation can be assessed during crying. The infant should be able to elevate the tongue blade more than half way to the palate with the mouth wide open (**Figure 8-4**). The exact degree of tongue elevation needed for comfortable, effective breastfeeding is still debated. Infants who can elevate the tongue tip to the palate with the mouth wide open are unlikely to have breastfeeding difficulties, but some who can bring the tongue tip to midmouth can breastfeed. Infants who cry with the tongue flat in the mouth or with just a small portion of the anterior tongue curled back are tongue-tied. The results of frenotomy seem to be proportional to the degree of restoration of normal tongue elevation. If no opportunity is found to observe crying (the author certainly is not in favor of stimulating it!), holding the alert infant in an en face position and talking to him or her will stimulate reciprocal mouth movements and allow visualization of the upper surface (dorsum) of the tongue. A dent or pulled-down area at the forward extent of the lingual frenulum may be noted as the infant talks back. Lifting the tongue with a grooved director, tongue depressor, or finger will generally reveal a restrictive frenulum, as will palpation under the tongue with a fingertip coming from the side toward midline (**Figures 8-5 and 8-6**).

The sides of the tongue need to elevate to groove the tongue longitudinally to help form a teat from the nipple and surrounding areola, to stabilize it in the mouth, and to help form milk into a bolus for a controlled swallow. The lateral edges of the tongue (sides) contact the palate to make a tunnel to control the milk bolus for a safe, controlled swallow (Yang, Loveday, Metreweli, & Sullivan, 1997). This may be more difficult in tongue-tied infants both because of their restrictive frenulum and the higher, more narrow palate that results from lack of normal tongue pressure in utero and during breastfeeding. In some tongue-tied infants, the frenulum is sufficiently elastic for the grooving to occur; in others grooving is weak (**Figure 8-7**). Grooving can be assessed by allowing the infant to suck a finger and assessing how well the sides of the tongue hug the finger.

Lateralization (the ability to move the tongue tip to the sides of the mouth) is more important in eating solids than during suckling, when lateralization moves food repeatedly to the chewing surfaces of the teeth and after the meal allows the tongue tip to remove food trapped between teeth (**Figure 8-8**). Nevertheless, the inability to lateralize the tongue tip to at least the corners of the mouth without twisting the body of the tongue is a good sign of ankyloglossia that requires treatment (**Figure 8-9**). Twisting of the tongue is a normal movement that is useful for pushing solids to the teeth during

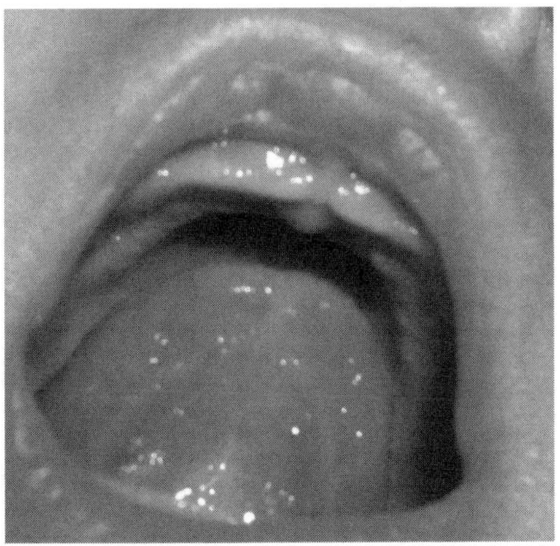

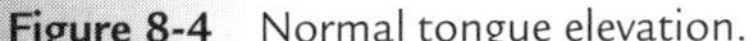

Figure 8-4 Normal tongue elevation.

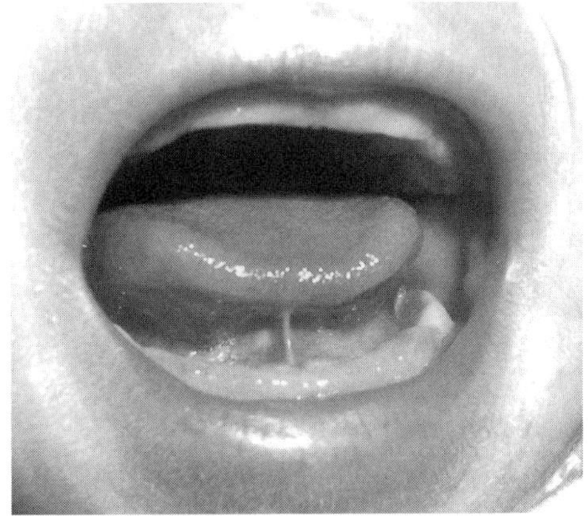

Figure 8-5 Restricted tongue elevation due to ankyloglossia (tongue-tie).

chewing (Hiiemae & Palmer, 2003), but it does not substitute for lateralization (**Figure 8-10**). Tongue-tied adults report that eating and swallowing are easier after frenotomy.

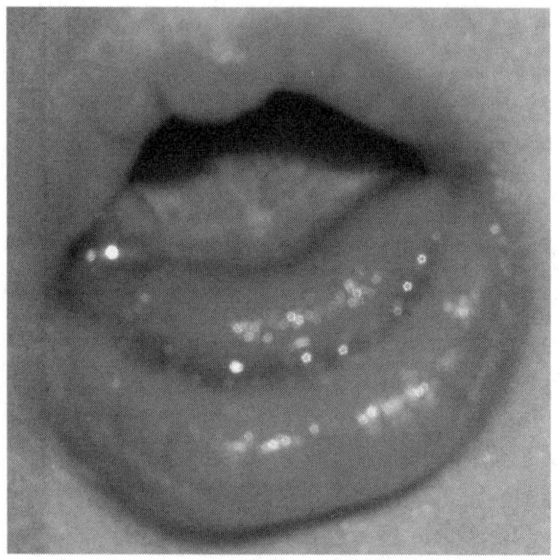

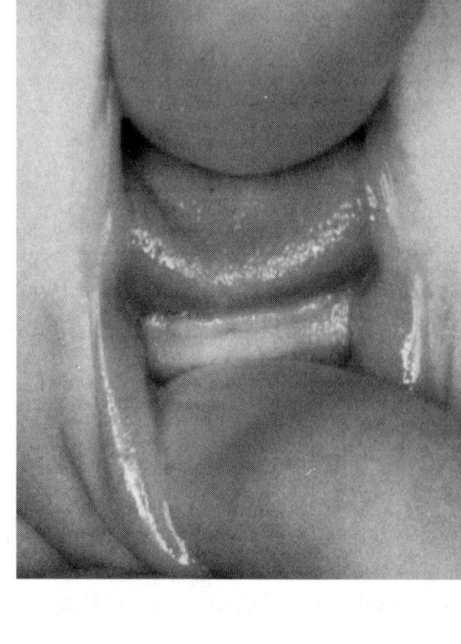

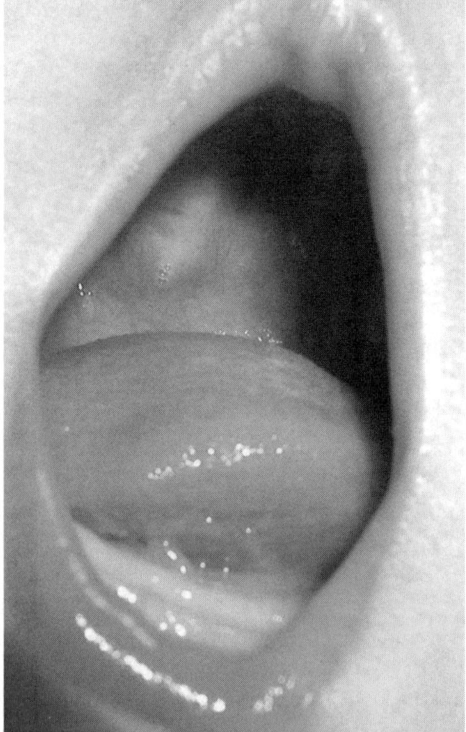

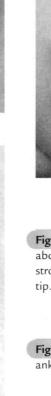

Figure 8-6 (top left) Posterior tongue-tie from above. Note how the tongue is pulled down strongly by the frenulum well behind the tongue tip.

Figure 8-7 (top right) Weak grooving due to ankyloglossia.

Figure 8-8 (left) Normal lateralization.

Lateralization is uncommonly observed spontaneously in young infants, but it can be stimulated by running a finger along the outside of the lower gum ridge from one side to the other. The tongue tip should be able to follow the finger at least to the corners of the lips with the body of the tongue held stationary in midline.

Examination of the hard palate may help to identify tongue-tied infants who require treatment. The palate forms from three plates, a small anterior midline primary palate and larger lateral palatine shelves. The shelves grow over the tongue and meet each other in midline, and they merge with the primary palate. Normal tongue movements in utero spread the forming palate into a broad U shape (**Figure 8-11**). Ankyloglossia prevents

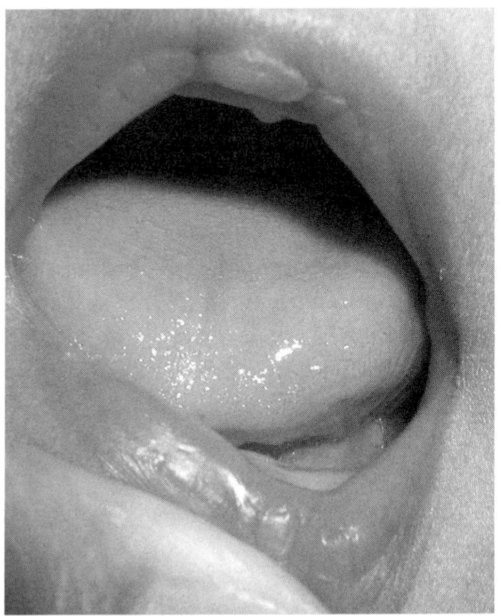

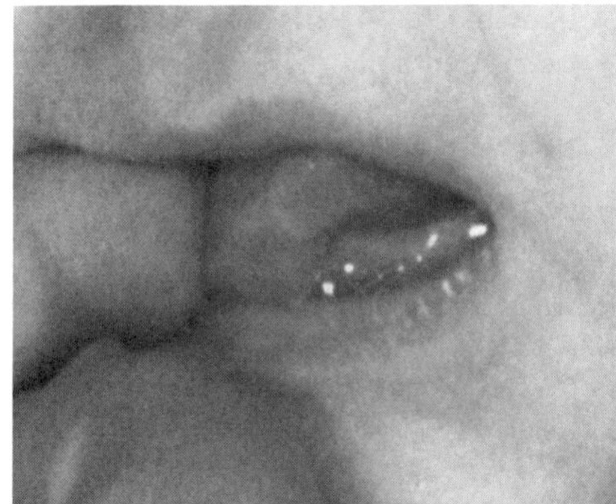

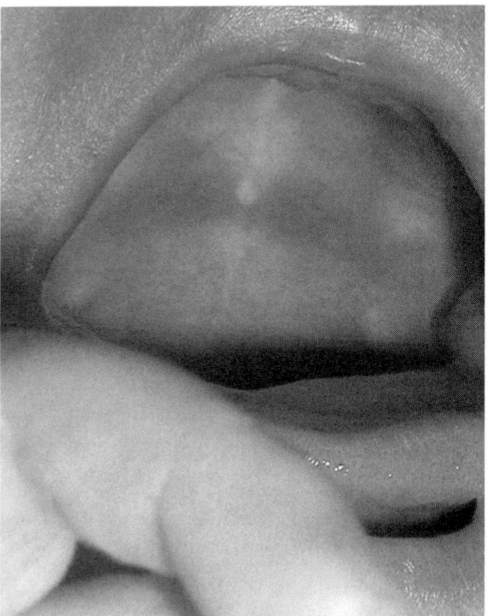

Figure 8-9 (top left) Restricted lateralization in complete tongue-tie. Note the large sucking blister on the upper lip.

Figure 8-10 (top right) Twisting on lateralization in posterior (submucosal) tongue-tie.

Figure 8-11 (left) Normal palate.

palatal spreading and will leave tongue-tied infants with a high, arched, and narrow palate (**Figures 8-12 and 8-13**). The severity of the palatal distortion is proportional to the degree of tongue restriction. Reduced tongue strength, tone, and range of motion due to neurological disorders can also lead to abnormal palate shape (Chapter 11).

Finally, allowing an infant to suck on a (suitably clean and covered) finger can be particularly helpful in assessing tongue mobility. Most infants will suck differently with and without fluid flow, so the use of an eyedropper or syringe of milk is important to get the true picture. Curved-tip syringes are particularly useful for this purpose because they are inexpensive and the tip can be inserted against the finger without disrupting the infant's lip seal. An infant with normal tongue mobility will use a biphasic pattern during sucking—a slow downward movement of the posterior tongue associated with a slight opening of the jaw while the anterior tongue and lips remain sealed on the finger (the suck) followed by a rapid backward wavelike movement along the anterior tongue with posterior and upward movement of the back of the tongue (the swallow). Graduation of pressure is normal; most infants will use progressively more positive and negative pressure until milk is delivered. Tongue retraction so that the lower gum ridge is felt; excessive negative pressure such that the sucking is uncomfortable; and chewing, sliding, thrusting, excessive humping, or bumping movements of the tongue are all abnormal. In some tongue-tied infants, tongue elevation is so restricted that the finger can be withdrawn from the mouth without any resistance. Infants who make no negative pressure in the mouth should also be examined for the presence of a submucosal or overt cleft of the hard or soft palate (which are discussed later in this chapter).

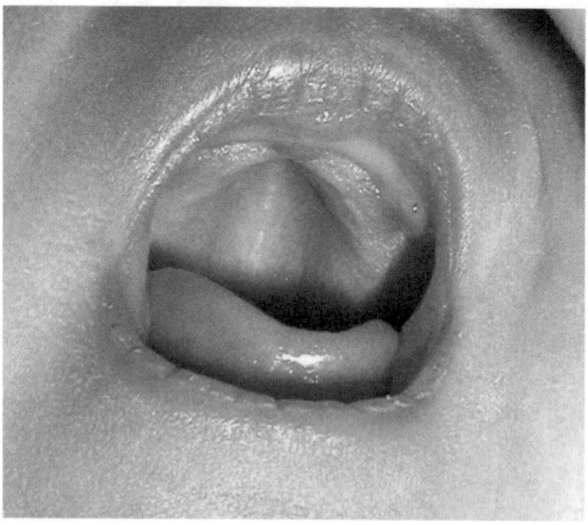

Figure 8-12 High, narrow, "V"-shaped palate in an infant with type 3 tongue-tie.

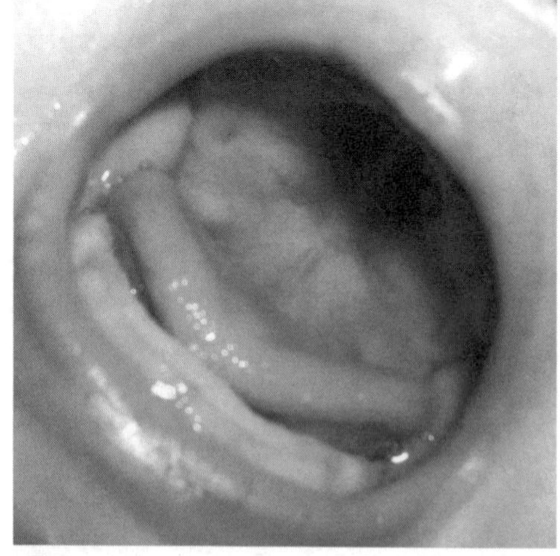

Figure 8-13 High, narrow palate in an infant with type 1 tongue-tie. Note the flat, retracted tongue.

Hazelbaker advocated the examination of multiple tongue movements in her Assessment Tool for Lingual Frenulum Function (ATLFF) (Hazelbaker, 1993). The ATLFF is a screening tool that identifies anterior ankyloglossia and has been used to identify infants requiring treatment in newborn nursery and lactation clinic settings (Ballard, Auer, & Khoury, 2002). Substantial interrater reliability was found in the function section for the characteristics of lift (elevation), extension, and lateralization (Amir, James, & Donath, 2006), with excellent agreement that frenotomy is indicated if the score on these three items is 4 or lower. Other authors have found that the sole reliance on this tool yielded a high rate of unclassified infants (Madlon-Kay, Ricke, Baker, & DeFor, 2008) and false negatives (Ricke, Baker, Madlon-Kay, & DeFor, 2005). The ATLFF was modified in 2010 to reflect recent research in an effort to better identify infants who require frenotomy.

The Frenotomy Decision Rule for Breastfeeding Infants is a simple tool for identifying dyads likely to benefit from tongue-tie treatment (Srinivasan, Dobrich, Mitnick, & Feldman, 2006). Dyads with nipple pain or trauma, unsustained latch, or inadequate infant weight gain coupled with a lingual frenulum that restricts either tongue elevation to the palate, grooving around a finger, or protrusion past the gum ridge were offered frenotomy. Frenotomy immediately improved LATCH scores (from 4–8 to 8–10), and at the 3-month follow-up, 92% of mothers were pain free, and 88% identified the procedure as having been helpful.

Effect on Breastfeeding

Tongue-tie often has a negative effect on latch, breastfeeding efficiency, and maternal comfort (Ballard et al., 2002; Buryk, Bloom, & Shope 2011; Dollberg, Botzer, Grunis, & Mimouni, 2006; Geddes, Langton et al., 2008; Griffiths, 2004; Hong et al., 2010; Klockars & Pitkaranta, 2009; Knox, 2010; Livingstone, Willis, Abdel-Wareth, Thiessen, & Lockitch, 2000). Some tongue-tied infants are able to latch and transfer milk (Geddes, Chadwick, Kent, Garbin, & Hartmann, 2009), though most are less efficient than their peers with unrestricted tongue motion (Ramsay et al., 2004a). Others are unable to attach to the breast at all. Some attach but fail to transfer enough milk to sustain growth (Forlenza, Paradise Black, McNamara, & Sullivan, 2010) and stimulate maternal supply, or they cause maternal nipple or breast damage. The presence of tongue-tie triples the risk of weaning in the first week of life (Ricke et al., 2005).

Some of the variability in breastfeeding effectiveness can be attributed to maternal breast characteristics. Elasticity, nipple protractility, and maternal motor skills are all important in allowing a tongue-tied infant to perform at his or her best. The more elastic the breast, the easier it is for the infant to grasp a good portion of the areolar tissue for good milk transfer. Nipples that retract when grasped make it more difficult for any infant to attach to the breast, but that may make it impossible for tongue-tied infants. Good maternal motor planning skills or previous breastfeeding experience improve the support and assistance the mother is able to give her infant to assist with obtaining an optimal latch. An optimal latch is vital to filling the mouth and stabilizing the tongue so it can function as well as possible during sucking.

Think of yourself with a rocket-shaped lollipop that has a narrow tip and widens toward the base. If you put only the slender tip of the rocket pop into your mouth, you need to lift your tongue tip to your upper gum ridge to press the pop there, and you have to purse your lips to hold it in. If you put the slender tip way back nearly to your soft palate, you have the much wider base at your lips, so you can hold onto it without pursing and your tongue can gently groove against the wide base of the lollipop without straining. Even if your tongue attachment is slightly tight, you should have enough give to press the lollipop farther up to your palate with your tongue. If your tongue is very tight and unable to lift off the floor of your mouth, your lips and jaws will have to do all the work of keeping the pop in your mouth.

Classification of Ankyloglossia

Ankyloglossia, or tongue-tie, can be classified according to the sites of attachment of the lingual frenulum on the tongue and the floor of the mouth (**Table 8-1**). Much of the disagreement in the literature on this subject is due to differing definitions of tongue-tie. It is generally more helpful to describe both the sites of attachment and the relative elasticity of the frenulum, as well as which specific tongue movements are restricted or altered. Griffiths (2004) classified tongue-tie by the proportion of the length of the tongue that was attached by the lingual frenulum. He found that even a thick, inelastic frenulum against the base of the tongue (0% tongue-tie) restricted tongue mobility and that treatment of these very posterior frenula had positive outcomes in at least 50% of infants (D. M. Griffiths, personal communication, 2004).

Tongue range of motion is the most important factor in an infant's ability to breastfeed with ankyloglossia. A thin, elastic frenulum will generally impact tongue movement less than a thick, fibrous one (**Figures 8-14 and 8-15**). Seventy-five percent of thick frenula were associated with breastfeeding difficulties in one case-control study (Messner, Lalakea, Aby, McMahon, & Bair, 2000). The elasticity of the floor of the mouth is another important component in tongue mobility. A very elastic mucosal floor may partially compensate for

Table 8-1 Classification of Ankyloglossia

Type	Superior Attachment	Inferior Attachment	Characteristics of Frenulum
1	Tip of tongue	Alveolar ridge	Often thin, may be elastic
2	2–4mm behind tongue tip	On or just behind alveolar ridge	Often thin, may be elastic
3	Mid-tongue	Middle of floor of mouth	Usually thicker, more fibrous, inelastic
4	Submucosal	Floor of mouth at base of tongue	Usually thick, fibrous, shiny, and inelastic

Source: Courtesy of Elizabeth V. Coryllos, MD, FAAP, FACS, IBCLC.

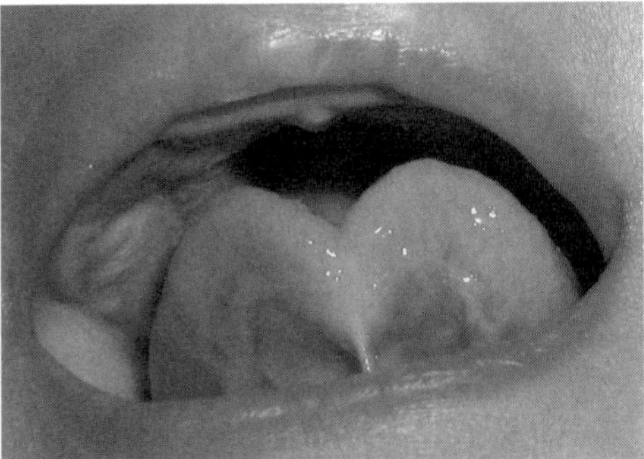

Figure 8-14 (left) "Classical" type 1 tongue-tie. Infant had sufficient tongue elevation to breastfeed after positioning was optimized. Bottle feeding was initially problematic as well.

Figure 8-15 (bottom left) Severe type 1 tongue-tie. This lingual frenulum is thick and inelastic, and required treatment.

Figure 8-16 (bottom right) Type 2 tongue-tie.

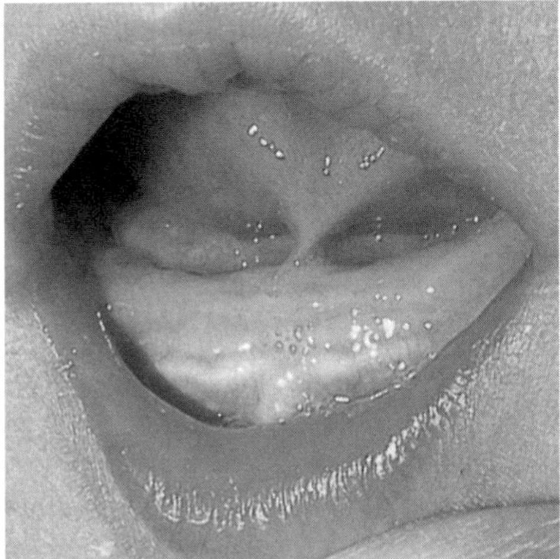

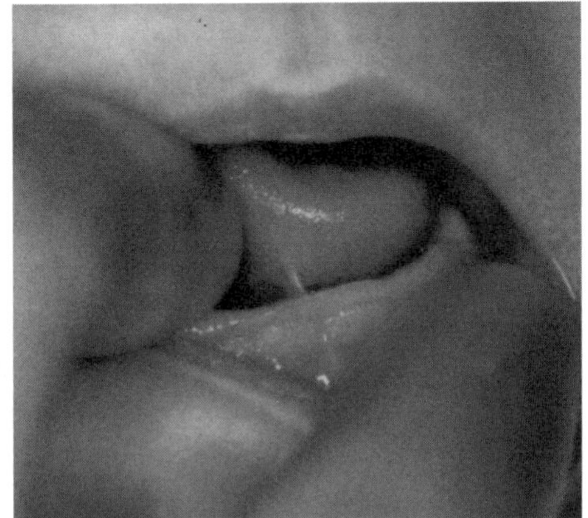

a restrictive lingual frenulum. If the floor of the mouth is tight and the frenulum is short and inelastic, the infant is at risk for very poor tongue function. The extent of the lingual frenulum along the underside of the tongue is another important determinant of function, with a longer attachment generally (but not always) restricting tongue elevation and extension more than a shorter one.

Often the most severe cases of ankyloglossia are not recognized because the infant has such limited ability to elevate the tongue that there is no tell-tale notching on the tongue tip, nor is there a heart-shaped anterior tongue. An infant with a severely restrictive lingual frenulum will usually keep the tongue behind the gum line, especially as the mouth opens (**Figure 8-16**). The tongue will appear flat or bunched into an unusual configuration. Touch to the future tooth-bearing surface of the exposed lower gum ridge triggers reflexive biting, which is normally inhibited by the presence of the tongue tip there. If the infant retracts the tongue during sucking, the lower gum is exposed to the breast, and a normal phasic bite (bite–release–bite) takes place. The upper gum may also damage the breast if the infant keeps the mouth tight in order to help maintain attachment or move milk when the tongue is not sufficiently mobile. The combination of inability to elevate the tongue for wavelike movements (**Figures 8-17 and 8-18**) and the triggering of the normal phasic bite reflex causes these infants to chew at the breast. Ultrasound studies are not capable of imaging the very front of the mouth because the sound waves bounce off the bone of the jaw, leaving a black shadow. The consistency of maternal reports and the bruising or skin injury seen on the areola from the infant's gums leave little doubt that biting is occurring, however.

Normal feeding requires the anterior tongue to cup (curve gently upward) to grasp the breast while the body of the tongue grooves and pulls the breast into the mouth. When the breast is in place, the baby begins to suck to stimulate a milk ejection reflex in the mother's breast, which increases the pressure differential between the breast and the mouth. While the tongue remains grooved around the teat and the anterior tongue remains elevated, the posterior tongue depresses and grooves to enlarge the volume of the oral cavity, creating negative pressure. This negative pressure opens the nipple pores, and milk flows from the area of higher pressure (breast) to lower pressure (mouth). Recent ultrasound studies have revealed that the degree of depression of the posterior tongue is extremely important to the quantity of milk transferred per suck (Geddes, Kent, Mitoulas, & Hartmann, 2008). The grooved tongue collects the milk into a bolus, which in young infants is delivered to the pharynx during every swallow (Geddes et al., 2009). Cineradiographic studies show that the anterior tongue presses against the breast in an anterior-to-posterior wave while the jaw assists by closing (Ardran, Kemp, & Lind, 1958), which was interpreted as providing positive pressure to strip milk from the breast and is now demonstrated to provide positive pressure for swallowing (Kennedy et al., 2010). The grooving of the posterior tongue and position of the lateral borders of the tongue against the palate are essential to controlled coordination of swallowing and breathing. Without this tunnel for milk transport, milk may overflow into the pharynx before the child is ready to close the airway. Hard swallowing

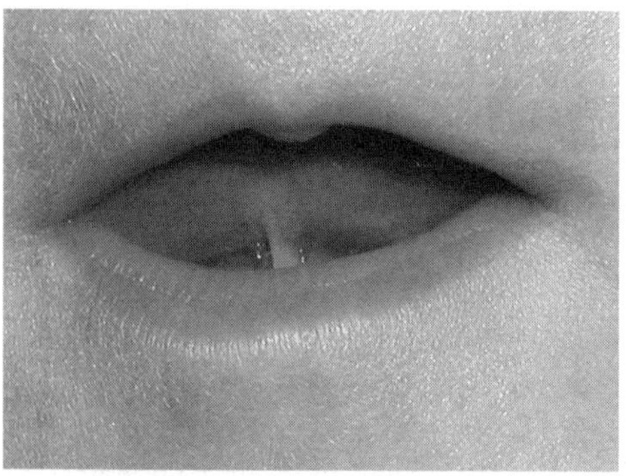

Figure 8-17 Type 3 tongue-tie. Tongue tip can elevate when mouth is not open widely.

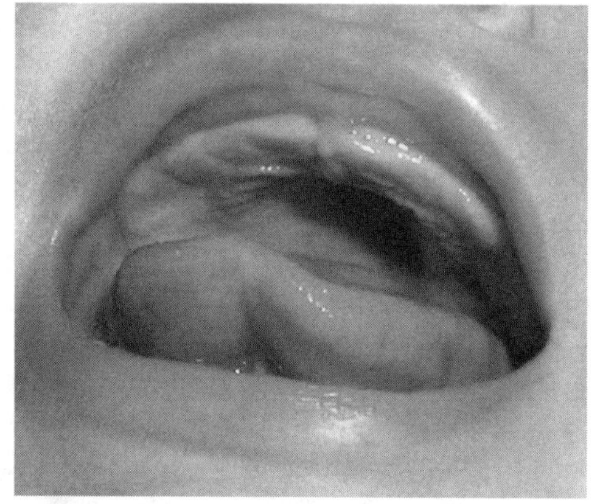

Figure 8-18 Type 3 tongue-tie. When the mouth is open, only the edges of the tongue are able to elevate.

(gulping) that is poorly coordinated with breathing, aerophagia (swallowing excessive air), laryngeal penetration (getting milk below the epiglottis but above the vocal folds), and even aspiration can result, making feeding uncomfortable, stressful, or scary for the infant. A poor ability to handle milk flow is a common cause of fussiness during feeding, or it can even result in feeding refusal.

The tongue is a bundle of muscles that is anchored to the floor of the mouth by the root of the genioglossus muscle at the posterior floor of the mouth, with fibers running under the floor of the mouth to the mandible. When it is anchored along much of its length by the midline frenulum, normal range of motion is not available, and the tongue is mainly able to redistribute its muscle mass backward or laterally. This results in a thick, bunched appearance of the tongue (**Figure 8-19**) that progresses into an elevation of the muscle mass of the tongue posteriorly, creating an unusually large hump in the posterior tongue (**Figure 8-20**). The repetitive stress of this piston movement against the breast or nipple can cause considerable trauma (**Figure 8-21**) and has been identified in ultrasound studies as being responsible for compression of the nipple tip (Geddes, Langton et al., 2008). The same researchers also observed that the midtongue can abnormally compress the base of the nipple in tongue-tied infants.

Another compensation for restrictive tongue attachment is the use of a sliding motion of the tongue from anterior to posterior. This was seen in the author's ultrasound studies when the geniohyoid and mylohyoid muscles overcontract to assist tongue elevation. As the tongue retracts, the posterior tongue elevates and rubs against the nipple.

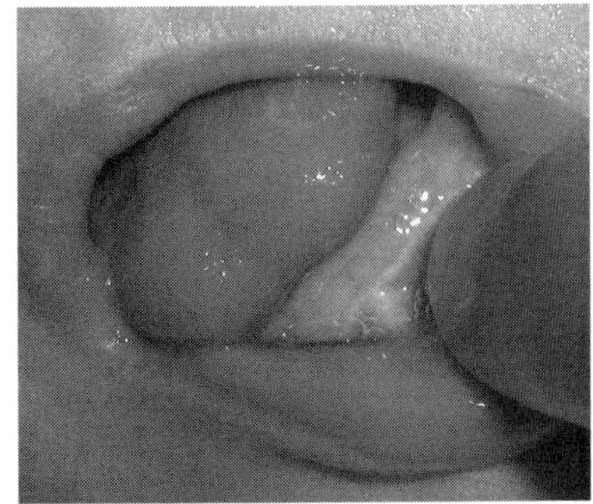

Figure 8-19 Attempts to mobilize the restricted tongue cause the thick, bunched configuration.

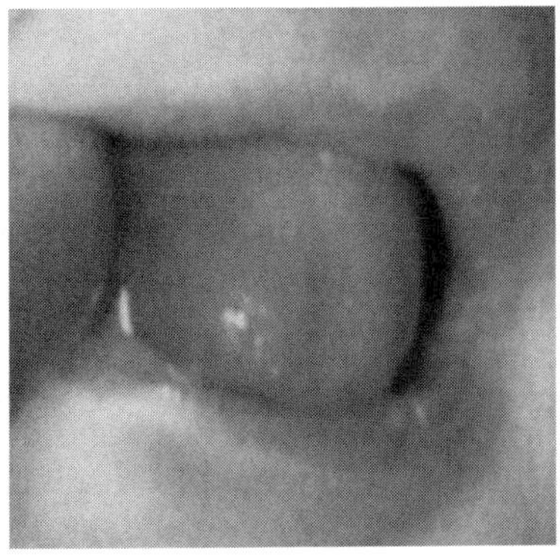

Figure 8-20 Posterior tongue elevation in type 3 tongue-tie.

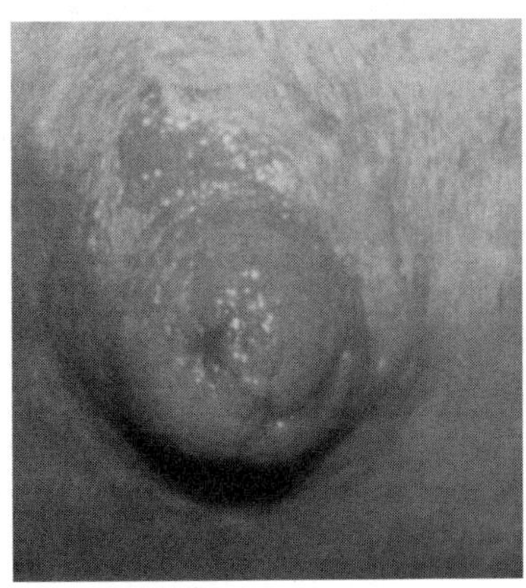

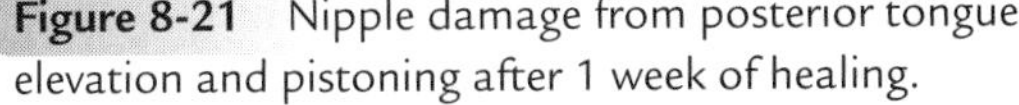

Figure 8-21 Nipple damage from posterior tongue elevation and pistoning after 1 week of healing.

Note the deep fissure at the nipple shaft just posterior to the face, and a compression fissure across the face of the nipple, leading to mastitis and candidiasis. Mother reported feeling the infant's tongue forcefully bumping into her nipple with each suck. Fingerfeeding with counterpressure on the posterior tongue helped the infant change her tongue movements so that feeding was then comfortable and more effective (see **Figure 12-41** in Chapter 12).

Mothers describe the sensation as feeling like sandpaper on their nipples. The infant can usually be observed to pull the breast in and out of the mouth when using this sucking pattern.

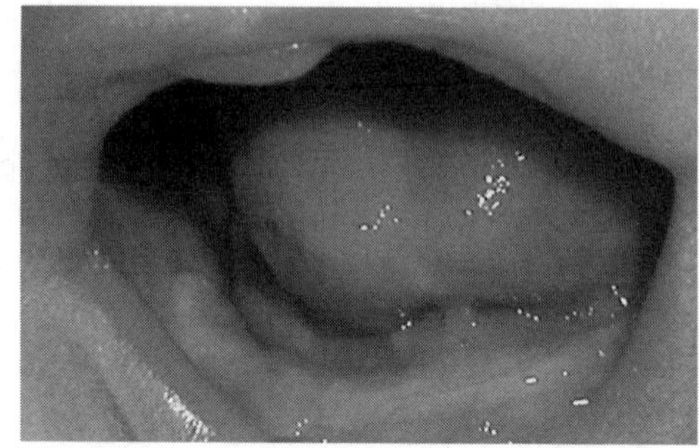

Figure 8-22 Infant with type 2 tongue-tie and large friction blister on upper lip. Compare the position of the blister in this photo and in Figure 8-24. This infant has a tight superior labial frenulum as well, so the blister is on the inner vermillion.

Infants with poor tongue function or a shallow latch may use a sweeping movement of the upper lip in an attempt to move milk from the breast with positive pressure or in an attempt to hold onto the breast while the tongue slides or slips. This strategy generally causes severe sucking blisters on the infant's lips (**Figures 8-22 through 8-24**). Ultrasound studies confirm that tongue-tied infants latch more shallowly than infants without a restrictive lingual frenulum (Geddes, Langton et al., 2008; Ramsay et al., 2004a). Lip sweeping is not specific to tongue-tie, and it is sometimes seen in infants with short mandibles as well.

Excessive jaw excursions are also seen in tongue-tied infants. The anterior tongue normally stays applied to the breast while the posterior tongue and mandible drop to make a small pocket of negative pressure in the mouth, which expands the nipple and pulls milk from the nipple pores. If the front of the tongue is not capable of elevating or remaining grooved around the breast as the back of the tongue drops, it is pulled by the frenulum to the floor of the mouth. Then the mandible must drop more in order to create negative pressure in the entire mouth, rather than in the small pocket behind the nipple. This increases the workload of the lips and cheeks; the cheeks may collapse or dimple (**Figure 8-25**), and the baby may fall off the breast if the lips are not sufficiently strong to maintain the latch. Some infants compensate by fixing the lips and overusing the orbicularis oris muscle (**Plate 3**). Tightening this circular sling of muscle around the lips often causes the baby to slide toward the nipple as the feed progresses, especially if the anterior tongue is not doing its part to help maintain attachment. Helping the mother recline so gravity holds the baby to her can improve the stability of the latch.

Treatment for Ankyloglossia

The obvious solution to symptomatic ankyloglossia is to divide the lingual frenulum against the underside of the tongue, releasing the restriction of tongue movements. Frenotomy was once routinely performed, until bottle feeding became the norm in Western culture. Now that breastfeeding initiation is increasing, articles advocating frenotomy for breastfeeding problems in infants with ankyloglossia are again appearing in the medical literature. Several randomized controlled trials have been conducted, indicating

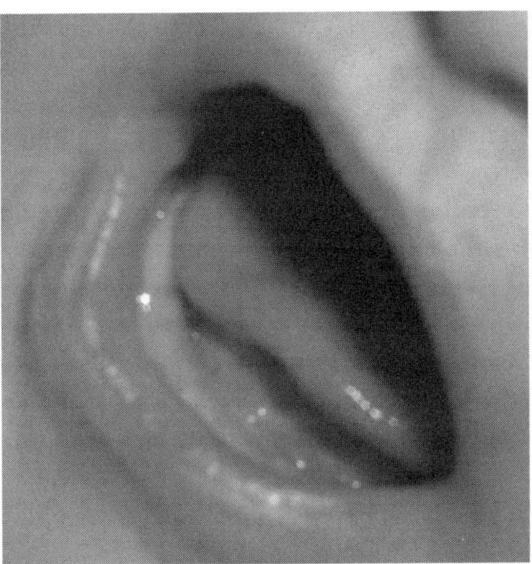

Figure 8-23 Type 4 tongue-tie is recognized by poor tongue mobility in a neurologically healthy infant with no visible frenulum.

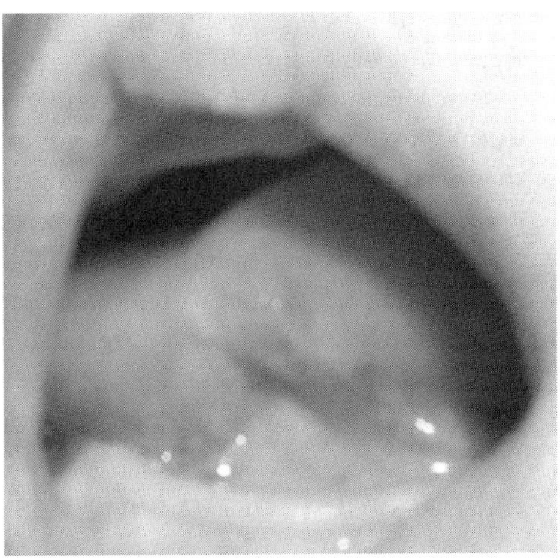

Figure 8-24 Infant with type 4 tongue-tie pulls up the floor of the mouth to elevate the tongue. Note the huge friction blister in the typical position in midline on the upper lip.

that 96% of infants who did not improve with intensive lactation consultant assistance substantially improved their feeding skills after frenotomy (Hogan, Westcott, & Griffiths, 2005), and that maternal pain and latch improve after frenotomy but not after a sham procedure (Dollberg et al., 2006).

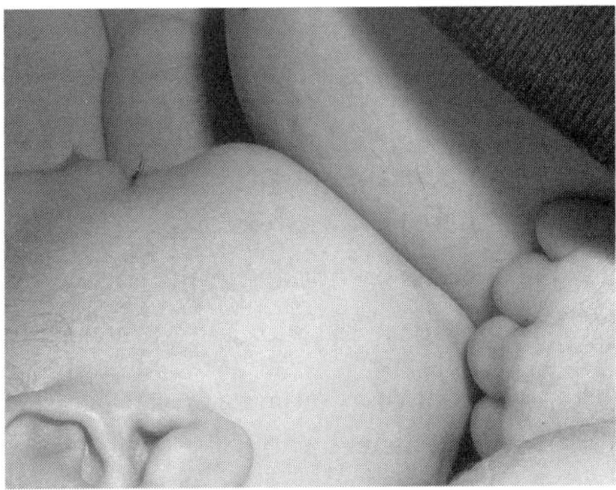

Figure 8-25 Excessive jaw excursion—note the flattened, dimpled cheek.

Frenotomy in young infants is generally an outpatient or office procedure. Some practitioners use flavored benzocaine gel as a topical anesthetic; others use no anesthesia. The infant is immobilized by an assistant, and the tongue is lifted either with gloved fingers or a grooved director, a tool designed for performing frenotomy. Surgical scissors or a surgical laser is used to cut the frenulum either in midline or at the underside of the tongue. Care is taken to avoid the orifices of the submandibular salivary glands on the floor of the mouth. The frenulum is usually avascular. If there is a blood vessel, it can be sutured above and below the frenotomy site and then the division is made between the two sutures. Pressure to the incision site with a gauze square is sufficient to prevent or stop bleeding in most cases. (See Chapter 9 for a detailed explanation of frenotomy procedures.)

After frenotomy, the majority of infants spontaneously correct their tongue movements during sucking. If improvement is not marked after 3–4 days, the infant should be reexamined to see if the tongue-tie was reduced but not eliminated. Further treatment is usually helpful in these cases. It is possible to perform simple frenotomy on infants with type 3 and 4 (posterior and submucosal) ankyloglossia. When the fibrous, posterior frenulum is snipped it opens up into a diamond shape, allowing more tongue movement in each direction. A more complex procedure, such as transverse-vertical frenuloplasty, is an option, though general anesthesia is required. For infants with very poor tongue motion, the lifelong benefits of improved tongue function can outweigh the risks of anesthesia.

Management of Ankyloglossia Without Frenotomy

Infants who do not self-correct their suck within 4–5 days, and those who are not treated, may benefit from exercises to help improve tongue extension and elevation to the extent possible. In the author's practice, a subset of infants with severe restriction of tongue movement were able to breastfeed by about 6–9 weeks of age without frenotomy. In these cases, infants were fed expressed milk by bottle or Hazelbaker FingerFeeder, and breastfeeding was attempted periodically until gradually the infant was able to transition to exclusive breastfeeding. If frenotomy is unacceptable or unavailable to the parents, they can be encouraged to

- maintain a full milk supply by pumping at least eight times each day with a rental-grade breast pump or efficient manual expression;
- maintain practice at breast by putting the baby to the breast after a partial alternate feeding (breast for dessert);
- focus on obtaining the deepest asymmetrical latch possible;
- reduce posterior tongue elevation and retraction with oral exercises.

Anticipatory guidance is important. Parents should be counseled to expect feedings to be less efficient and to be patient if their infant needs to feed more often or for longer periods of time.

Even in tongue-tied infants who are able to breastfeed without maternal pain, feeding is less efficient. The infant may fatigue before being satiated, and the milk supply will calibrate downward if mom fails to pump or express. Tremors of the tongue and/or mandible are common in tongue-tied infants, due to the fatigue involved in using less ergonomic compensatory tongue, jaw, and lip movements. This enhanced physiologic tremor is a reliable sign that the infant is working too hard. If tremor is seen in a neurologically healthy infant, oral anatomy and oral motor function should be assessed, and the infant's growth should be followed closely. If growth is suboptimal, supplementation with expressed milk fed in a way that supports breastfeeding (Chapter 12) is important.

Latch Alterations

Attachment to the breast requires the tongue tip to be down in the mouth and in contact with the breast. This is more difficult for infants with tongue-tie, who generally gape less well and may retract the tongue more as they open wider (**Figure 8-3**). Several management alterations can help improve a tongue-tied infant's ability to latch. Giving good positional stability and shaping the breast to help the infant get a larger mouthful are covered in Chapter 5. Several additional strategies are helpful for tongue-tied infants.

Healthy, neurotypical infants with ankyloglossia may attach better if they are simply given optimal positioning and allowed to self-attach. This gives them more time to organize their tongue movements so they can drop the tongue and grasp the breast. Optimal positioning includes holding baby diagonally against mom, with the baby's belly snuggled to mom's ribcage, hips flexed around mom's side, chest brought to mom's breast, chin on the areola, and philtrum to the nipple (**Figure 8-26**). Mom should be encouraged to support baby's shoulders and back, and keep her fingers off the head and neck to allow the head to extend as the baby gapes widely and lunges for the breast (**Figure 8-27**). Mom supports baby's movements by snuggling the baby straight toward her as the baby grasps the breast (**Figure 8-28**). If the mother takes a semireclined position, gravity can help keep the baby close to her body.

If the baby is unable to bring the tongue down sufficiently and repeatedly fails to grasp the breast, the baby's entire body can be slid slightly toward the other breast, exposing a larger and easier-to-grasp circle

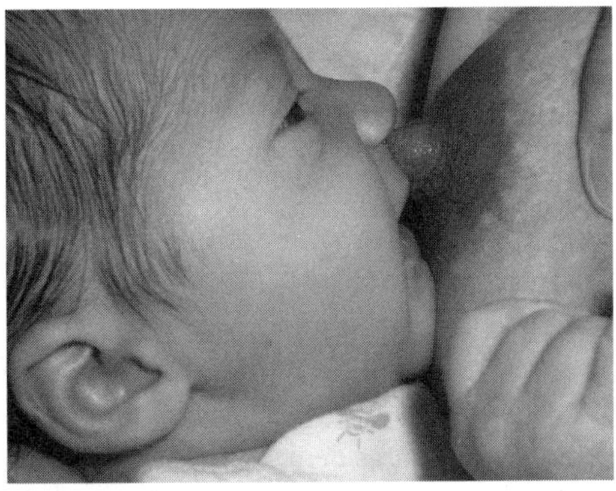

Figure 8-26 Asymmetrical attachment: chin on breast, philtrum to nipple.

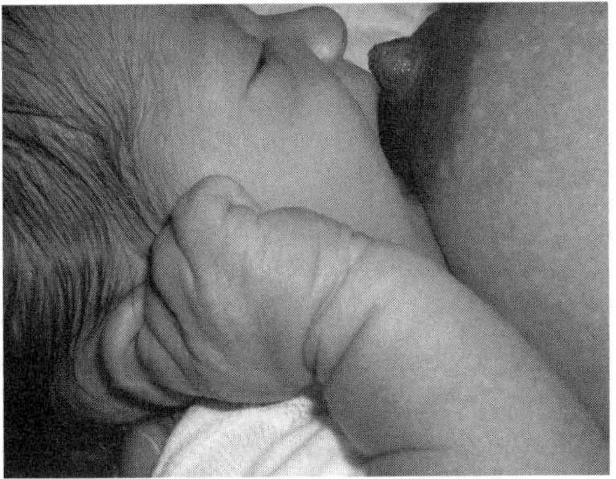

Figure 8-27 Asymmetrical attachment: allows baby to gape.

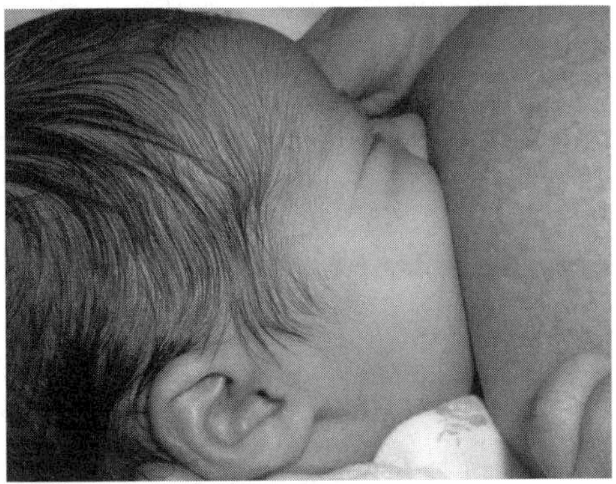

Figure 8-28 Asymmetrical attachment: baby snuggled in for a deep latch.

of breast to the infant's tongue tip. The shoulders can also be pressed in during this maneuver to bring the chin and tongue tip closer to the breast.

Another strategy that is particularly useful, if the baby slides the lower lip and tongue tip toward the nipple during latch, is to dent the breast at or just beyond the margin of the areola with one finger to form a firmed, billowed-out area of breast for the baby to grasp. The baby's chin is snuggled in the hollow created by the denting finger, which helps prevent the lower lip from sliding toward the nipple as the baby latches. Denting the breast to provide an exaggerated mouthful is particularly helpful when mothers have flat or inverted nipples. Compressing the breast between two fingers makes a tethered nipple retract; whereas denting the breast with one finger does not retract the nipple.

Fingerfeeding Tongue-Tied Infants

The most important consideration for a tongue-tied infant who will not be treated is to help reduce some of the negative effects of sucking compensations. For infants who retract the tongue tip and/or use forceful posterior elevation, modified finger feeding can be helpful in reducing the excessive shifting of the tongue mass toward the back of the mouth. The finger and tube are held across both of the infant's lips with a well-filed fingernail on the philtrum to simulate the feeling of the breast on the lower lip and the nipple touching the philtrum (**Figure 8-29**). When the infant gapes widely, the fingertip is slid against the palate to reduce the chance of stimulating the gag reflex. Ideally, the infant will grasp the finger with the tongue and suck it deeply into the mouth until the finger pad rests on the back of the hard palate and the nail side of the finger is against the tongue in midline. Good contact with tongue and palate and alignment of the finger in midline is important to model the position of the teat in breastfeeding, and it helps to stimulate central grooving of the tongue, which is so important in both stabilizing the teat and bolus control for safe swallowing (**Figure 8-30** and **Figure 8-31**).

When the infant begins to suck, milk is delivered either by the infant's efforts (Hazelbaker FingerFeeder or feeding tube in a bottle) or by the feeder (curved tip syringe or syringe and feeding tube). Feeder-controlled methods are particularly effective for operant conditioning. Milk delivery is stopped when the tongue retracts or the posterior tongue is pistoned against the finger, and it is resumed when the tongue tip is brought back over the gum ridge and the posterior tongue drops slightly. A slight reduction of the excessive posterior elevation may be enough to keep mom comfortable. The goal is not to completely flatten the tongue, but to help the infant maintain the tongue tip over the gum ridge to inhibit the bite reflex. It is important to remember that posterior tongue elevation is an important part of normal sucking; it is the degree to which the mass of the tongue is distributed backward and the force of the elevation that are abnormal in ankyloglossia.

Counterpressure from the feeder's finger can also be used to discourage excessive posterior tongue elevation or tongue retraction. If there is posterior elevation but the tongue tip stays over the lower gum ridge, the feeder can simply angle the fingertip down against the over-elevated tongue until it drops slightly. Usually the tongue is retracted as well, and a slight traction toward the front of the mouth is helpful. The finger is angled downward against the humped tongue, and the humped area is pushed slightly toward the front of the mouth. The corrective force is provided with minimal finger movement to avoid disrupting the infant's attachment to the finger.

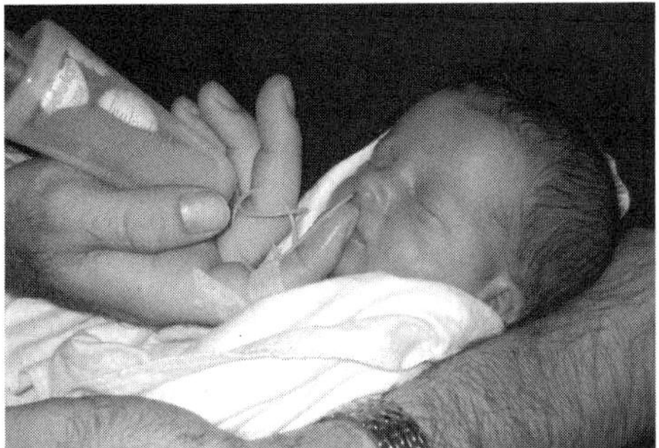

Figure 8-29 Presenting finger for fingerfeeding.

Tongue Exercises

No oral exercise is capable of curing ankyloglossia, but specific targeted interventions may help reduce maladaptive or limiting compensations. With knowledge of tongue movements during normal suckling and infant sensory reflexes, exercises can be easily constructed to address each infant's needs. It is vital to respect the infant's autonomy and body integrity and to make the exercise a game that the infant enjoys and actively participates in. Therefore, the infant should be in a receptive (quiet alert or early active alert) state. The more predictable the sequence of stimuli and elicited movements, the more the infant is likely to tolerate and even enjoy the exercise.

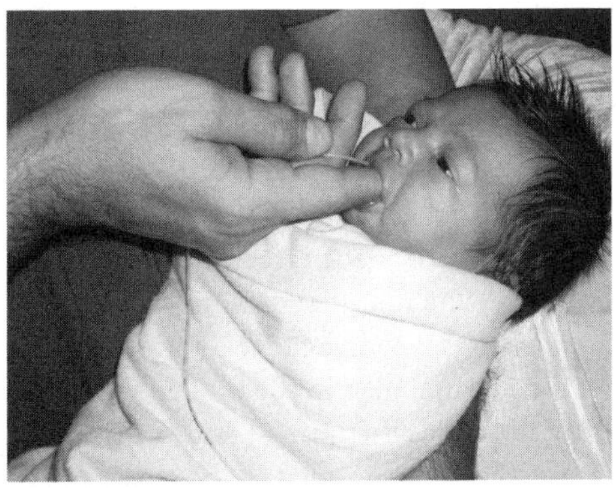

Figure 8-30 Fingerfeeding with head extended over arm in infant with respiratory disorder.

Any exercise should show some signs of effectiveness in early trials. If the infant rejects it or it is ineffective in changing tongue movements even slightly, a different exercise or strategy should be used. Ideally, an infant with oral motor issues will be working with both a lactation consultant and a speech or occupational therapist with expertise in feeding.

Press-Down Exercise

This exercise was designed for an infant with a short mandible who was still using excessive posterior tongue elevation after frenotomy but did not like having a finger

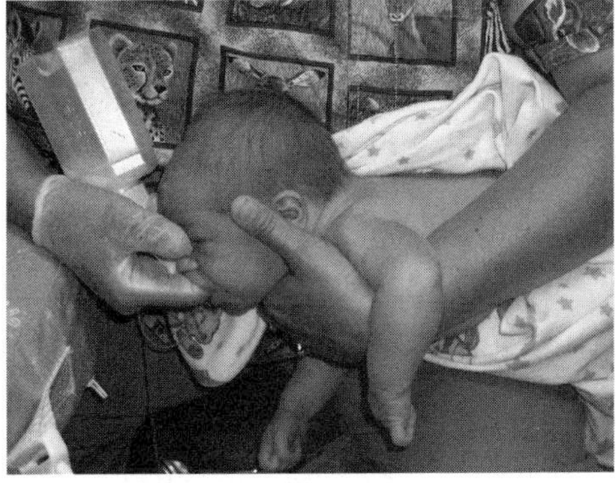

Figure 8-31 Fingerfeeding in prone position for infant with severe laryngomalacia.

in her mouth. Touch stimulation was given to the chin, nose, and philtrum, and when the baby opened in response to touch on the philtrum, brief fingertip pressure was applied to the humped area of the tongue and the finger was quickly withdrawn. A different sound was made with each touch, but the sound and tone for each specific touch was kept consistent, further adding to the predictability (and tolerability) of the stimulation. The sounds were silly (beep, bip, bop, boop) to help make it fun for the infant and to provoke cross-modal processing to reinforce the effectiveness of the sequence. The adult performing the sequence smiled and made eye contact with the baby to reinforce the playfulness of the interaction. As soon as the baby failed to play along and open her mouth, the exercise was terminated for that session. After a few repeats, the baby was starting to drop her posterior tongue slightly when she opened her mouth. Her mother was encouraged to try this game very briefly before feedings, or between breasts if the baby was too hungry to tolerate delaying the feeding a few seconds (**Figure 8-32A through 8-32E**).

Tongue Massage

Infants with severe tongue retraction may respond to a small amplitude circular massage on the anterior tongue. The baby is stimulated to open the mouth by touch to the philtrum, and the finger pad is placed on the surface of the tongue just behind the tongue tip. The fingertip is rotated in a small circle without losing contact with the tongue (**Figure 8-33**). The infant should improve the shape and extension of the tongue at least slightly during this massage. The infant will generally attempt to suck the finger; the finger can then be upended in the mouth so the finger pad is on the palate, and massage can continue with the (well-trimmed and filed) nail side of the finger on the posterior tongue. Forward traction can be added to the massage by accentuating the portion of the circular movement that is moving anteriorly. Massage can precede finger feeding in an infant who is unable to latch onto the breast due to the severity of the tongue-tie. Sometimes just one brief session of tongue massage with or without finger feeding is sufficient to improve tongue extension enough for the baby to be able to attach to the breast, though it might take many weeks before the infant is able to latch consistently and suckling is painless for the mother and efficient for the infant.

Increasing Tongue Lateralization

After frenotomy, the infant may need some assistance to extend and lateralize the tongue. This exercise helps to stimulate the transverse tongue reflex, where the tongue tip follows a fingertip around the gum from center to side. The baby is stimulated to open the mouth by touching the philtrum or lips. When the infant opens, the fingertip is placed on the center of the lateral surface (outside) of the lower gum ridge and, maintaining contact with the gum ridge, moved around to the side, then slid back to the front and returned to center (**Figure 8-34**). This is repeated three times in the same quadrant and then repeated in the other quadrants of the mouth, lower gums first and then upper gums. The immediate repetition in each quadrant gives the infant time to anticipate and follow the finger.

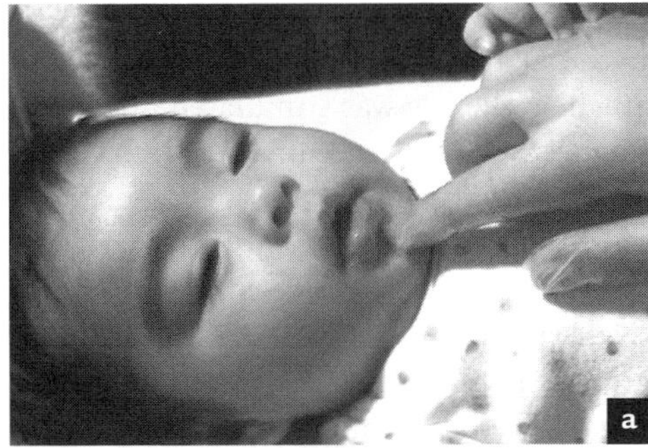

Figure 8-32 Press-down exercise.

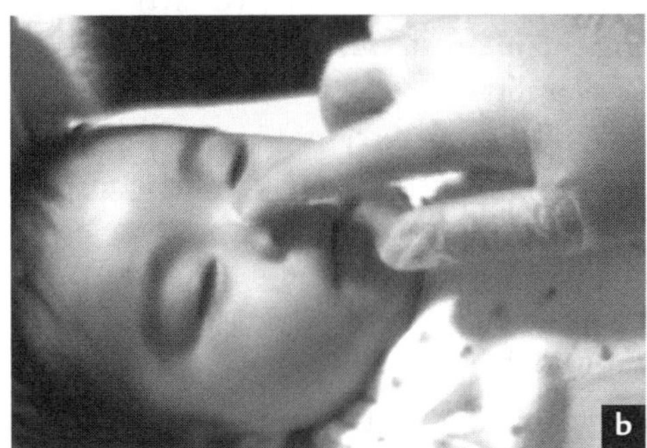

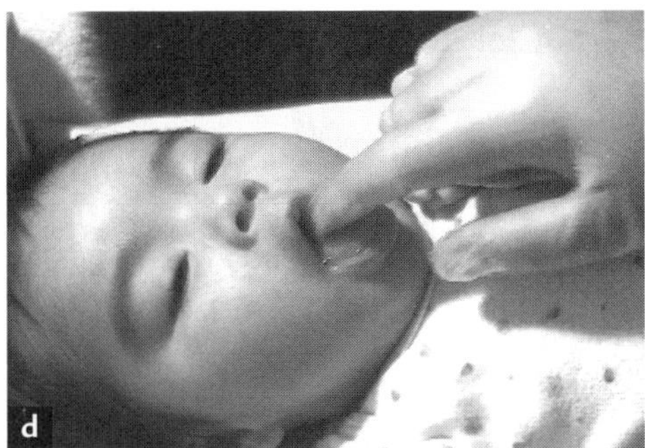

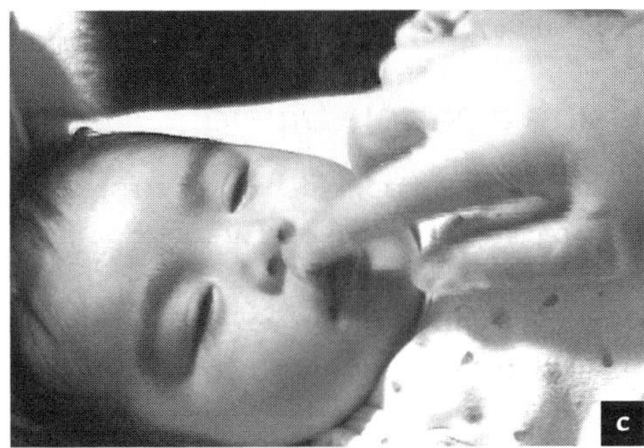

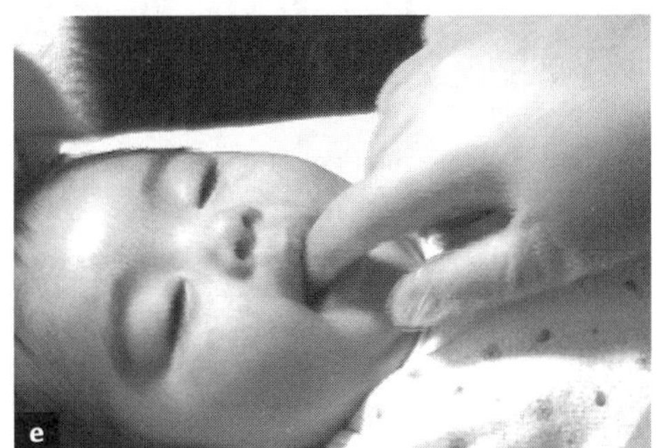

Desensitizing the Palate

Infants with high palatal arches occasionally resist a deep latch because stimulation to the relatively naïve apex of the palate stimulates their gag reflex. Many tongue-tied infants have strong and more anteriorly provoked than usual gag reflexes. The sensory characteristics of the soft breast and the provision of milk allow many infants to inhibit the gag. For infants with a gag that is difficult to inhibit, systematic desensitization may be helpful.

The infant is stimulated to open with touch to the philtrum or upper lip, and the fingertip touches the anterior hard palate in midline. The finger is gently slid back along the

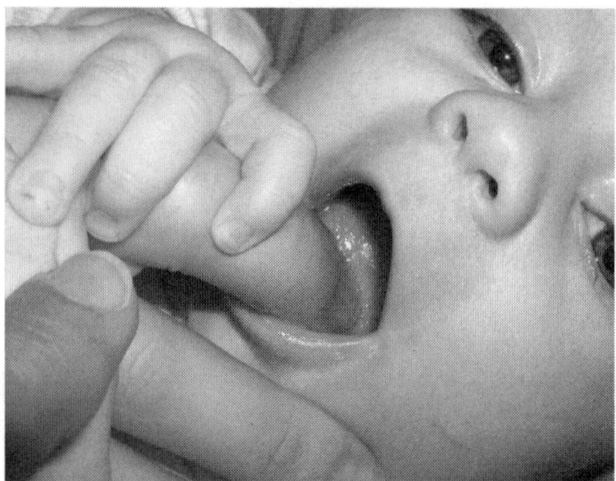

Figure 8-33 Tongue massage.

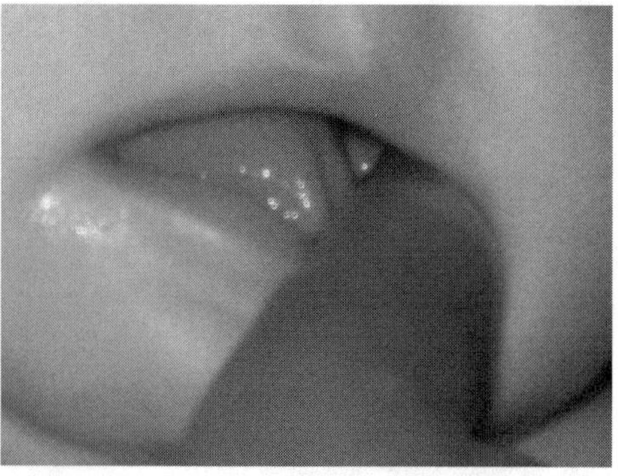

Figure 8-34 Stimulating tongue lateralization

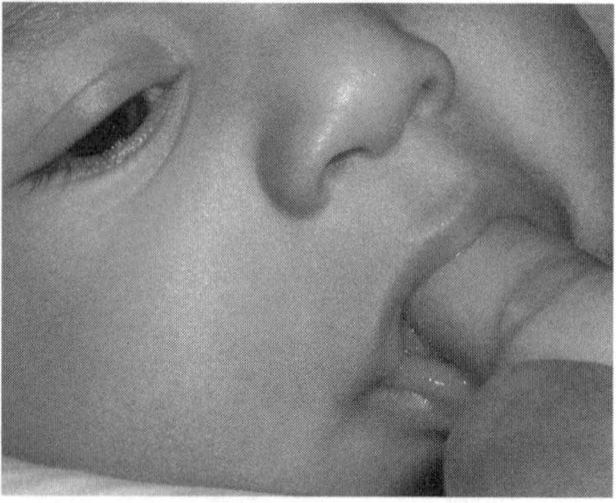

Figure 8-35 Pressure on the anterior palate helps desensitize a hypersensitive gag response.

hard palate, stopping just before the spot at which the gag was stimulated previously (**Figure 8-35**). (If the infant begins to gag as soon as the finger presses the anterior palate, firm pressure from the finger may help inhibit it.) Over several sessions or days, the infant generally learns to tolerate normal touch pressure to the palate. Desensitization requires finesse to find the right balance of gentle challenge to help the infant tolerate touch yet avoid pushing the infant too far and reinforcing the discomfort.

Oral motor exercises designed for neurologically impaired infants can sometimes be useful for improving sucking in tongue-tied infants. These are found in Chapter 12. In choosing or designing exercises, it is important to identify the normal movements that are not being produced and encourage those, while discouraging the compensatory movements that are inefficient for the infant or painful for the mother.

Using a Nipple Shield

A thin silicone nipple shield used to preform the breast may assist infants with significant tongue retraction who are otherwise unable to latch. For tongue-tied infants, the widest diameter nipple shield teat that will fit completely in the mouth is optimal because their restricted tongue grooving makes a narrow teat difficult to grasp. It is important to draw the entire nipple and significant areola into the shield teat. A particularly effective method of applying a nipple shield was innovated by professional engineer and International Board Certified Lactation Consultant (IBCLC) Linda Pohl (personal communication, July 24, 2002). The nipple shield is held on the fingers of both hands, with the thumbs on either side of the teat. The teat is partially inverted by bringing the thumbs toward the fingers and rotating the hands slightly away from each other. The shortened teat is placed over the nipple, and two fingers from each hand press into the folded area of the teat, first back toward the chest wall, and then outward toward the sides of the breast. The nipple and much of the surrounding tissue is drawn into the teat as it everts.

The breast should be presented as much as if the nipple shield were not there as possible, to preserve oral searching and gaping behaviors for eventual direct breastfeeding. Presenting the tip of the teat to the infant's philtrum helps create an asymmetrical latch and assists the infant in taking some of the area surrounding the teat, at least in the lower part of the mouth. (See **Figures 11-11 and 11-12** in Chapter 11.)

There are potential pitfalls of using a nipple shield in this population. For infants with significant tongue retraction, the shield becomes a stimulus for the bite reflex and may actually increase maternal pain. Tongue-tied infants with high palates generally have an accentuated gag response, which may be stimulated by the shield. Expressing a few drops of milk into or onto the shield may help the infant inhibit the gag. Tongue-tied infants are less effective feeders, and the nipple shield may not allow good milk transfer. Whenever possible, test weights should be performed when trying a nipple shield, and the shield should be abandoned if milk transfer is problematic. If milk transfer is substantial but still suboptimal, brief breastfeeding for practice combined with pumping and alternate feeding may be the best use of the mother's time until the baby's sucking improves.

> Restricted tongue movements due to an anteriorly placed, short, or inelastic lingual frenulum can cause infants to use alternate, and less efficient, movements during feeding. Common movement patterns include posterior tongue elevation (humping) and pistoning, excessive compression and chewing, upper lip sweeping, and anterior-posterior sliding of the tongue. Each of these patterns has specific disadvantages to both mother and infant during feeding and can usually be eliminated by frenotomy.

Superior Labial Frenulum

The lips are attached to the gum ridge in midline by frenula as well. If the superior (upper) labial frenulum is very tight, it might interfere with the infant's ability to maintain attachment to the breast. Generally, increasing head extension will allow the infant to grasp the breast sufficiently. If the labial frenulum is inserted into the upper gum ridge, it will cause a gap between the central incisors. Treatment in infancy can improve breastfeeding (Wiessinger, 1995) and can cause the frenulum to regress by interrupting its blood supply. Treatment in adulthood is much more difficult and involves dissecting the labial frenulum from the gum ridge.

Hemangioma

Hemangiomas are the most common tumor in infancy. They are benign and may be present at birth or appear during the early weeks of life. Hemangiomas grow rapidly and then regress by about age 9 years (Smolinski & Yan, 2005). However, hemangiomas of the face may cause distortion of form and function, and those on mucosal areas such as the lip may ulcerate and cause pain, bleeding, and feeding difficulties (Band, 2000). The use of a topical anesthetic before feeding along with pain-relieving medication can help infants with an ulcerated hemangioma to breastfeed. Asymmetrical latch with head extension will help reduce upper lip stress and make feeding as comfortable as possible. If breastfeeding is temporarily impossible, the infant may be more comfortable with cup or syringe feeding to avoid contact with the ulcerated lip (**Plate 2**).

Micrognathia and Mandibular Hypoplasia

There is no standard definition of what constitutes micrognathia (unusually short lower jaw). Clinically, if the infant's lower lip and jaw are completely subsumed by the maxillary (upper) gum ridge, the difference in jaw lengths is relevant. Newborns normally have recessed mandibles, partially due to in utero positioning with their head flexed into the chest. Breastfeeding provides normal muscular stresses on the jaws and may improve mandible growth (Page, 2001, 2003). However, Luz, Garib, and Arouca (2006) failed to find a difference in the persistence of a short mandible in 5- to 11-year-old children who breastfed for greater than, versus less than, 6 months.

Infants with shorter than usual lower jaws are likely to have feeding difficulties related to displacement of the tongue, reduced mechanical advantage, and restricted tongue movements. When the mandible is short, the tongue attachment is generally closer to the gum ridge, restricting elevation of the mid- to posterior tongue. The habitual position of the tongue tip is often elevated and held to the palate, perhaps due to lack of space for the normal resting posture of the tongue tip over the lower lip. Micrognathia is associated with a narrower upper airway (Gunn, Tonkin, Hadden, Davis, & Gunn, 2000). A recent study found shorter mandibles as measured by a higher mandibular index in infants who had suffered an apparent life-threatening event versus controls (Horn, 2006). Infants with short or retroplaced mandibles generally extend their heads and fix their tongues to the palate to help stabilize and enlarge the airway. (Compare **Plates 6 and 7** of tongue tip elevation and tongue fixing; the excessive muscle activity of fixing is obvious.) If the tongue is particularly long, it may be curled or humped in the mouth. These abnormal positions can be a poor basis for normal muscle strength and activation during sucking. Some infants with relatively long tongues have difficulty with coordination and may use a tongue thrust pattern that pushes the breast out of the mouth. The use of a thin silicone nipple shield may help the infant maintain a deep attachment while tongue movements improve. If the infant cannot feed even with the shield, fingerfeeding can help strengthen the tongue and improve anticipatory tongue positioning for feeding.

Asymmetrical attachment to the breast is essential for infants with short jaws. Positioning the infant with the head well extended and the body snuggled under the mother's contralateral breast is often sufficient to improve feeding efficiency (**Figure 8-36A and B**, and **Figure 8-37A and B**). Side-lying or prone positioning on a reclined mother may

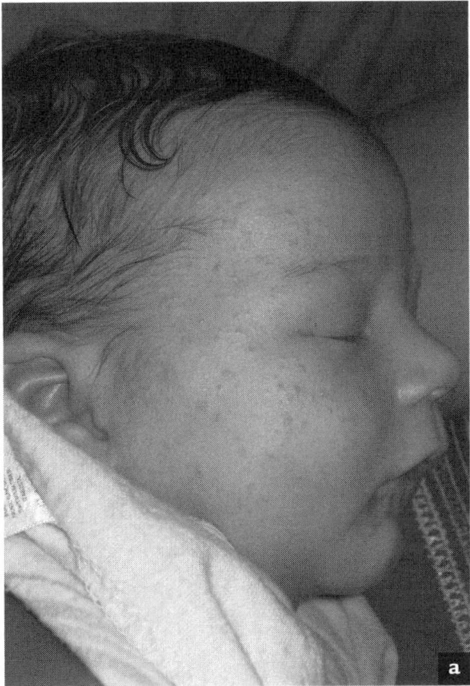

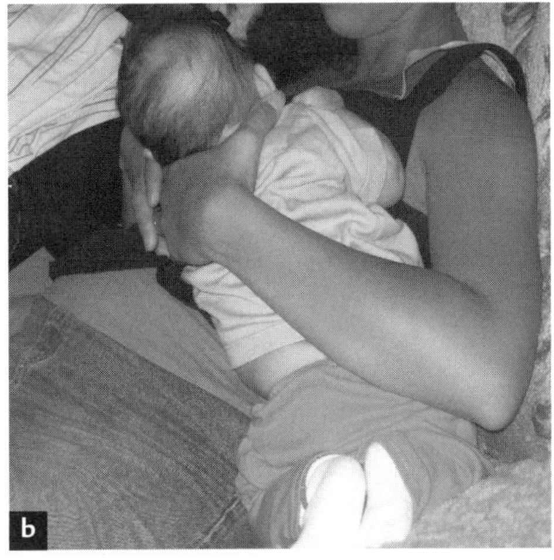

Figure 8-36a and 8-36b A modified kneeling prone position brought this baby's short jaw forward and improved baby's ability to manage milk flow.

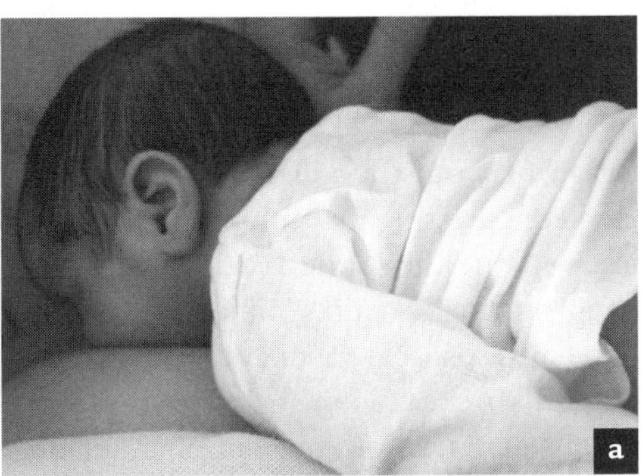

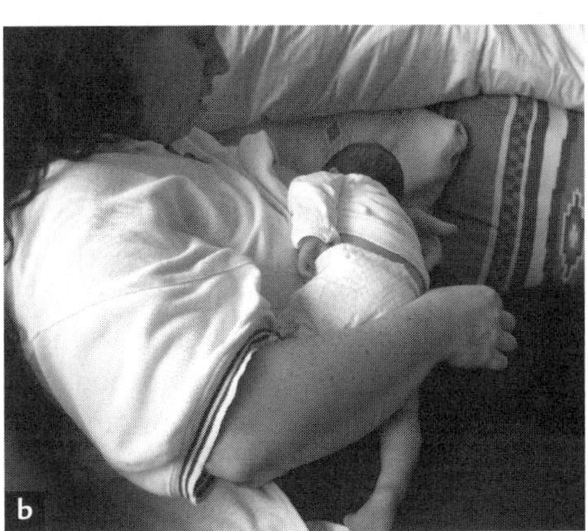

Figure 8-37a and 8-37b Prone positioning improves ability to manage milk flow in micrognathic infants with respiratory instability.

allow better head extension, depending on the mother and baby's geometry (**Figure 8-38**). Concerns about hyperextension of the neck in infants may be overstated; for at least the first 3 months of life, the epiglottis and soft palate are in contact, and swallowing is not stressed by extension (Takagi & Bosma, 1960). Of course, the effect of every intervention needs to be observed and evaluated to avoid destabilizing the infant.

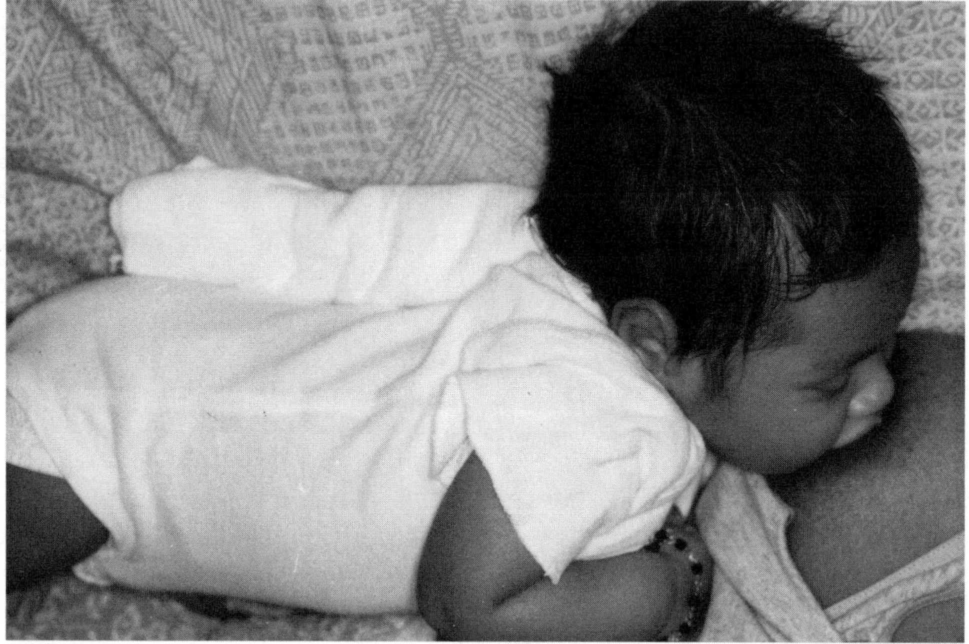

Figure 8-38 Sidelying allows greater head extension. This much head extension was required for painless feeding in the early weeks in this dyad.

The combination of a short tongue and lower jaw may cause the infant to use excessive suction pressure during suckling. Consistent unrelieved pressure may interfere with nipple perfusion and stimulate nipple vasospasm (blanching of the nipple due to vasoconstriction), which is usually accompanied by stabbing, shooting, or stinging pain. Chilling of the nipple or evaporative cooling may increase the severity of reflex vasospasm and may even trigger it in women with Raynaud phenomenon. Wool nursing pads in the bra have helped reduce spontaneous nipple vasospasm in women with a previous diagnosis of Raynaud phenomenon. For feeding-related vasospasm, drying the nipple immediately after the baby releases it and providing a dry heat source (a hot water bottle or a rice sock—raw rice microwave heated in a cotton sock) may relieve pain and stimulate the constricted arterioles to dilate. Vitamin B6 or calcium-magnesium supplements help some women. Diana West, IBCLC, recommends teaching mothers to massage blood back into the nipple with their fingertips (personal communication, February 24, 2009). Pharmacologic treatment with calcium channel blockers can help reduce the incidence and pain of vasospasm in mothers with significant difficulty. Visible blanching of the nipple may continue for some months after the pain resolves.

Impeccable attention to attachment along with infant growth usually improves the situation. If extreme asymmetrical latch with head extension does not markedly improve maternal comfort, tongue mobility should be assessed because tongue-tie can and does co-occur with micrognathia. If pain remains problematic, milk expression and alternate feeding may need to be used for several feedings per day to preserve the mother's ability to continue breastfeeding. In the author's clinical practice, most infants with shorter than average mandibles were breastfeeding without maternal discomfort by 12 weeks of age.

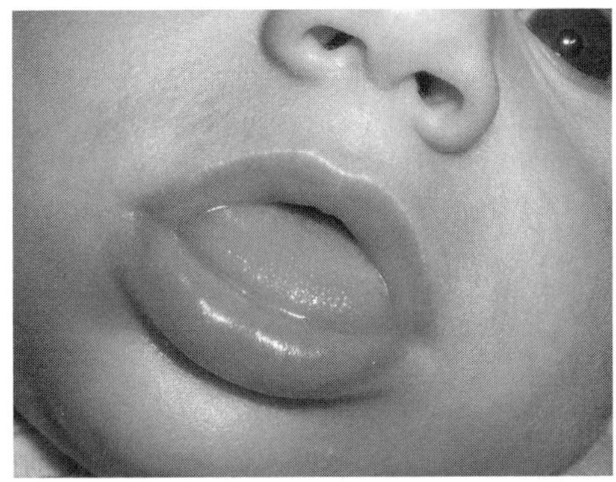

Figure 8-39 Mild macroglossia.

Macroglossia

Macroglossia (large tongue) can occur in isolation or as part of a genetic overgrowth disorder such as Beckwith-Wiedemann syndrome (**Figures 8-39 and 8-40**). There is no standard definition of macroglossia, which is usually diagnosed clinically when the infant has difficulty keeping the tongue in the mouth, function is affected, or the jaw is distorted by pressure from the large tongue.

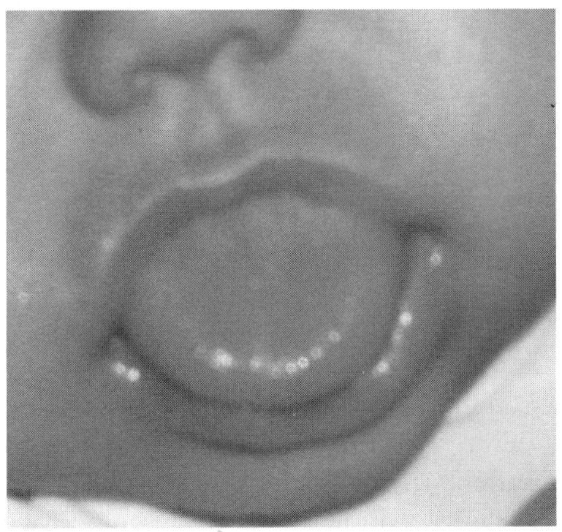

Figure 8-40 Macroglossia associated with Beckwith-Wiedemann syndrome (BWS).

Infants with macroglossia may be inefficient feeders, perhaps due to insufficient room in the mouth for normal posterior tongue depression during suckling, even with wide jaw excursions. Pre- and postfeeding test weights can be used to determine whether maternal accommodations, such as increasing frequency and duration of feeds, are likely to be sufficient. Maintaining generous milk production by brief postfeed pumping may increase the speed of maternal milk flow and will provide human milk for alternative feedings. Surgical reduction of the tongue may improve feeding ability in infants with severe macroglossia (Kveim, Fischer, Jones, & Gruer, 1985; Maturo & Mair, 2006) (**Figure 8-41**). Maintenance of milk production and allowing the baby to breastfeed for dessert, even if little milk is transferred, helps protect feeding skills until tongue reduction can be attempted. If bottle feeding is used, it is important to use the widest based teat possible to allow the use of the entire tongue.

Anatomical variations of the tongue and jaw reduce feeding efficiency and predispose infants to reduced milk transfer. Careful monitoring of the infant for sufficient milk intake, and encouraging the mother to express milk and use alternative feeding methods when needed, can help maintain breastfeeding until growth or treatment improves feeding abilities.

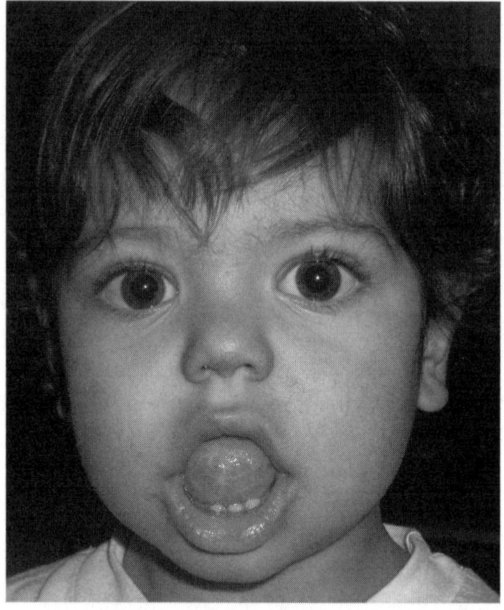

Figure 8-41 Child with BWS after tongue reduction surgery. Breastfeeding ability improved markedly after tongue reduction surgery.

Breastfeeding and Oral Clefts

Although clefts of the lip are obvious, lactation consultants may be the first professional to identify a cleft of the palate. A study conducted in the United Kingdom (Habel, Elhadi, Sommerlad, & Powell, 2006) identified a 28% incidence of delayed detection of overt clefts. Even relatively large clefts of the hard palate were not identified, in several cases for years after birth, especially if the physicians who examined the infants after birth performed only digital examination and were not specifically instructed in cleft detection. The authors recommend visual inspection with a light and a tongue depressor in addition to a digital exam. It is important to either wait for the baby to depress the tongue or to gently press it down or stimulate the gag reflex in order to examine the soft palate. Soft palate clefts are often missed due to the large size of the newborn's tongue.

Overt Clefts

Infants with hard palate clefts tend to rest their tongue tip in the defect, which can influence the development of tongue movements (**Figure 8-42**). Another major issue in breastfeeding an infant with a cleft is the inability to produce negative pressure in the mouth unless the cleft can be occluded. Mild negative pressure helps to hold the breast in the mouth during sucking. More importantly, negative pressure is necessary for normal milk removal from the breast. Previously, wavelike tongue movements were thought to strip or press milk from the breast. Recent ultrasound studies have suggested that the negative pressure generated by depression of the posterior tongue and mandible at the end of the peristaltic wave is most important to the amount of milk transferred (Geddes, Kent, Mitoulas, & Hartmann, 2008; Ramsay & Hartmann, 2005). If the hard palate is not intact, and the soft palate is not able to seal with the back of the tongue, no negative pressure can be created in the mouth. Infants with only a small soft palate cleft may be able to produce suction pressure, but they may or may not be able to sustain vacuum sufficiently to transfer milk from a bottle (Reid, Reilly, & Kilpatrick, 2007).

Infants move milk from the breast by compartmentalizing the oropharynx (mouth) from the nasopharynx (nasal air space) and the hypopharynx (the area above the esophagus). The soft palate behaves like a hinged flap attached to the posterior hard palate. It flips downward to lie against the back of the tongue, isolating the oropharynx. The anterior tongue cups and compresses the breast; the posterior tongue then depresses while the mandible drops slightly. This enlarges the space in the mouth. As long as the anterior tongue stays sealed on the breast and the cheeks are able to resist collapsing inward, the pressure in the mouth is reduced and milk flows from the breast along the pressure gradient onto the depressed grooved tongue until a sufficient bolus size is reached for swallowing. Then the soft palate elevates to seal off the nasopharynx, the vocal folds adduct (pull together), the epiglottis depresses to direct milk around the vocal folds and add another layer of protection for the airway, and the swallow is initiated by movements of the tongue and the muscles of the floor of the mouth.

Feeding difficulties contribute to a higher risk of growth deficiencies in cleft-affected infants (Montagnoli, Barbieri, Bettiol, Marques, & de Souza, 2005). Clefts provide an alternate route for air to enter the oropharynx, potentially preventing the isolation necessary for the production of negative pressure (**Figure 8-43**). If the cleft is confined to the lip and

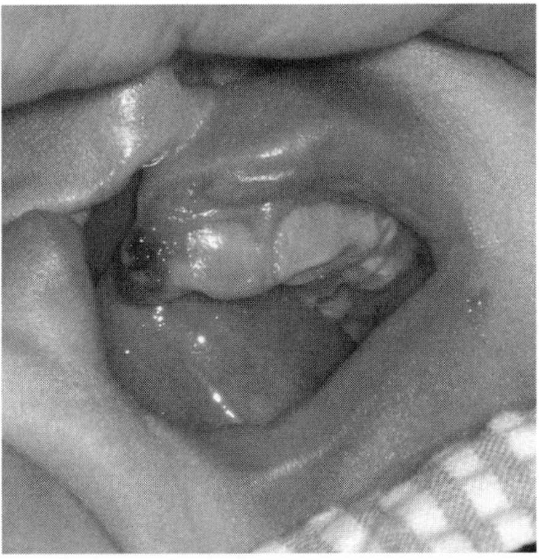

Figure 8-42 Infants with unilateral clefts frequently press the tongue tip into the cleft, distorting normal tongue movement patterns.

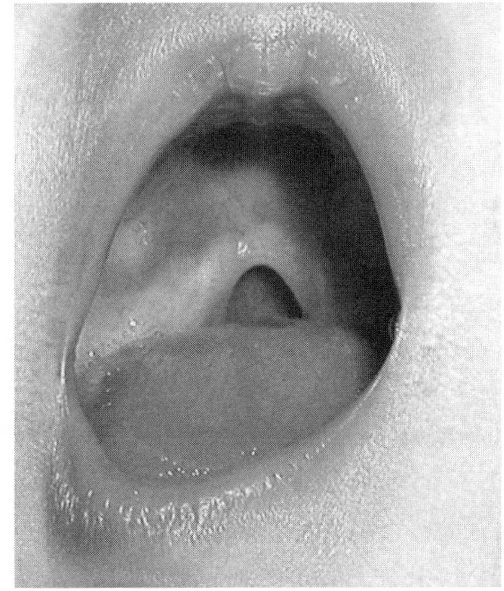

Figure 8-43 Cleft of the soft palate.

the tongue incompletely seals the breast, then the breast tissue or the mother's finger can occlude the cleft sufficiently to prevent air from rushing into the mouth. If there are small clefts in the anterior hard palate, breast tissue or a thin silicone nipple shield may provide sufficient surface to occlude the cleft and allow near normal suction levels. If the cleft extends farther than the breast tissue can reach, an obturator (an acrylic prosthesis that covers the palate) can be made. Kogo et al. (1997) reported successful partial breastfeeding with a Hotz-type plate modified to include a posterior ridge to seal with the tongue and replace the function of the soft palate. If an obturator is used, it should be smoothed on the oral side to avoid irritating the breast.

If the nares are occluded, negative pressure can be created throughout the nasopharynx, oropharynx, and hypopharynx together. Because this creates so large a volume of airspace, it would take a greater deflection of the tongue and mandible to pull milk from the breast. It is unknown if anatomic limits allow enough range of movement to provide appropriate negative pressure in so large a volume. There is evidence that some cleft-affected infants are able to transfer some milk from the breast (Garcez & Giugliani, 2005), but the mechanisms have not been studied. When bottle-fed, cleft-affected infants chew or bite instead of sucking, producing positive pressure (Masarei, Sell, et al., 2007).

Some infants with clefts are able to maintain attachment to the breast if they are held snugly by the shoulders and the mother uses one hand to hold the breast in the mouth. This hand can be used to compress the breast or to manually express milk into the infant's mouth. If the cleft is small and the infant's major issue is maintaining attachment, firming the anterior breast with two adjacent fingers (scissors hold) may help. The mother needs to be cautious to keep the fingers sufficiently far back on the breast to avoid blocking the infant's access to the areola and creating a shallow latch.

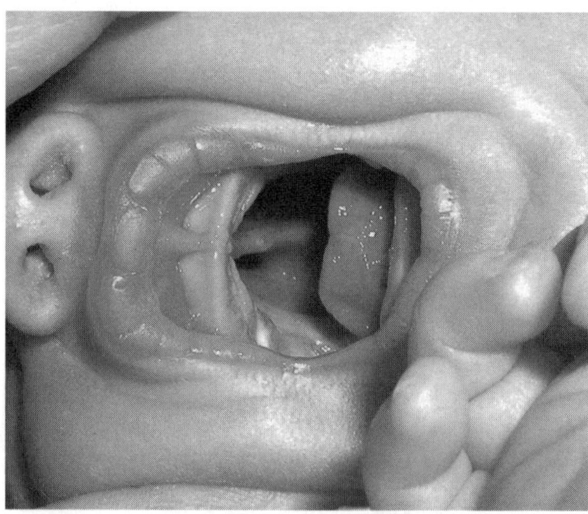

Figure 8-44 "Complete "U"-shaped cleft palate in an infant with Pierre Robin sequence. Note the short mandible and retroplaced tongue.

Pierre Robin Sequence

Pierre Robin sequence (PRS) consists of micrognathia, retroplaced tongue, and a high or U-shaped cleft palate (**Figure 8-44**). It is called a malformation sequence because the extremely small mandible causes the other features. The small jaw causes the tongue to be placed more posteriorly and hump up more in the mouth, preventing the palatal shelves from closing or causing a very high palate. The major difficulty in PRS is the infant's inability to maintain an airway, particularly during feeding. Some researchers believe the anatomical changes are insufficient to cause the airway obstruction and postulate a brainstem abnormality (Abadie, Morisseau-Durand, Beyler, Manach, & Couly, 2002), but a large prospective study showed four different anatomical mechanisms of obstruction (Marques et al., 2001), as well as poor function of the genioglossus muscle. Marques et al. found that feeding difficulties were proportional to airway instability; infants with the most difficulty breathing were the poorest feeders. Abnormalities of the facial nerve have been found in the majority of autopsies of infants with PRS (Gruen, Carranza, Karmody, & Bachor, 2005). Because the facial nerve innervates some of the facial muscles used during feeding, this compounds the feeding problems.

Feeding in a prone or semiprone position with head extension can be helpful for infants with PRS (Takagi & Bosma, 1960). Infants with PRS without a cleft may be able to breastfeed, but it will likely be inefficient and growth may be poor. Infants with clefts will usually need alternative feeding, along with the use of special positioning strategies.

Breastfeeding Cleft-Affected Infants

Active supplementation at breast can also be used to give infants with cleft palates the experience of breastfeeding even if they are unable to transfer milk. This can help to normalize tongue movements and provide traction on the palate for normal spreading. Commercial or homemade supplementer devices that rely on negative pressure (Medela Supplemental Nursing System [SNS], Lact-Aid Nursing Trainer, or a feeding tube in a bottle of milk) may not work for infants with cleft palates, unless the tube end can be placed between the tongue and the breast and the breast occludes the cleft sufficiently or the device is modified so that milk flows with gravity. For the Lact-Aid Nursing Trainer, removing the larger diameter tube and upending the device provides this free flow (Genna, 2009). The SNS can be similarly modified by making a pinhole and occluding it with a finger to stop the flow (Guóth-Gumberger, 2008). A feeding tube (5 French or finer) or a butterfly catheter with the needle cut off on a syringe full of milk can supply milk during suckling (**Figure 8-45**). The tube is best taped or held to the breast with the end of the tube at the tip of the nipple, with the tube

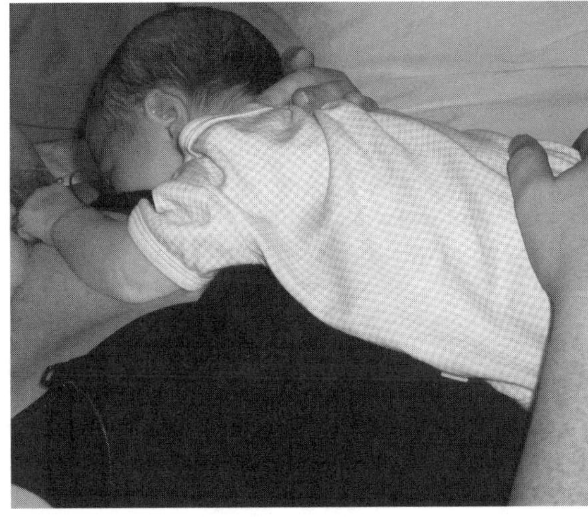

Figure 8-45 Active supplementation at breast with syringe and feeding tube.

running along the breast where the center of the infant's lower lip will contact it during latch and direct it into the mouth, between the tongue and breast. Alternatively, a periodontal syringe (a syringe with a curved, tapered tip) can be used, but care must be taken to direct the milk where it will not enter the cleft. The Lactation Institute sells flexible tip covers for curved tip syringes used in infants' mouths if the rigid tip is a concern. Most lactation consultants who use them rest the tip of the periodontal syringe against the breast rather than the infant's oral mucosa.

During active supplementation, the mother synchronizes the delivery of milk from the syringe with the infant's suckling. When the infant lowers the mandible and posterior tongue, the feeder presses the plunger of the syringe to deliver a small bolus (approximately 0.5 ml, or as much as the infant can safely swallow) into the infant's mouth. The goal is to achieve a normal sucking pattern if possible: a 1:1 suck–swallow ratio for bursts of 10–20 sucks, followed by a 5- to 6-second respiratory pause, for at least the initial 5–10 minutes of the feeding. Thereafter, pauses will likely increase in length as the infant fatigues. Lack of swallowing is a sign that boluses are too small, and loss of milk from the lips or uncoordinated swallowing sounds are signs that the bolus is too large. Finger splaying, eye widening, or avoidance responses are signs that pacing is too rapid. The mother is supervised until she correctly synchronizes milk delivery with the infant's sucking and stops delivering milk during respiratory pauses. This process can be particularly tricky with cleft-affected infants who have been using alternate swallowing movements in utero.

Positioning may prevent the loss of milk into the nasopharynx during sucking and swallowing. Use a reclining maternal position so the infant is prone on the mother's chest and the throat is uphill from the breast, or use a straddle position where the infant's legs straddle the mother's thigh and the infant rests upright along the mother's trunk to reach the breast.

Alternate Feeding for Cleft-Affected Infants

If active supplementation during breastfeeding is insufficient to provide for optimal growth, alternate feeding will be necessary. The goal of any alternate feeding method is to provide as close to the normal sensory motor experience of feeding as possible, particularly to promote normal tongue movements, including normal coordination of swallowing and breathing, which is often deficient in these infants (Masarei, Wade, Mars, Sommerlad, & Sell, 2007).

Mothers who are breastfeeding or using alternate human milk feeding techniques for cleft-affected infants will need information about maintaining milk production. Early initiation of milk expression, choice and fitting of breast pump equipment, and management of milk expression are all important issues to cover. It can be helpful to recommend overexpressing milk at first (8–10 times per day) to calibrate high milk production. Mothers might also need help problem solving ways to fit expression into their day. Many mothers find it is easier to follow a goal for the number of pumpings than a schedule of exactly when to pump. When milk production is well established, mothers with larger milk storage capacities can reduce the number of daily pumpings and maintain overall milk production.

The Haberman Feeder (SpecialNeeds Feeder)

The Haberman Feeder (marketed in the United States as the SpecialNeeds Feeder by Medela) was designed by the mother of an infant with Stickler syndrome. The teat is isolated from the bottle by a one-way valve, which allows the infant to use compression alone to move milk. The feeder can squeeze the teat to assist the infant's efforts. In addition, the nipple has a slit design that allows the feeder to control the bolus size by the orientation of the nipple in the baby's mouth. If the slit is parallel to the plane of the tongue, the flow is slowest; if the slit is perpendicular, the flow is fastest. The teat is molded with three raised lines to indicate the flow. The relative length of the line that points to the nose indicates the flow setting. The teat comes in a long (regular) version intended to promote central grooving of the tongue and a shorter (mini) version that is useful for tiny preterm infants or infants with strong gag reflexes. The Haberman teat has a narrow base and promotes a tighter lip seal than breastfeeding does, but no wide-based teat exists for cleft-affected infants at this time.

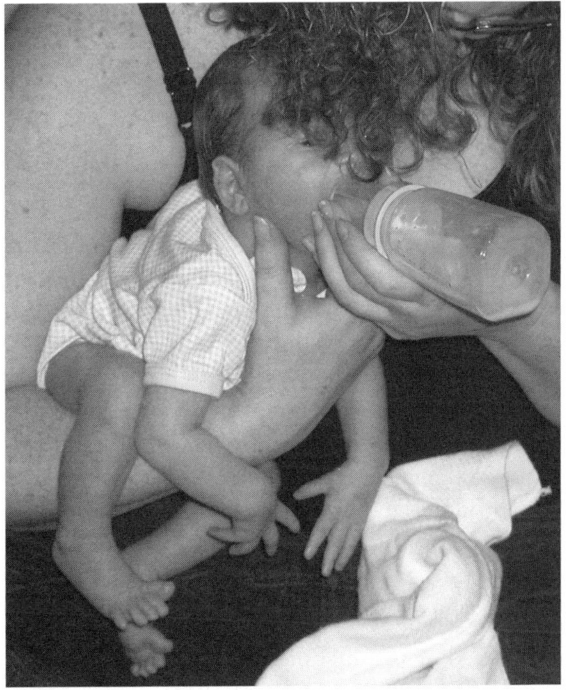

Figure 8-46 Using a Haberman feeder in a semiprone position with head extension to feed an infant with PRS and airway instability. Note splayed fingers and toes.

Using the Haberman Feeder

The feeder should help the infant preserve the gape response (a wide open mouth) by presenting the teat to the upper lip or philtrum, or crossing the teat across both lips, so the tip rests on the philtrum. When the infant opens wide, the feeder can touch the base of the feeder nipple to the tongue and then tip the feeder into the mouth, allowing the baby to assist with the tongue (**Figure 8-46**). These two nuances help simulate drawing the breast into the mouth to preserve normal feeding behaviors. It can be helpful to begin with the slowest flow (shortest line on the teat pointing to the infant's nose) and rotate the feeder in the infant's mouth until a 1:1:1 suck-swallow-breathe ratio, with good coordination of swallowing and breathing, is achieved. If the infant is not able to handle that rapid a flow, the flow is reduced until the infant feeds without signs of stress (splayed fingers, widened eyes, furrowed forehead, worried expression, color changes) or dysphagia (coughing, congestion that increases as the feeding progresses, gulping, or other poorly coordinated swallowing sounds).

If the teat is squeezed to assist the infant's tongue movements, care should be taken to coordinate the pressure with the infant's feeding efforts to avoid overwhelming the capacity to coordinate swallowing and breathing.

The Pigeon Feeder

The Pigeon feeder is a pliable plastic bottle with a valved teat marketed in the United States by Respironics. The teat looks like a normal silicone bottle nipple, but it has a softer side and a firmer side. The softer side is placed against the tongue, and milk streams from the nipple in response to compression of the teat by the tongue. The teat is narrow based, which uses a mouth position unlike breastfeeding and necessitates more activation of the orbicularis oris than breastfeeding does. The flow is rather high from the Pigeon feeder, so the baby's ability to safely swallow this flow should be assessed. For infants who can handle the flow rate, the Pigeon feeder can allow the infant more autonomy than using a squeeze feeder. Mizuno and colleagues (Mizuno, Ueda, Kani, & Kawamura, 2002) found that infants with clefts fed more effectively using the Pigeon teat than a standard teat.

The Mead Johnson Feeder

This feeder consists of a soft, squeezable bottle with a tip shaped like a short plastic straw. The feeder squeezes the container to direct milk into the infant's mouth. If it is skillfully used in synchrony with the infant's feeding efforts, milk can be delivered without causing respiratory stress, but this is rarely the case in practice. The feeder does not promote normal tongue movements, is extremely narrow, promotes feeding with an open mouth, and does not allow the infant much participation in feeding other than swallowing milk that is delivered into the mouth. The outlet tends to migrate toward the front of the mouth in use, making it more difficult for the infant to keep milk from leaking into the nasopharynx through the cleft. In general, this device provides nutrition but little normal feeding development.

Fingerfeeding

Fingerfeeding is sometimes useful for cleft-affected infants, particularly those with Pierre Robin sequence, who may have difficulty maintaining airway patency with other feeding devices even when fed in a semiprone position. An active flow device, such as a syringe and feeding tube, is needed for these infants, who cannot create negative intraoral pressure. The infant can be held sitting or prone, with the head extended to improve airway patency (Takagi & Bosma, 1960) (**Figure 8-47**). The feeder should stimulate the gape response. The

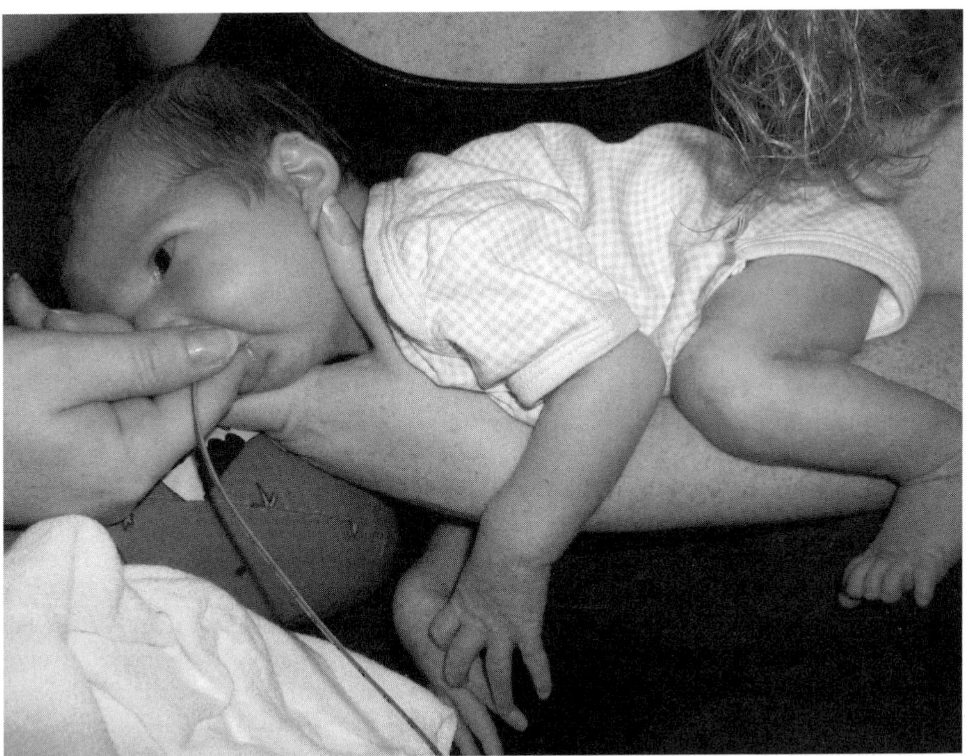

Figure 8-47 Fingerfeeding a prone infant with mild head extension can provide slow pacing and encourage improved tongue movements.

parent can slide a clean finger, or the therapist can slide a gloved finger, along the palate when the infant opens wide. The infant will soon learn to use the tongue to draw the finger deep into the mouth to where the junction of the hard and soft palate would be if there were no cleft. The infant's sucking efforts determine the pace of feeding. The feeder delivers small boluses of milk when the infant sucks, and stops when the infant pauses.

Submucous Clefts and Velopharyngeal Inadequacy

Submucous clefts of the junction of the hard and soft palate (velum) can disrupt the normal arrangement of the muscles of the soft palate, causing prolonged feeding (consistently greater than 40 minutes) and nasal regurgitation (loss of milk through the nose during quiet feeding) (Moss, Jones, & Pigott, 1990). Submucous clefts are uncommon in the general population, but they occur in 36% of children with cleft lip (Gosain, Conley, Santoro, & Denny, 1999). One result of submucous clefting is velopharyngeal inadequacy (inability of the soft palate and pharyngeal muscles to close off the nasopharynx). Neurological mechanisms (poor strength, timing, or coordination of muscular contractions) can also cause velopharyngeal incompetence, as can other anatomical issues such as hypoplasia (undergrowth) of the velum.

Infants with velopharyngeal inadequacy can usually breastfeed, but they may become irritated by milk loss from the nose (**Figure 8-48**). Some infants suffer nasal regurgitation after or between feedings or seem inexplicably unable to breastfeed well (**Figure 8-49**). Suspicion of velopharyngeal inadequacy is raised when the infant displays short sucking bursts, has harsh sounding respiration during feeding without cyanosis, and at least occasional nasal regurgitation. Positional changes (straddle, side-lying, or prone) can reduce milk loss through the nose. Exercises to improve bolus handling by stimulating better tongue grooving are recommended by feeding therapists (Morris & Klein, 2000).

Physical signs of submucous cleft palate include bifid uvula, notching at the junction of the hard and soft palate, absence of the posterior nasal spine at the posterior hard palate, a prominent midline palatal suture, and paranasal bulging (Stal & Hicks, 1998). If a light is shined in the infant's nostril, a translucent area in the central palate may be visible as well. Occult submucous cleft occurs without a bifid uvula and can be difficult to detect without magnetic resonance imaging (MRI). Velopharyngeal inadequacy can be diagnosed by nasal endoscopy. The physician may discourage the mother from breastfeeding, but infants in the author's practice with this condition were better able to breastfeed than bottle feed, even with the use of a Haberman Feeder and careful pacing (**Figure 8-50**). The Haberman Feeder can be used in addition to breastfeeding until the infant is able to meet all the feeding needs at the breast. Feeding resistance may occur at about the third month of life due to discomfort or stress of having milk penetrate the nasopharynx. Gentle encouragement

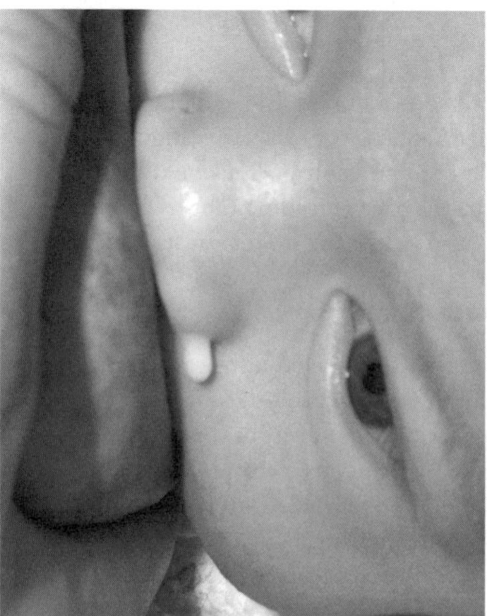

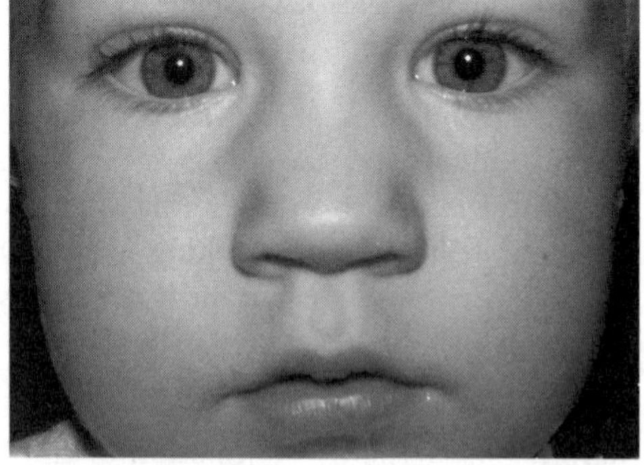

Figure 8-48 Nasal regurgitation due to velopharyngeal inadequacy.

Figure 8-49 Child with velopharyngeal insufficiency and subtle signs of submucous cleft, including paranasal bulges and "gull wing" upper lip.

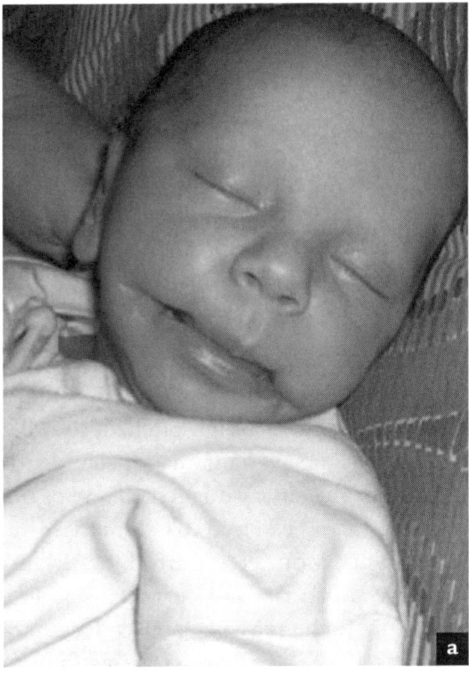

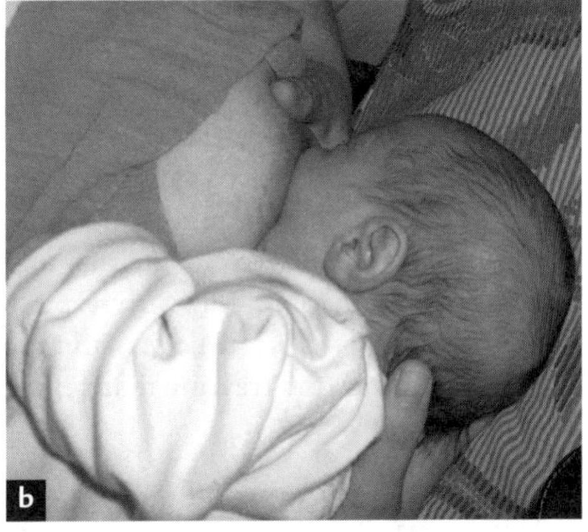

Figure 8-50a and 8-50b Bilateral transverse facial clefts (macrostomia). This condition can be isolated, or can occur with hemifacial microsomia, or undergrowth of the mandible and midface. This infant breastfed well by taking a large mouthful of breast, but was unable to seal on the bottle.

and distraction of the infant during feeding is usually helpful. Some infants respond well to having a toy to hold during feeding, others respond to the mother walking around while feeding in a sling.

Infants with overt or submucous clefts may feed less efficiently than necessary, and maternal milk supply may decline over time if pumping or expression is not maintained. Infant growth should be monitored frequently, and expression and supplementation with mother's milk by alternate feeding methods should be instituted if necessary. Alternate feeding should have the dual goal of providing nutrition and normalizing oral motor skills. It is important that the infant participate as fully as possible in feeding, that milk is not simply squeezed into the infant's mouth. Normal tongue movements should be encouraged and required by the feeding method to provide a good basis for future tongue functions.

Congenital Abnormalities of the Airway

The work of feeding requires an increase in oxygen intake, and the intermittent presence of food in the shared areas of the pharynx requires intricate coordination of swallowing and breathing. Healthy infants given a normal flow of milk are up to the challenge. Infants who are working harder to breathe at rest due to instability or malformation of their respiratory tract have less reserve of energy and oxygen to devote to feeding and may require more calories to support the increased work of breathing (Goberman & Robb, 2005). When the baseline respiratory rate is high, there are fewer spaces available between breaths for safe swallowing. Feeding refusal or failure to thrive result when the infant is forced to choose between inhibiting breathing in order to swallow or going hungry (see Chapter 6). The increased intrathoracic pressures generated by the respiratory efforts predispose infants with airway anomalies to gastroesophageal reflux (GER) (Bibi et al., 2001). In addition to the loss of milk that the infant obtained at high cost, GER causes pain and increased risk of aspiration (Suskind et al., 2006) that may lead to increased feeding resistance. The management of feeding for infants with respiratory issues involves modifying flow, improving the infant's ability to handle flow, maintaining airway patency by positioning the infant with head extension, and treating reflux if present (**Figure 8-51**).

Laryngomalacia

Laryngomalacia is the most common cause of neonatal stridor, a high-pitched, squeaky sound during breathing that indicates a narrow airway. Three variants have been identified (Kay & Goldsmith, 2006), but all cause narrowing of the airway due to collapse of the epiglottis and/or related structures (Daniel, 2006). Severe cases can lead to failure to thrive, usually between 2 and 4 months of age (Manning, Inglis, Mouzakes, Carron, & Perkins, 2005). About half of infants with laryngomalacia have another area of airway instability, typically subglottic stenosis or tracheomalacia (Dickson, Richter, Meinzen-Derr, Rutter, & Thompson, 2009). Lactation consultants can generally reduce the risk for growth failure by providing compensatory strategies for feeding that can allow the infant to get sufficient calories despite increased difficulty coordinating swallowing and breathing (Glass & Wolf, 1994).

Symptoms of laryngomalacia include inspiratory stridor (stridor when the infant breathes in) that appears or worsens during supine positioning, feeding, or crying, and suprasternal retractions (sucking in of the suprasternal notch immediately above the breastbone). During feeding, sucking bursts are likely to be very short (3–5 sucks per burst) and respiratory pauses significantly longer than the average 3–5 seconds. The child may have a worried expression and pallor or cyanosis (blueness) of the hands and feet or around the mouth and orbits. Difficulty coordinating swallowing and breathing manifesting as coughing occurred in 40% of 22 infants with laryngomalacia during breastfeeding (Avelino, Liriano, Fujita, Pignatari, & Weckx, 2005). Holding the infant in a side-lying or prone position with the head extended can help reduce respiratory distress.

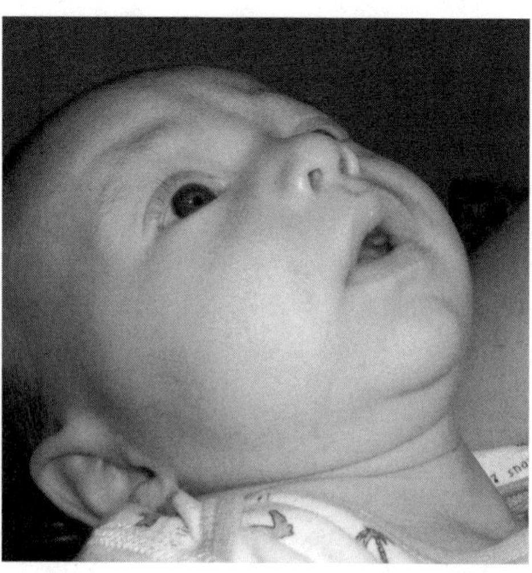

Figure 8-51 Worried expression and preferred posture of head extension in an infant with a respiratory issue.

Head extension during feeding helps to elevate the larynx and reduce airway resistance, and it may ease coordination of swallowing and breathing. Head extension can be increased in response to stridor by snuggling the infant's shoulders and sliding slightly toward the infant's feet. The mother can recline while feeding, allowing the infant to be in a prone position during feeding to help increase head extension and ease coordination of swallowing and breathing. Brief, frequent feedings are generally helpful, but some infants prefer to take longer, more leisurely feedings with long respiratory pauses. If the milk flow is rapid, the infant should be free to release the breast and rest. Holding the baby by the shoulders rather than the head and neck allows both head extension and self-pacing.

Milk expression may temporarily be necessary if the infant is an inefficient feeder. Expressed milk can be fed to the infant with a Haberman Feeder used at the lowest setting or by fingerfeeding. Infants with severe respiratory instability may fingerfeed best in a prone position with the head extended. Laryngomalacia generally begins to improve by 4–6 months of age, and it resolves by 9–18 months in most infants (Thompson, 2007). Supplemental feedings can be gradually phased out as respiratory capacity and coordination of sucking, swallowing, and breathing improve. Infants who are unable to grow well with feeding compensations should be referred to a specialist (ear, nose, and throat [ENT], or otorhinolaryngologist) to rule out vascular malformations, webs, or masses that can cause the same symptoms and to assess the need for surgery.

Tracheomalacia

Although it is far less common than laryngomalacia, tracheomalacia is the most common malformation of the lower airway. In this condition, the cartilage rings that maintain the stiffness of the trachea during airflow are abnormally shaped and/or weak. The Bernoulli principle states that rapid air movement decreases the surrounding air pressure. The strength of this pressure differential allows airplanes to fly and partially collapses the trachea as the infant breathes. Airflow through the narrowed trachea causes stridor. Adults with tracheomalacia exhibit expiratory stridor. Infants with tracheomalacia generally have expiratory stridor and cough if the intrathoracic trachea is affected, and they have inspiratory stridor if the cervical trachea is affected (Carden, Boiselle, Waltz, & Ernst, 2005). The use of accessory muscles to attempt to move air past the obstructed area (Altman, Wetmore, & Marsh, 1999) pulls the sternum, intercostal (rib) muscles, or abdomen in, resulting in a retracted appearance (**Figure 8-52**).

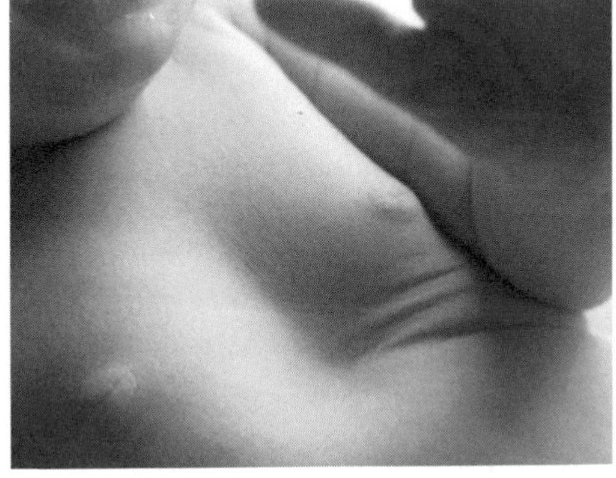

Figure 8-52 Sternal retraction in an infant with tracheomalacia.

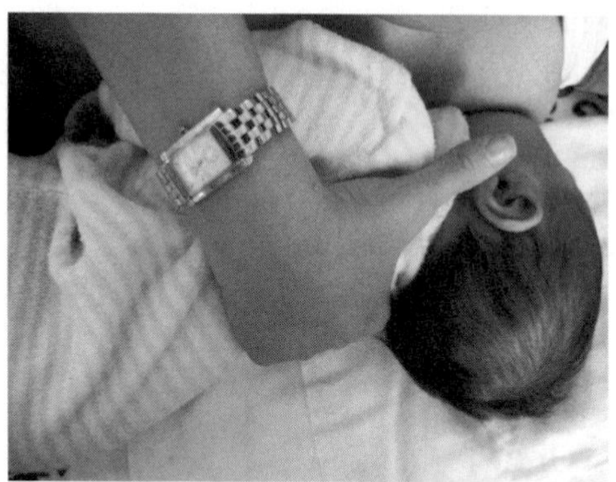

Figure 8-53 Strong head extension can help infants with respiratory malformations by reducing airway resistance to airflow.

Feeding concerns are similar to those with laryngomalacia, as are interventions. Head extension, prone positioning for feeding, allowing the infant to self-pace, and offering frequent feedings to compensate for reduced efficiency are all helpful (**Figure 8-53**). Infants with sternal or intercostal retractions and biphasic stridor (stridor with both inhalation and exhalation) should receive a medical workup because they are more likely to have compression of the trachea from a tumor or vascular ring (Spencer, Yeoh, Van Asperen, & Fitzgerald, 2004).

Vocal Fold (Cord) Paralysis

Stridor and hoarse cry are signs of vocal fold paralysis (VFP) or paresis (weakness) in infants (Daniel, 2006). Paralysis can be either unilateral or bilateral. The etiology (cause) can be neurological, structural, or due to birth trauma. Most infants recover from VFP within 24–36 months. Bilateral VFP in the adducted (closed) position can be life threatening and requires intubation (Kaushal, Upadhyay, Aggarwal, & Deorari, 2005). In the past, tracheostomy was performed to open the airway for adducted vocal folds. Partial removal of the arytenoid cartilage with a surgical laser restores the airway and often allows the tracheotomy tube to be removed (Bower, Choi, & Cotton, 1994; Brigger & Hartnick, 2002; Hartnick, Brigger, Willging, Cotton, & Myer, 2003). When the VFP is in the abducted position (open) bilaterally, the airway is unprotected during swallowing and the infant is at risk for aspiration. Many different surgical techniques are possible for abducted VFP. Infants with unilateral abducted VFP feed best with the undamaged cord downward (dependent) for best airway protection (Tunkel, 1994).

Subglottic Stenosis

Subglottic stenosis, or narrowing of the lumen of the cricoid cartilage, causes excessive work of respiration and biphasic stridor (stridor during both inhalation and exhalation) (Daniel, 2006). This condition is usually self-limiting and resolves as the child grows, but during early infancy feeding can be difficult. Breastfeeding can be particularly important both in providing optimal pacing of feeding and to help prevent airway inflammation that would exacerbate the condition.

Nasal Blockages

Choanal atresia (blockage of the posterior nasal opening in the skull) can be unilateral or bilateral. When it is bilateral, it can cause severe breathing difficulties and cyanosis that are relieved by crying (Daniel, 2006). An infant with reduced nasal airway patency from any cause will release the breast repeatedly during a feeding to breathe through the mouth. Short, frequent feedings and referral for medical evaluation are warranted. Other causes of nasal obstruction include small nares and nasopharyngeal tumors. One case of mouth breathing and breastfeeding difficulties in a young infant resolved when a salivary gland tumor in the nasopharynx was identified and removed (Cohen, Yoder, Thomas, Salerno, & Isaacson, 2003).

Congenital Heart Disease

Although there are many types of malformations of the heart, they are currently classified as those that reduce pulmonary blood flow, those that increase it, and those that obstruct it. Infants with congenital heart disease (CHD) have reduced energy and endurance, increased hypoxia with effort, and breathlessness. There is generally a higher metabolic need for calories; at the same time fluids may need to be restricted in order to prevent congestive heart failure. The appropriate renal solute load of human milk is particularly advantageous for infants with CHD. Children with CHD are particularly prone to infections and need the anti-infective properties of human milk even more than their well peers.

In the past, breastfeeding was thought to be too much effort for infants with CHD, but studies have shown better growth and shorter hospitalization (Combs & Marino, 1993) and better oxygen saturation during feeding (Marino, O'Brien, & LoRe, 1995) for breastfed versus bottle-fed infants with heart defects. Support, staff education, and accessibility of breast pumps and lactation consultants increased the rate of breastfeeding among infants with CHD in one institution (Barbas & Kelleher, 2004). Feeding compensations recommended for infants with CHD include short, very frequent feeding and supplementation at the breast with hindmilk, which is high-fat milk expressed at the end of feedings, if additional calories are needed to support growth (Lambert & Watters, 1998). Minimal mother-baby separation may reduce infant stress and increase the percentage of calories that can go toward growth.

> Feeding is aerobic exercise and requires normal cardiorespiratory function. Infants with airway anomalies or cardiac issues are vulnerable to failure to thrive if their need to feed frequently for short durations is not accommodated. Depending on the severity of the condition, feeding compensations may be insufficient to allow the infant to meet caloric needs, and alternative feeding may be necessary. Careful pacing of the feeding will help avoid hypoxia and reduce the risk of aspiration. Infants who are unable to feed without substantial accommodations should be referred for medical evaluation because delayed identification of cardiorespiratory malformations is not uncommon.

Other Structural Issues

Congenital Muscular Torticollis

The etiology of torticollis is still debated, but it is thought to result from either restricted intrauterine positioning or vascular injury to one sternocleidomastoid (SCM) muscle before or during birth (Do, 2006). A contracted SCM muscle causes the head to be rotated to the contralateral (opposite) side and tilted to the ipsilateral (same) side. There are associated facial asymmetries, including changes in eye height and size, unequal mandible opening (Wall & Glass, 2006), and lowering and posterior rotation of the ear on the same side as the muscle imbalance. The contralateral ear is usually flattened. If untreated, progressive fibrosis (replacement of muscle tissue with inelastic fibrous tissue) may occur (Hsu et al., 1999). Treatment consists of stretching exercises performed by the parents under direction of a physician, chiropractor, or therapist and is most effective if started before 1 year of age (Cheng et al., 2001). The neck movement deficits in persistent cases are treated surgically or, more recently, by injections of botulinum toxin (Joyce & de Chalain, 2005; Oleszek, Chang, Apkon, & Wilson, 2005).

Breastfeeding issues posed by torticollis include difficulty attaching and transferring milk due to the asymmetrical mandible and twisted neck position (**Figure 8-54** and **Figure 8-55**). The infant should be positioned at the breast in a way that maintains the preferred head position until therapy begins to yield results (**Figure 8-56**). Milk transfer should be assessed to ensure that the infant is able to drive milk production, and pumping and alternate feeding should be used if necessary. Two infants in Wall and Glass's case series (2006) and several in the author's practice showed improved milk transfer and ease of attachment with a nipple shield. Sublingual support (fingertip pressure directed upward toward the

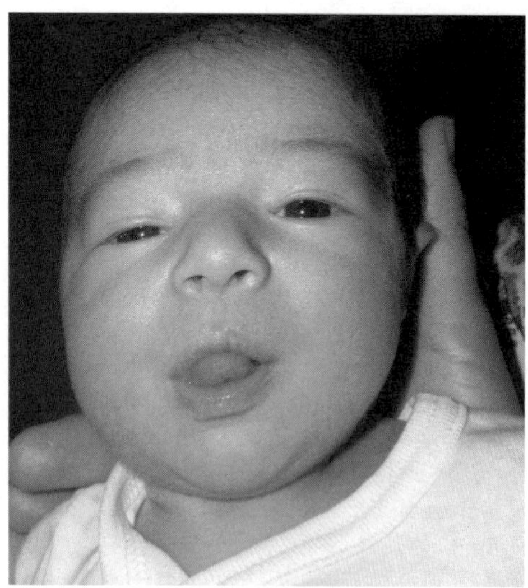

Figure 8-54 Infant with torticollis. Note the rotated and tipped head, and asymmetrical face and eyes.

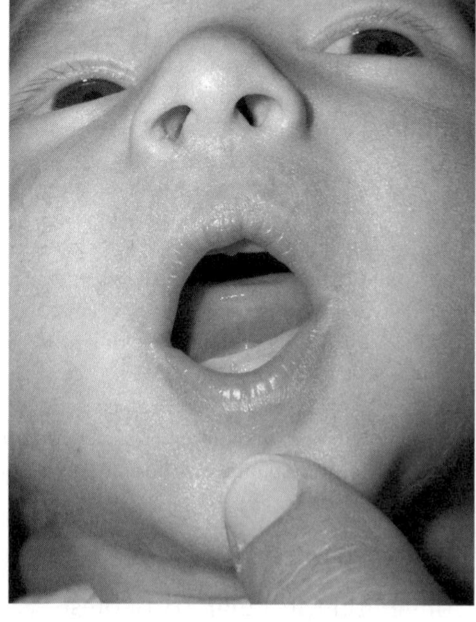

Figure 8-55 Asymmetrical mandibular opening in torticollis.

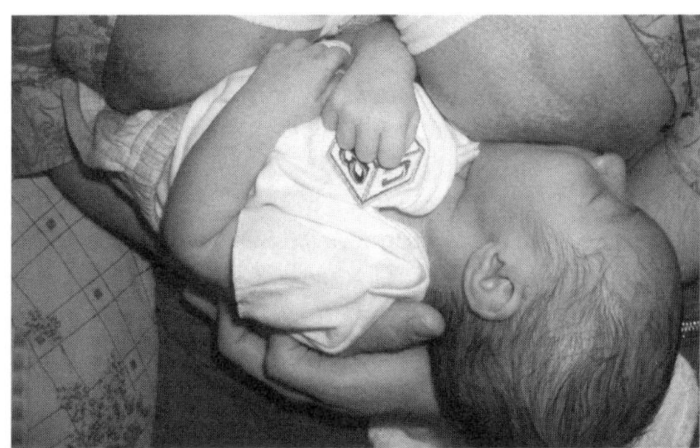

Figure 8-56 Allowing infant to latch with head rotated to the preferred side.

mouth and forward toward the jaw bone on the underside of the chin, to support the musculature of the tongue) may assist tongue movements in babies with torticollis and jaw asymmetry (see Chapter 12, **Figure 12-15**).

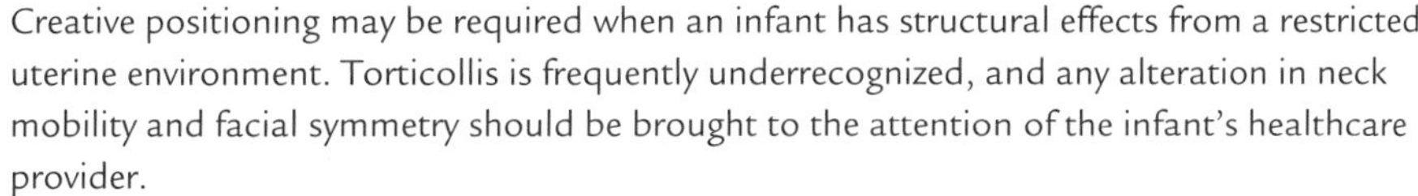

Creative positioning may be required when an infant has structural effects from a restricted uterine environment. Torticollis is frequently underrecognized, and any alteration in neck mobility and facial symmetry should be brought to the attention of the infant's healthcare provider.

Developmental Dysplasia of the Hip

Although hip dysplasia does not affect the mouth directly, instability of the hips reduces stability of the jaw and tongue. Treatment consists of a rigid metal frame that immobilizes the legs from the pelvis to the feet, which can make positioning for feeding a challenge. The mother may need protection from the brace in the form of a towel or pillow between the metal and her body. One option for feeding an infant in a hip brace is to lay the infant's trunk and legs on a pillow placed next to the mother's thigh, and bring the infant's chin to the breast at the lateral (outer) side of the nipple.

Conclusion

The structure and function of the body are intimately intertwined. Anatomical variations and anomalies of the tongue and jaw have the most obvious effects on feeding, but alterations of other parts of the body may also be relevant due to their effect on stability. Anomalies that affect cardiorespiratory function leave less energy and oxygen for feeding. Breastfeeding is the easiest method of feeding for infants with reduced aerobic capacity because they are in control of pacing.

References

Abadie, V., Morisseau-Durand, M. P., Beyler, C., Manach, Y., & Couly, G. (2002). Brainstem dysfunction: A possible neuroembryological pathogenesis of isolated Pierre Robin sequence. *European Journal of Pediatrics, 161*(5), 275–280.

Altman, K. W., Wetmore, R. F., & Marsh, R. R. (1999). Congenital airway abnormalities in patients requiring hospitalization. *Archives of Otolaryngology—Head and Neck Surgery, 125*(5), 525–528.

Amir, L. H., James, J. P., & Donath, S. M. (2006). Reliability of the Hazelbaker assessment tool for lingual frenulum function. *International Breastfeeding Journal, 1*(1), 3.

Ardran, G. M., Kemp, F. H., & Lind, J. (1958). A cineradiographic study of breast feeding. *British Journal of Radiology, 31*(363), 156–162.

Avelino, M. A., Liriano, R. Y., Fujita, R., Pignatari, S., & Weckx, L. L. (2005). Treatment laryngomalacia: Experience with 22 cases. *Brazilian Journal of Otorhinolaryngology, 71*, 330–334.

Ballard, J. L., Auer, C. E., & Khoury, J. C. (2002). Ankyloglossia: Assessment, incidence, and effect of frenuloplasty on the breastfeeding dyad. *Pediatrics, 110*(5), 63.

Band, C. (2000). Breastfeeding an infant with an ulcerated hemangioma on the lip. *Current Issues in Clinical Lactation, 1*, 68–71.

Barbas, K. H., & Kelleher, D. K. (2004). Breastfeeding success among infants with congenital heart disease. *Pediatric Nursing, 30*(4), 285–289.

Bibi, H., Khvolis, E., Shoseyov, D., Ohaly, M., Ben Dor, D., London, D., & Ater, D. (2001). The prevalence of gastroesophageal reflux in children with tracheomalacia and laryngomalacia. *Chest, 119*(2), 409–413.

Bower, C. M., Choi, S. S., & Cotton, R. T. (1994). Arytenoidectomy in children. *The Annals of Otology, Rhinology, and Laryngology, 103*(4 Pt. 1), 271–278.

Brigger, M. T., & Hartnick, C. J. (2002). Surgery for pediatric vocal cord paralysis: A meta-analysis. *Archives of Otolaryngology—Head and Neck Surgery, 126*(4), 349–355.

Buryk, M., Bloom, D., & Shope, T. (2011). Efficacy of neonatal release of ankyloglossia: A randomized trial. *Pediatrics, 128*(2), 280–288.

Carden, K. A., Boiselle, P. M., Waltz, D. A., & Ernst, A. (2005). Tracheomalacia and tracheobronchomalacia in children and adults: An in-depth review. *Chest, 127*, 984–1005.

Cheng, J. C., Wong, M. W., Tang, S. P., Chen, T. M., Shum, S. L., & Wong, E. M. (2001). Clinical determinants of the outcome of manual stretching in the treatment of congenital muscular torticollis in infants. A prospective study of eight hundred and twenty-one cases. *Journal of Bone and Joint Surgery, American, 83-A*(5), 679–687.

Cohen, E. G., Yoder, M., Thomas, R. M., Salerno, D., & Isaacson, G. (2003). Congenital salivary gland anlage tumor of the nasopharynx. *Pediatrics, 112*(1 Pt. 1), 66–69.

Combs, V. L., & Marino, B. L. (1993). A comparison of growth patterns in breast- and bottle-fed infants with congenital heart disease. *Pediatric Nursing, 19*(2), 175–179.

Daniel, S. J. (2006). The upper airway: Congenital malformations. *Paediatric Respiratory Review, 7*(Suppl. 1), 260–263.

Dickson, J. M., Richter, G. T., Meinzen-Derr, J., Rutter, M. J., & Thompson, D. M. (2009). Secondary airway lesions in infants with laryngomalacia. *Annals of Otology, Rhinology, and Laryngology, 118*, 37–43.

Do, T. T. (2006). Congenital muscular torticollis: Current concepts and review of treatment. *Current Opinions in Pediatrics, 18*(1), 26–29.

Dollberg, S., Botzer, E., Grunis, E., & Mimouni, F. B. (2006). Immediate nipple pain relief after frenotomy in breast-fed infants with ankyloglossia: A randomized, prospective study. *Journal of Pediatric Surgery, 41*(9), 1598–1600.

Forlenza, G. P., Paradise Black, N. M., McNamara, E. G., & Sullivan, S. E. (2010). Ankyloglossia, exclusive breastfeeding, and failure to thrive. *Pediatrics, 125*, e1500–e1504.

Garcez, L. W., & Giugliani, E. R. (2005). Population-based study on the practice of breastfeeding in children born with cleft lip and palate. *Cleft Palate-Craniofacial Journal, 42*, 687–693.

Geddes, D. T., Chadwick, L. M., Kent, J. C., Garbin, C. P., & Hartmann, P. E. (2009). Ultrasound imaging of infant swallowing during breast-feeding. *Dysphagia*, 25(3), 183–191.

Geddes, D. T., Kent, J. C., Mitoulas, L. R., & Hartmann, P. E. (2008). Tongue movement and intra-oral vacuum in breastfeeding infants. *Early Human Development, 84*, 471–477.

Geddes, D. T., Langton, D. B., Gollow, I., Jacobs, L. A., Hartmann, P. E., & Simmer, K. (2008). Frenulotomy for breastfeeding infants with ankyloglossia: Effect on milk removal and sucking mechanism as imaged by ultrasound. *Pediatrics, 122*, e188–e194.

Genna, C. W. (2009). *Selecting and using breastfeeding tools improving care and outcomes*. Amarillo, TX: Hale.

Glass, R. P., & Wolf, L. S. (1994). Incoordination of sucking, swallowing, and breathing as an etiology for breastfeeding difficulty. *Journal of Human Lactation, 10*(3), 185–189.

Goberman, A. M., & Robb, M. P. (2005). Acoustic characteristics of crying in infantile laryngomalacia. *Logopedics, Phoniatrics, Vocology, 30*(2), 79–84.

Gosain, A. K., Conley, S. F., Santoro, T. D., & Denny, A. D. (1999). A prospective evaluation of the prevalence of submucous cleft palate in patients with isolated cleft lip versus controls. *Plastic and Reconstructive Surgery, 103*(7), 1857–1863.

Griffiths, D. M. (2004). Do tongue ties affect breastfeeding? *Journal of Human Lactation, 20*(4), 409–414.

Gruen, P. M., Carranza, A., Karmody, C. S., & Bachor, E. (2005). Anomalies of the ear in the Pierre Robin triad. *Annals of Otology, Rhinology, and Laryngology, 114*(8), 605–613.

Gunn, T. R., Tonkin, S. L., Hadden, W., Davis, S. L., & Gunn, A. J. (2000). Neonatal micrognathia is associated with small upper airways on radiographic measurement. *Acta Paediatrica, 89*(1), 82–87.

Guóth-Gumberger, M. (2008). Making a supplemental feeding tube device work for a baby with a cleft palate. In M. Guóth-Gumberger (Ed.), *A world wide view on breastfeeding* (pp. 94–95). Vienna, Austria: European Lactation Consultant Association.

Habel, A., Elhadi, N., Sommerlad, B., & Powell, J. (2006). Delayed detection of cleft palate: An audit of newborn examination. *Archives of Disease in Childhood, 91*(3), 238–240.

Hartnick, C. J., Brigger, M. T., Willging, J. P., Cotton, R. T., & Myer, C. M., III. (2003). Surgery for pediatric vocal cord paralysis: A retrospective review. *Annals of Otology, Rhinology, and Laryngology, 112*(1), 1–6.

Hazelbaker, A. K. (1993). *The assessment tool for lingual frenulum function (ATLFF): Use in a lactation consultant private practice*. Unpublished master's thesis, Pacific Oaks College, Pasadena, CA.

Hiiemae, K. M., & Palmer, J. B. (2003). Tongue movements in feeding and speech. *Critical Reviews in Oral Biology and Medicine, 14*(6), 413–429.

Hogan, M., Westcott, C., & Griffiths, M. (2005). Randomized, controlled trial of division of tongue-tie in infants with feeding problems. *Journal of Paediatrics and Child Health, 41*(5–6), 246–250.

Hong, P., Lago, D., Seargeant, J., Pellman, L., Magit, A. E., & Pransky, S. M. (2010). Defining ankyloglossia: A case series of anterior and posterior tongue ties. *International Journal of Pediatric Otorhinolaryngology, 74*, 1003–1006.

Horn, M. H. (2006). Smaller mandibular size in infants with a history of an apparent life-threatening event. *Journal of Pediatrics, 149*(4), 499–504.

Hsu, T. C., Wang, C. L., Wong, M. K., Hsu, K. H., Tang, F. T., & Chen, H. T. (1999). Correlation of clinical and ultrasonographic features in congenital muscular torticollis. *Archives of Physical Medicine and Rehabilitation, 80*(6), 637–641.

Joyce, M. B., & de Chalain, T. M. (2005). Treatment of recalcitrant idiopathic muscular torticollis in infants with botulinum toxin type A. *Journal of Craniofacial Surgery, 16*(2), 321–327.

Kaushal, M., Upadhyay, A., Aggarwal, R., & Deorari, A. K. (2005). Congenital stridor due to bilateral vocal cord palsy. *Indian Journal of Pediatrics, 72*(5), 443–444.

Kay, D. J., & Goldsmith, A. J. (2006). Laryngomalacia: A classification system and surgical treatment strategy. *Ear, Nose and Throat Journal, 85*(5), 328–331.

Kennedy, D., Kieser, J., Bolter, C., Swain, M., Singh, B., & Waddell, J. N. (2010). Tongue pressure patterns during water swallowing. *Dysphagia, 25*, 11–19.

Klockars, T., & Pitkaranta, A. (2009). Pediatric tongue-tie division: Indications, techniques and patient satisfaction. *International Journal of Pediatric Otorhinolaryngology. 71*(8), 1321–1324.

Knox, I. (2010). Tongue tie and frenotomy in the breastfeeding newborn. *NeoReviews, 11*, e513–e519.

Kogo, M., Okada, G., Ishii, S., Shikata, M., Iida, S., & Matsuya, T. (1997). Breast feeding for cleft lip and palate patients, using the Hotz-type plate. *Cleft Palate-Craniofacial Journal, 34*(4), 351–353.

Kveim, M., Fischer, J. C., Jones, K. L., & Gruer, B. (1985). Early tongue resection for Beckwith-Wiedemann macroglossia. *Annals of Plastic Surgery, 14*(2), 142–144.

Lambert, J. M., & Watters, N. E. (1998). Breastfeeding the infant/child with a cardiac defect: An informal survey. *Journal of Human Lactation, 14*(2), 151–155.

Livingstone, V. H., Willis, C. E., Abdel-Wareth, L. O., Thiessen, P., & Lockitch, G. (2000). Neonatal hypernatremic dehydration associated with breast-feeding malnutrition: A retrospective survey. *Canadian Medical Association Journal, 162*(5), 647–652.

Luz, C. L., Garib, D. G., & Arouca, R. (2006). Association between breastfeeding duration and mandibular retrusion: A cross-sectional study of children in the mixed dentition. *American Journal of Orthodontics and Dentofacial Orthopedics, 130*(4), 531–534.

Madlon-Kay, D. J., Ricke, L. A., Baker, N. J., & DeFor, T. A. (2008). Case series of 148 tongue-tied newborn babies evaluated with the assessment tool for lingual frenulum function. *Midwifery, 24*, 353–357.

Manning, S. C., Inglis, A. F., Mouzakes, J., Carron, J., & Perkins, J. A. (2005). Laryngeal anatomic differences in pediatric patients with severe laryngomalacia. *Archives of Otolaryngology—Head and Neck Surgery, 131*(4), 340–343.

Marino, B. L., O'Brien, P., & LoRe, H. (1995). Oxygen saturations during breast and bottle feedings in infants with congenital heart disease. *Journal of Pediatric Nursing, 10*(6), 360–364.

Marques, I. L., de Sousa, T. V., Carniero, A. F., Barbieri, M. A., Bettiol, H., & Gutierrez, M. R. (2001). Clinical experience with infants with Robin sequence: A prospective study. *Cleft Palate and Craniofacial Journal, 38*(2), 171–178.

Masarei, A. G., Sell, D., Habel, A., Mars, M., Sommerlad, B. C., & Wade, A. (2007). The nature of feeding in infants with unrepaired cleft lip and/or palate compared with healthy noncleft infants. *Cleft Palate-Craniofacial Journal, 44*, 321–328.

Masarei, A. G., Wade, A., Mars, M., Sommerlad, B. C., & Sell, D. (2007). A randomized control trial investigating the effect of presurgical orthopedics on feeding in infants with cleft lip and/or palate. *Cleft Palate-Craniofacial Journal, 44*, 182–193.

Maturo, S. C., & Mair, E. A. (2006). Submucosal minimally invasive lingual excision: An effective, novel surgery for pediatric tongue base reduction. *Annals of Otology, Rhinology, and Laryngology, 115*(8), 624–630.

Messner, A. H., Lalakea, M. L., Aby, J., McMahon, J., & Bair, E. (2000). Ankyloglossia: Incidence and associated feeding difficulties. *Archives of Otolaryngology—Head and Neck Surgery, 126*(1), 36–39.

Mizuno, K., Ueda, A., Kani, K., & Kawamura, H. (2002). Feeding behaviour of infants with cleft lip and palate. *Acta Paediatrica, 91*, 1227–1232.

Montagnoli, L. C., Barbieri, M. A., Bettiol, H., Marques, I. L., & de Souza, L. (2005). Growth impairment of children with different types of lip and palate clefts in the first 2 years of life: A cross-sectional study. *Journal de Pediatrica, 81*(6), 461–465.

Morris, S. E., & Klein, M. D. (2000). *Pre-feeding skills.* San Antonio, TX: Therapy Skill Builders.

Moss, A. L., Jones, K., & Pigott, R. W. (1990). Submucous cleft palate in the differential diagnosis of feeding difficulties. *Archives of Disease in Childhood, 65*(2), 182–184.

Oleszek, J. L., Chang, N., Apkon, S. D., & Wilson, P. E. (2005). Botulinum toxin type A in the treatment of children with congenital muscular torticollis. *American Journal of Physical Medicine and Rehabilitation, 84*(10), 813–816.

Page, D. C. (2001). Breastfeeding in early functional jaw orthopedics (an introduction). *The Functional Orthodontist, 18*(3), 24–27.

Page, D. C. (2003). "Real" early orthodontic treatment. From birth to age 8. *The Functional Orthodontist, 20*(1–2), 48–54.

Ramsay, D. T., et al. (2004a). Ultrasound imaging of the effect of frenulotomy on breastfeeding infants with ankyloglossia. Abstracts of the Proceedings of the 2004 International Society for Research in Human Milk and Lactation Conference (ISRHML). Queens' College Cambridge, UK, September 10–14, 2004.

Ramsay, D. T., et al. (2004b). Ultrasound imaging of the sucking mechanics of the breastfeeding infant. Abstracts of the Proceedings of the 2004 International Society for Research in Human Milk and Lactation Conference (ISRHML). Queens' College Cambridge, UK, September 10–14, 2004.

Ramsay, D. T., & Hartmann, P. (2005). Milk removal from the breast. *Breastfeeding Review, 13*(1), 5–7.

Reid, J., Reilly, S., & Kilpatrick, N. (2007). Sucking performance of babies with cleft conditions. *Cleft Palate-Craniofacial Journal, 44*, 312–320.

Ricke, L. A., Baker, N. J., Madlon-Kay, D. J., & DeFor, T. A. (2005). Newborn tongue-tie: Prevalence and effect on breast-feeding. *Journal of the American Board of Family Practice, 18*(1), 1–7.

Smolinski, K. N., & Yan, A. C. (2005). Hemangiomas of infancy: Clinical and biological characteristics. *Clinical Pediatrics, 44*(9), 747–766.

Spencer, S., Yeoh, B. H., Van Asperen, P. P., & Fitzgerald, D. A. (2004). Biphasic stridor in infancy. *Medical Journal of Australia, 180*(7), 347–349.

Srinivasan, A., Dobrich, C., Mitnick, H., & Feldman, P. (2006). Ankyloglossia in breastfeeding infants: The effect of frenotomy on maternal nipple pain and latch. *Breastfeeding Medicine, 1*, 216–224.

Stal, S., & Hicks, M. J. (1998). Classic and occult submucous cleft palates: A histopathologic analysis. *Cleft Palate and Craniofacial Journal, 35*(4), 351–358.

Suskind, D. L., Thompson, D. M., Gulati, M., Huddleston, P., Liu, D. C., & Baroody, F. M. (2006). Improved infant swallowing after gastroesophageal reflux disease treatment: A function of improved laryngeal sensation? *Laryngoscope, 116*(8), 1397–1403.

Takagi, Y., & Bosma, J. F. (1960). Disability of oral function in an infant associated with displacement of the tongue: Therapy by feeding in prone position. *Acta Paediatrica Scandinavia, 49*(Suppl.), 62–69.

Thompson, D. M. (2007). Abnormal sensorimotor integrative function of the larynx in congenital laryngomalacia: A new theory of etiology. *Laryngoscope, 117*, 1–33.

Tunkel, D. E. (1994). Surgical approach to diagnosis and management: Otolaryngology. In D. N. Tuchman & R. S. Walter (Eds.), *Disorders of feeding and swallowing in infants and children* (pp. 131–152). San Diego, CA: Singular.

Wall, V., & Glass, R. (2006). Mandibular asymmetry and breastfeeding problems: Experience from 11 cases. *Journal of Human Lactation, 22*(3), 328–334.

Wiessinger, D. (1995). Breastfeeding difficulties as a result of tight lingual and labial frena: A case report. *Journal of Human Lactation, 11*(4), 313–316.

Yang, W. T., Loveday, E. J., Metreweli, C., & Sullivan, P. B. (1997). Ultrasound assessment of swallowing in malnourished disabled children. *British Journal of Radiology, 70*, 992–994.

CHAPTER 9

Minimally Invasive Treatment for Posterior Tongue-Tie (The Hidden Tongue-Tie)

Elizabeth V. Coryllos, Catherine Watson Genna, and Judy LeVan Fram

The need for frenotomy when infants are unable to breastfeed effectively or without causing maternal pain is increasingly well recognized (Geddes et al., 2008; Griffiths, 2004; Hong et al., 2010; Khoo, Dabbas, Sudhakaran, Ade-Ajayi, & Patel, 2009; Kupietzky & Botzer, 2005; Messner, Lalakea, Aby, Macmahon, & Bair, 2000; Ricke, Baker, Madlon-Kay, & DeFor, 2005). Improvements in breastfeeding ability and maternal comfort after frenotomy have been confirmed in randomized controlled trials (Buryk, Bloom, & Shope 2011; Dollberg, Botzer, Grunis, & Mimouni, 2006; Hogan, Westcott, & Griffiths, 2005; Srinivasan, Dobrich, Mitnick, & Feldman, 2006).

Since the publication of our article in the American Academy of Pediatrics Section on Breastfeeding newsletter (Coryllos, Genna, & Salloum, 2004) and our presentations of our ultrasound research on more subtle cases of ankyloglossia, we have been contacted by women throughout the world who have had difficulty obtaining treatment for their infants who are struggling to latch, maintain attachment, or transfer milk. We hope to remedy this situation by detailing the conservative management (modified frenotomy in early infancy without general anesthesia) reintroduced and expanded by Coryllos.

Recognition

The first step toward treating any issue is recognition of the problem. Practitioners who merely look for a heart-shaped tongue tip are likely to miss restrictive frenula that restrict only the mid- or posterior tongue. Frenula that extend the entire length of the tongue or are particularly tight can completely impede tongue elevation, preventing the elevation of the sides of the tongue that produces the heart shape. Frenula remnants that extend along the posterior half of the tongue, or that are buried behind the oral mucosa, reduce tongue mobility without producing an indentation in the tongue tip. Normal tongue mobility includes elevation of the tongue tip to the palate with the mouth fully open, extension of the tongue tip over the lower lip without pulling down the tongue tip, and lateralization of the tongue tip to the corners of the mouth without twisting the body of the tongue (Chapter 8).

In addition to observing tongue movement, elevation of the tongue and palpation of the base of the tongue are necessary to avoid missing submucosal frenula.

Breastfeeding History and Assessment

The breastfeeding history can help determine the need for a frenotomy. If positioning and management are optimal, yet the dyad is frustrated by poor milk transfer, prolonged feeding, difficulty coordinating swallowing and breathing, or maternal pain, frenotomy may be indicated. The presence of compensatory tongue movements during breastfeeding can be observed on ultrasound with a transducer placed submentally (beneath the baby's chin). Nipple compression and distortion is readily visible, which is one mechanism by which milk flow is obstructed.

The clinical breastfeeding assessment should focus on attachment, milk transfer, ability to sustain attachment, and efficiency of bolus handling (soft, rhythmic swallowing without gulping, mistimed swallows, coughing, milk loss from the lips or stress signs). An entire feeding should be observed because some infants with posterior ankyloglossia are able to feed well for short periods of time and then become fatigued and display fasciculations (tremors) of the tongue and jaw or push off the breast and cry or fall asleep without getting sufficient calories. Subtle signs of sucking difficulties related to tongue-tie include dimpling of the cheeks with excessive jaw excursions, upper lip sweeping, or movement of the breast into and out of the mouth.

A family history of problems related to ankyloglossia is also explored. The need for speech therapy, orthodontia, or sleep apnea treatment in family members may expose previously unrecognized tongue-tie. More subtle indicators in families include parental complaints of excessive snoring in the nonobese, jaw fatigue issues (often noted by singers and professional speakers), and dental crowding requiring orthodontia. Bleeding disorders and allergies to topical anesthetic agents should be ruled out before performing a frenotomy. Relative contraindications to frenotomy include Pierre Robin sequence, congenital amyotonia, or macroglossia, where it might increase the risk of upper airway obstruction.

The Frenotomy Procedure and Modifications for Posterior Tongue-Tie

The baby is observed lying down on his or her back, then swaddled, and gently but firmly restrained at the head and shoulders. It is usually best if someone other than the family performs this task so the parent is in the baby's line of sight and can provide reassurance. Swaddling and being held still will generally elicit crying. Although it is troubling for parents, this enables the doctor to better visualize the tongue and nearby structures.

The physician looks for the presence of a white cord of tissue or a membranous film that attaches along the midline of the underside of the tongue to the floor of the mouth. The baby then is offered a gloved finger to suck, which will provide soothing and more information about tongue mobility. Starting in midline at the tip of the tongue, the finger is then slid along the underside of the tongue until it presses against the leading edge of the tissue where the tongue base meets the floor of the mouth (**Figure 9-1**). If there is resistance, a tongue-tie is present. A restrictive residual frenulum indicates an incomplete separation between the tongue and the floor of the mouth. If reduced tongue mobility suggests tongue-tie but nothing is visualized, the examination is repeated with the tongue elevated with a grooved director or notched tongue depressor or two gloved fingers under the tongue, one on either side of the midline. The presence of a faint white line from the base of the tongue to the floor of the mouth that resists when pressed indicates the presence of a submucosal (type 4) tongue-tie (**Figures 9-2 through 9-5**). A residual frenulum may cause a deep crease down the middle of the tongue's underside at the base of the tongue, extending forward between the anterior fibers of the genioglossus muscle (**Figure 9-6**). Rather than the resilient feel of the muscle fibers, the practitioner feels a resistant string that prevents the tongue from elevating.

The diagnosis of ankyloglossia, especially the posterior variants, is based more on lack of normal function of the tongue than appearance. The tongue's normal range of motion includes extension over the lower gum ridge and lip, lateralization to each corner of the

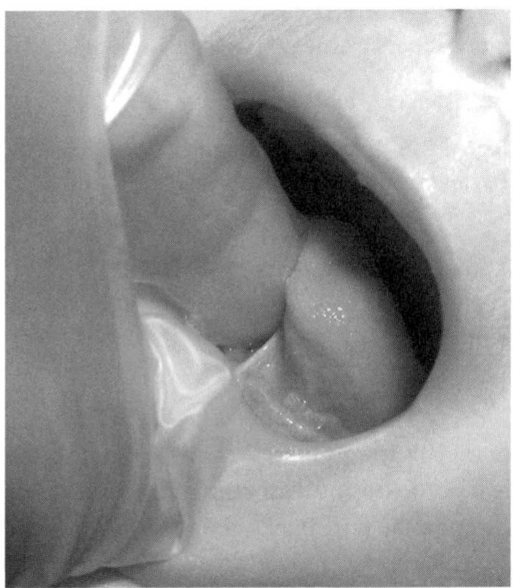

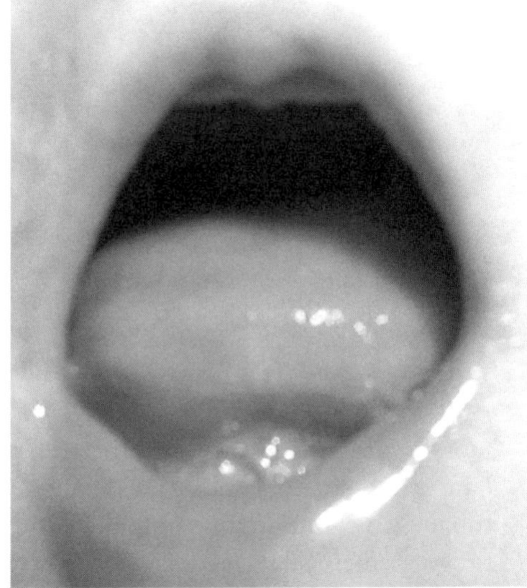

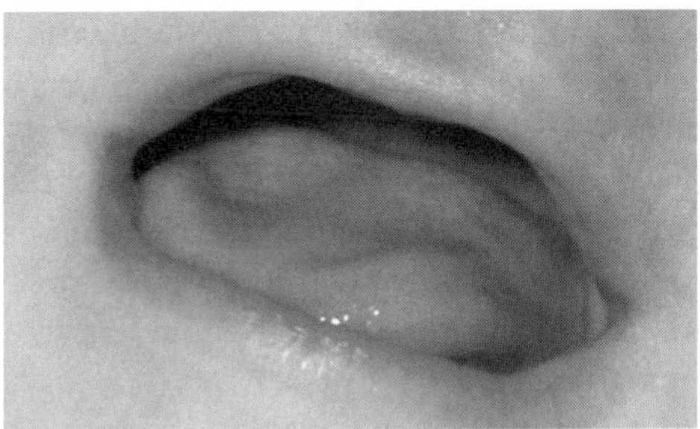

Figure 9-1 (top left) Identifying a posterior frenulum by palpation.

Figure 9-2 (top right) Submucosal tongue-tie makes the tongue appear short or the floor of the mouth webbed.

Figure 9-3 (right) Asymmetrical, limited tongue elevation due to submucosal tongue-tie.

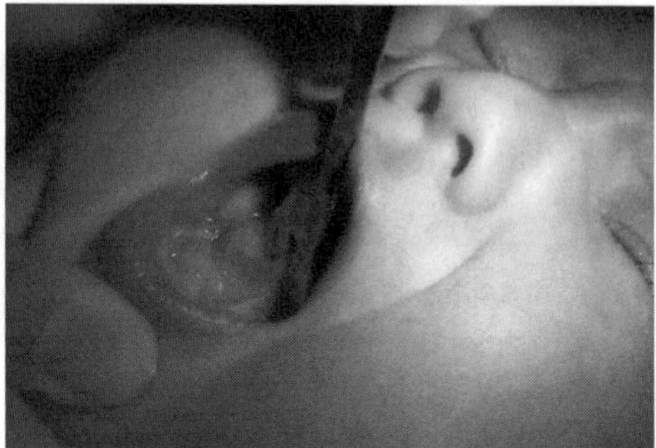

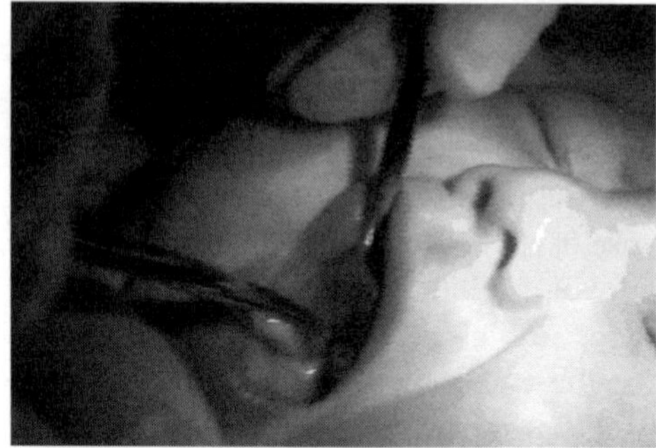

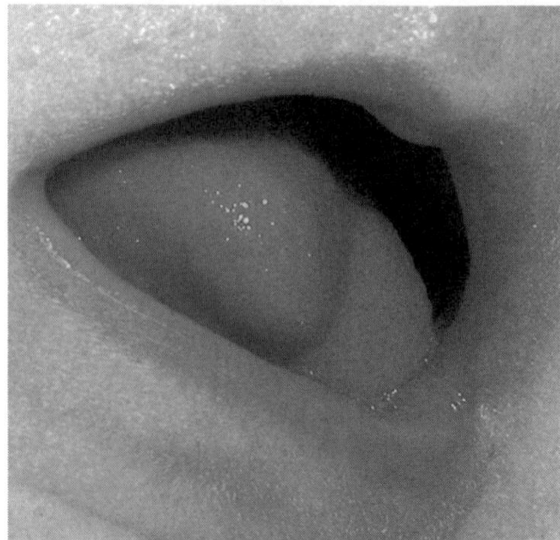

Figure 9-4 (top left) The faint white string of a submucosal tongue-tie.

Figure 9-5 (top right) The string becomes more apparent when the tongue is stretched.

Figure 9-6 (right) Restriction along midline by the lingual frenulum distorts tongue shape.

mouth without twisting, and the ability to elevate the tongue more than halfway to the hard palate with the mouth wide open. Infants with posterior tongue-tie may have some tongue tip elevation, but only the tip of the tongue may curl back while the bulk of the tongue remains flat (**Figure 9-7**). The tongue may extend, even over the lip, but the tip of the tongue will be pulled down, causing the tongue tip to look rolled under. As the infant gapes, the tongue generally retracts in tongue-tied infants. A wide gape is critical for optimal attachment to the breast, as is the ability of the tongue edges to stabilize the breast in the mouth. Therefore, all functions should be tested with the mouth wide open.

Unless the frenulum is a thin, avascular transparent web, a topical anesthetic (benzocaine gel) is applied to both sides of the lingual frenulum with a cotton swab, and the infant is held and comforted while the anesthetic is given time to numb the tissues. The infant is returned to the treatment table or parent's lap and is firmly restrained, with one adult holding the sides of the head over the ears, and another holding the shoulders with their hands and immobilizing the body with their arms.

When performing frenotomy, it is important to get as close as possible to the tongue without cutting into the tongue itself. During the release, the tongue is lifted as high as possible to make the tissue as taut as possible—this makes the clipping more accurate and allows the scissors to be further from the floor of the mouth. This allows the physician to avoid injury to the orifices of the submandibular glands at the floor of the mouth. The use of a grooved director stabilizes the tongue and provides a better field of view, but practitioners may instead use their fingers to elevate the tongue while a parent stabilizes the baby's head.

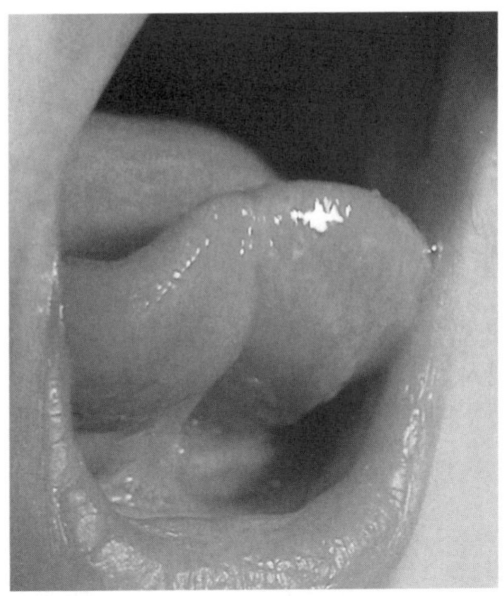

Figure 9-7 Limited elevation due to type 3 tongue-tie.

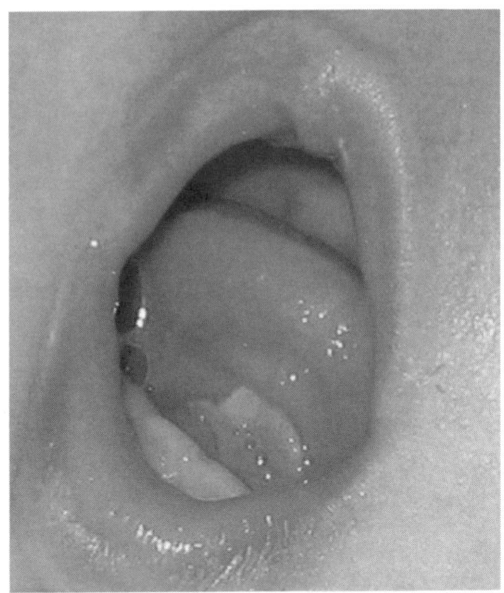

Figure 9-8 Healing eschar 1 week postfrenotomy.

Posterior tongue-ties tend to bleed more than the simple, thin, more anterior restrictions because the physician is clipping through a thicker frenulum remnant, or in the case of submucosal restrictions, through a small area of the oral mucosa itself. The incision is continued posteriorly until a popping sensation occurs and the tissue opens into a diamond shape, providing the tongue a greater freedom of motion in all planes and more functional length. Linear incisions are expected to heal within 24 hours, but the diamond-shaped opening may take 3–4 days, with a white to yellow eschar persisting for a week (**Figure 9-8**). When treating submucosal (type 4) frenula, it is sometimes necessary to clip more than once (**Figure 9-9**). The first snip just releases the soft mucosal covering over the leading edge of the frenulum, and there may be a less noticeable pop during the release (**Figure 9-10**). A white strip may still remain that may be visible only when the tongue is elevated strongly, and it will require a second snip. A partial release that frees the soft tissue but not the tighter cord in midline may not improve tongue function sufficiently or at all (**Figure 9-11**). After a successful release, the tongue should elevate to the palate and reveal the new diamond-shaped opening at the base of the tongue when the infant cries (**Figure 9-12**). Close collaboration between treating practitioners and feeding specialists is vital to ensure that normal function is restored.

Bleeding is controlled with direct pressure for about 2 minutes using sterile gauze. The infant's sucking efforts usually signal the cessation of bleeding. The baby can be immediately offered the breast to ensure that sufficient release was performed to improve attachment, milk transfer, and maternal comfort. The first feeding postfrenotomy is usually a good indicator of the degree of eventual improvement. Soreness may impede feeding for 24 hours or more and can be managed with analgesics.

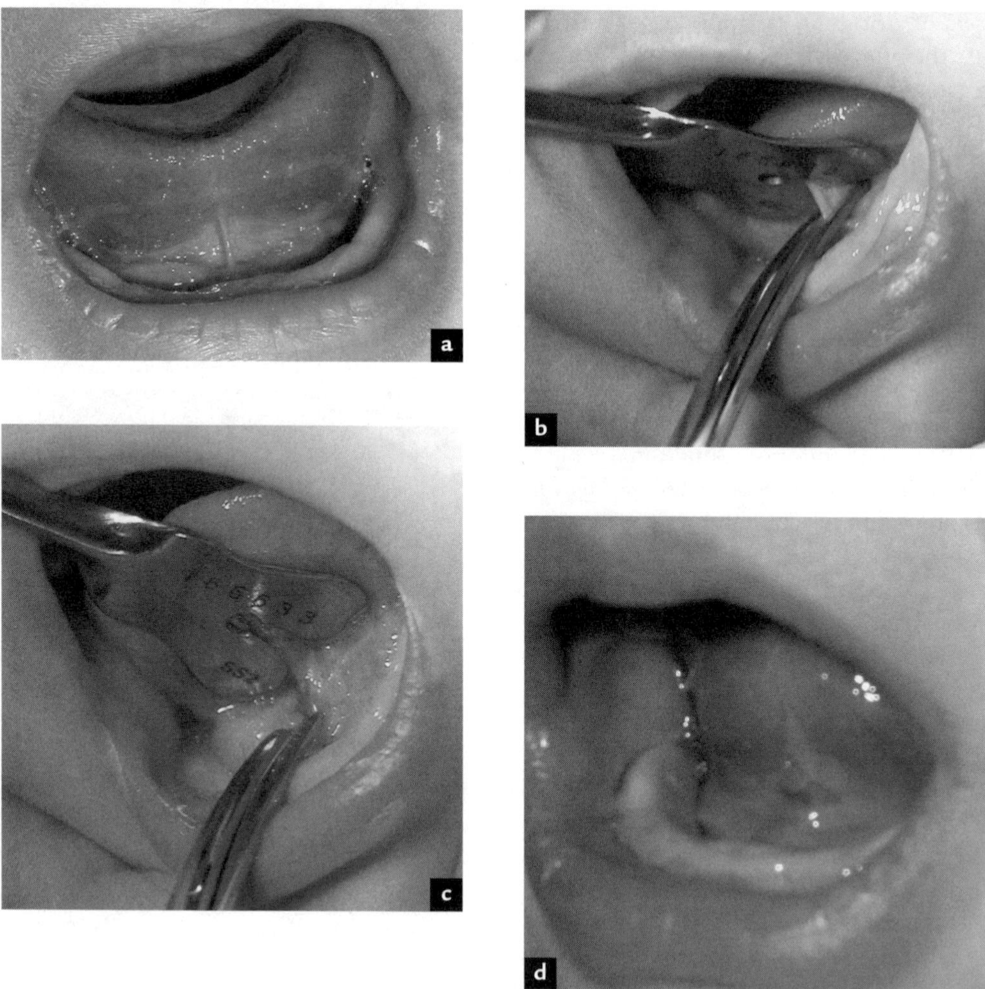

Figure 9-9a–9-9d Treatment of type 3 tongue-tie requiring two snips to release the tongue sufficiently.

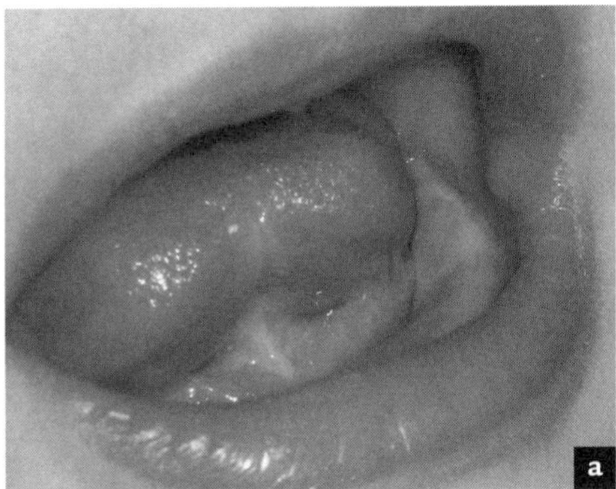

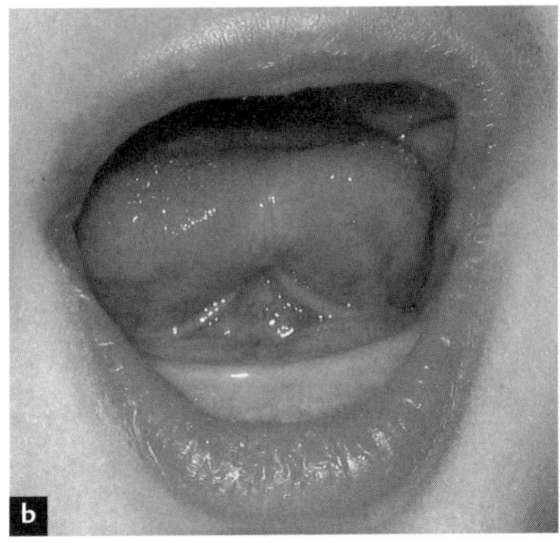

Figure 9-10a–9-10b This posterior frenulum required only one snip. There is still some submucosal restriction, but release was sufficient for breastfeeding to become comfortable and effective.

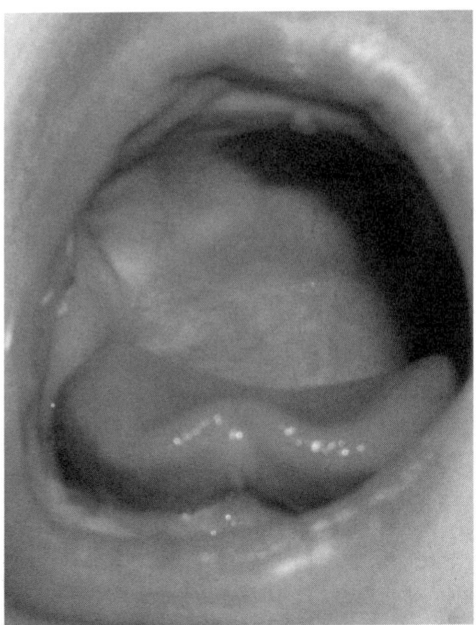

Figure 9-11 Incompletely treated tongue-tie increased maternal pain during feeding.

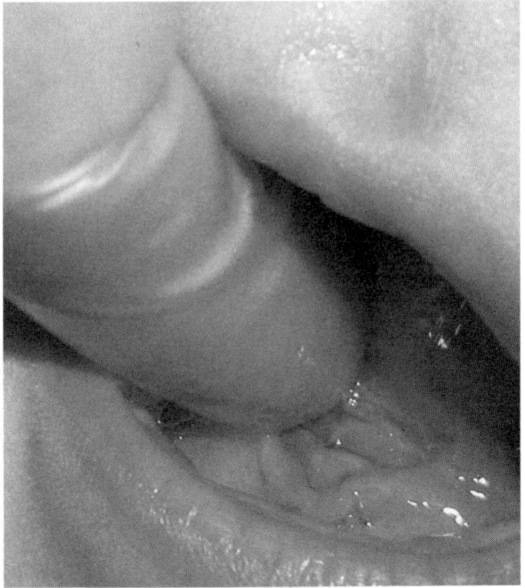

Figure 9-12 Postoperative appearance of infant in **Figure 9-3**: Note the folds of the mucosa that were attached to the tongue lateral to the midline frenulum. Treatment consisted of one snip to open the mucosa to expose the frenulum, snipping the frenulum, and spreading of the mucosa with blunt Metzenbaum scissors.

Laser Frenotomy

Increasing numbers of practitioners are using lasers to perform frenotomy under light sedation or local anesthesia (Aras, Goregen, Gungormus, & Akgul, 2010; Kotlow, 2004, 2008). Lasers vaporize tissue and provide immediate hemostasis, and there may be less pain. Laser treatment takes longer than sharp frenotomy, so light sedation is often used. Especially in cases where sharp frenotomies need revision, laser treatment has been extremely useful.

Postoperative Care and Expectations

A common concern about office frenotomy is that retreatment may be necessary due to healing or scarring. Indeed, Klockars and Pitkaranta (2009) found that almost one-third of their patients (but none of the infants) treated under local or no anesthesia required revisions. They still recommended office frenotomy as the first-line treatment due to safety and cost-effectiveness. Hong et al. (2010) also found a higher revision rate for posterior ankyloglossia than anterior ankyloglossia (21% versus less than 4%, respectively) in their large case series of infants treated with frenotomy for breastfeeding difficulties. Recently, the International Affiliation of Tongue-tie Professionals (IATP) has experimented with elevating the tongue 5–8 times daily in the week after the procedure to prevent and disrupt re-adhesion, particularly in posterior tongue-ties.

Expectations

The newly released tongue may initially be weak. If frenotomy is delayed until the second half of the first year, rehabilitation of tongue movements may take longer than in newborns. The more limiting a tongue-tie has been and the longer the infant has tried to compensate with limited tongue movements, the longer it may take the baby to be able to use the new range of motion with full strength, coordination, and stamina. Chapter 8 contains suggestions for oral exercises if feeding issues do not resolve spontaneously.

Conclusion

Many sucking problems that make breastfeeding difficult, painful, or frustrating are due to variable degrees of restricted tongue movement secondary to tongue-tie. Effective, minimally invasive treatment is possible in infancy, without general anesthesia.

References

Aras, M. H., Goregen, M., Gungormus, M., & Akgul, H. M. (2010). Comparison of diode laser and Er:YAG lasers in the treatment of ankyloglossia. *Photomedicine and Laser Surgery, 28*, 173–177.

Buryk, M., Bloom, D., & Shope, T. (2011). Efficacy of neonatal release of ankyloglossia: A randomized trial. *Pediatrics, 128*(2), 280–288.

Coryllos, E., Genna, C. W., & Salloum, A. C. (2004, Summer). Congenital tongue-tie and its impact on breastfeeding. *Breastfeeding: Best for Baby and Mother*. Retrieved from http://www.aap.org/breastfeeding/files/pdf/BBM-8-27%20Newsletter.pdf

Dollberg, S., Botzer, E., Grunis, E., & Mimouni, F. B. (2006). Immediate nipple pain relief after frenotomy in breast-fed infants with ankyloglossia: A randomized, prospective study. *Journal of Pediatric Surgery, 41*(9), 1598–1600.

Geddes, D. T., Langton, D. B., Gollow, I., Jacobs, L. A., Hartmann, P. E., & Simmer, K. (2008). Frenulotomy for breastfeeding infants with ankyloglossia: Effect on milk removal and sucking mechanism as imaged by ultrasound. *Pediatrics, 122*, e188–e194.

Griffiths, D. M. (2004). Do tongue ties affect breastfeeding? *Journal of Human Lactation, 20*(4), 409–414.

Hogan, M., Westcott, C., & Griffiths, M. (2005). Randomized, controlled trial of division of tongue-tie in infants with feeding problems. *Journal of Paediatrics and Child Health, 41*(5–6), 246–250.

Hong, P., Lago, D., Seargeant, J., Pellman, L., Magit, A. E., & Pransky, S. M. (2010). Defining ankyloglossia: A case series of anterior and posterior tongue ties. *International Journal of Pediatric Otorhinolaryngology, 74*, 1003–1006.

Khoo, A. K., Dabbas, N., Sudhakaran, N., Ade-Ajayi, N., & Patel, S. (2009). Nipple pain at presentation predicts success of tongue-tie division for breastfeeding problems. *European Journal of Pediatric Surgery, 19*, 370–373.

Klockars, T., & Pitkaranta, A. (2009). Pediatric tongue-tie division: Indications, techniques and patient satisfaction. *International Journal of Pediatric Otorhinolaryngology, 73*(10), 1399–1401

Kotlow, L. A. (2004). Oral diagnosis of abnormal frenum attachments in neonates and infants: Evaluation and treatment of the maxillary and lingual frenum using the erbium: YAG laser. *Journal of Pediatric Dental Care, 10*, 11–13.

Kotlow, L. (2008). Lasers and soft tissue treatments for the pediatric dental patient. *Alpha Omegan, 101*, 140–151.

Kupietzky, A., & Botzer, E. (2005). Ankyloglossia in the infant and young child: Clinical suggestions for diagnosis and management. *Pediatric Dentistry, 27*(1), 40–46.

Messner, A. H., Lalakea, M. L., Aby, J., Macmahon, J., & Bair, E. (2000). Ankyloglossia: Incidence and associated feeding difficulties. *Archives of Otolaryngology—Head and Neck Surgery, 126*(1), 36–39.

Ricke, L. A., Baker, N. J., Madlon-Kay, D. J., & DeFor, T. A. (2005). Newborn tongue-tie: Prevalence and effect on breast-feeding. *Journal of the American Board of Family Practice, 18*(1), 1–7.

Srinivasan, A., Dobrich, C., Mitnick, H., & Feldman, P. (2006). Ankyloglossia in breastfeeding infants: The effect of frenotomy on maternal nipple pain and latch. *Breastfeeding Medicine, 1*(4), 216–224.

CHAPTER

10

Hands in Support of Breastfeeding: Manual Therapy

Sharon A. Vallone

Breastfeeding is an elegant symphony of movements orchestrated by the newborn's brain, eliciting responses via the nervous system and the hormones of the mother. This innate relationship can be disrupted for either member of the breastfeeding dyad, resulting in what appears to be a failure to bond and nurture, yet it may be corrected and supported by the detection of any abnormal function of the nervous, muscular, or skeletal systems that interferes with the goals of production, ejection, extraction, or removal and utilization of mother's milk.

As we provide support to the breastfeeding mother and her baby, we are witness time and again to an amazing phenomenon of the human brain. The brain possesses an ability to seek new avenues of adaptation. The brain's ability to create new pathways to learn or overcome obstacles is called *plasticity*. In this case, newborns relearn (or devise their own unique, ingenious method) how to accomplish the life-sustaining activity of emptying the breast when something is interfering with the usual strategies. When the door is locked, an open window will be swiftly recognized as an alternate route of entry. Soon a path will be well worn to the open window from constant use, although the possibility that someone will produce the key to open the door still remains. How soon that key is produced will determine how easily traffic can be rerouted through the door.

Tow and Vallone (2009) observed that the success of the breastfeeding dyad may ultimately depend on collaboration between the lactation consultant and a professional trained in manual therapy. They suggest that cultivating an appreciation of form versus function (or, said another way, our body versus how our body works) can help the lactation consultant make an appropriate referral for early intervention. Hopefully, the early intervention will facilitate a faster resolution of the challenges that are interfering with successful breastfeeding. Specifically, the lactation consultant should be able to recognize alterations in the symmetry of the bones of the skull or features of the face (Do the bones of the skull overlap and form a ridge? Is one eye larger or more open than the other? Is one ear higher than the other?), restricted ranges of motion of the spine and limbs, and the appearance of behavior patterns that are repeated over and over again. It can also help if the manual therapist understands the expertise and enlists the support of the lactation consultant to support reeducation of the infant after the problem has been corrected and normal function has been restored. Clear, prompt, and continuous inter-professional communication improves outcomes for dyads and practitioners.

Biomechanics

Biomechanics is the study of the mechanical principles of physics and engineering as they apply to the motion, structure, and function of living systems (Hoffman & Harris, 2000). In the context of lactation, we will look at how structure and function affect endocrine and neurologic function. In the context of breastfeeding, we are interested primarily in the biomechanics that affect the motions required for the infant to successfully latch on and efficiently empty the breast. This will include identifying (1) the structures involved, (2) how those structures move in an integrated fashion, and (3) how, when the structures are altered through injury or constraint (limited by space during development or the presence of tension in the soft tissue structures around a joint that restrains its movement), dysfunction is replaced with compensating behaviors arising from the powerful, overriding innate drive to survive. These compensations may present to the lactation consultant as simple, unusual behaviors, like a head nod at each suckle, or more complex behaviors that might make one think the baby is uncomfortable, in pain, overstimulated, or dealing with sensory integration dysfunction.

Movement is vital to brain development and precedes cognition (Joseph, 2000), driving the development of synaptic connections. The movements of the fetus in the womb drives not only the expanding neuronal network, but it also affects normal anatomic development of osseous and soft tissue structures (Pecka & Hannamb, 2006). Hall (2010) describes how the lack of craniofacial movement and muscular action can result in ear curling, a small open mouth, microretrognathia, a small tongue, and an abnormal palate.

Neurologically mature movement is controlled by muscles of the body when instructed to act by the brain via the nervous system. The parts of the body that are involved in motion are the joints, which consist of two or more adjoining bone surfaces, the ligaments that bind the bones together, tendons that attach the muscle to the bone, and the muscles themselves. Surrounding each of these structures and binding them together is connective tissue called *fascia*, which can be delicate or thick depending on its function in that location. For example, strong, fibrous ligaments keep two bones in alignment at a joint, despite the power of the muscles that move the bones versus the delicate layer that surrounds it, called the periosteum, from which living cells produce more bone. Fascia is not only the defining outline or border of all the tissues mentioned, but it is continuous and contiguous (it has no beginning and no end) throughout the body (Ward, 1993). For those who quarter and prepare chicken for the oven or skillet, careful observation may help you visualize different types of fascia. The thin yellow tissue often removed and discarded and the thick band of tissue securing the leg to the thigh are both examples of fascia in various forms.

Along with all these important body parts are the more delicate nerves, blood vessels, and lymphatic vessels that the tissues rely on for innervation, oxygen and nutrient supply, immunity, and the removal of waste and excess fluid. All of these may influence function at the joint level. For example, edema (excess fluid) surrounding a joint may decrease the ability to move that joint freely.

Under normal circumstances, these individual components function together smoothly, regulated by independent nerve pathways already laid down in the brain during fetal development. If that independent circuitry (the brain) experiences interference by drugs administered during labor and delivery, oxygen deprivation, or trauma, the newborn's normal function could appear disorganized, erratic, and inefficient, or, in the worst-case scenario, the systems would simply cease to function and there would be a failure to thrive.

If the structure itself were abnormal or injured, even under the best neurologic direction the action of the structures would be altered or would fail altogether. If your leg is shattered in a bad fall, no matter how the brain directs you to get up and walk, it is unlikely that you would be able to do so.

If a structure prevents the body from functioning properly, *neuroplasticity* allows exploration of alternate methods of, in this case, life-sustaining activities. Neuroplasticity is the ability to create new problem-solving nerve pathways by adding or removing connections among neurons (LeDoux, 2002). The brilliance of the neonate's neurologic system is that it has a preprogrammed directive to survive, and this will lead to creative compensations (using other methods or techniques) to attempt to achieve that end. If you did not have feet to walk with, then you might learn to walk upside down on your hands. If an infant cannot create a seal around the nipple with the lips and tongue, her or she will clamp down to hold it with the jaw.

How do these structures become deranged, misaligned, or dysfunctional? As early as life in the womb, the lack of space can be the source of problems. This can be the result of the mother having adhesions from previous trauma or surgery, a fibroid tumor, a congenital anomaly (like a heart- or T-shaped [bicornuate] uterus or a septate uterus with a connective tissue membrane dividing it completely into two chambers), misalignment of the pelvis resulting in uneven traction of the ligaments that support the pelvis, and/or multiple in utero residents. This less-than-optimal environment can result in anything from club foot to plagiocephaly (flattening or deforming of the head shape) (Graham, Miller, Stephan, & Smith, 1980; Lajeunie, Crimmins, Amaud, & Renier, 2005; Leon, 2008; Littlefield, Kelly, Pomatto, & Beals, 1999). Although club foot will most likely not interfere with breastfeeding, flattened or deformed bony plates of the skull may result in decreased ability to move the head and neck into positions needed to breastfeed efficiently, or it can interfere with the movement of the jaw (mandible) by altering its position and/or the position of the temporal bone (which together make up the temporomandibular joint, or TMJ), preventing the infant from opening the mouth widely enough (gape) to latch well.

The journey of birth is the next potential source of structural derangements or soft tissue injury (Laroia, 2010; Mathai et al., 2000). As an example, a presentation of the fetal head in an *asynclitic* position (a less than desirable presentation of the fetal head at the cervix, with the widest diameter rather than the narrowest diameter of the head) can slow down or prevent the progress of cervical effacement and dilation and can also result in excessive force from the contractions of the uterus acting on the head of the fetus as it fails to progress down the canal (repeated microtrauma to the head and neck with each contraction). Another example is the fetus presenting with the brow (forehead) or face against the cervix.

In this position, in what is often a prolonged labor, the fetus can suffer injuries to the neck because it is placed in a hyperextended position (tipping of the head back so far that the back of the head might lay against the spine right above the shoulder blades). This type of trauma, repeated with each contraction, could possibly result in diminished, or a complete absence of, specific reflexes, like suckling and rooting. This trauma might affect (1) the individual segments of the bones of the skull or bones of the neck, (2) the nerves from the brain (cranial nerves) that exit the skull close to the first vertebrae, or (3) the soft tissue covering of the brain and spinal cord (meninges or, collectively, the dura). Or the trauma could simply decrease the range of motion of the head and neck, which may prevent the infant from putting the chin to the chest. This is often seen in babies who appear arched at the breast while held in their parents' arms or lying in the crib (**Figure 10-1**).

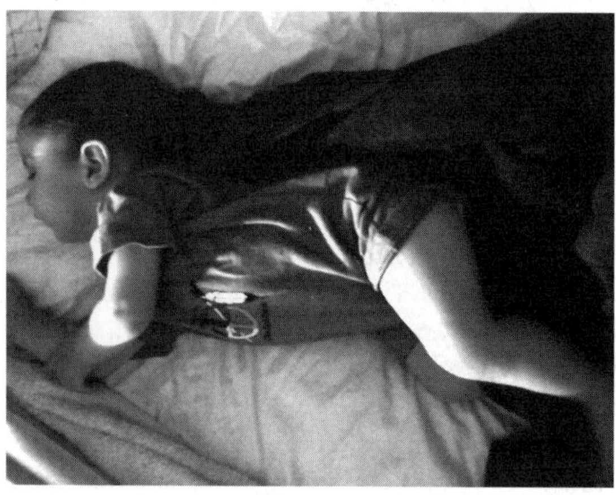

Figure 10-1 Baby arching during sleep.

This type of presentation at birth (brow or facial) can also result in injuries to the nose (which can affect the infant's breathing while at the breast) or to the TMJ and, once again, potentially interfere in the movement of the jaw up and down or side to side or causing it to be retracted (a sunken chin) (**Figures 10-2A** and **B**).

Any or all of these factors—in utero posture during gestation (the position the fetus maintained in the womb during the 10 months of pregnancy); the force of the contractions of the uterus during labor and delivery; the

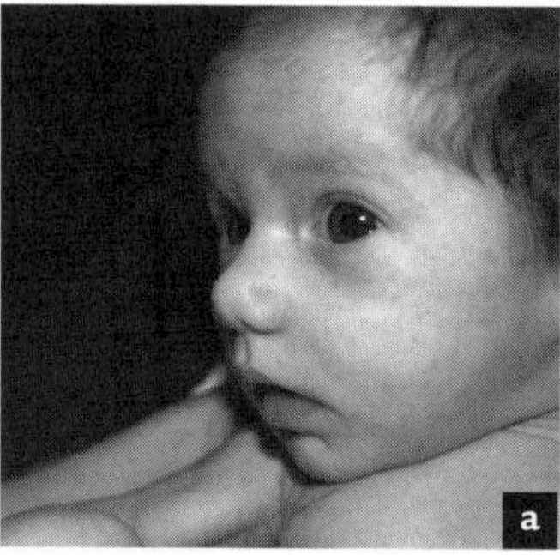

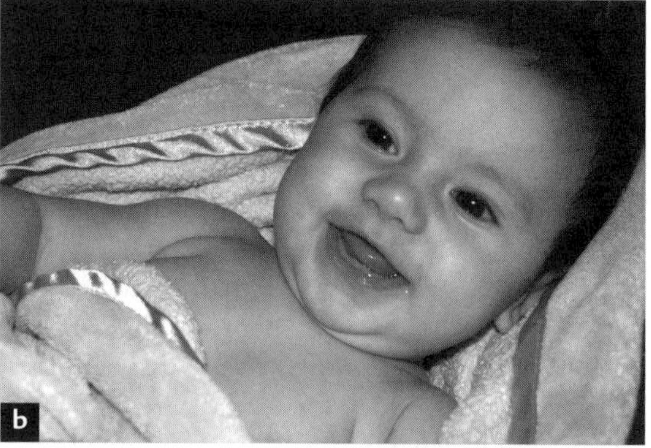

Figure 10-2 Retracted chin, before (A) and after (B) manual therapy.

speed of the journey down the birth canal and the position (or presentation) in which the fetus traverses the birth canal; and the mother's position during labor and delivery, which can affect the size of the pelvic inlet and outlet—can potentially play a role in determining the structural integrity of the neonate.

The neonate has an astounding built-in system of correction when function is normal. For example, the neonatal cranium molds and overlaps its plates to accommodate the difference in size between the head and the cervix. Changes in atmospheric pressure from inside the womb to outside the womb, the initiation of the cerebrospinal fluid pumping from the ventricles of the brain to the sacrum, and the gentle stroking of the nipple and tongue along the hard palate all serve to open the overlapped plates and reshape the infant's skull. It is only when the integrity of the cranial system has been impaired, by things like excess force of uterine contractions, assistive devices (such as forceps or a ventouse, or vacuum extractor) (Putta & Spencer, 2000), or the rapid decompression of a precipitous labor, that intervention might be required. The most effective form of intervention this author has experienced is manual therapy.

What Is Manual Therapy?

We have previously discussed the tissues of the body that enable us to function through motion. Manual therapy is a hands-on method of treating those tissues to support and normalize function when there has been an injury or derangement of any of the components involved. The cultivation of a broad understanding of anatomy and physiology as well as developing specific and effective manual techniques provides the practitioner with a means of reducing inefficient compensations to restore full normal function. For example, a nursing neonate can burn more calories feeding inefficiently than taken in during the feeding. A qualified manual therapist could help the baby suckle more effectively, thus encouraging the body to use those calories for growth, rather than suckling.

In western Europe, North America, and Australasia, manual therapy is practiced by members of many of the healthcare professions, including chiropractors, naturopaths, physiotherapists and physical therapists, occupational therapists, osteopaths, and physiatrists, as well as acupuncturists, massage therapists, and bonesetters, who also provide techniques that fall within the scope of manual therapy.

Manual therapy may be defined differently within the context of the profession describing it. For example, professions like chiropractic (DC), naturopathy (ND), or osteopathy (DO) define their systems more holistically, where physical therapists and physiatrists concentrate specifically on functional movement patterns as they are affected by structure.

Chiropractic translates from Greek as "done by hand." Chiropractic is defined by the World Federation of Chiropractic as "a health profession concerned with the diagnosis, treatment and prevention of mechanical disorders of the musculoskeletal system, and the effects of these disorders on the function of the nervous system and general health. *There is an emphasis on manual treatments including spinal adjustment and other joint and soft-tissue manipulation* [emphasis added]" (World Federation of Chiropractic, 2009). Similarly, it is defined by the World Health Organization as "a health care profession concerned with the diagnosis, treatment and prevention of disorders of the neuromuscular system and the effects of these disorders on general health. *There is an emphasis on manual techniques, including joint adjustment and/or manipulation with a particular focus on subluxations* [emphasis added]" (World Health Organization, 2005, as cited in World Federation of Chiropractic, 2009). The relationship between structure and function, especially as coordinated by the nervous system, is central to the profession's approach to treatment, health, and well-being. Philosophically there is an emphasis on the mind–body relationship in health and the natural healing powers of the body. This represents a biopsychosocial philosophy of health rather than a biomedical one.

Management with the goal of optimizing the body's innate ability to heal or find homeostasis includes manual techniques with particular competency in joint adjustment and manipulation, supported by rehabilitation exercises, patient education, and lifestyle modification. The profession makes no use of prescription drugs or surgery, and patients requiring these interventions are referred for medical care (Keating, 2005; Mootz & Phillips, 1997).

A consensus study of US chiropractors (Gatterman & Hanson, 1994) defined manual therapy as "procedures by which the hands directly contact the body to treat the articulations and/or soft tissues." This said, there are several effective techniques devised by chiropractors that utilize mechanical instruments, like the Activator Technique (Fuhr, 2005; Fuhr, 2011) to perform effective low-force treatments. Other chiropractors have devised specific ancillary methods to support the neuromuscular system's rehabilitation after an adjustment that have proven effective when working with both neonates and infants (Kase, 2010). All specific chiropractic techniques, whether by performed by hand or by instrument, should be modified based on the age and anatomy of the pediatric patient. It is this author's opinion that techniques in chiropractic that utilize low-force adjustments and soft-tissue contacts to achieve structural biomechanical change to deal with the components of the biomechanical lesion, including but not limited to, reflex contacts, sacro-occipital technique (SOT) (Howat, 2000; Sacro-Occipital Research Society International, 2011), applied kinesiology (Frost, 2002; International College of Applied Kinesiology, 2005), Logan Basic technique (Hutti & Montgomery, 2006), directional nonforce technique (John, 2003), bioenergetic synchronization technique (BEST) (Morter, 2011), Nimmo receptor tonus technique (Nimmo, 2011), specific fingertip thrusts and pressures (often falling in the broad category of diversified technique), and mechanical adjusting apparatus (such as the activator method) upon the spine and tissues adjacent to the spine, are the most appropriate for this age group.

Retrospective reviews of available data on the safety and effectiveness of chiropractic treatment for pediatric patients has been outlined by several authors (Humphreys, 2010; Miller, 2009; Vohra, Jonston, & Humphreys, 2007). Although pediatric education is a component of the required undergraduate curriculum for all chiropractors, advanced education is available on a postgraduate basis. In the United States, those practitioners who pursue this educational track will become a Diplomate in Clinical Chiropractic Pediatrics (DICCP). Doctors with the DICCP credential are doctors who have completed a postgraduate clinical specialist level training cosponsored by a CCE-accredited (or international equivalent) chiropractic institution and demonstrated competency in both the written and oral examinations administered by the International College of Chiropractic Pediatrics (ICCP). In Europe, the current postgraduate specialist training includes a strong emphasis on research and will confer a Master's degree on their graduates. Any of these specialists may be identified for consultation on more complex clinical cases (ICCP, 2011; Anglo-European College of Chiropractic, 2010).

Naturopathic medicine is also based on the belief that the human body has an innate healing ability. Naturopathy consists of traditional healing methods, principles, and practices focusing on holistic, proactive prevention and comprehensive diagnosis and treatment. By using protocols that minimize the risk of harm, the naturopathic physician helps to facilitate the body's inherent ability to restore and maintain optimal health. Naturopathic doctors (NDs) teach their patients to use diet, exercise, lifestyle changes, and natural therapies to enhance their bodies' ability to prevent and cure disease. Their comprehensive treatment plan includes not only treatment of disease but restoration of health. The training and scope of practice of licensed naturopathic physicians in the United States and Canada includes the use of physical medicine. Naturopathic physicians may include a wide variety of diagnostic and treatment modalities, including naturopathic manipulative therapies (Chaitow, 2006).

Osteopathy is another established, recognized system of allopathic health care that includes manual techniques for diagnosis and treatment in its holistic approach to the patient. Osteopathic physicians are taught to respect the relationship of body, mind, and spirit in health and disease and emphasize the structural and functional integrity of the body and the body's intrinsic tendency for self-healing. Osteopathic manipulative medicine (OMM) is viewed as a facilitative influence to encourage this self-regulatory process (Peppin, 1993). Pain and disability experienced by patients are viewed as resulting from a reciprocal relationship between the musculoskeletal and visceral components of a disease or strain. Korr (1978) described manual therapy as techniques in which specific forces are applied by hand to structures of the body (connective tissue, skeletal muscles, joints) to increase mobility in areas of restriction.

The American Academy of Orthopedic Manual Physical Therapists' *Orthopaedic Manual Physical Therapy: Description of Advanced Specialty Practice* (2008) includes a description of manual physical therapy. *Manual therapy techniques* consist of a broad group of skilled hand movements comprising a continuum of skilled passive movements to the joints and/or soft tissues that are applied at varying speeds and amplitudes, including a small amplitude/high velocity therapeutic movement intended to improve tissue extensibility; increase range of motion; induce relaxation; mobilize or manipulate soft tissues and joints; modulate pain; and reduce soft tissue swelling, inflammation, or restriction (p. 51).

Cranial Techniques

Cranial manipulation was practiced by the ancient Egyptians, members of the Paracas culture in Peru (2000 BC to 200 AD), and in India for centuries (American Physical Therapy

Association, 1999). In the 18th century, Emanuel Swedenborg, a philosopher and scientist, described a rhythmic expansion and contraction of the brain (American Physical Therapy Association, 1999; Swedenborg, 1882). Italian anatomists, in the early 1900s, taught that cranial suture ossification was pathological in the mature human adult. These teachings contradicted the British anatomists who taught that suture ossification and cranial immobility was a normal condition (Sperino, 1939).

Manipulative techniques involving the cranium have been controversial since the 1920s when they were pioneered by individuals in the fields of chiropractic and osteopathy. The first to develop cranial adjusting (craniopathy) was Nephi Cottam, DC, followed by William G. Sutherland, DO, who is considered the father of cranial osteopathy (Sutherland, Adah, & Wales, 1967).

Cranial osteopathy is a set of hypotheses and techniques using Sutherland's observations that the plates of the cranium permit microscopic movement or force dissipation and that there is a force, or rhythm, that is operating in moving the plates of the skull. Cranial osteopathy is said to be based on a *primary respiratory mechanism*, a rhythm that can be felt with a very finely developed sense of touch. The craniosacral approach includes a structured diagnostic process that evaluates the mobility of the osseous cranium, the skull as it relates to the sacrum and the craniosacral rhythmic impulse (CRI) throughout the body. Craniosacral osteopathic manipulative techniques attempt to restore motion to restrictions within individual sutures of the skull, the skull as a total entity, and the skull in relation to the sacrum, and they apply inherent force to the articulations of the vertebral axis, rib cage, and extremities (Greenman & McPartland, 1995). A large cohort of osteopaths contend that improving dysfunctional cranial rhythmic impulses not only enhances cerebrospinal fluid flow to peripheral nerves, thereby enhancing metabolic outflow and nutrition inflow, but it also can be measured manually and by instrumentation (Moskalenko & Kravchenco, 2004; Nelson, Sergueef, & Glonek, 2004; Nelson, Sergueef, & Glonek, 2006; Nelson, Sergueef, Lipinski, Chapman, & Glonek, 2001; Sergueef, Nelson, & Glonek, 2002; Upledger, 1977, 1995). Detractors cite studies demonstrating that interrater reliability in assessing cranial rhythms is extremely poor (Hartman & Norton, 2002; Moran & Gibbons, 2001; Rogers, Witt, Gross, Hacke, & Genova, 1998; Wirth-Pattulo & Hayes, 1994) and that biological plausibility seems low (Green, Martin, Bassett, & Kazanjian, 1999). The main plausibility concern based on observations, which may be considered dated, is that the sutures close and ossify in adulthood (Todd & Lyon, 1924), but this does not apply to infants, whose skull plates indeed are free to move. Craniosacral therapy has become particularly popular in treating babies and young children (Upledger, 2003) and demonstrates pain management applications in fibromyalgia (Castro-Sanchez et al., 2011). The craniosacral therapy practitioner works to release adverse mechanical tension in the meninges and connective tissue to restore the normal cranial rhythms and cerebrospinal fluid flow (Upledger & Vredevoogd, 1983).

Sacro-occipital technique (SOT) was discovered and developed by Major Bertrand DeJarnette. SOT became an integration of engineering, osteopathic, and chiropractic principles honed by clinical research. It was designed to assist the chiropractor in locating and correcting the primary subluxation, which is accomplished through evaluation of indicators relating to specific category subluxation complexes. Using a category system of analysis and treatment, SOT seeks to peel off the layers of distortion to uncover the causative subluxation pattern and remove it (Howat 2000; Unger, 1995).

Craniosacral therapy is based on the same principles as cranial osteopathy, but the practitioners are not necessarily licensed osteopaths (Retzlaff, Michael, Roppel, & Mitchell, 1976; Upledger & Vredevoogd, 1983). Instruction in craniosacral therapy is offered to nonhealthcare providers and healthcare providers (MDs, osteopaths, chiropractors, naturopaths, dentists, RNs, physical therapists, occupational therapists, massage therapists, lactation consultants, etc.).

What Is the Subluxation or the Mechanical Lesion/Somatic Dysfunction?

When external forces impact any joint, it can result in a subluxation (historically, chiropractic nomenclature) or manipulable lesion, mechanical lesion (historically, osteopathic nomenclature), somatic dysfunction, or motion dysfunction. The Association of Chiropractic Colleges defines a subluxation as "a complex of functional and/or structural and/or pathological articular changes that compromise neural integrity and may influence organ system function and general health (Association of Chiropractic Colleges, 1996). In the World Health Organization's *Benchmarks for Training in Osteopathy*, somatic dysfunction is described as "impaired or altered function of related components of the somatic (body framework) system; skeletal, arthrodial [joint] and myofascial structure and their related vascular, lymphatic, and neural elements" (2010, p. 1).

Either definition serves to help us understand that there are both specific and broad ramifications to joint dysfunction. If the TMJ is edematous or swollen, its range of motion will be impaired (the specific ramification being a change in the ability to drop the jaw). But at the same time, the TMJ may be the source of nociceptive (painful!) input to the brain, which increases the activity of the sympathetic nervous system (fight or flight), resulting in an irritable or colicky infant (broad ramification). According to a published randomized controlled trial (RCT), osteopathic manual therapy (OMT) was found to decrease the need for pain medication in adults with TMJ dysfunction, which might allow us to predict some success in infants with TMJ dysfunction (Cuccia, Caradonna, Annunziata, & Caradonna, 2010).

The Breastfeeding Dyad

The Mother

The conception and development of life in the womb is dependent on a synchronized cascade of hormonal activity that is subject to a woman's emotional and physical state of well-being. Her nutrition, her ergonomics, her rest and exercise habits, and her stress levels and state of mind have all been shown to have a potential effect on the health and well-being of the developing fetus and on her ability to sustain its life both in and outside of the womb, intra- and extrauterine life (Kinsella & Monk, 2009; Leung et al., 2010; Makino et al., 2009; Wadhwa, 2005). Although the focus of our discussion should remain on the infant, some maternal issues, such as those that will be outlined here, can be confused with suckling problems in an infant. We must be thorough in taking the history of both the mother and the neonate when evaluating breastfeeding dysfunction as it may relate to mother's milk production because any alteration in homeostasis for either member of the dyad can result in lactation disruption.

During puberty, a woman's breasts grow in response to hormones. These hormones include prolactin, estrogen, progesterone, cortisol, insulin, thyroid hormones, and growth hormone. The release of these hormones during puberty causes proliferation of the lactiferous ducts and the development of breast tissues. Many factors, including stress levels, nutritional deficits or excesses, structural faults (including mechanical lesions or subluxations), or organic pathology, can potentially interfere with hormone production at this time and, as a result, disrupt the body's preparation for lactation long before the woman may even be considering pregnancy.

During pregnancy, the breasts increase in size due to an increase in duct branching and the formation of alveoli. The release of estrogen and progesterone from the placenta and prolactin from the adenohypophysis causes the breast development. Therefore, placental and pituitary integrity are essential to develop the breasts and prepare them for the production and delivery of milk. When the neurohormonal axis is intact, women's breasts are prepared to produce milk as early as the 16th to 20th week of gestation; human milk production is inhibited during pregnancy by the effect of progesterone on prolactin (O'Connor, 2011; Riordan & Auerbach, 1998).

If a woman's pregnancy and birth experience was stressful (Dewey, Nommsen-Rivers, Heinig, & Cohen, 2003) or resulted in acute or chronic pain (like the acute pain of an episiotomy or the chronic pain of adhesions from a cesarean section), then this nociceptive input can trigger a dominance of the sympathetic nervous system, which might hinder or suppress hormone production, resulting in an alteration in milk production, or hypolactation (Almeida, Yassouridis, & Forgas-Moya, 1994; Dewey, 2001; Lau, 2001). Pain may also result in a mother putting her baby to the breast less often.

Because stress or pain can trigger the fight-or-flight response, the presence of a mechanical lesion or subluxation can interfere with the integrity of the neurohormonal axis at the cranial or vertebral level. The uterus, cervix, and vaginal canal are innervated by afferent nerve fibers traveling in the hypogastric and pelvic nerves (Berkley, Robbins, & Sato, 1993). Afferent nerves are those that bring information into the spinal cord and brain for information processing. Subluxation at the vertebral levels from which these branches originate could interfere with the function of the placenta and its important hormonal role in the maintenance of pregnancy, the onset and progress of labor and delivery, and the development of breast tissue.

Another potential disruption of the neurohormonal axis could be dysfunctional motion among the cranial bones. The cranium (or skull) houses both the main frame of the nervous system (the brain) and the very important endocrine organs, the hypothalamus and pituitary. The sphenoid is an unpaired cranial bone shaped remarkably like a butterfly or a bat with its wings extended. The sphenoid passes through the center of the cranium, at the base of the skull in front of the paired temporal bones, and behind the orbits of the eyes (near the apex of the orbits, the superior wall is formed by the lesser wing of the sphenoid). The sphenoid articulates with the anterior or basilar portion of the occipital bone (the occipital bone makes up the base and back of the head) (Frey, 1999). The pituitary sits in a bony saddle (the sella turcica) on the superior aspect of the sphenoid bone (**Figures 10-3 and 10-4**).

The movement between the sphenoid and the occiput is a primary focus in manual craniosacral therapy and chiropractic and osteopathic techniques. The sphenoid and occiput, located at the base of the cranium, are points of attachment for important connective tissue or fascial layers that divide the individual lobes of the brain (the cerebrum and the cerebellum). These are the falx cerebri, falx cerebelli, and tentorium cerebelli, folds of the dura mater (**Figure 10-5**). Problems may arise in this area associated with some obstetric interventions (forceps, ventouse) or when there is excessive or rapid molding during the birth process. There is a risk of a tear, which can lead to cerebral bleeding (Areya & Dent, 1953; Holland, 1922; Reichard, 2008; Siu & Kwong, 2006).

The falx and tentorium are continuous with the fascial layers that make up the three connective tissue layers that cover the brain and the descending spinal cord. These meninges include the dura mater, arachnoid mater, and pia mater (often referred to in manual therapy collectively as *the dura*). They also connect to the temporal bones bilaterally. The meninges contain foramina (openings) for blood vessels and cranial nerves to pass through (Williams, Gray, Warwick, & Bannister, 1989). Both osteopathic and chiropractic craniosacral techniques theorize a variety of movements that occur between the sphenoid and occiput near or at the sphenobasilar junction (**Figure 10-6**).

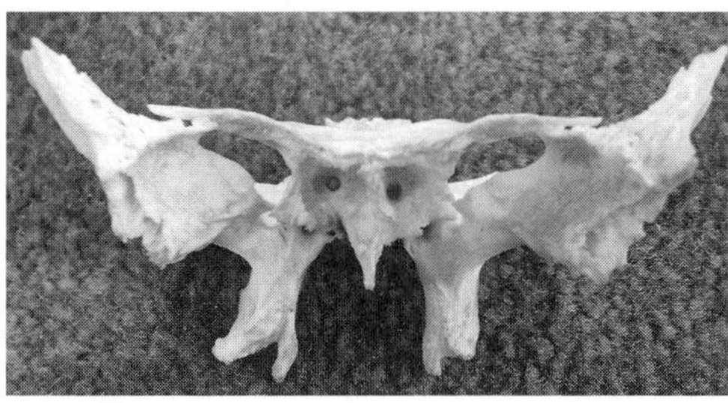

Figure 10-3 (Above) The sphenoid bone.

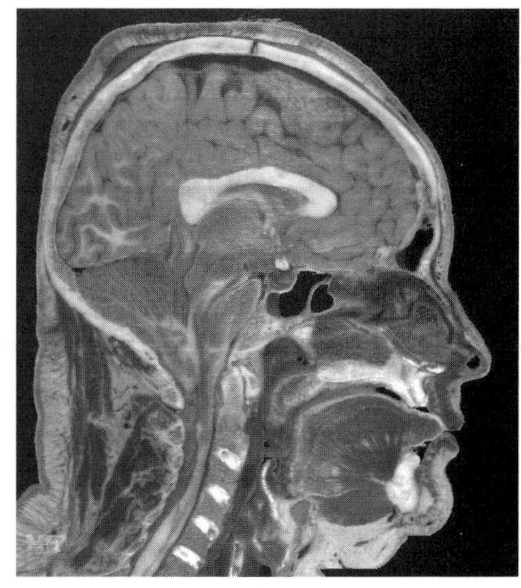

Figure 10-4 (Right) Sagittal section of the brain.

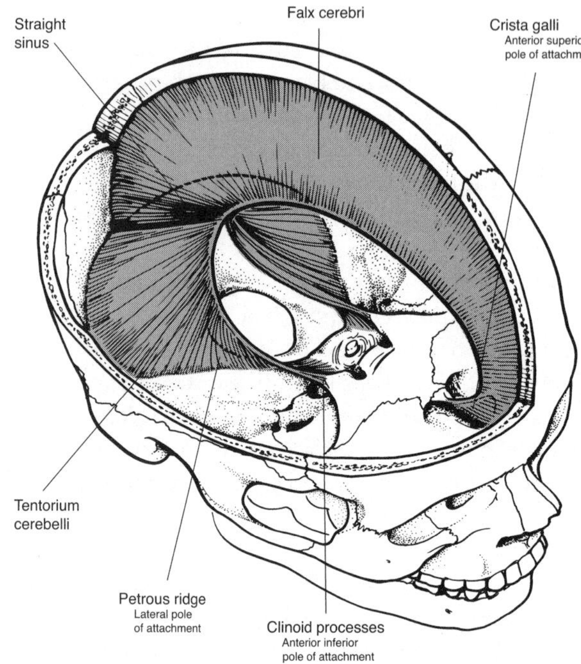

Figure 10-5 (Left) The "tent" and "falx" (brain cut-away).

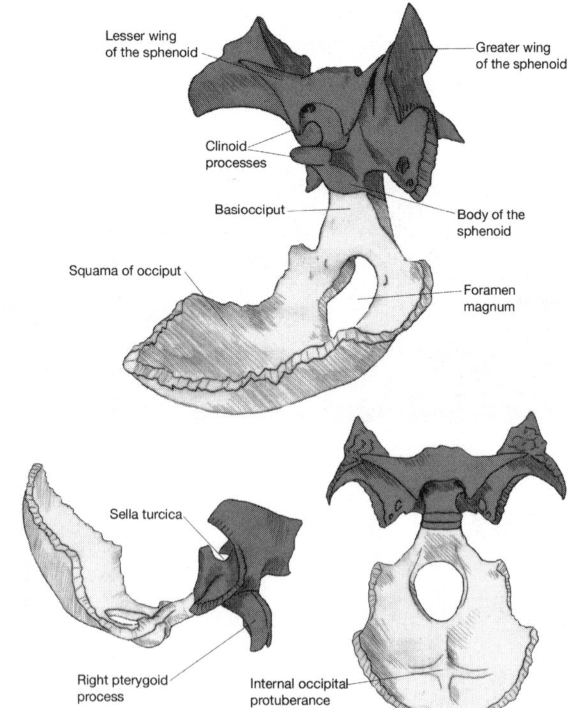

Figure 10-6 (Right) The sphenobasilar junction.

A manual therapist palpates movement throughout the cranial bones by locating and palpating specific landmarks. In testing for sphenobasilar movement, or the movement of any cranial bone, gentle pressure is applied to the cranium in each direction of movement. The testing is performed in opposing directions (for example, flexion and extension or right rotation and left rotation) to determine any restrictions. The amount, length, and degree of movement is evaluated. The movement will reflect tissue resistance or compliance to the force put into the body by the practitioner. When functional, this compliance to an initiating force should be balanced in all directions throughout the cranium, specifically as related to the sphenobasilar junction.

How might structure or alteration of functional mechanics at the sphenobasilar junction affect physiology? Let us consider the relationship of the pituitary with this junction. Anatomically, the pituitary has two main parts, posterior (neurohypophysis) and anterior (adenohypophysis). Between the two, a specialized vascular (portal) system allows communication from the brain to peripheral endocrine organs and other systems (Hill, 2010). Documented reasons for failure to secrete pituitary hormones include pathologies ranging from tumors, infections, and post- or intrapartum hemorrhage to congenital abnormalities (Melmed & Jameson, 2005). Some authors in the field of manual therapies have controversially hypothesized that when a subluxation or mechanical lesion of the cranium occurs at the sphenobasilar junction, the normal flexion and extension of the sphenobasilar junction is restricted, and this in turn may have an influence on pituitary function (Dobson, 1994; Upledgwer, 1987). The reasoning follows that pituitary dysfunction related to a cranial lesion could potentially affect the onset and progress of labor and delivery and the involution of the postpartum womb, and it could affect lactation via hormonal inadequacy of prolactin (affecting milk production) or oxytocin (affecting milk ejection).

Other disruptions could occur at various points in the nervous system. The nerve supply of the breast is derived from the nerves of the fourth, fifth, and sixth intercostal spaces. The fourth intercostal nerve penetrates the posterior aspect of the breast (4 o'clock on the left breast and 8 o'clock on the right breast) and supplies the greatest amount of sensation to the nipple and to the areola. This sensory function is the direct feedback mechanism to the mother's posterior pituitary, instructing it to release oxytocin, which in turn regulates the milk ejection reflex (MER), also known as the milk letdown (Riordan & Auerbach, 1998). Vertebral subluxations at these thoracic levels could interfere with the appropriate responsiveness of these important sensory nerves, disrupting the feedback cycle to the posterior pituitary and preventing efficient release of milk when the infant goes to breast. These vertebral subluxations could be preexisting conditions related to chronic postural strain, scoliosis, pulmonary compromise (asthma, chronic obstructive pulmonary disease, smoking), ergonomics, or breast mass, or they could be the result of subluxations induced injuriously during the postures and physical activity associated with labor and delivery. Multiple contributing factors could lead to this situation (adolescent scoliosis, breast mass, strain during labor).

Milk production is initiated in the breasts in the postpartum period due to prolactin production and decreased estrogen and progesterone after delivery of the placenta. The onset of lactogenesis II (the copious production of human milk) has been shown to be delayed by stressful events around delivery. Dewey found that women who underwent an urgent cesarean section or had a long duration of labor before vaginal delivery were more likely to have a delayed onset of breast fullness in the first days after delivery (2001). By the third or fourth postpartum day, stimulation of the breast by milk removal is required to continue milk production. Mothers produce milk between feedings at a rate based on breast drainage. The prolactin surges initiated by sucking are vital to the maintenance of lactation (Lawrence & Lawrence, 2005). As stated earlier in this discussion, an interference with the sensory feedback from the nipple due to subluxations of the thoracic spine or costal elements could reduce this prolactin surge and prevent the release of adequate levels of oxytocin, resulting in a poor MER and emphasizing the need for manual therapy in breastfeeding success.

During continued lactation, milk production is based on infant demand. The average mother's ability to produce milk is much greater than the average infant's appetite (Daly & Hartmann, 1995). The rate of milk production varies during the day. The speed of milk production is highest in a mostly empty breast and slowest in a mostly full breast; this speed makes the difference in production over time. Suckling or any nipple or breast manipulation should stimulate sensory nerves in the areola and nipple if the integrity of these nerves are intact. These nerves stimulate the pituitary gland to release oxytocin along with prolactin. A conditioned milk ejection can occur when a woman hears her baby cry. This is due to a conditioned release of oxytocin without the release of prolactin; this conditioning can occur very rapidly upon return of sensory integrity.

Another example of a mechanical problem resulting in disruption of the mother's ability to breastfeed is the occurrence of pain as a result of Raynaud phenomenon. Although Raynaud phenomenon is known to occur and cause problems for mothers who attempt to breastfeed, the following case illustrates the importance of discerning whether the patient's pain is Raynaud phenomenon or if there is a neuromusculoskeletal derangement resulting in vasospasm and pain.

A 28-year-old Caucasian female presented 3 weeks postpartum complaining of vasospasm, hyperventilation, and intrascapular and deep breast pain thought to be caused by her daughter's painful latch and dysfunctional breastfeeding. The patient was originally referred to our office by a physician for an evaluation of the infant, who was diagnosed with dysfunctional breastfeeding, but in listening to the history, some interesting facts about the mother's pregnancy came to light.

In the second trimester, she slipped and fell on a wet kitchen floor, striking her back on the edge of the kitchen counter, which resulted in localized acute pain over the seventh rib head on the right between the spine and the shoulder blade. The pain was constant and unremitting, but the localized paraspinal pain decreased in intensity as she approached 40 weeks gestation.

Since giving birth and attempting to breastfeed her daughter, the patient had suffered damage to her nipples, which were blistered, cracked, and bleeding with residuals from resolving mastitis. She had been advised to substitute a bottle for the breast until her nipples could heal. The patient related that there was some recent relief of nipple pain and breakdown since following that advice. She had also heard someone describing similar pain in a woman who had Raynaud phenomenon, but her physician did not think she met all of the criteria for this diagnosis.

An evaluation of the functional motion integrity of her spine and rib cage was recommended. The patient was found to have a decrease in the normal front-to-back curve of the spine between the scapulae (thoracic kyphosis) and faulty motion between the spine and the sixth and seventh thoracic vertebrae and the seventh rib on the right when she was breathing (the normal movement of the ribs when breathing is similar to a bucket handle being lifted and lowered with each inspiration and expiration).

According to Holmen and Backe (2009), nipple pain is a common cause of weaning, second only to low milk production. The most common causes of nipple pain are poor positioning and improper latch. Blanching of the nipple may be caused by mechanical pressure, so additional symptoms (such as biphasic or triphasic color changes, precipitation by cold stimulus, bilateral involvement, and occurrence of symptoms when the patient is not breastfeeding) should therefore be present before a diagnosis of Raynaud phenomenon of the nipple is made. It is also important to not confuse pain and whitish coloration of the nipple with candida, resulting in an inappropriate course of antifungals. In general, Raynaud phenomenon occurs when the ambient temperature drops below a certain threshold; this threshold is specific to each individual. Patients with Raynaud phenomenon are usually advised to avoid medications or substances such as caffeine, nasal vasoconstrictors, and tobacco, which induce vasoconstriction (Anderson, Held, & Wright, 2004; Holmen & Backe, 2009).

Our patient's symptoms did not match the prerequisites for the diagnosis of Raynaud phenomenon. Most importantly, the patient's symptoms were not recreated when exposed to cold or at times other than when she was breastfeeding. Rather, it was possible that the perpetuation of mechanical trauma to the nipple, as a result of the poor latch, resulted in a sensitization of the mother to any of the multiple noxious stimuli. A painful latch or even the contact of an infant's hand on her mother's breast could result in vasospasm and be at the root of her complaint.

The patient continued to follow the acute care instructions and interventions that were put in place to restore the integrity of the injured nipple and to correct mechanical problems with the neonate, which had resulted in a tight and abrasive latch. These suggestions had allowed significant improvement in the integrity of the nipple, but the patient's deep chest pain had not subsided. The patient therefore began a simultaneous protocol of chiropractic adjustments of the joint between the sixth and seventh thoracic vertebrae and seventh rib on the right three times in six days, resulting in abatement of vasospasm and intrascapular pain.

Vasospasm is a frequent complaint among postpartum women who are having difficulty breastfeeding due to their infants' inability to latch properly. Dysfunctional biting, clamping, chewing, or licking of the nipple can result in loss of tissue integrity (bleeding, cracking, blistering, and infection). In this clinical situation, there was no question of injury to the nipples. This injury could result in painful stimuli traveling via efferent nerve endings from the nipple to the respiratory center of the brain each time it was touched. This could then result in an alteration of breathing patterns leading to hyperventilation (even at the anticipation of a painful latch).

The painful stimuli that the patient's brain received directly from the nerve endings of the breast during a feeding also appeared to be compounded (meaning there was more than just one thing going on) by the preexisting mechanical problem at T6–T7 and the seventh rib. This dysfunctional motion resulted in excitation of the nerve that runs between each rib (intercostal nerves) as well as the thoracic sympathetic chain, which lies along both sides of the thoracic spine. The compression of the nerve root, or any nerve in the periphery, by a mechanical lesion initially results in facilitation or increased firing of the nerve (and in chronic conditions, decreased firing of the nerve). In this case, the initial increased firing could have contributed to hyperventilation and vasospasm (as a result of neural dysregulation). If the nerves are irritated and the mother is in pain, her respiratory rate increases, her heart rate increases, her blood pressure might elevate, and she might experience vasospasm in the afflicted area (or, as with Raynaud phenomenon, in a variety of areas), resulting in breast and intrascapular pain.

Structural dysfunction as a result of posture, ergonomics, strain, or trauma can result in a disruption in the neural competency of a mother to successfully breastfeed her infant. Nociceptive stimulus from a musculoskeletal source, as well as from an outside source (rough clothing or the neonate's fingernails or clenched jaw), can then be hypothesized to result in an alteration in respiratory and circulatory patterns in the breastfeeding female. As this author has previously related (Vallone, 2007), structural dysfunction as a result of posture, ergonomics, strain, or trauma can also result in a disruption in the neural competency of a mother to successfully breastfeed her infant. A specific example is when cranial lesions of the sphenoid could potentially result in an alteration in pituitary function, or a thoracic lesion results in decreased sensory input from the nipple to the hypothalamus and alters oxytocin and prolactin release. This suggests that chiropractic evaluation for subluxations would be a key element in the holistic assessment of the failure to establish a milk supply in a postpartum patient. As seen in this author's clinical practice, reduction of subluxations (mechanical lesions) in the cranium and vertebral segments associated with the neurohormonal axis governing lactation can be successful in promoting successful lactogenesis and galactopoiesis.

It is this author's hope that the case studies within this text demonstrate the merit of chiropractic care for the mother, along with other established interventions, and encourage further observation and data collection in this population of patients.

The Infant

As outlined by Tow and Vallone (2009), it is appropriate to make a referral when the history and visual observation includes the following:

- Constraint during pregnancy or difficult labor and delivery
- Visual craniofacial asymmetry or abnormal head shape (see **Figure 10-7**), including palatal anomalies, such as the following:
  - Extremely high rather than gently domed hard palate
  - Anteriorly or posteriorly pitched hard palate with a broad alveolar ridge
  - Narrow palate
- Bruising or swelling around the head
- Asymmetric muscular recruitment
- Apparent discomfort when being held in a specific reproducible position
- Inability to move the head and neck or limbs in all ranges of motion
- Inability to hold the head in a neutral posture
- Absence or exaggeration of infantile reflexes (rooting, suckling, biting)
- Demonstration of a variety of ineffective or inefficient behaviors at the breast, such as the following:
  - Inability to latch efficiently, with symptoms of clicking, slurping, or leaking milk
  - Biting the nipple
  - Walking up the nipple (incremental latch)
  - Tongue thrusting
  - Pushing off the breast or arching away from the breast
  - Lack of endurance at the breast (falling asleep after moments at the breast)

A chiropractor may also provide a second diagnostic opinion when there are concerns of ankyloglossia, or tongue-tie.

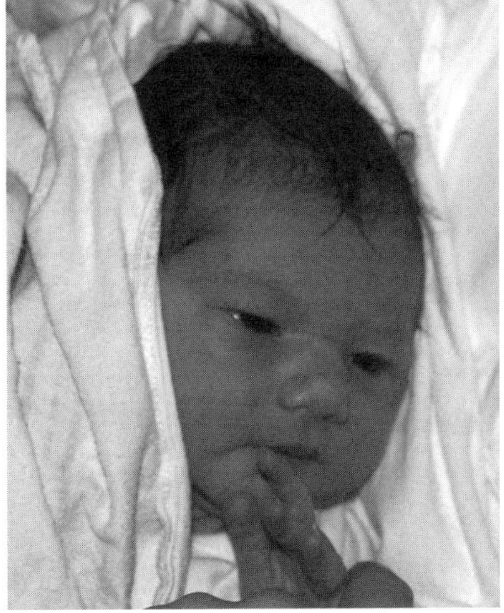

Figure 10-7 Asymmetrical head shape and facial compression.

Chiropractic Care of the Infant

In utero constraint, the birth process, interventions, and birth trauma and early handling of the neonate may all contribute to alterations in structure that affect normal function. The chiropractor will assess the infant's neurologic integrity, including infantile reflexes like rooting and suckling, the coordinated suckle, swallow and breathe, and other neurologic milestones (eye contact, response to sensory stimuli, etc.). An assessment will also be made of the cranial, spinal, and extraspinal joints (for example, the elbow or knee joint or the joint where the ribs or clavicle meet with the sternum) for stability and range of motion, as well as cerebrospinal fluid rhythm and muscle length, tone, and symmetry or asymmetry. In conjunction with the detailed history and observations by the lactation consultant and chiropractor of the infant at breast, rest, and play, a thorough neuromusculoskeletal examination may indicate concomitant neurologic, genetic, or structural problems that could impede breastfeeding, including ankyloglossia, temporomandibular injury, fracture (most frequently cranial or clavicular), avulsion (brachial plexus), hypotonicity (pharmacologically induced, neurodevelopmental delay, or cerebral palsy), diaphragmatic dysfunction resulting in a hiatal hernia (and reflux), or a genetic syndrome, to name a few.

Any impediment to the normal initiation of the hardwired program to seek sustenance will result in strong compensatory behaviors in the neurotypical neonate. Early detection of dysfunction and early, aggressive intervention is critical to prevent infant weight loss or failure to thrive, damage to mother's nipple, decreased stimulus for milk production, or failure to bond. The longer and more vital the compensation is to the neonate, the more deeply the impressionably plastic brain will imprint the behavior. That said, and not to soften the directive to intervene early and aggressively, this same neural plasticity is what creates the possibility of correcting dysfunction even when it has existed for many months, sometimes years. In many cases, the infant brain can continue to adapt to corrective changes made in the structure to promote appropriate function.

The process of suck and swallow has been well defined in several other chapters of this text. But it remains critical to understand that each of the phases of feeding at the breast (oral, pharyngeal, and esophageal) rely on specific biomechanics. These biomechanics will be influenced by cranial nerve function, joint integrity, and muscles weakness or strength. For example, making a seal around the nipple requires closure of the jaw and sealing of the lips. Closure of the jaw requires use of the masseter, temporalis, and medial pterygoid, and it is controlled by the motor portion of the trigeminal nerve (cranial nerve V). Sealing of the lips requires the buccinators and orbicularis oris, which are both controlled by the facial nerve (cranial nerve VII) (Lund et al., 2011). It is necessary for practitioners of manual medicine to fully understand the anatomy and physiology, as well as the biomechanics, of breastfeeding when there is feeding dysfunction in order to differentiate and treat the involved structures and potential lesion or subluxation.

Trauma or physical limitations can result in interference with this process or any normal physiologic process involved in feeding (at breast or bottle). For example, prolonged labor with the fetus in an asynclitic presentation can result in a hyperflexion subluxation at C0 (the occipitoatlantal junction) or molding of the cranium in an attempt to narrow the diameter of the skull as it passes through the birth canal. A hyperflexion subluxation will restrict the normal extension or tipping of the head back at the cranial base on the atlas or first cervical vertebrae (C1), which is necessary for the infant to gape widely and encompass the nipple and areola in the mouth to suckle. An examination may reveal hypertonicity of the anterior cervical and submandibular muscles and compensatory behaviors, which may manifest as arching away from the breast using the lower cervical and upper thoracic spine and larger muscles of the neck and back (levator scapulae and trapezius). This is just one of the many characteristics of a fussy, crying, colicky baby (Browning & Miller, 2008; Miller, 2007; Miller & Phillips, 2009). Molding of the cranium could result in a derangement of the normal motion of the parietal and temporal bones, which could in turn affect the motion at the TMJ and alter the mandibular excursion or the ability to open the mouth widely.

Another example of subluxation, as a result of a presenting congenital physical limitation resulting in compensation, would be a submucosal tongue-tie, which causes abbreviated tongue action (extension, elevation, and lateral deviation) and mandibular excursion by tethering the mandible sublingually. The compensatory behaviors may include excessive hyperextension at C1 in an attempt to gape more widely, as well as overdevelopment of submandibular muscles. This hyperextension can result in inflammation, increased arousal due to sensitivity and pain, or muscle spasm and subluxation, which again results in a fussy or crying baby. An examination may also reveal more developed musculature or hypertonicity (high muscle tone or muscle spasm) of the muscles of mastication as the infant attempts behaviors to get the nipple into the mouth and hold it there (such as an incremental latch, which looks like the infant is walking up the nipple with the lips and gums and clamping or biting the nipple, or grinding the nipple, by moving the mandible from right to left) (Tow & Vallone, 2009).

Dysfunctional presentations are as numerous as there are children who present with a posterior tongue-tie (PTT) or any other biomechanical restriction or structural alteration. The presentation is unique for each child, but there are threads of similarity. For example, a PTT is considered a midline defect that often restricts the tongue in all ranges of motion. Yet it has been my experience that all PTTs are not tethered symmetrically, which can be observed by differences in restriction on the right and left sides (the infant might have the ability to laterally deviate the tongue to one side or elevate one side more than the other). Sometimes the asymmetry is a natural occurrence, and sometimes it is due to a previous incomplete frenotomy or revision. That is why one must observe and think functionally rather than statically to devise the best therapeutic approach. A few descriptive examples of infant compensations one might see are as follows:

- A tethered tongue may require the child to tilt (posterior and medial scalenes for lateral flexion, sternocleidomastoid muscle for lateral flexion with rotation), flex (anterior scalenes, platysmas), or extend (suboccipital and splenii muscles) the head in a direction that allows the most control of the tongue during nursing attempts (usually inefficiently), or the child must passively receive a strong milk flow without gagging, choking, or aspirating milk.

- An infant might tilt the head to be more in control of mom's flow and bite down on the nipple (the compression results in a changed nipple shape when the infant is finished nursing). The direction in the infant tilts may be secondary to how the tongue is tethered (which is not always symmetrical) or the shape of mom's nipple or how mom holds the infant. The infant may flex the head while chomping or biting down on mom in an attempt to hang on to the nipple, or the infant may even crawl up the nipple (like using your lips to get a full piece of spaghetti in your mouth, again, an incremental latch).
- The mandible follows the tethered tongue, resulting in repeated nodding during sucking. If the infant lifts the tongue to encompass the nipple, the mandible (lower jaw) follows and snaps the jaw shut. The infant will extend the head at C1 in an attempt to open the mouth again, and the same sequence will follow, resulting in repeated extension and closure. This results in hypertonic occipital musculature and sometimes even inflammation of the C1 junction and its associated musculature.
- A tethered tongue results in recruitment of submandibular muscles to move the tongue. After they are clipped, ultrasound has shown these muscles to be at rest while nursing (before clipping, ultrasound shows gross contraction of those muscles) (Genna, 2008).
- A tethered tongue results in poor milk flow control if mom has a fast MER or if her supply is engorged or she simply has a heavy flow. If biting is used, then the muscles of mastication become more developed and active. If the infant is choking and pulling off, the trapezius and levator scapulae (and sometimes the splenii) are overactive.

Whether or not it is established that any of these cases require comanagement with an additional specialist (pediatric surgeon, otolaryngologist, dentist or oral surgeon, orthopedist, neurologist), treatment planning by the manual therapist to address these issues usually consists of several visits in rapid succession (1–2 days apart) to help facilitate a successful latch because further weight loss or failure to gain weight has a more dramatic consequence at this young age. Further, premature weaning may be avoided when the mother experiences rapid, noticeable improvement in breastfeeding.

Treatment consists of myofascial release of associated soft tissue structures (cranial and submandibular, cervical and tongue muscles), adjustments (by a chiropractor) or manipulation (by an osteopath) of the individual cranial bones and spinal vertebrae, lymphatic drainage and light massage techniques, and specific stretches or range of motion exercises as indicated.

The frequency and length of care is predicated on the preexisting factors. For example, severe cranial molding from in utero constraint will respond more slowly than an infant whose cranial molding was due to a prolonged labor. The treatment plan may require multiple weekly visits (progressively becoming less frequent) over 1 to 12 weeks. This plan may be tempered by other interventions. For example, if an infant requires a frenotomy or laser revision, it would be most efficacious to see the child as soon as possible after the procedure to assure structural integrity secondary to the restraint of the infant's cranium during the procedure (fix any structural alterations that may have occurred during the procedure) and to facilitate integration of the increased range of motion of the tongue by reducing the interference of any residual structural compensations. Home care protocols should be available for parents to continue to work with the neonate between visits, and recommendations should be given for ongoing lactation and peer support. Although successful breastfeeding may be the most immediate goal, the long-term goal is structural normalization that can potentiate neurologic competency and appropriate development of oral facial structures and oral motor skills and, in some cases, respiratory skills.

A large percentage of the infants I have seen in the past 15 years with difficulty breastfeeding have had PTTs and, although a few have declined, most parents have chosen to have their infants undergo a revision procedure. It is also very possible that my population of patients is skewed because more manual therapists (chiropractors, physical therapists, occupational therapists, osteopaths, massage therapists, craniosacral therapists) are now treating these neonates, and I receive referrals of the more difficult cases that are not resolving.

That said, as important as it is to educate lactation consultants, MDs, osteopaths, obstetrical nursing staff, midwives, advanced practice nurses, and physician assistants in pediatrician's offices how to recognize PTT and how it interferes with breastfeeding (among many important developmental processes, including dentition and speech), it is important to not immediately assume every dysfunctional breastfeeding situation has a PTT at its root. It is important to evaluate for fascial, muscular, or articular constraint or dysfunction and any related potential neurologic deficit. This dysfunction (whether caused by in utero constraint, birth trauma, postpartum trauma, or ergonomics) could be the root of a neonate's inability to root, latch, suckle, sustain the suckle, or efficiently empty the breast and may be the cause of damage to mother's nipple.

If the TMJ is injured and the mandibular excursion is restricted, that is a straightforward mechanical disruption of the normal biomechanics of breastfeeding. If the fetus presented in a facial presentation during a long labor, resulting in an injury and spasm of the musculature of the occipitoatlantal junction (the junction between the base of the skull and the first vertebrae of the neck) and the cervical spine, restricting the cervical range of motion, that could be a straightforward mechanical disruption of the normal biomechanics of breastfeeding. If there is also a displacement of one of the segmented bones at the base of the skull (the occiput), it could result in an alteration in the function of the cranial nerves that exit the skull nearby, thus dampening the normal infantile reflexes associated with breastfeeding (**Figure 10-8**).

A mechanical disruption of the normal biomechanics may also be at the root of a variety of compensatory behaviors that develop in a healthy, neurotypical (or neurologically

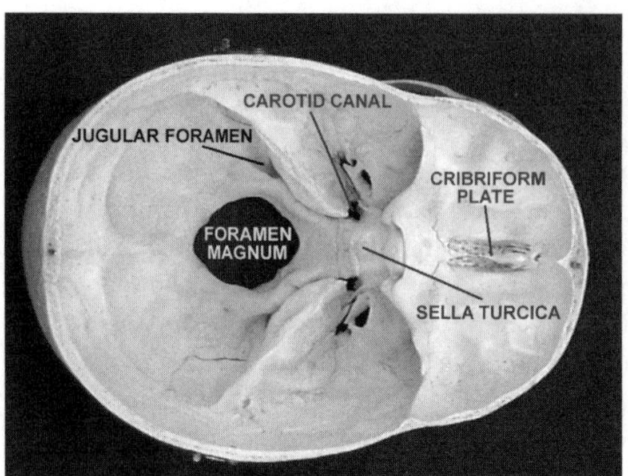

Figure 10-8 Foramina of the skull for the exit of cranial nerves.

competent) neonate to overcome whatever is preventing successful breastfeeding (or in some cases, even bottle feeding when breastfeeding fails). The challenge is to sort out whether there is a mechanical issue (fascial, muscular, articular) at the root of those compensations or whether a true developmental anomaly, like ankyloglossia or developmental delay, is interfering with the ability to breastfeed and resulting in compensatory behaviors.

If the disruption is purely mechanical, manual therapy (depending on the age of the infant) coupled with retraining exercises (such as stretching a tight sternocleidomastoid muscle in a torticollis or teaching a child not to bunch up the tongue to protect the airway) will correct the problem (Miller, 2009; Vallone, 2004). If the mechanical problems are a result of the neonate's compensations for something like PTT, then the neonate might require some manual therapy after surgical or laser revision to assure the ability to override or dampen the compensatory neurology and retrace to the original, prewired circuitry that was intact at birth but limited by the anomalous tissue.

The most complex cases in my practice are those that involve children who have multiple issues or experiences contributing to their presentation. A child with PTT might also have experienced constraint in the womb and as a result had a difficult birth experience resulting in the need for assistive maneuvers (forceps, vacuum, cesarean section, etc.). I have seen three infants who have experienced all these situations and presented on nasogastric or gastric feedings at 4, 6, and 7 months old. A careful unraveling of all the contributing factors along with a board-certified lactation consultant has resulted in complete resolution (and removal of tubes) for two of the children and partial resolution for one child (Tow & Vallone, 2009).

The full success of the latter case was possibly hindered by the family's experience with a manual therapist who worked with one of their older children in whom the breastfeeding dysfunction had not improved. They initially did not follow-up on the referral for the new child because of this experience. Although they reconsidered when the child had reached age 7 months and was on a gastric feeding tube, the family's fear of deviating from the advised medical course when the child had been failing to thrive for so many months and had gone through extensive medical interventions may have influenced their compliance to the suggested treatment plan and the outcome of the limited ensuing treatment.

Case Studies

Case 1

A 4-day-old female presents with her parents who, despite their best attempts, could not wake her to feed by breast or bottle. The infant failed to respond to stroking of the face by finger or with the nipple (no rooting response) and would not suckle when the finger or nipple of the bottle was placed in her mouth. There was no known history of trauma (8-hour labor and delivery, home birth, midwives in attendance), and her Apgar scores at birth were 9/10 (1 min/5 min). She initially went to breast but quickly fell asleep and has been difficult to arouse since. An examination revealed all passive ranges of motion of the head and neck within normal limits except for rotation of the occiput (base of the skull) on the atlas (first vertebra).

At birth, the occiput, or base of the skull, is in four individual pieces instead of a solid ring (solidification occurs later in life as the bone ossifies). The two lateral pieces have a knob, or condyle, that fits perfectly into a matching indentation on the first vertebra (like a cup in a saucer), which allows articulation in all directions, allowing the skull to move freely on that first vertebra. In this infant's case, the occipital condyles had both been compressed and moved toward the midline, both limiting the full range of motion and potentially decreasing the patency of the foramen where the cranial nerves that influence rooting and suckling exit the skull. Correction of the condylar position with cranial techniques consisted of gentle fingertip contact acting as a fulcrum for the neonate to self-mobilize the joints by active range of motion of the head and neck. In this case, the correction resulted in arousal and immediately going to breast for 20 minutes. There was no need for further treatment.

Case 2

A mother and neonate presented with a chief complaint of inability to latch and suckle successfully since birth, despite lactation support. The child had been born 6 days earlier and delivered with the assistance of forceps application to the head due to failure to progress in labor. There was a visible crescent of bruising on the left temporal bone above the ear and on the right side of the jaw at the angle of the mandible. Observation of an attempt to latch revealed mild left head tilt (flexing laterally) and right rotation of the head and neck with asymmetry in the excursion of the jaw. As the jaw opened, the right TMJ popped with a visible, transient lump over the joint (directly in front of the ear). Only the left side of the mouth opened. The neonate could neither open her mouth sufficiently to encompass the nipple and areola, nor could she create a seal. In cross-cradle hold, the neonate would attempt to latch at the right breast but would arch and cry at the left breast. She would cry if held in the football hold at either breast.

Palpation revealed dysfunctional motion at the junction of the occiput (base of the skull) and the first moveable vertebra (atlas or C1). Gentle palpation also elicited discomfort, as noted by the infant's attempting to reflexively withdraw from the touch and crying.

The neonate was not able to hold the head in a neutral posture, laterally flex to the right, or rotate the head to the left. The muscles on the left side of the neck (left sternocleidomastoid muscle and the anterior scalene) were taut, which restricted these movements, creating a mild torticollis. There was also reduced motion at the right TMJ, which resulted in excessive movement at the left TMJ when attempting to open the mouth.

The mechanism of injury could be hypothesized to be a result of a restricted position in the womb, but based on the location of the bruising on the skull and jaw, the injury was more likely associated with presentation during birth and the placement and direction of traction that was used during the forceps extraction.

Treatment was directed to the dysfunctional motion at the base of the skull to allow full range of motion. The head was turned to the right and left, and it was tilted to the right and left, as well as to the TMJ, to increase the motion on the right side and decrease the range of motion on the left side. This allowed the jaw to drop evenly and the mouth to open widely to fully encompass the nipple and areola. The treatment consisted of soft tissue release and mobilization of the joints that were not moving within their normal range of motion.

After the first treatment, the infant was able to latch and suckle successfully on the right breast, but she was still arching and protesting at the left breast. It took two more treatments until she was comfortably nursing at both breasts.

Case 3

A mother presents her male infant at 3 months of age with the chief complaint of not sustaining a latch, failing to empty the breast, gastroesophageal reflux, and biting at the breast, all accompanied by failure to thrive. Hers was a prolonged labor with the infant in an asynclitic presentation, ultimately resulting in a cesarean section. The infant had swelling over the parietotemporal suture on the right and a parallelogram head shape (with the elevated peak being over the same parietotemporal suture). This was accompanied by the eyes and ears appearing uneven when observing the face (see **Figure 10-7**).

The evaluation revealed a retracted mandible, decreased excursion of the jaw, and flexion of the head on the chest with limited extension (the infant would push up from the mother instead of tipping the head backward). The intraoral evaluation was normal except for bilaterally taut pterygoid muscles resulting in tautness and retraction of the mandible, as well as an elevated and fixed hyoid bone accompanied by increased tension in all the attaching submandibular muscles. The respiratory diaphragm was taut, and the junction of the esophagus and stomach was being tractioned by the connective tissue-holding elements. Myofascial release of all connective tissue and muscular components and cranial adjustment of the C1 junction and parietal, temporal, and sphenoid bones resolved the breastfeeding issues after four treatments. Ten treatments continued over a period of 1 month, resulting in 75% correction of the craniofacial asymmetry and resolution of the reflux as a result of releasing the connective tissue traction and promoting normal peristalsis initiated by more functional oral biomechanics.

Case 4

In this compound case, a mother presented with her 10-week-old female infant with a chief complaint of an inability to nurse without compression of the nipple, which caused the mother pain and breakdown of the integrity of the nipple (bleeding, cracking, blistering). The birth had been challenging, with the umbilical cord wrapped twice around the infant's neck and once around her abdomen. After birth, the neonate was immediately put to breast, and she began suckling. There was pain from the first latch, and after the first feed the mother's nipples were cracked and bleeding. It was more difficult to feed on the left breast, and there was more damage to that nipple. Despite the pain, the mother had persevered and the infant had only been breastfed until recently, when it was suggested that the mother should attempt to pump and bottle feed so her nipples could heal. When bottle feeding, the infant chewed the nipple, leaking milk from either side of her mouth and pushing the bottle out of her mouth with her tongue. The infant's weight gain had been slow but did not fall below the 25th percentile. She was frequently troubled with gas, and although she initially moved her bowels with each feeding, she was now stooling only twice a day.

The physical exam revealed a healthy, nourished Caucasian female with cranial molding. The cranium, in aerial view, was diamond-shaped with several cranial bones overlapping—the base of the skull, or occiput, was compressed under the parietal (top) and temporal (side) bones bilaterally. The posterior skull had an elongated, horizontal indentation, most likely where the umbilical cord wrapped twice around the head and neck. The ears both protruded from the pull of the anterior neck muscles and without opposition from the posterior muscles, which did not appear to be engaging. This was possibly due to restriction of the C1 junction (base of the skull and first vertebra), which was fixed in forward flexion (chin to chest) and unable to extend. When attempting to lift her head, the infant arched from the midback and lifted the head and neck as a single unit. When on her stomach, she could not lift her head without arching her thoracic spine, and she became frustrated easily (it looked as if she was attempting to accomplish a push-up).

Palpation of the cranial base revealed that the occipital condyles had both migrated toward the midline. The mandible's excursion (opening of the mouth) was limited due to the flexion of the chin onto the chest and the tension of the anterior neck muscles. The hyoid was retracted due to the tension of the attached muscles. There was visible recruitment of the submandibular muscles and the muscles of mastication while nursing, and an obvious chewing motion could be observed.

An intraoral evaluation revealed that the right pterygoid muscle was extremely tight (resulting in lateral movement of the jaw and retraction), restricting the movement of the right TMJ. The left mandible dropped more easily than the right. The palate was gently domed but narrow in width. The tongue did not extend easily past the gum line, nor did it elevate or laterally deviate easily. The posterior tongue elevated, or bunched, when the infant yawned or opened her mouth widely. It formed a shallow bowl when she cried or laid completely flat. It was difficult to manually lift the tongue from the floor of the mouth, but when she cried, one could visualize a transverse membranous attachment with a midline, dense white vertical ligamentous frenum just posterior to the first half of the tongue. The lips did not appear to be restricted by any tissue, and the circular muscle around the mouth (orbicularis oris) was relaxed. The infant's gag reflex was easily elicited, and she did not appear to be able to normally coordinate swallowing during rapid milk ejection.

The treatment consisted of extensive mobilization of the cranial plates, including decompression of the lambdoidal suture, spreading of the occipital condyles and maxilla, restoration of C1 into extension, relaxation of the submandibular muscles, and mobilization of the hyoid, the muscles of mastication, and the pterygoids, as well as myofascial release to the underside of the tongue and the cervical spine. Treatment consisted of gentle fingertip application to the aforementioned joints acting as fulcrum to allow the neonate to mobilize the joint or stretch the soft tissue using the action of her own muscles and only the amount of force that felt comfortable to her.

The mother was instructed on how to support the head while allowing the infant to extend the head and neck by placing her hand at the nape of the neck with her fingers in a V shape. This technique is often more successful for mother and infant rather than holding and pushing the infant's head onto the nipple, which a mother will often be instructed to do when an infant cannot support and position his or her own head. It was also suggested to allow the infant to find the nipple (which the mother correctly directed asymmetrically toward the palate). In addition, the parents were instructed to massage the infant's muscles, stretch the pterygoids, and stretch the tongue manually at home 6 to 10 times per day for only 1 to 2 minutes each time. A consultation for a frenotomy was recommended.

After the initial treatment, the parents noted greater range of motion of the head and neck, and the infant was lifting her head without elevating her shoulders during "tummy time." But there was no improvement in breastfeeding, and about 72–96 hours after the treatment, she showed signs of being sensitive to touch when holding the back of her head and neck. She also began to become more irritable lying on her stomach and began to demonstrate a decrease in range of motion in that same position, reverting back to lifting her head by recruiting the large muscles (trapezius and levator scapulae) and extending from the waist to the tip of her head as one solid unit. A return visit confirmed inflammation and fixation at the C1 junction, which most likely occurred from the repetitive microtrauma of extending at C1 when attempting to open the mouth. When she attempted to open the mouth and encompass the nipple and areola, the infant would rock the head back and drop the jaw. But each time she tried, the mandible would elevate and close the gap, following the tethered tongue as it attempted elevate to the nipple. She was treated again and regained full cervical range of motion.

A pediatric consult resulted in a surgical release of the lingual frenulum. There was no immediate change in her ability to latch and suckle, and over the course of the next 3 days she became more irritable and disorganized at the breast and with the bottle. The parents performed a digital sweep under the tongue several times a day as instructed by the surgeon and continued to feel a "speed bump" as they moved from right to left.

An evaluation 48 hours after the frenotomy revealed a more posterior residual vertical midline attachment continuing to restrict elevation and lateral deviation of the tongue. Although the extension had greatly improved while at rest and playing with her tongue in imitation of her mother sticking her tongue out, when she yawned or cried, the tongue continued to retract and elevate posteriorly. A second surgical release was performed on the revealed tissue. Once more, there was no immediate change when put to breast, and she appeared to remain disorganized.

The patient was treated on several more occasions, and the parents were given support to continue to work with their daughter with patience and gentle encouragement, continuation of the facial and intraoral massage, and mimicry. With the addition of an exercise to train the tongue to lie flat and extend, she was able to successfully latch and suckle after 3.5 weeks. Her colicky symptoms resolved, and she was stooling several times a day.

Conclusion

As seen in these case studies, children, like snowflakes, will each present with their own unique set of issues and compensations. It is our responsibility to be thorough in our assessment and well educated in the possible causes of their presenting complaint and to be familiar with the most effective ways of addressing the root cause. Collegial communication with a wide variety of healthcare practitioners expands our value to our patients and clients by opening the door to possibilities that might be overlooked if we remain in isolation.

Dedication

With gratitude and my deepest respect to my mentor, Jennifer Tow, whose thoughts, words, and brilliant insights are so deeply reflected in this chapter because she is the one who most influenced me professionally as she fearlessly advocated for these mothers and children. She not only taught me a holistic view of the neurology and physiology of breastfeeding and its relationship to form, but the comprehensive benefit of early intervention. And to Dr. Betty Corrylos, whose gentle conviction and incredible skill has opened the eyes of many healthcare providers and turned the tide for so many children, and Cathy Watson Genna, who walked the walk with Dr. Coryllos and so many others and manifested this venue to bring into perspective the many facets of breastfeeding, our ability to understand and support, and our desire to communicate professionally to expand our ability to make changes for the better. And to my dedicated and brilliant proofreader, JRP, without whom this would not have been completed.

References

Almeida, O. F., Yassouridis, A., & Forgas-Moya, I. (1994). Reduced availability of milk after central injections of corticotropin-releasing hormone in lactating rats. *Neuroendocrinology, 59*(1), 72–77.

American Academy of Orthopaedic Manual Physical Therapists. (2008). *Orthopaedic manual physical therapy: Description of advanced specialty practice.* Tallahassee, FL: Author. Retrieved from http://www.aaompt.org/publications/dasp.cfm

Anderson, J. E., Held, N., & Wright, K. (2004). Raynaud's phenomenon of the nipple: A treatable cause of painful breastfeeding. *Pediatrics, 113*, e360–e364.

Anglo-European College of Chiropractic. (2010). *Master of Science in Advanced Professional Practice (Chiropractic Pediatrics)*. Retrieved from http://www.aecc.ac.uk/cms/site/docs/MSc%20APP%20Chiropractic%20Paediatrics.pdf

Areya, J. B., & Dent, J. (1953). Causes of fetal and neonatal death with special reference to pulmonary and inflammatory lesions. *Journal of Pediatrics, 42*(2), 205–227.

Berkley, K. J., Robbins, A., & Sato, Y. (1993). Functional differences between afferent fibers in the hypogastric and pelvic nerves innervating female reproductive organs in the rat. *Journal of Neurophysiology, 69*(2), 533–544.

Browning, M., & Miller, J. E. (2008). Comparison of the short-term effects of chiropractic spinal manipulation and occipito-sacral decompression in the treatment of infant colic: A single-blinded, randomised, comparison trial. *Clinical Chiropractic, 11*(3), 122–129.

Castro-Sanchez, A. M., Matarán-Peñarrocha, G. A., Sánchez-Labraca, N., Quesada-Rubio, J. M., Granero-Molina, J., & Moreno-Lorenzo, C. (2011). A randomized controlled trial investigating the effects of craniosacral therapy on pain and heart rate variability in fibromyalgia patients. *Clinical Rehabilitation, 25*(1), 25–35. Retrieved from http://www.ncbi.nlm.nih.gov/pubmed/20702514

Chaitow, L. (2006). What is naturopathic physical medicine? *Journal of Bodywork and Movement Therapies, 2007*(10), 1016.

Cuccia, A. M., Caradonna, C., Annunziata, V., & Caradonna, D. (2010). Osteopathic manual therapy versus conventional conservative therapy in the treatment of temporomandibular disorders: A randomized controlled trial. *Journal of Bodywork and Movement Therapies, 14*(2), 179–184.

Daly, S. E. J., & Hartmann, P. E. (1995). Infant demand and milk supply. Part 1: Infant demand and milk production in lactating women. *Journal of Human Lactation, 11*(1), 21–26.

Dewey, K. G. (2001). Maternal and fetal stress are associated with impaired lactogenesis in humans. Symposium: Human lactogenesis II: Mechanisms, determinants and consequences. *The Journal of Nutrition, 131*, 30128–30158.

Dewey, K. G., Nommsen-Rivers, L. A., Heinig, M. J., & Cohen, R. J. (2003). Risk factors for suboptimal infant breastfeeding behavior, delayed onset of lactation, and excess neonatal weight loss. *Pediatrics, 112*, 607–619.

Dobson, J. (1994). *Baby beautiful: A handbook of baby head shaping*. Carson City, NV: Heirs Press.

Educational Council on Osteopathic Principles of the American Association of Colleges of Osteopathic Medicine. (2009). *Glossary of osteopathic terminology*. Retrieved from http://www.aacom.org/resources/Documents/Downloads/GOT2009ed.pdf

Frey, K. I. (1999). Craniosacral therapy and the visual system. *Journal of Behavioral Optometry, 10*(2), 31–35.

Frost, R. (2002). *Applied Kinesiology: A Training Manual and Reference Book of Basic Principles and Practices.* Berkeley, California: North Atlantic Books. (p. 4).

Fuhr, A. W., & Menke, J. M. (2005). Status of activator methods chiropractic technique, theory and practice. *Journal of Manipulative Physiologic Therapeutics, 28*(135), e1–e20.

Fuhr, A.W. (2011). *Activator methods.* Retrieved from http://www.activator.com/about

Gatterman, M., & Hanson, D. (1994). Development of chiropractic nomenclature through consensus. *Journal of Manipulative Physiological Therapeutics, 17*(5), 302–309.

Genna, C. W. (2008). Partial ankyloglossia: Ultrasound examination of breastfeeding before and after treatment for posterior tongue-tie. VELB/ILCA Conference: A Worldwide View on Breastfeeding, Vienna, Austria.

Graham, J. M., Miller, M. E., Stephan M. J., & Smith, D. W. (1980). Limb reduction anomalies and early in utero limp compression. *Journal of Pediatrics, 96*(5), 1052–1056.

Green, C., Martin, C. W., Bassett, K., & Kazanjian, A. (1999). A systematic review of craniosacral therapy: Biological plausibility, assessment reliability and clinical effectiveness. *Complementary Therapies in Medicine, 7*(4), 201–207.

Greenman, P. E., & McPartland, J. M. (1995). Cranial findings and iatrogenesis from craniosacral manipulation in patients with traumatic brain syndrome. *Journal of the American Osteopathic Association, 95*(3), 182–188.

Hall, J. G. (2010). Importance of muscle movement for normal craniofacial development. *Journal of Craniofacial Surgery, 21*, 1336–1338.

Hartman, S. E., & Norton, J. M. (2002). Interexaminer reliability and cranial osteopathy. *The Scientific Review of Alternative Medicine, 6*(1), 23–34.

Hill, M. (2010). *UNSW embryology: Endocrine development—pituitary*. Retrieved from http://embryology.med.unsw.edu.au/Notes/endocrine7.htm

Hoffman, S., & Harris, J. (2000). *Introduction to kinesiology: Studying physical activity*. Champaign, IL: Human Kinetics.

Holland, E. (1922). *The causation of foetal death. Reports on public health and medical subjects* (No. 7 Ministry of Health). London, England: His Majesty's Stationery Office.

Holmen, O. L., & Backe, B. (2009). An underdiagnosed cause of nipple pain presented on a camera phone. *British Medical Journal, 339*, b2553.

Howat, J. (2000). The philosophy of sacro-occipital technique. *The British Journal of Chiropractic, 4*(4), 75.

Humphreys, K. (2010). Possible adverse events in children treated by manual therapy: A review. *Chiropractic and Osteopathy, 18*, 12.

Hutti, L., & Montgomery, P. (Eds.). (2006). *Textbook of Logan basic methods and Logan basic technique* (4th ed.). Chesterfield, MO: LBM.

International College of Applied Kinesiology. (2005). *What is applied kinesiology?* Retrieved from http://www.icak.com

John, C. (2003, March/April). Directional non-force technique. *Today's Chiropractic*, 20–23.

John, C. (2011). *Directional non-force technique* .Retrieved from http://www.nonforce.com

International College of Chiropractic Pediatrics. (2011). *Homepage*. Retrieved from http://internationalcollegeofchiropracticpediatrics.org/index.htm

Joseph, R. (2000). Fetal brain behavior and cognitive development. *Developmental Review, 20*(1), 81–98.

Kase, K. (2010). *Kinesio taping method*. Retrieved from http://www.kinesiotaping.com

Keating, J. C., Jr. (2005). Philosophy in chiropractic. In S. Haldeman et al. (Eds.), *Principles and practice of chiropractic* (3rd ed., pp. 77–98). New York, NY: McGraw-Hill.

Kinsella, M. T., & Monk, C. (2009). Impact of maternal stress, depression and anxiety on fetal neurobehavioral development. *Clinical Obstetrics and Gynecology, 52*(3), 425–440.

Korr, I. M., & Peterson, B. (Eds.). (1978). *The collected papers of Irvin M. Korr*. Colorado Springs, CO: American Academy of Osteopathy.

Lajeunie, E., Crimmins, D. W., Amaud, E., & Renier, D. (2005). Genetic considerations in nonsyndromic midline craniosynostoses: A study of twins and their families. *Journal of Neurosurgery: Pediatrics, 103*(4), 353–356.

Laroia, N. (2010). *Pediatric cardiac birth trauma*. Retrieved from http://emedicine.medscape.com/article/980112

Lau, C. (2001). Effects of stress on lactation. *Pediatric Clinics of North America, 48*, 221–234.

Lawrence, R. A., & Lawrence, R. M. (2005). *Breastfeeding: A guide for the medical profession* (6th ed.). Philadelphia, PA: Elsevier Mosby.

LeDoux, J. (2002). *Synaptic self: How our brains become who we are*. New York, NY: Penguin.

Leon, D. (2008). Commentary: The development of the Ounsteds' theory of maternal constraint—a critical perspective. *International Journal of Epidemiology, 37*(2), 255–259.

Leung, E., Tasker, S. L., Atkinson, L., Vaillancourt, T., Schulkin, J., & Schmidt, L. A. (2010). Perceived maternal stress during pregnancy and its relation to infant stress reactivity at 2 days and 10 months of postnatal life. *Clinical Pediatrics, 49*(2), 158–165.

Littlefield, T., Kelly, K. M., Pomatto, J. K., & Beals S. P. (1999). Multiple-birth infants at higher risk for development of deformational plagiocephaly. *Pediatrics, 103*(3), 565–569.

Lund, G. C., Edwards, G., Medlin, B., Keller, D., Beck, B., & Carreiro, J. E. (2011). Osteopathic manipulative treatment for the treatment of hospitalized premature infants with nipple feeding dysfunction. *Journal of the American Osteopathic Association, 111*(1), 44–48.

Makino, I., Matsude, Y., Yoneyama, M., Hirasawa, K., Takagi, K., Ohta, H., & Konishi, Y. (2009). Effect of maternal stress on fetal heart rate assessed by vibroacoustic stimulation. *Journal of International Medical Research, 37*(6), 1780–1788.

Mathai, M., Sanghvi, H., Guidotti, R., Broekhuizen, F., Chalmers, B., Johnson, R., . . . Zupan, J. (2000). *Managing complications in pregnancy and childbirth: A guide for midwives and doctors.* Geneva, Switzerland: World Health Organization.

Melmed, S., & Jameson, J. L. (2005). Disorders of the anterior pituitary and hypothalamus. In D. L. Kasper et al. (Eds.), *Harrison's principles of internal medicine* (16th ed., pp. 2076–2097). New York, NY: McGraw-Hill.

Miller, J. E. (2007). Cry babies: A framework for chiropractic care. *Clinical Chiropractic, 10*(3), 139–146.

Miller, J. E. (2009). Safety of chiropractic manual therapy for children: How are we doing? *Journal of Clinical Chiropractic Pediatrics, 10*(2), 655–660.

Miller, J. E., & Phillips, H. L. (2009). Long-term effects of infant colic: A survey comparison of chiropractic treatment and nontreatment groups. *Journal of Manipulative and Physiologic Therapeutics, 32*(8), 635–638.

Mootz, R. D., & Phillips, R. B. (1997). Chiropractic belief systems. In D. C. Cherkin & R. D. Mootz (Eds.), *Chiropractic in the United States: Training, practice, and research.* Rockville, MD: Agency for Health Care Policy and Research.

Moran, R., & Gibbons, P. (2001). Intraexaminer and interexaminer reliability for palpation of the cranial rhythmic impulse at the head and sacrum. *Journal of Manipulative and Physiological Therapeutics, 24*(3), 183–190.

Morter, M. (2011). *Bioenergetic synchronization technique (BEST).* Retrieved from http://www.morter.com/what_is_best.php

Moskalenko, Y. E., & Kravchenko, T. I. (2004). Wave phenomena in movements of intracranial liquid media and the primary respiratory mechanism. *American Academy of Osteopathy Journal, 14,* 29–40.

Nelson, K. E., Sergueef, N., & Glonek, T. (2004). Cranial manipulation induces sequential changes in blood flow velocity on demand. *American Academy of Osteopathy Journal, 14,* 15–17.

Nelson, K. E., Sergueef, N., & Glonek, T. (2006). Recording the rate of the cranial rhythmic impulse. *The Journal of the American Osteopathic Association, 106*(6), 337–341.

Nelson, K. E., Sergueef, N., Lipinski, C. L., Chapman, A., & Glonek, T. (2001). The cranial rhythmic impulse related to the Traube-Hering-Mayer oscillation: Comparing laser-Doppler flowmetry and palpation. *The Journal of the American Osteopathic Association, 101,* 163–173.

Nimmo, R. (2011). *Nimmo Educational Foundation.* Retrieved from http://nimmoed.org/history.shtml

O'Connor, M. (2011). *Breastfeeding basics* [Lecture notes]. Retrieved from http://www.breastfeeding-basics.org

Pecka, C. C., & Hannamb, A. G. (2006). Human jaw and muscle modeling. *Archives of Oral Biology, 52*(4), 300–304.

Peppin, J. F. (1993). The osteopathic distinction: Fact or fancy. *Journal of Medical Humanities, 14*, 203–222.

Putta, L., & Spencer, J. (2000). Assisted vaginal delivery using the vacuum extractor. *American Family Physician, September 2000,* 1269. Retrieved from http://www.aafp.org/afp/20000915/1316.html

Reichard, R. (2008). Birth injury of the cranium and central nervous system. *Brain Pathology, 18*(4), 565–579.

Retzlaff, E. W., Michael, D., Roppel, R., & Mitchell, F. (1976). The structures of cranial bone sutures. *Journal of the American Osteopathic Association, 75*(6), 607–608.

Riordan, J., & Auerbach, K. (1998). *Breastfeeding and human lactation* (2nd ed.). Sudbury, MA: Jones and Bartlett.

Rogers, J. S., Witt, P. L., Gross, M., Hacke, T., & Genova, P. A. (1998). Simultaneous palpation of the craniosacral rate at the head and feet: Intrarater and interrater reliability and rate comparisons. *Journal of the American Physical Therapy Association, 78*(11), 1175–1185.

Sacro Occipital Research Society International. (2011). *About SORSI.* Retrieved from http://www.sorsi.com/about-us.html

Sergueef, N., Nelson, K. E., & Glonek, T. (2002). The effect of cranial manipulation upon the Traube Hering Meyer oscillation. *Alternative Therapies in Health and Medicine, 8*, 74–76.

Siu, S. L. Y., & Kwong, K. T. S. (2006). A 10 year review of intracranial hemorrhage in term neonates. *Hong Kong Journal of Pediatrics, 11*(2), 140–146.

Sperino, G. (1939). *Anatomia umana* (Vol. 1, pp. 203, 342). Torino, Italy: Unione Tipografico-Editrice Torinese.

Sutherland, W. G., Adah, S., & Wales, A. L. (1967). *Collected writings of William Gamer Sutherland 1914–1954.* Yakima, WA: The Sutherland Cranial Teaching Foundation.

Swedenborg, E. (1882). *The cerebrum and its parts: The brain considered anatomically, physiologically and philosophically.* London, England: James Speirs.

The Association of Chiropractic College. (1996) *Issues in chiropractic, position paper 1.* Retrieved from http://www.chiro.org/chimages/chiropage/acc.html

Todd, T. W., & Lyon, D. W., Jr. (1924). Endocranial suture closure, its progress and age relationship. *American Journal of Physical Anthropology, 7*(3), 325–384.

Tow, J., & Vallone, S. (2009). Development of an integrative relationship in the care of the breastfeeding newborn: Lactation consultant and chiropractor. *Journal of Clinical Chiropractic Pediatrics, 10*(1), 626–632.

Unger, J. F. (1995, September). The legacy of a chiropractor, inventor and researcher: Dr. Major Bertrand DeJarnette. In *Conference Proceedings of the Chiropractic Centennial Foundation.* Davenport, IA.

Upledger, J. E. (1977). The reproducibility of craniosacral examination findings: A statistical analysis. *Journal of the American Osteopathic Association, 76*, 890–899.

Upledger, J. E. (1987). *Craniosacral therapy II—beyond the dura.* Seattle, WA: Eastman Press.

Upledger, J. E. (1995). Craniosacral therapy: Response to Virginia Wirth-Pattullo and Karen W. Hayes, *Physical Therapy, 75*, 328–330.

Upledger, J. E. (2003). Applications of craniosacral therapy in newborns and infants, part I. *Massage Today, 3*(5), 1–4. Retrieved from http://www.massagetoday.com/archives/2003/05/08.html?no_b=true

Upledger, J. E., & Vredevoogd, J. D. (1983). *Craniosacral therapy.* Seattle, WA: Eastland Press.

Vallone, S. (2004). Chiropractic evaluation and treatment of musculoskeletal dysfunction in infants demonstrating difficulty breastfeeding. *Journal of Clinical Chiropractic Pediatrics, 5*(1), 349–368.

Vallone, S. (2007). Role of subluxation and chiropractic care in hypolactation. *Journal of Clinical Chiropractic Pediatrics, 8*(1, 2), 518–524.

Vohra, S., Jonston, B., & Humphreys, K. (2007). Adverse events in the manipulation of pediatric patients: Flaws in a systematic review. *Pediatrics, 119*(6), 1266–1267.

Wadhwa, P. H. (2005). Psychoneuroendocrine processes in human pregnancy influence fetal development and health. *Psychoneuroendocrinology, 30*(8), 724–743.

Ward, R. C. (1993). *Myofascial release concepts*. In J. V. Basmajian & R. Nyberg (Eds.), *Rational manual therapies* (pp. 223–240). Philadelphia, PA: Lippincott Williams and Wilkins.

Williams, P. L., Gray, H., Warwick, W., & Bannister, D. (1989). *Gray's anatomy* (37th ed.). New York, NY: Churchill Livingstone.

Wirth-Patullo, V., & Hayes, K. (1994). Interrater reliability of craniosacral rate measurements and their relationship with subjects' and examiners' heart and respiratory rate measurements. *Physical Therapy, 74*(10), 908–916.

World Federation of Chiropractic. (2009). *Definitions of chiropractic*. Retrieved from http://www.wfc.org/website/index.php?option=com_content&view=article&id=90&Itemid=110&lang=en

World Health Organization. (2010). *Benchmarks for training in osteopathy*. Geneva, Switzerland: Author.

CHAPTER 11

Sensory Integration and Breastfeeding

Catherine Watson Genna and Diklah Barak

What Is Sensory Integration?

Sensory integration (SI) is the process by which the brain coordinates all the information coming in from the senses in order to plan and execute appropriate and responsive (adaptive) behavior. This theory of brain-behavior relationships was posited by occupational therapist A. Jean Ayres (1979) from careful observation and testing of young children with learning disabilities. SI theory continues to be refined by both therapists and scientists. It is important for professionals working with infants to understand the principles of SI because feeding difficulties can result from or be exacerbated by poor sensory processing.

The Process of Sensory Integration: Important Concepts

Registration is the intake and noting of sensory information. If information is not registered, it cannot be acted on. Each person has an individual threshold for sensory intake. Stimuli falling below the threshold intensity are not taken in; those above it are. A hungry infant who ignores touch from the nipple could be displaying poor registration due to an unusually high threshold or deliberately withdrawing from too much incoming traffic due to a low threshold. Hunger itself is an alerting state, lowering motor and sensory threshold (Berg, Pangborn, Roessler, & Webb, 1963) to improve the ability to find food. For already challenged infants, the lowering of the threshold might be disorganizing, reducing feeding ability.

Next, information needs to be modulated. In the process of *modulation,* the neural signals are strengthened (facilitated) or weakened (inhibited). Useful information is normally facilitated, and extraneous, repetitive stimulation, such as the feeling of clothing on the body, is usually inhibited. Selection of stimuli for facilitation is a vital step in this process. If extraneous detail is focused on, the important stimuli that guide feeding are going to get lost in the static. The balance between excitatory (norepinephrine, serotonin, and dopamine) and inhibitory (GABA) neurotransmitters provides the mechanism for accommodation, the ability to stop responding to repetitive stimuli while retaining sensitivity to novelty.

Comparison is the next step in sensory processing. The cortex is arranged in layers and tracts. This arrangement allows an organized, three-dimensional association of information because it can travel both up and down and side to side through the brain.

New sensory information is compared to previous experience in the associative cortex, and emotional nuances are added by the limbic system. Imagine you are preparing to cross the street. You will see the cars coming, hear the air they displace, and make a judgment based on past experience about whether or not it is safe to cross, decide how fast you need to walk, then implement that speed. This *cross-modal* processing of visual and auditory cues improves your accuracy. If you've previously had a close call while crossing the street, your limbic system will add some fear to encourage you to either speed up or to wait for a safer opportunity to cross. This process of association may lead infants who are frustrated with past difficulties to refuse to feed even though they are hungry. One toddler in the author's practice who was diagnosed with leukemia refused to breastfeed or take milk in any form during chemotherapy, though she would eat other foods. It took some detective work to reveal the association she formed between exacerbated nausea from moving into a breastfeeding position with the taste of her mother's milk. When given antiemetic medication that eliminated her nausea, she returned to breastfeeding.

The Special Senses

Children are traditionally taught that there are five senses: visual (sight), auditory (hearing), tactile (touch), olfactory (smell), and gustatory (taste). There are actually several more special senses that are important to our sense of the body and its orientation and movement in space. These include the vestibular (balance and gravity), kinesthetic (joint movement), and proprioceptive (body position) senses.

The *vestibular* apparatus is located in the inner ear. Information from the otoliths and semicircular canals is used to sense head orientation and movement and to subtract out the static effects of gravity while allowing changes in orientation to gravity (falling or tilting) to be noted. The ability to hold a steady gaze uses similar mechanisms derived from the vestibular sense (Green & Angelaki, 2003). Infants with difficulty processing vestibular information may be terrified of movement due to gravitational insecurity, and they may flail and startle when moved toward the breast.

Kinesthesia and *proprioception* likewise interact with the tactile system to form the *body schema,* which maps the position of the body and its movement in space. The proprioceptive sense delivers information from stretch receptors in joint capsules and muscle spindles to be processed into a global sense of body position. The kinesthetic sense uses similar information to identify the movement of each individual joint. Neonates are dealing with unrestricted movement after having been constrained snugly in the uterus and with gravity after having lived in a fluid, low-gravity environment. These factors along with neurological immaturity and inexperience with the postbirth environment lead infants to have poorly graded (jerky) movement.

Work on tactile extinction (Vaishnavi, Calhoun, & Chatterjee, 2001) reveals that there are actually three mental representations or maps that are formed and refined by cross-modal processing between tactile–proprioceptive–kinesthetic and visual input:

- Personal space is from the skin inward.
- Peripersonal space is from the skin surface to the surrounding space within the reach of one's limbs.
- Extrapersonal space is out of reach but within visual range.

The existence of these maps explains the disorienting, closed-in feeling that a nearsighted person gets when removing eyeglasses or contact lenses because the extrapersonal space no longer agrees with the brain's map. It seems reasonable that children with poorly constructed maps will feel similar disorientation when their maps and reality fail to coincide perfectly.

Accurate modeling of the body is required for *praxis.* Praxis is the ability to conceive of, plan, and execute novel motor tasks. Infants and children with poor praxis are said to have dyspraxia, whereas adults who have lost this ability are diagnosed with apraxia. The difficulty in motor planning can occur in any of the three components. The child may lack the ability to think about new ways to use the body, may be unable to plan a sequence of movements, and/or may have difficulty performing the movements. Dyspraxic children are clumsy and require more environmental stability and practice to develop good motor skills. For breastfeeding infants with dyspraxia, keeping the environment as simple and similar as possible for each feeding will facilitate feeding.

Forward Modeling

When the motor system is activated, a neural signal called a *corollary discharge* is sent to sensory areas in the brain, forming a prediction of the sensations resulting from the action. This prediction is called a *forward model.* The refinement of movement is dependent on rapid comparison of the model with actuality in the cerebellum. The greater the difference between the predicted and actual sensation, the more the incoming sensations will be amplified (facilitated) so the conflict can be resolved. (For example, if you are walking down stairs, and a step is missing, you'd suddenly be very aware of your body and where it is in space.) If a movement produces self-touch, the forward model is likely to be quite accurate, and the tactile sensations are attenuated (muted). This explains both why we cannot tickle ourselves (Blakemore, Wolpert, & Frith, 2000) and why children with oral defensiveness can better tolerate mouthing an object voluntarily than having the same object introduced into their mouths. Letting the infant maintain control allows him or her to more accurately predict the sensations resulting from the action. Conversely, seeing a touch occur that is not felt actually increases tactile sensitivity. Subjects tricked with mirrors into seeing the opposite hand brushed reported feeling touch to both hands and experienced increased sensitivity to touch in the unbrushed hand for several minutes after the experiment (Ro, Wallace, & Hagedorn, 2004). This phenomenon may be responsible for the crawling sensation one feels after brushing away a seen but unfelt insect.

It is postulated that an *efference copy* of motor commands remains in the brain for each movement. An efference copy is a complete copy of the outgoing (efferent) signals from the brain to the muscles, analogous to how outgoing e-mail is copied to the sent folder. This system allows rapid changes in motor responses to be guided by the cerebellum if physical conditions change and disrupt the goal, since relying on the entire sensory feedback loop would result in delay (Shadmehr, Smith, & Krakauer, 2010). Efference copies may provide templates to guide future repetitions of the same movement and may help explain the automatic, subconscious nature of well-practiced movements. The efference copy may be sufficient to produce correct movements, even when feedback is disrupted (Lewis, Gaymard, & Tamargo, 1998).

Putting It All Together: Sensory Integration

Constant refinement of these processes occurs with practice. The first time one picks up a heavy object, the amount of force needed may be misjudged, leading to the object not moving or moving too quickly. The brain must then adjust the instructions to the muscles after taking in the feedback received from the senses to show that the action is not occurring as intended (when compared with the forward model). The circular process of SI—consisting of sensory intake and registration, modulation and association, adaptive motor behavior with forward modeling, and finally sensory feedback, which provides more input—becomes more rapid and more finely tuned over time.

The process of SI is important to maintaining a learning-ready state. Williamson and Anzalone (2001) explain how SI maintains the four As: arousal, attention, affect, and action (or adaptive behavior). *Arousal* is the balance of excitatory and inhibitory transmission in the brain. Too much arousal, and the child is jittery or jumpy and can't settle down to feed. Too much inhibition, and the baby may not even notice that a feeding opportunity exists. *Attention* requires sensory filtering; it needs to be focused on the sensations that are relevant or changing rather than on the static ones. A baby who is paying too much attention to clothing brushing the face may root toward the collar rather than toward the breast, whereas a baby with low attention will filter out the sensations of the breast and not respond to them. *Affect* is the emotional state related to mood. A relatively positive, stable affect is best for feeding. Too low an affect is often associated with passiveness and happy-to-starve behavior in infants, and too high an affect may lead to disorganization and make it more difficult for the baby to produce feeding-directed behavior.

Cross-modal processing, or the use of several senses together, is important in correcting and refining adaptive behavior. It also allows us to have a *gestalt* (sense of the totality or multisensory synthesis) of objects in the environment. For example, if you see an unopened can of a familiar soft drink, you know without touching it just how much it will weigh, how much you will have to open your hand to enclose it, how the aluminum will feel smooth and cool, how much grip strength you will need to hold the can without crushing or dropping it, how fast you can lift it to your lips without spilling it, how fast it will flow when you tip it toward you, and what it will smell and taste like. You can judge its temperature from the presence or absence of condensation on the can. You remember to expect the feeling of bubbles in your nose from the carbonation, so you are not startled into sneezing.

Studies of stroke patients with deficits in a single sensory system reveal that combining information from different senses can help restore the injured system. In patients with impaired tactile sense in the fingers, seeing the touch occur allowed them to actually feel it (Vaishnavi et al., 2001). In patients with visual field defects, an auditory cue spatially coordinated with the visual cue improved visual functioning (Frassinetti, Bolognini, Bottari, Bonora, & Ladavas, 2005). A baby who responds poorly to tactile cues may function better if he or she can see and smell the nipple.

Sensory Processing Disorder

Imagine that you have poor sensory processing and some of your maps are out of sync with one another, like anaglyphs (3-D pictures) viewed without colored glasses. If you were trying to pick up that soft drink can, the can might not be exactly where you see it to be, and you might knock it over rather than picking it up. You might grab it too hard and squeeze out some fluid onto your hand, or not grab hard enough and the can may slip right out of your grip. You might tip it too far, get a too-fast flow, and feel as if a fire hose is spraying into your mouth. Even a normal flow might feel that way as your brain and tongue take longer to communicate about what to do about the liquid in your mouth.

Other abilities would be affected as well. Moving around would be scary. Ladders and stairs might be terrifying because you would not be confident of locating the steps properly. (We've probably all experienced the jarring sensation of descending a staircase, mistakenly thinking there was another step and putting a foot down too hard.) This is how the environment seems to someone with a sensory processing disorder (SPD). Every behavior takes more effort because the first attempt is rarely correct. Information coming in is fuzzy and provides poor feedback for your efforts. Sensations are poorly modulated and might overwhelm you. If you were a breastfeeding baby, you might not notice that soft breast nipple in your mouth at all, or it might trigger your gag reflex. However, if your parents are sensitive to your state and needs and offer appropriate support for your efforts, your coping abilities increase. Let's look at some of the specific sensory tasks that breastfeeding entails and how to help infants and mothers who have SPDs.

The Role of Sensory Integration and Sensory Processing in Breastfeeding

Intact sensation and sensory processing are important for breastfeeding. The infant must be able to tolerate touch and movement through space to be positioned at the breast, and the infant must be able to respond to touch and smell cues from the breast to orient to the nipple, gape appropriately, and grasp a sufficient amount of breast tissue to transfer milk. The infant must modulate muscle tone appropriately and maintain sufficient arousal to facilitate the work of feeding. The infant needs to respond to the tactile and proprioceptive input of the soft breast in the mouth and use this information to cup and groove the tongue to form a teat and stabilize it in the mouth. Sequential activation of small bundles of the genioglossus and the transverse intrinsic tongue muscles are required for wavelike movements of the tongue. The posterior half of the tongue must depress to pull milk from the breast while the soft palate seals the mouth from behind, and the cheek and lip muscles must have sufficient tone to resist the intraoral negative pressure. Tactile and kinesthetic sensory registration and fine control of tongue, velar (soft palate), and pharyngeal muscles is necessary for coordination of swallowing and breathing.

The innate behavioral program (Chapter 2) helps to provide a template so that feeding behavior does not have to be learned from scratch, but modifications need to be made on the fly to compensate for fit and flow. Variables include infant mandible length and tongue mobility, maternal breast and nipple characteristics, and milk flow dynamics. The relatively low volumes and high viscosity of colostrum reduce the consequences of imperfect ability to coordinate swallowing and breathing in the inexperienced infant. Learning must occur quickly as milk volume increases rapidly over the first week postpartum.

Neuroscience research (Diedrichsen, Verstynen, Hon, Lehman, & Ivry, 2003) demonstrates that for muscle adjustments to be made properly to compensate for a changing load (the removal of a weight from the palm), the participant must perform a muscle action that leads to the load change. Just knowing the weight is going to be lifted is not enough to guide these *anticipatory adjustments.* For breastfeeding infants, this research suggests that the baby must be an active participant in feeding to produce the correct changes in muscle activity to anticipated changes in the feeding task. This is why pushing the infant's head into the breast does not facilitate latch. Being fed passively without sucking (tube feeding) or having a nipple placed in the mouth are not as good for learning fine control of feeding as active practice at sucking and swallowing and grasping the breast. Likewise, prodding does not help the baby become more skilled at feeding, and instead may make coordination of swallowing and breathing more difficult (Lefton-Greif, 1994).

Infants have poorer SI than older children by virtue of their immaturity, inexperience, more rapid cycling through states of arousal, and difficulty resisting the disorganizing effects of stress, hunger, and pain. Neurobehavioral organization is vital to the ability to handle all the incoming sensations and plan and execute the necessary motor responses (Als, 1991). Quiet alert and active alert are the most organized infant neurobehavioral states; crying and conservation withdrawal are the most disorganized. Infants are more likely to have feeding problems in less organized states. In some infants, organization can be improved through vestibular and tactile-proprioceptive input. Preterm, ill, or otherwise stressed infants may need to sleep to allow them to reorganize.

Skin-to-skin contact with mother is the most organizing input for most infants. Some infants respond to rhythmic rocking or swaying while held snuggled firmly against an adult's chest, gentle swinging from head to toe in a gathered-up blanket (**Figure 11-1**), or swaddling with the hands placed near the face (**Figure 11-2**). Some infants respond to repetitive sound, such as the traditional shushing sound, during these vestibular-tactile stimulation activities. Sucking is organizing for infants, and brief nonnutritive sucking on an adult finger (with appropriate infection control practices) or a pacifier or dummy may be used to help an infant achieve an organized state. The increased sensory input due to lowered thresholds during hunger can be disorganizing for infants, and giving a small

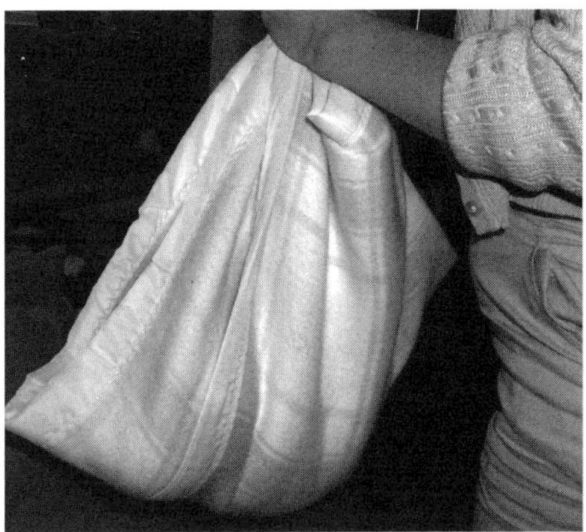

Figure 11-1 Swinging infant from head to toe in a blanket is organizing.

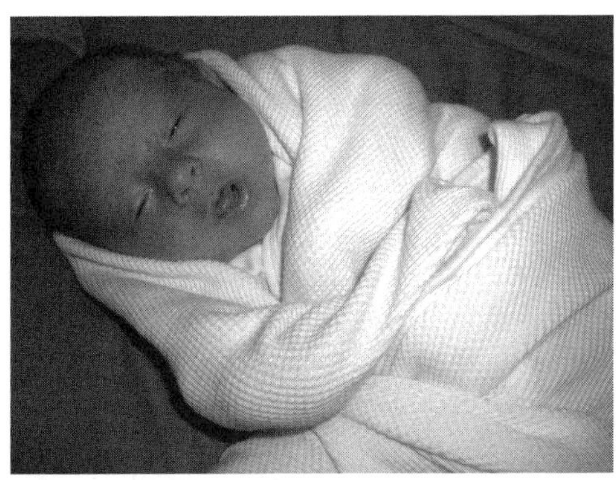

Figure 11-2 Swaddling in flexion—bringing the arms across the chest abducts the shoulders—stabilizes neck and jaw.

amount of milk in a way that is workable for the infant (spoon, cup, finger feeding, bottle) may allow the baby to settle and work at breastfeeding.

Infants give very clear signs of sensory stress (Als, 1991). Adults working with infants should be aware of these stop signs so that stimulation can be reduced to prevent the infant from becoming disorganized. Particularly in preterm or ill infants, stop signs may be subtle: an averted gaze, a single raised finger, or a sign of autonomic instability, such as increased respiratory rate, color changes, or yawning. In more vigorous infants, a grimace, finger splaying, or hands held up in a warding-off gesture are more easily observed (**Figure 11-3**). It is

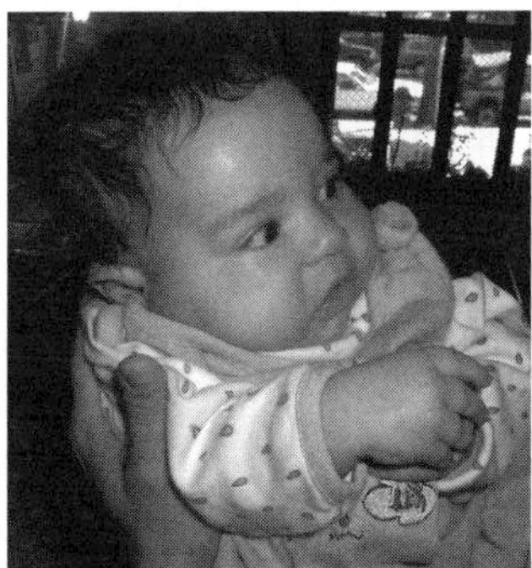

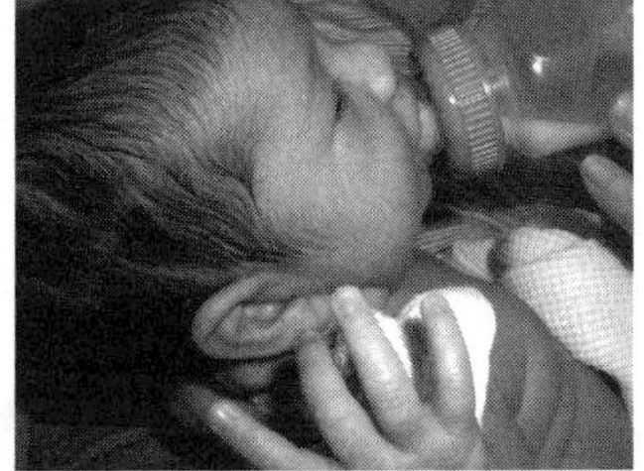

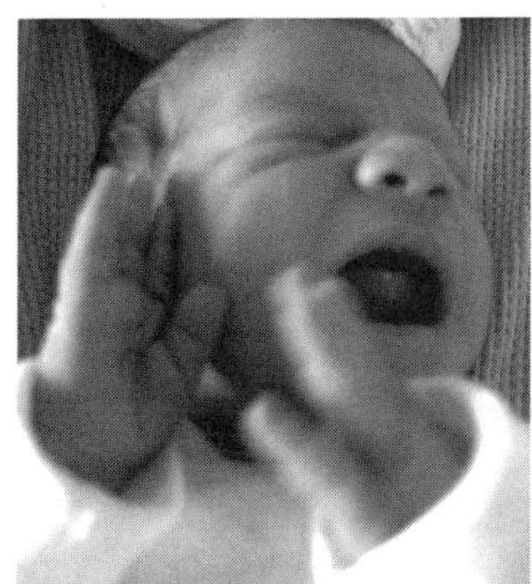

Figure 11-3 Some stress signals in infants are (from left to right) gaze aversion, splayed fingers, and warding off.

important to recognize that infants who are overstimulated can close down in an attempt to shut out additional input. A closed-down infant holds the eyes shut and is very still but may display tightened muscles and color changes that distinguish this overaroused state from sleep (see **Figure 11-4** in contrast with the sleeping baby in **Figure 11-5**). Alerting activities that are appropriate for sleepy babies just make a closed down infant more stressed. As a general rule, when a baby shows stress cues, stimulation should cease until the baby stops signaling, and a gentler, organizing stimulus should be applied. Environmental alterations, such as placing the baby skin to skin with mom and perhaps reducing light and noise, may be all that are needed to allow the baby to enter a more receptive state for feeding.

Mothers generally respond appropriately to infant stress cues without necessarily being conscious of them. Acknowledging these interactions when they occur can reinforce the mother's sensitivity to her infant and increase her confidence. If mother is not well integrated herself, her inability to correctly modulate her responses to her infant can cause feelings of rejection as the infant becomes overwhelmed and cries or closes down (Williamson & Anzalone, 2001). Teaching her how to recognize her own infant's cues and modulate her approach accordingly can improve both the infant's functioning and the maternal-child relationship.

Parents may interpret stress behaviors of their infants in different ways. *Reframing* the infant's behavior by voicing the infant's communication may help the parents to care for their child more appropriately. For example, saying in a high-pitched baby voice, "Mommy, I'm hungry, my hands don't have any milk in them!" when a baby is observed mouthing his hands can be a humorous way to draw parental attention to an important hunger cue. Interpreting frequent infant feeding requests or fussiness as manipulative or spoiled is counterproductive but rampant in Western culture. Brief education about breastfeeding

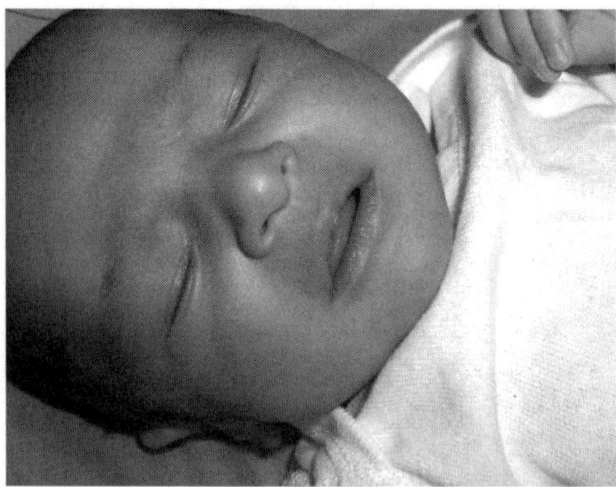

Figure 11-4 Closed down infant; note the muscle tension around the bridge of the nose and the tightly closed eyelids. Compare to **Figure 11-5**.

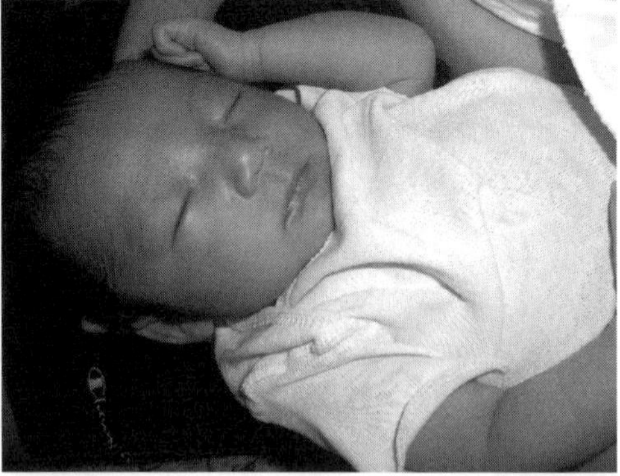

Figure 11-5 Sleeping infant; note the smooth forehead and relaxed hand.

physiology and the ability of maternal adaptation to help compensate for infant feeding deficiencies (Lau & Schanler, 1996) may be helpful, as may a review of infant feeding cues or behaviors (licking and mouthing movements, rooting, hand to mouth, squirming, throwing the body down from an adult's shoulder to the chest, or scanning and searching for a breast with the cheeks). Demonstrating ways to help infants reduce arousal levels such as rocking, colic hold (**Figure 11-6**), carrying in a baby sling, and so on can help parents to scaffold their infant's developing coping skills (**Figure 11-7**).

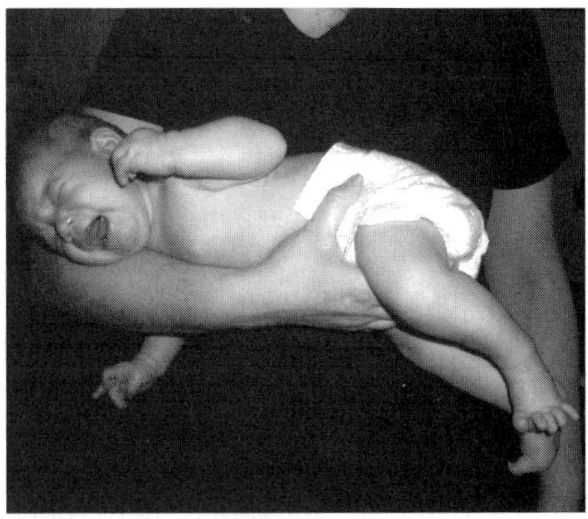

Figure 11-6 Colic hold.

Breastfeeding Infants with Sensory Processing Difficulties

SPDs currently are classified as either sensory modulation disorder, sensory discrimination disorder, or sensory-based motor disorder (Lane, Miller, & Hanft, 2000). Sensory modulation disorder has three subtypes:

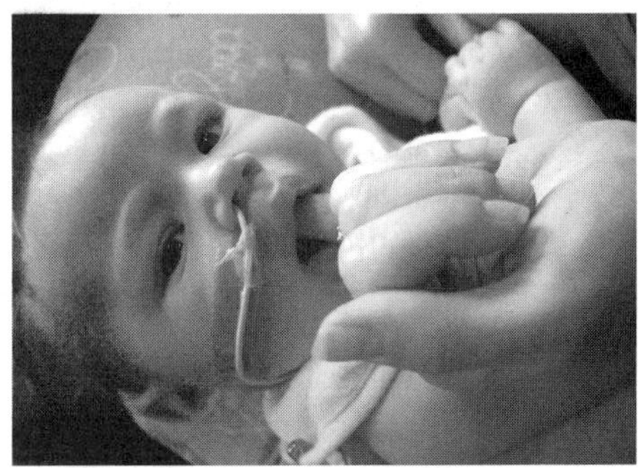

Figure 11-7 Firm pressure to the anterior palate helped this easily disorganized infant with feeding difficulties to reorganize and prepare for breastfeeding. The infant's mother discovered and reinforced this scaffolding technique.

- Sensory overresponsivity, in which ordinary sensations are overfacilitated and may feel painful and dangerous. Babies who overrespond may have difficulty choosing the important input during feeding attempts and may be distracted by their clothing, their hands, or other irrelevant stimuli.
- Sensory underresponsivity, in which the threshold is abnormally high.
- Sensory seeking, in which a child who registers sensation poorly seeks strong sensation in order to provide sufficient input to the nervous system.

In her sensory profile model, Dunn (1997) offers a fourth behavioral option:

- Sensory avoidance, in which an abnormally low threshold leads to avoidance of sensory input whenever possible.

In this way, children can either work in accordance with or to counteract their sensory thresholds. It is important for parents and caregivers to understand both the threshold and the behavioral results so they can support the child's needs. Children can either be passive in accepting sensory input according to their thresholds, or be active in striving for more normality. For example, an infant with a low threshold can either cry to avoid the environment or work to shut it out. It's important to realize that the child is actively avoiding sensation, not looking for more sensation. A sensitive caretaker may shut off extraneous lights or noise sources, or go into a quiet room to feed. A high-threshold infant might also seem to be shutting out sensation, but the infant needs the environment to be more stimulating to wake up. The infant might generate this sensation by making noises or, later, making movements such as rocking or head banging.

Sensory discrimination disorder is related to poor processing of sensation. A person with sensory discrimination disorder may be unable to identify an object by feel or may have difficulty localizing touch sensation on the body. An infant with this disorder may have difficulty responding to touch from the breast and nipple or may have swallowing difficulties due to poor ability to sense milk in the mouth.

Sensory-based motor disorder is caused by poor sensory processing. *Postural disorders* are an inability to hold the body properly against gravity due to poor integration of vestibular and proprioceptive information. *Dyspraxia,* another disorder in this category, is a sensory-based impairment of motor planning and is related to poor tactile processing.

It is rare for infants with SPDs to have difficulty with only one sensory modality. They will likely have difficulty with related sensory systems, such as the vestibular, proprioceptive, kinesthetic, and visual systems. The suspicion of an SPD is raised when the infant's responses to sensory stimuli are frequently and intensely unusual. These can include avoidance reactions, self-stimulatory behaviors such as head banging, difficulties with arousal, deficient control of autonomic functions including low or variable muscle tone, and irritability. Poor regulation is a common feature of SPDs (DeGangi & Laurie, 1991), making these infants difficult to parent. Increased fussing, but not crying, was associated with SPD diagnoses in childhood in a prospective study by DeSantis, Coster, Bigsby, and Lester (2004).

Early intervention services can improve the infant's ability to function and meet developmental tasks. Breastfeeding usually can't wait for referral, testing, and treatment to be completed, so lactation consultants need to know how to assist infants with SPDs.

Gravitational Insecurity

Gravity can be frightening for newborns when they are laid or held supine. Infants have antigravity reflexes that are active in feeding, but these work best in prone positions, when the baby is lying on a semireclined mother (Colson, Meek, & Hawdon, 2008). As discussed in Chapter 5, neonates derive their stability from positional support. Infants vary in their ability to tolerate reduced support and the stimulation of movement when being positioned at the breast. An infant with gravitational insecurity will flail, startle, and become disorganized when moved with the head dependent. Turning the infant on his side before lifting him off a surface increases neck control and allows him to stabilize his own head, even in newborns. Lifting from a side-lying position, firmly containing the baby with the head and shoulders aligned (Creger, 1995), preparing for movement with verbal cues, moving slowly, and allowing her to see where she is going are all helpful interventions for infants with gravitational insecurity. When the baby is in a breastfeeding position, he or she will be most secure and better able to attend to feeding if his or her body is actively snuggled against mom by gravity or her arms rather than passively resting on a pillow. Alternatively, the baby can be picked up while still asleep but displaying early feeding behaviors, placed skin to skin with mom, and allowed to self-attach to the breast.

Muscle Tone

Muscle tone is a reflection of the level of activation of muscles by the brain to provide the right amount of support for the body against gravity and provide a stable base for movement (Chapter 12). Decreased activation of muscles (hypotonia) can also be associated with decreased activation of affect, arousal, and attention.

Infants with hypotonia (low muscle tone) can benefit from *alerting* stimulation prior to feeding. Hypotonia and low alertness can be increased by stimulation that requires active postural adjustments by the baby (Lefton-Greif, 1994). Upright rocking while grasping the infant's shoulders, neck, and buttocks (Karl, 2004) or snuggling the infant and bouncing gently in an irregular rhythm both fulfill this requirement. Firm but gentle massage, if the infant tolerates touch, and applying vibration to low tone areas may also be helpful. Several vibrating teething toys are available; these are useful for increasing oral tone before feeding. Vibration can also be applied by rapidly wiggling a fingertip in place, or a battery-operated vibrator can be held in the palm and a finger used to massage the infant's tongue, cheeks, and lips. Any oral stimulation must be carefully applied and the infant's consent obtained. The infant consents by opening his mouth and engaging with active attention and wide, bright eyes; he withdraws consent by pursing his lips, turning his eyes or head away, or showing stress signs (**Figures 11-8 and 11-9**).

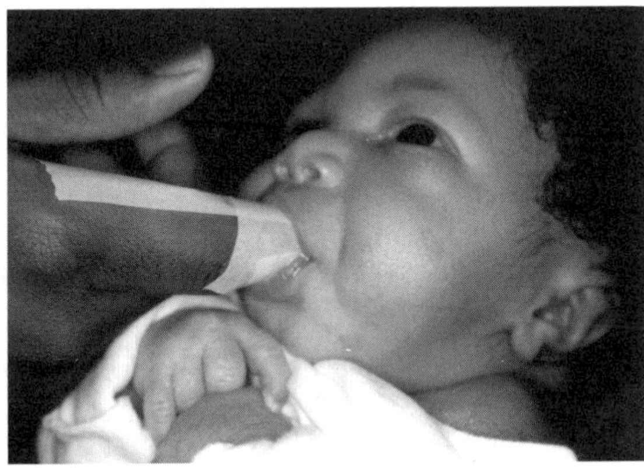

Figure 11-8 En face attention, hands in midline, show this infant is enjoying finger feeding.

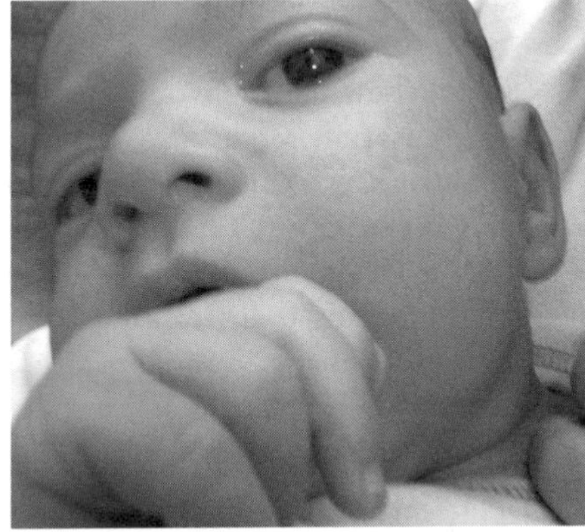

Figure 11-9 Babies are most organized if fed when feeding behaviors are first observed.

High tone (*hypertonia*) can be temporarily reduced by massage as well, or by rhythmic vestibular stimulation, including rocking and swinging from head to toe. A blanket can be used as a low-tech swing and can provide full body flexion at the same time. The infant is placed diagonally in a strong blanket, and the ends are gathered up in the adult's hand. The infant is swung from head to toe until her muscle tone is reduced and her body flexion increases. Gravitationally insecure infants may not tolerate swinging. As with any intervention, infant stress or distress cues should be respected.

It is important to distinguish hypertonia from both fixing and motoric stress and avoidance behaviors. *Fixing* is abnormal muscle contraction in compensation for low tone. The fixed muscle is tightened and held firmly in place to help provide artificial stability. Fixing interferes with normal range of motion. *Arching*, or extending the head, neck, and trunk backward, can be due to hypertonia if it is part of whole body extension and is the baby's habitual posture, but it can also be a communication that the baby is frustrated and wants to avoid the breastfeeding position, part of the infant's attempt to push away from the breast to visualize the nipple for latch (Colson et al., 2008; Genna & Barak, 2010), or it can be an attempt to elongate the esophagus in response to the pain of gastroesophageal reflux (Sandifer sign). A frustrated baby will usually become calm when lifted away from the nipple and placed with his face touching the upper breast. An infant with reflux will show other symptoms, including cud chewing or reswallowing refluxed milk, preference for low-volume feeds, fussiness, and often frequent vomiting or spitting.

Tactual Defensiveness

Infants with hyperregistration of tactile input may act as if touch is painful and dangerous. Indeed, a tactile-defensive child feels touch more acutely and attempts to avoid it. Pain processing to pinprick and prickly sensations are rated as more painful, and the pain lasts longer in children with sensory modulation disorders, showing that processing is affected and not just threshold (Bar-Shalita, Vatine, Seltzer, & Parush, 2009). Generally, firmer touch is more tolerable than light touch. Vision predominates over the tactile sense, so touching the infant only where your hands can be seen may allow the infant to modulate the sensation better. Also, self-touch is much more tolerable due to the ability to attenuate sensations when the forward model matches actual input well (Voss, Bays, Rothwell, & Wolpert, 2007). Placing a tactually defensive infant prone on mom's trunk so the baby can self-attach to the breast is sometimes more tolerable for him than all the stimulation of trying to actively latch him on. Soft, smooth-textured cotton clothing may help reduce distractibility and irritation, or the infant may be more comfortable skin to skin. A few tactually defensive infants have been willing to breastfeed only when placed at breast height on a nursing pillow and allowed to approach and self-attach. Some defensive infants prefer the containment of being swaddled below the waist with the hips in a flexed position for breastfeeding, and some enjoy the firm proprioceptive input of a baby sling.

Oral stimulation should be used cautiously in tactually defensive infants. Providing textured toys for the baby to voluntarily explore may be helpful. Infants with tactile processing issues generally tolerate sensation they apply to themselves much better than sensation that is imposed on them. It is best to place the toy near the baby's lips and invite her to mouth it. Slightly older infants can hold and help control the adult's finger in her mouth. Infant toothbrushes worn on an adult finger can be used this way. Discontinuous stimuli like tapping are often poorly tolerated because of their unpredictable nature, whereas touch that remains in contact with the infant's body (long or circular massage strokes) may be better accepted. Using a steady rhythm in the massage movements will also help with predictability.

Infants with poor tactile processing may also exhibit an elevated sensory threshold. These infants seem not to notice the breast or nipple and may fail to root well. If firm containment against mom and chin to breast positioning does not trigger rooting, or if the baby attempts to take the breast and pulls away after an abortive attempt to suck as if she has not even noticed the nipple is in her mouth, a nipple shield may amplify the tactile input from the breast. (High-threshold or tongue-tied infants may fail to root when the nipple is already in the mouth. Sliding the baby along the mom's body to bring the tongue tip further from the nipple may allow her to locate the breast with the tongue and grasp the breast properly.)

Thin silicone nipple shields with a teat of a sufficient diameter to fit the maternal nipple and some of the surrounding breast, but short enough to fit the entire teat and some of the flat portion of the shield in the infant's mouth, are best. The shield is shortened (folded back like a turtle's neck) and placed on the nipple, then the mother presses into the fold with two fingers from each hand and moves the fingers outward slightly so the breast pops into the shield as it everts (**Figure 11-10**). The shield should be presented the same way the bare breast would be, with the nipple to the baby's philtrum or at the least to the upper lip, to facilitate

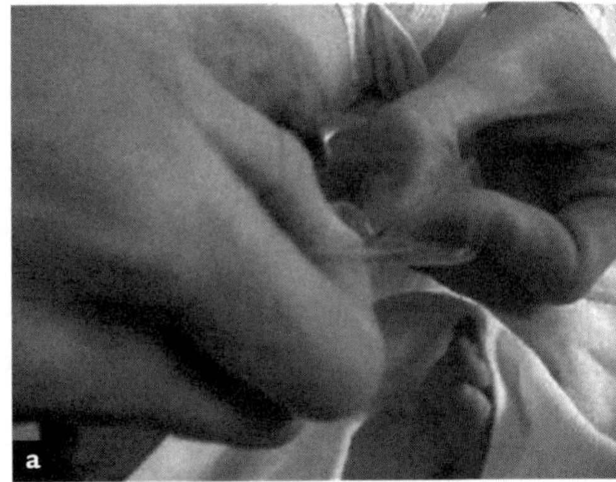

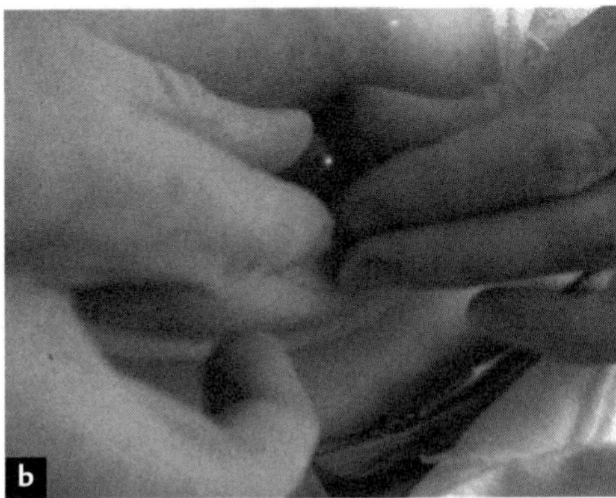

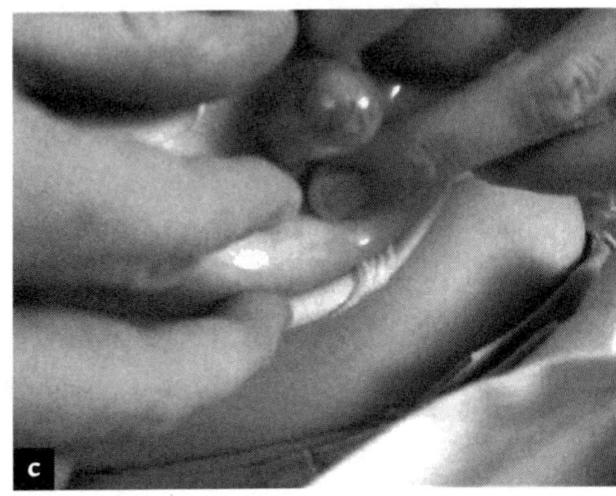

Figure 11-10 Inverting and applying a thin silicone nipple shield.

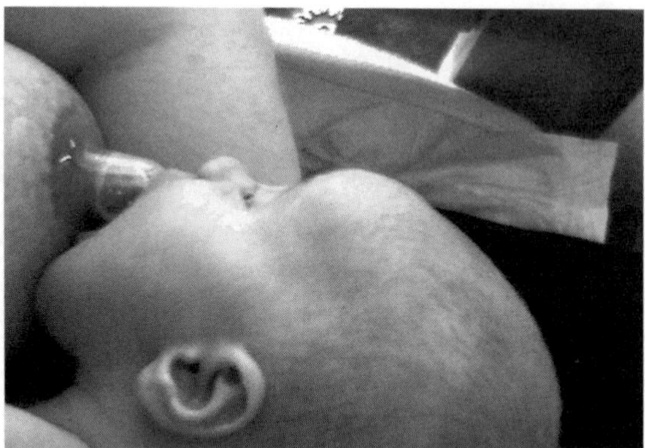

Figure 11-11 Align the infant as if she were latching to the bare breast, with chin on breast and philtrum as close to the tip of the nipple shield teat as possible.

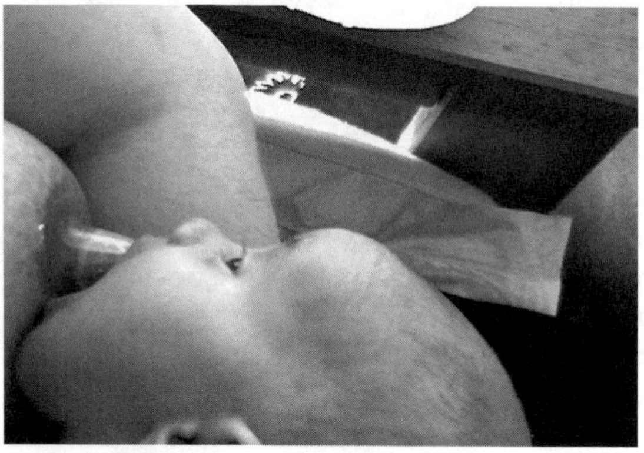

Figure 11-12 Infant grasps both nipple shield teat and some of the breast below it.

the transition to direct breastfeeding (**Figures 11-11 and 11-12**). It is important not to allow the infant to slide the lips down the shield teat when latching because this strategy used at the bare breast would push the maternal nipple out of the infant's mouth. When latching on chin to breast, the height of currently manufactured shield teats can be difficult for some infants to clear with their upper lips. Hopefully the development of a variety of teat heights will solve this dilemma. In the meantime, the greater tactile quality of the shield will often allow the infant to latch when it is presented to the lips, even if the chin is not able to contact the breast.

Massage Therapy

Massage therapy is a powerful tool for parents of infants and children with sensory, neurological, or medical challenges. Massage therapy improves neurobehavioral organization and growth in high-risk infants (Dieter, Field, Hernandez-Reif, Emory, & Redzepi, 2003; Feijo et al., 2006; Ferber et al., 2002; Field, 1998, 2002; Field, Diego, Hernandez-Reif, Deeds, & Figuereido, 2006). Moderate touch massage by mothers improved maternal infant attachment (Ferber et al., 2005) and improved growth in preterm infants (Field et al., 2006), whereas light pressure massage did not. Parents can learn appropriate infant massage techniques from occupational therapists, massage therapists, infant massage instructors, and books.

Maternal Sensory Processing

Mothers with poor sensory processing are likely to have difficulty with breastfeeding, as with any new skill. Like infants, adults perform better when they are in an optimal state of neurobehavioral organization than when they are disorganized. Organization is a challenge for individuals with sensory processing problems. A basic assessment of physical organization (which can reflect neurological organization) can be made when you first see a mother or her home. Meeting mom's emotional needs will help improve her organization by lowering unusually strong affect and arousal. She might need empathy about the difficulty of the transition to motherhood, she may need to talk about the birth, or she may need to assess your professional competence by asking some questions.

It is helpful if mom's best sensory modality can be identified and used. Sometimes it is obvious from the language she uses which is her dominant learning modality: "I see what you mean" (visual), "I hear you" (auditory), "That feels right" (kinesthetic). If the dominant modality is not obvious, a brief discussion about how she prefers to learn physical skills is in order. One dyspraxic mom said she felt like she was hopeless in aerobics class and needed things to be slowed down and repeated in order to not feel like she was three steps behind everyone else. This information allowed the consultation to focus on practicing one feeding position in which the mother could see the baby's face and repeating it in slow motion several times.

If the mother is a visual learner, a small mirror can be placed at her side to allow her to see the baby's approach to the breast, or the baby's body can be tipped so that the lower shoulder and hip are slightly closer to mom's chest than the upper ones, particularly if the nipple points downward at rest. Instant print or digital photos can be provided of the process of latch or the baby positioned at the breast for her to use to consolidate her new skill of providing proper support and alignment for the baby. Visual demonstrations with a doll or a stuffed animal are also helpful to a visual learner.

An auditory learner may prefer to be talked through procedures a step at a time, and a kinesthetic learner may appreciate the consultant's hands being placed over hers to guide her movements. For most mothers, a multisensory (cross-modal) approach will lead to the best learning, but when mothers get overwhelmed easily, choosing her one best modality and using it more intensively can reduce overstimulation.

Mothers can be tactually defensive as well. One mother needed to have a thin cloth between her arm and her infant's skin to tolerate feeding. A rules-based approach to breastfeeding management would dictate removing the cloth due to the importance of skin-to-skin contact, but this would have made breastfeeding unworkable for this mother. Creativity and flexibility are needed when assisting mothers with SPDs.

When working with a tactually defensive mother, it is important to avoid accidental touch. The fear of touch will increase physiologic arousal and activate the defense program. (Nils Bergman, MD, reports that defense and feeding are mutually exclusive; see Chapter 2.)

Staying just out of arm's reach from her, remaining within her visual field, and keeping your hands either in her sight or clasped behind your back may help reduce her level of arousal and defensiveness and allow her to attend to feeding her infant. Encouraging her to snuggle her baby closely not only will provide deeper, more tolerable touch, but it also will constrain the baby's movements somewhat and make them feel more predictable. Explaining the tactile cues that baby needs during a shortcut latch (arms hugging breast, chin to areola, nipple at philtrum, tongue on areola) and movements the baby uses when attaching (scan, gape, head extension, lunge, and grasp) will help her prepare for them.

Reiterating her baby's competence and discouraging her from fighting with him can also be helpful. For example, allowing him to suck his hands rather than trying to take them away, and bringing him closer to the breast when he realizes that hands don't make milk and releases them, can reduce everyone's frustration (Genna & Barak, 2010). Again, sight attenuates touch sensation by increasing the accuracy of modeling, so using a mirror for mom to visualize the baby's mouth with may help her better tolerate her baby's touch and latch.

Tactually defensive mothers may also have a heightened pain threshold. She might interpret sensations as painful that would be merely annoying to another mother. This does not mean that her pain is not real and can be dismissed. She needs help to make the feeding perfect so that she has no discomfort, and she needs to be believed about her degree of pain. Examine the breast and nipple to rule out painful inflammation or infection. If normal management techniques (positioning and latch) are not helpful or are already correct and mom still has discomfort, the infant should be examined for a subtle tongue-tie or dysfunctional sucking, and any problems should be addressed. Recent studies using ultrasound and pressure catheters have identified several invisible sources of pain during breastfeeding, including nipple base compression (Geddes et al., 2008) and high vacuum during sucking (McClellan et al., 2008).

Dyspraxic moms need simplicity and repetition. Realistic goals should be set for the consultation, such as making feeding comfortable and effective in one position. Minimizing environmental distractions is helpful for moms with any SPD, but it is particularly important for moms with dyspraxia. Try turning down lights and shutting off televisions and telephones. Modifying mom's technique to make it workable may be more tolerable for her than doing something completely different. Practice is vital for dyspraxic individuals. Sufficient practice changes breastfeeding from a novel, difficult task to an automatic one, at least in the current environment.

If breastfeeding tools are needed (nipple shields, supplementers, pillows), carefully assess their effect on the mother's organization and coping skills. Mothers with SPD may have more difficulty than neurotypical mothers with these added complications. Good instruction and practice can moderate the disorganizing effect of new tools, but sometimes not sufficiently to allow the mother to continue efforts to breastfeed. It is better to supplement in a less optimal way than to overwhelm the mother to the point that she weans. A little creativity will usually allow you to come up with an acceptable and effective plan B.

Parents with SPD may unwittingly disorganize their infants by their poor modulation of stimulation. Infants communicate by their behavior when their ability to maintain homeostasis (a smoothly functioning nervous system) is compromised by overstimulation. These include gaze aversion (looking away), yawning, increased motor activity, or autonomic changes such as color changes or changes in respiratory patterns. When the infant communicates impending overstimulation, the adults need to back off, reduce or eliminate stimulation, allow the baby to recover, then use more gentle stimulation that helps baby organize. It is vital to point out the baby's cues and reframe the infant's withdrawal as self-protection rather than rejection of mom. When parents or other caretakers have SPD, they will likely need active instruction on helping the baby stay organized. Demonstrating sensitive interactions is sufficient for neurotypical parents, but poorly organized parents need more help.

Occupational and physical therapists with SI training are vital team members when there are SPDs in the family. Early intervention programs will generally cover these services for infants with feeding problems and regulatory issues. The lactation consultant or feeding specialist should work with the infant's intervention team to advocate for goals that will facilitate normal feeding (i.e., breastfeeding).

Conclusion

Recent neuroscience research has illuminated the processes that human beings use to interact meaningfully with their environment. Consistent interactions help to hone SI over time. Newborns have less developed sensory processing due to inexperience, immaturity, and rapid cycling through neurobehavioral states, and some individuals have SPDs that disadvantage them further. Promoting neurobehavioral organization, using the sensory modality that functions best and enhancing predictability of stimulation, can improve the breastfeeding abilities of dyads affected by these issues.

References

Als, H. (1991). Neurobehavioral organization of the newborn: Opportunity for assessment and intervention. *NIDA Research Monograph, 114,* 106–116.

Ayres, A. J. (1979). *Sensory integration and the child.* Los Angeles, CA: Western Psychological Services.

Bar-Shalita, T., Vatine, J. J., Seltzer, Z., & Parush, S. (2009). Psychophysical correlates in children with sensory modulation disorder (SMD). *Physiology and Behavior, 98,* 631–639.

Berg, H. W., Pangborn, R. M., Roessler, E. B., & Webb, A. D. (1963). Influence of hunger on olfactory acuity. *Nature, 197,* 108.

Blakemore, S. J., Wolpert, D., & Frith, C. (2000). Why can't you tickle yourself? *Neuroreport, 11*(11), R11–R16.

Colson, S. D., Meek, J. H., & Hawdon, J. M. (2008). Optimal positions for the release of primitive neonatal reflexes stimulating breastfeeding. *Early Human Development, 84,* 441–449.

Creger, P. (Ed.). (1995). *Developmental interventions for preterm and high-risk infants.* San Antonio, TX: Therapy Skill Builders.

DeGangi, G. A., & Laurie R. S. (1991). Assessment of sensory, emotional, and attentional problems in regulatory disordered infants: Part 1. *Infants and Young Children, 3,* 1–8.

DeSantis, A., Coster, W., Bigsby, R., & Lester, B. (2004). Colic and fussing in infancy, and sensory processing at 3 to 8 years of age. *Infant Mental Health Journal, 25*(6), 522–539.

Diedrichsen, J., Verstynen, T., Hon, A., Lehman, S. L., & Ivry, R. B. (2003). Anticipatory adjustment in the unloading task: Is an efference copy necessary for learning? *Experimental Brain Research, 148,* 272–276.

Dieter, J. N., Field, T., Hernandez-Reif, M., Emory, E. K., & Redzepi, M. (2003). Stable preterm infants gain more weight and sleep less after five days of massage therapy. *Journal of Pediatric Psychology, 28,* 403–411.

Dunn, W. (1997). The impact of sensory processing abilities on the daily lives of young children and their families: A conceptual model. *Infants and Young Children, 9,* 23–35.

Feijo, L., Hernandez-Reif, M., Field, T., Burns, W., Valley-Gray, S., & Simco, E. (2006). Mothers' depressed mood and anxiety levels are reduced after massaging their preterm infants. *Infant Behavior and Development, 29*, 476–480.

Ferber, S. G., Feldman, R., Kohelet, D., Kuint, J., Dollberg, S., Arbel, E., & Weller, A. (2005). Massage therapy facilitates mother-infant interaction in premature infants. *Infant Behavior and Development, 28*, 74–81.

Ferber, S. G., Kuint, J., Weller, A., Feldman, R., Dollberg, S., Arbel, E., & Kohelet, D. (2002). Massage therapy by mothers and trained professionals enhances weight gain in preterm infants. *Early Human Development, 67*, 37–45.

Field, T. M. (1998). Massage therapy effects. *American Psychologist, 53*, 1270–1281.

Field, T. (2002). Massage therapy. *Medical Clinics of North America, 86*, 163–171.

Field, T., Diego, M. A., Hernandez-Reif, M., Deeds, O., & Figuereido, B. (2006). Moderate versus light pressure massage therapy leads to greater weight gain in preterm infants. *Infant Behavior and Development, 29*, 574–578.

Frassinetti, F., Bolognini, N., Bottari, D., Bonora, A., & Ladavas, E. (2005). Audiovisual integration in patients with visual deficit. *Journal of Cognitive Neuroscience, 17*(9), 1442–1452.

Geddes, D. T., Langton, D. B., Gollow, I., Jacobs, L. A., Hartmann, P. E., & Simmer, K. (2008). Frenulotomy for breastfeeding infants with ankyloglossia: Effect on milk removal and sucking mechanism as imaged by ultrasound. *Pediatrics, 122*, e188–e194.

Genna C. W., & Barak, D. (2010). Facilitating autonomous infant hand use during breastfeeding. *Clinical Lactation, 1*, 15–21.

Green, A. M., & Angelaki, D. E. (2003). Resolution of sensory ambiguities for gaze stabilization requires a second neural integrator. *The Journal of Neuroscience, 23*(28), 9265–9275.

Karl, D. J. (2004). Using principles of newborn behavioral state organization to facilitate. *The American Journal of Maternal Child Nursing, 29*(5), 292–298.

Lane, S. J., Miller, L. J., & Hanft, B. E. (2000). Towards a consensus in terminology in sensory integration theory and practice: Part 2: Sensory integration patterns of function and dysfunction [*Special interest section*]. *Sensory Integration, 23*(2), 1–3.

Lau, C., & Schanler, R. J. (1996). Oral motor function in the neonate. *Clinics in Perinatology, 23*(2), 161–178.

Lefton-Greif, M. A. (1994). Diagnosis and management of pediatric feeding and swallowing disorders: Role of the speech-language pathologist. In D. N. Tuchman & R. S. Walter (Eds.), *Disorders of feeding and swallowing in infants and children* (pp. 97–113). San Diego, CA: Singular Publishing Group.

Lewis, R. F., Gaymard, B. M., & Tamargo, R. J. (1998). Efference copy provides the eye position information required for visually guided reaching. *Journal of Neurophysiology, 80*, 1605–1608.

McClellan, H., Geddes, D., Kent, J., Garbin, C., Mitoulas, L., & Hartmann, P. (2008). Infants of mothers with persistent nipple pain exert strong sucking vacuums. *Acta Paediatrica, 97*, 1205–1209.

Ro, T., Wallace, R., & Hagedorn, J. (2004). Visual enhancing of tactile perception in the posterior parietal cortex. *Journal of Cognitive Neuroscience, 16*(1), 24–30.

Shadmehr, R., Smith, M. A., & Krakauer, J. W. (2010). Error correction, sensory prediction, and adaptation in motor control. *Annual Review of Neuroscience, 33*, 89–108.

Vaishnavi, S., Calhoun, J., & Chatterjee, A. (2001). Binding personal and peripersonal space: Evidence from tactile extinction. *Journal of Cognitive Neuroscience, 13*(2), 181–189.

Voss, M., Bays, P. M., Rothwell, J. C., & Wolpert, D. M. (2007). An improvement in perception of self-generated tactile stimuli following theta-burst stimulation of primary motor cortex. *Neuropsychologia, 45*, 2712–2717.

Williamson, G. G., & Anzalone, M. E. (2001). *Sensory integration and self regulation in infants and toddlers: Helping very young children interact with their environment.* Washington, DC: Zero to Three.

Additional Resources

Baranek, G. T., Foster, L. G., & Berkson, G. (1997). Tactile defensiveness and stereotyped behaviors. *American Journal of Occupational Therapy, 51*(2), 91–95.

Biel, L., & Peske, N. (2005). *Raising a sensory smart child: The definitive handbook for helping your child with sensory integration issues.* New York, NY: Penguin.

Blanche, E., Botticelli, T., & Hallway, M. (1995). *Combining neuro-developmental treatment and sensory-integration principles: An approach to pediatric therapy.* San Antonio, TX: Therapy Skill Builders.

Capra, N. F. (1995). Mechanisms of oral sensation. *Dysphagia, 10,* 235–247.

Dowling, D., Danner, S., & Coffey, P. (1997). *Breastfeeding the infant with special needs.* New York, NY: March of Dimes Birth Defects Foundation.

Fisher, A., Murray, E., & Bundy, A. (Eds.). (1991). *Sensory integration: Theory and practice.* Philadelphia, PA: F. A. Davis.

Gaebler, C. P., & Hanzlik, J. R. (1996). The effects of a prefeeding stimulation program on preterm infants. *American Journal of Occupational Therapy, 50*(3), 184–192.

Lundqvist-Persson, C. (2001). Correlation between level of self-regulation in the newborn infant and developmental status at two years of age. *Acta Paediatrica, 90*(3), 345–350.

Palmer, M. M. (1998). Weaning from gastronomy tube feeding: Commentary on oral aversion. *Pediatric Nursing, 23*(5), 475–478.

Palmer, M. M., & VandenBerg, K. A. (1998). A closer look at neonatal sucking. *Neonatal Network, 17*(2), 77–79.

Royeen, C. B. (1986). The development of a touch scale for measuring tactile defensiveness in children. *American Journal of Occupational Therapy, 40*(6), 414–419.

Stevenson, R. D., & Allaire, J. H. (1991). The development of normal feeding and swallowing. *Pediatric Clinics of North America, 38*(6), 1439–1453.

Weiss-Salinas, D., & Williams, N. (2001). Sensory defensiveness: A theory of its effect on breastfeeding. *Journal of Human Lactation, 17*(2), 145–151.

Wolf, L., & Glass, R. (1992). *Feeding and swallowing disorders in infancy: Assessment and management.* San Antonio, TX: Therapy Skill Builders.

Zeskind, P. S., Marshall, T. R., & Goff, D. M. (1992). Rhythmic organization of heart rate in breast-fed and bottle-fed newborn infants. *Early Development and Parenting, 1,* 79–87.

Zeskind, P. S., Marshall, T. R., & Goff, D. M. (1996). Cry threshold predicts regulatory disorder in newborn infants. *Journal of Pediatric Psychology, 21*(6), 803–819.

CHAPTER

12

Neurological Issues and Breastfeeding

Catherine Watson Genna, Judy LeVan Fram, and Lisa Sandora

The nervous system is the director for other body systems, with stacked layers of control systems that interact in complex ways to help infants meet their needs and maintain homeostasis. Brainstem centers contain central pattern generators for breathing and sucking, providing basic programs for these functions. Chemoreceptors for carbon dioxide regulate respiratory rate; water receptors in the airway provoke apnea to limit aspiration of fluids (Thach, 2001). Higher brain centers modify the basic programming based on input from these receptors, the cranial nerves (particularly the vagus), and the special senses, and they also exert control on autonomic functions through feedback loops. Abnormal development of the brain or injury as it develops can have significant consequences on the infant's ability to perform the many movements that need to be coordinated in feeding and swallowing.

Causes of Neurological Disability in Newborns

Brain Bleeds

Bleeding or insufficient blood flow in the brain is a common cause of temporary or permanent neurological disability in the fetus or infant. Preterm infants are more vulnerable to cell death from brain bleeds due to the following:

- Deficient control of cerebral blood flow under conditions of hypoxia or changes in peripheral blood pressure
- Underdevelopment of the vasculature between the main arteries of the brain
- Increased vulnerability of some cell populations (particularly oligodendrocyte precursors, which differentiate into myelin-producing cells) (Volpe, 2001)
- Underdeveloped antioxidant protection against free radical damage due to hemorrhage, ischemia, or infection

Full-term infants are less vulnerable to intracranial bleeds, but these can occur in cases of blood vessel malformations, mutations in clotting factor genes, cardiorespiratory disorders that cause extremes of blood pressure, and cytokine release in response to infection. Though they can also be caused by reduced oxygen transfer through the placenta before or during birth, it is now recognized that a wide variety of mechanisms can disrupt brain blood flow, including intense crying (Ludington-Hoe, Cong, & Hashemi, 2002). The narrow-term *hypoxic–ischemic brain injury* has therefore been replaced with *newborn or neonatal encephalopathy*.

Neonatal Encephalopathy

Newborn encephalopathy is defined as depression of the central nervous system as revealed by decreased level of consciousness and impaired control of breathing. Feeding difficulty requiring tube or intravenous feeding is the sign of cerebral depression most likely to correlate with later minor neurological dysfunction. The next most likely correlation is the presence of neonatal seizures and the need for mechanical ventilation (Moster, Lie, & Markestad, 2002). Apgar scores at 1 and 5 minutes after birth grade infant autonomic functions on a scale of 0–10, providing a simple way to differentiate infants who are making their postbirth physiological transitions well from those who require further observation or immediate intervention. Though Apgar scores have not been shown to have a linear relationship with neurological risk, low 5-minute Apgar scores (less than 5) were associated with increased risk of infant death and cerebral palsy (Moster, Lie, Irgens, Bjerkedal, & Markestad, 2001) in full-term, low-risk infants.

Developmental Structural Issues

Neuronal Proliferation Disorders

Brain structure is integrally connected with function. Errors in prenatal development can affect the brain either in isolation or in addition to other organs. An unusually large (macrocephaly) or small (microcephaly) head can be a marker for abnormal brain cell proliferation during gestation. Errors in differentiation and overproliferation are associated with a large brain (megalencephaly, or hemimegalencephaly if mainly one hemisphere is involved) that is poorly organized, with abnormal cells and masses of abnormally placed, disorganized gray matter (heterotopia). Motor, cognitive, and behavioral deficits are noted when the brain is improperly organized. Microencephaly can be caused by reduced brain cell proliferation due to infections during pregnancy, maternal alcohol use (Gohlke, Griffith, & Faustman, 2005), metabolic disorder, or other toxic exposures including drugs of abuse and radiation. Genetic causes can be familial or sporadic. Microencephalic infants usually have below-average intelligence, and many have motor difficulties and seizures.

Fetal Alcohol Spectrum Disorders

Alcohol exposure in utero is the most prevalent preventable cause of developmental disability. Fetal alcohol syndrome (FAS) is diagnosed by a cluster of typical facial features, growth restriction, and central nervous system abnormalities (Bertrand, Floyd, & Weber, 2005). In infants with FAS, the severity of the typical facial features (shortness of palpebral [eye] fissures, flatness of the philtrum, and thinness of the upper lip) correlates well with neurological deficits measured by brain imaging and psychometric testing (Astley & Clarren,

2001). However, alcohol-related neurodevelopmental disorder (ARND) can exist without tell-tale facial features. Even low levels of ethanol (drinking alcohol) exposure during pregnancy can affect neurobehavioral functioning of newborns, decreasing arousal and operant learning, which is important to feeding, and increasing habituation (Streissguth, Barr, & Martin, 1983). Infants with FAS suffer from growth retardation, are frequently hypotonic, have reduced fine and gross motor skills, and may have small upper jaws.

Neuronal Migration Disorders

Abnormal brain structure can occur with or without changes in brain size. The organized, layered, networked structure of the normal brain is due to carefully timed migration of new neurons during fetal development from the center of the brain outward along glial (support cell) pathways to form the layers of the cortex. A minority of neurons travel orthogonally (across the normal radial lines of migration) to become the interneurons that connect different brain structures. Some of these interneurons become GABA-ergic (using gamma-aminobutyric acid as their neurotransmitter) (Gressens, 2005). GABA is the chief inhibitory neurotransmitter, responsible for modulation of input and responses, and seems important in reducing seizure susceptibility.

Disorders of neuronal migration lead to a variety of structural brain disorders with functional consequences. If the disordered area is small, the disorder may not even be diagnosed until the infant's development begins to lag or seizures occur. If there is a more extensive area of involvement, the infant may have greater difficulty with the activities of everyday life, such as maintaining appropriate alertness, interacting with mother and the environment, and coordinating sucking, swallowing, and breathing.

Lissencephaly is a severe failure of neuronal migration that reduces gyrus formation, leading to a smooth brain surface. Because neurons do not reach their appropriate destination, the brain structure may be very abnormal. The severity can vary from agyria (lack of brain convolutions with immature brain structure) to variable degrees of pachygria (decreased gyrus formation with shallow sulci). Lissencephalic infants usually fail to thrive and have a high risk of pneumonia (Pavone, Rizzo, & Dobyns, 1993), generally from aspiration (Ashwal, 1999). Microcephaly and seizures develop during the first year of life, initial hypotonia may give way to spasticity, and mental retardation is moderate to profound. Infants with syndromic forms of lissencephaly have small mandibles (lower jaws), which can further impact feeding ability.

Subcortical band heterotopia is now considered part of the lissencephaly spectrum and consists of normal to reduced convolutions, with a thickened cortex and a band of white matter just below the cortex and above a layer of misplaced gray matter (Guerrini, 2005). Five genes that normally code for the cytoskeleton that neurons migrate on, including LIS1 and DCX, are responsible for the agyria-pachygyria-band spectrum (Kato & Dobyns, 2003); mild (missense) mutations cause less severe cases, whereas deletions or truncating mutations cause more severe lissencephaly with proportional cognitive and motor deficits. Infants with classical lissencephaly have indentations at the temples and small mandibles, and they may have a weak suck. Swallowing difficulties, aspiration, severe reflux, and feeding refusal may become apparent after a few months as hypotonia gives way to spasticity (abnormal muscle stiffness). Human milk is particularly important to these infants, who are at high risk of aspiration pneumonia.

Cortical Dysplasia

Cortical dysplasias are abnormalities of the layered structure of the cerebral cortex that are caused by disordered neuronal migration. The most common cortical dysplasia is polymicrogyria, or small, closely packed convolutions of the cerebral cortex that can occur in one of several brain areas. Some microgyria have no layering at all; in others, only four of the six cortical layers are present. Recent genetics research reveals that the defects in the genes coding for the microtubules or glial support cells that guide neuronal migration cause overmigration of cortical neurons, leading to the abnormal brain structure (Bahi-Buisson et al., 2010; Poirier et al., 2010). Bilateral perisylvian polymicrogyria is associated with pseudobulbar palsy, causing weakness or diplegia (bilateral paralysis) of the facial, tongue, masticatory (jaw closing), and palatal muscles, which obviously impacts feeding. Tongue movements, particularly protrusion (extension) and lateralization, were restricted; the orbicularis oris was often weak; and the gag reflex was absent in the majority of 31 children studied (Kuzniecky, Andermann, & Guerrini, 1993). Swallowing problems are prominent in this disorder (Kim, Palmini, Choi, Kim, & Lee, 1994), probably due to weakness and poor motor control of the tongue and pharyngeal muscles. Half the babies in a recent report on polymicrogyria caused by TUBA1a mutations had sucking problems during breastfeeding and hypotonia as presenting symptoms (Bahi-Buisson et al., 2008). Nevertheless, there is a wide range of severity of this disorder, and one author (Genna) is aware of several children with bilateral perisylvian polymicrogyria who were able to breastfeed.

Effect of Seizures and Anticonvulsants

Seizures (abnormal synchronization and proliferation of electrical impulses in the brain) are commonly associated with neurological dysfunction in newborn infants. Seizures can be generated by the brain's attempt to make working connections in the presence of abnormal neural migration or brain injury (symptomatic), or they can be the result of genetically based dysfunction of ion channels involved in the firing of neurons (idiopathic). Seizures can be difficult to identify in young infants because the well-defined patterns that occur in older children are not usually seen. Any recurrent, stereotyped motor or sensory event that cannot be interrupted by stimulating or distracting the child may be the result of seizure activity. Infants who have been diagnosed with seizures may have special feeding concerns.

Seizures can affect the infant's arousal level, making them functionally unavailable for feeding. Some seizures produce a *postictal* (after the seizure) reduced level of consciousness. Auras, or partial seizures that presage a wider spread of abnormal electrical activity in the brain, may be disconcerting or disorienting to the child, reducing the ability to attend to hunger or work at attaching to the breast. Even seizures that remain localized without changes in consciousness (simple partial seizures) can reduce a child's motivation to eat.

Seizures can cause perception of a bad taste or smell (parietal lobe), strong unprovoked fear (limbic system), paroxysmal stomach pain, nausea, or the feeling of rising stomach contents (temporal lobe). It is unknown if infants experience these sensory seizures, but careful observation of the infant for behavioral signs of distress may help identify optimal states for feeding.

Anticonvulsant side effects can cause significant feeding issues. Phenobarbital is often the first-line medication for newborns because it can be rapidly titrated, but it is very sedating and may contribute to developmental delay. Benzodiazepines are useful for stopping prolonged seizures, but they are also sedating and may accumulate in newborns due to reduced breakdown by immature liver enzyme systems (Mandelli, Tognoni, & Garattini, 1978). Anticonvulsants can also greatly increase (valproate) or decrease (topiramate or zonisamide) appetite. Adrenocorticotropic hormone (ACTH) is used for infantile spasms and can cause irritability. Close monitoring of the infant and the presentation of frequent feeding opportunities when the baby seems comfortable and alert can help overcome some of these issues.

The ketogenic diet is a high-fat, low-carbohydrate diet that helps a significant portion of children with medication-resistant seizures. Until recently, breastfed infants were weaned before starting the diet, but a recent case series reported successful seizure reduction with partial breastfeeding in addition to ketogenic formula (Cole, Pfeifer, & Thiele, 2010; Poirier et al., 2010).

Hydrocephaly

The brain is cushioned by cerebrospinal fluid (CSF) that circulates through and around the brain and spinal cord. If there is a blockage in the circulatory path for CSF, it can build up in the ventricles, or if there is oversecretion or reduced absorption, CSF can build up throughout the head. In young infants, the increased pressure in the head causes the fontanelles to bulge and/or causes the sutures to separate. Frequent vomiting, irritability, and unusual eye movements are early effects of the increased intracranial pressure (**Figure 12-1**). The infant's primary physician should be alerted to vomiting that interferes with growth or is associated with infant distress so the cause can be sought and treated. Feeding ability deteriorates rapidly as CSF pressure builds. When the pressure is relieved by surgical installation of a shunt to drain excess CSF into the peritoneum, feeding abilities generally recover. Shunts have a high failure rate in infants younger than 1 year of age and those born preterm (McGirt et al., 2002) and require revision if symptoms recur.

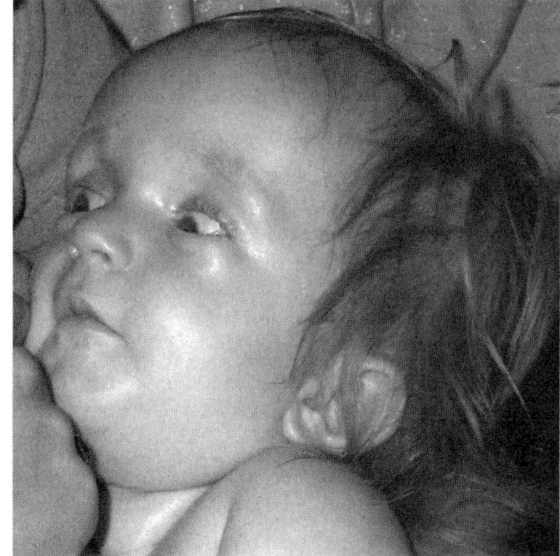

Figure 12-1 Rapid head growth with rotation of eyes downward (sunset sign) increases suspicion of hydrocephalus.

Autistic Spectrum Disorders

Children with autism or pervasive developmental disorder have deficits in reciprocal social interactions, nonverbal and verbal communication, and behavioral flexibility. Various theories exist about the reasons for these deficits, including an extreme manifestation of sensory processing disorder, generally disordered information processing, increased testosterone exposure in utero (Knickmeyer & Baron-Cohen, 2006), and a defect in mirror neuron function that reduces the ability to empathize and imitate behaviors and cognitive-emotional states (Dapretto et al., 2006). Children with autism seem to extract less information from complex stimuli, and it is possible that differences in memory function prevent autistic children from extracting information from the environment to guide adaptive behavior (Williams, Goldstein, & Minshew, 2006). Genetic research has identified a number of genes associated with small numbers of autism cases, and many scientists are beginning to believe that there are a number of genetic defects that cause slightly different autistic symptomatology (Cusco et al., 2009). Looking at the genetics of a single symptom is one way to tease out some of these genes. Chapman and colleagues (2011) focused on increased scores on performance versus verbal IQ and found a small region on chromosome 10 that has been implicated in autism through other means.

There is evidence for genetic differences in the innate immune system (Grigorenko et al., 2008), with autistic children having twice the blood levels of macrophage migration inhibitory factor as their unaffected siblings. Exclusivity of breastfeeding in the first months of life may affect the development of the innate immune system through activation of toll-like receptors in the intestine (LeBouder et al., 2006). A case-control study of autistic and neurotypical children showed a more than threefold risk of weaning in the first week of life for the autistic children (Tanoue & Oda, 1989). The study's authors discuss whether this difference is due to a potentially protective effect of breastfeeding or increased difficulty initiating breastfeeding on the part of autistic infants.

Breastfeeding is a prototypical reciprocal social interaction and depends on consistent infant cueing, maternal response (making the breast available), infant response to the breast by attaching and feeding, and releasing the breast when sated. Although autism is generally not diagnosed until preschool age, examination of home movies generally shows that the reduced facial expression and eye contact, lack of joint attention (looking at what caregivers look at, and later bringing their attention to items of interest), difficulty tolerating environmental change, and stereotypical play are present from early infancy. Infant-related questions on the Pervasive Developmental Disorders Screening Test-II include unpredictability in sleep patterns or short sleeping bouts, staring or tuning out, ignoring most toys in favor of a few favorites, disinterest in learning to talk, and enjoyment of chasing and tickling but not interactive lap games such as peek-a-boo and pat-a-cake (Siegel, 1996). Tuning out the unfamiliar often extends to people as well as to objects; the infant may respond to family members and may ignore others.

Symptoms that are most often seen in newborns include reduced facial expression and eye contact and an increased propensity to shut down and tune out. Newborns in the author's practice who were later diagnosed with autistic spectrum disorders were under-responsive to normal feeding stimuli and needed to be taught to feed in a step-by-step manner by stimulating individual steps in the feeding sequence with a finger and providing milk upon completion of the sequence, then generalizing the feeding movements to the breast. Sequential stimulation of feeding-related reflex movements is one method of doing this (see the oral exercises in the Oral Stimulation section later in this chapter).

Genetic Neurological Conditions

Genetic syndromes can cause neurological dysfunction by interfering with brain structure or function. *Down syndrome* (trisomy 21) is the most common of these, causing variable degrees of cognitive disability, hypotonia (low muscle tone, **Figure 12-2**), a small mandible, and reduced energy and alertness (**Figure 12-3**). The frequent presence of cardiac malformations in infants with Down syndrome further impacts their feeding ability. Feeding problems may include difficulty with attachment due to the relatively large tongue for the small jaw, decreased stability and increased work expended during feeding due to the low muscle tone, and impaired coordination of sucking movements (**Figure 12-4**). Allowing the infant to learn to breastfeed immediately after birth, if stable, seems to be important. Stabilizing the head and neck is particularly important in infants with Down syndrome because there might be malformation or laxity of the ligaments of the first two cervical vertebrae (atlantoaxial instability) that can put pressure on the brainstem or spinal cord with head flexion or excessive extension. Laid-back (biological

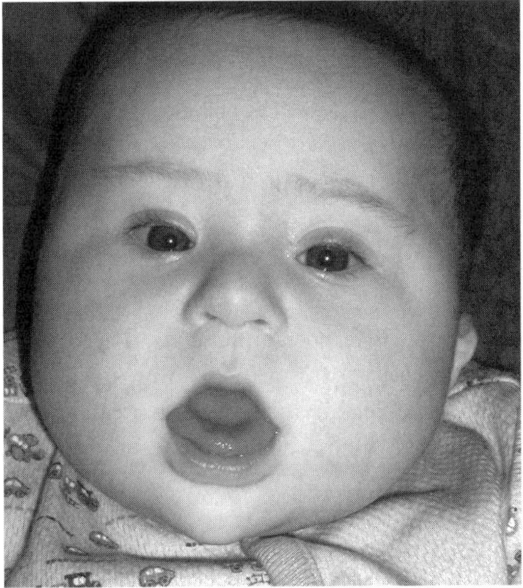

Figure 12-2 Well-nourished breastfed infant with Down syndrome. Note the effects of hypotonia—mouth hangs open, mild tongue protrusion, and reduced facial creases.

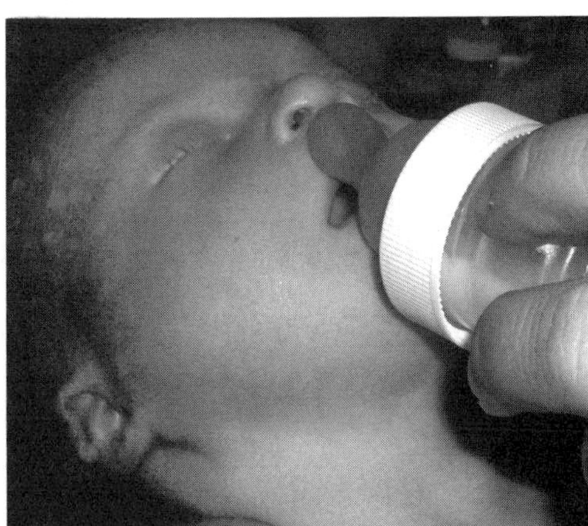

Figure 12-3 Presenting a bottle across the lips helps preserve normal gape response. Note the low alertness and energy in this young infant with Down syndrome.

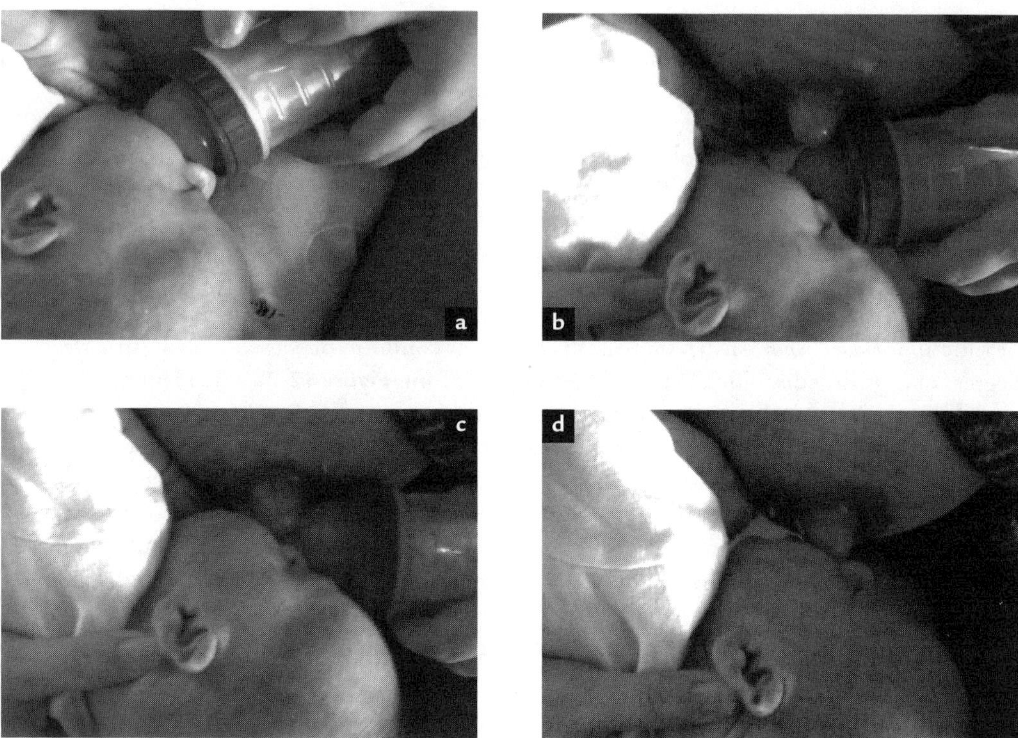

Figure 12-4 Bait and switch technique to move from bottle to breast with nipple shield. Infant is fed from a wide-based bottle near breast, and is moved into alignment for good attachment as the bottle is removed. Baby latches onto breast and continues sucking. Use of the nipple shield can be continued if it helps the infant maintain attachment and transfer milk, or it can be eliminated once breastfeeding becomes familiar.

nurturing) positions can provide support from gravity that helps infants with hypotonia and small mandibles to feed more effectively.

For some genes, a parent of origin effect exists due to differential inactivation according to parental sex. *Prader-Willi syndrome (PWS),* which causes hypotonia and feeding difficulties in the first years of life (**Figure 12-5**), can be caused by deletion (loss) of the paternal chromosome 15 long arm bands 11-13 (abbreviated 15q11-13−), maternal uniparental disomy (two of chromosome 15 from mom, none from dad), or errors of inactivation in the paternal chromosome 15. Errors of imprinting, where one parent's DNA is not properly inactivated, causing an effective double dose of the gene's protein product, are becoming more common due to assisted reproductive technologies (Niemitz & Feinberg, 2004). Feeding difficulties in this syndrome stem from incoordination of oral motor movements, significant hypotonia, and impaired hypothalamic control of satiety (**Figures 12-6 through 12-9**). There is a high incidence of laryngomalacia/tracheomalacia in infants with PWS, which

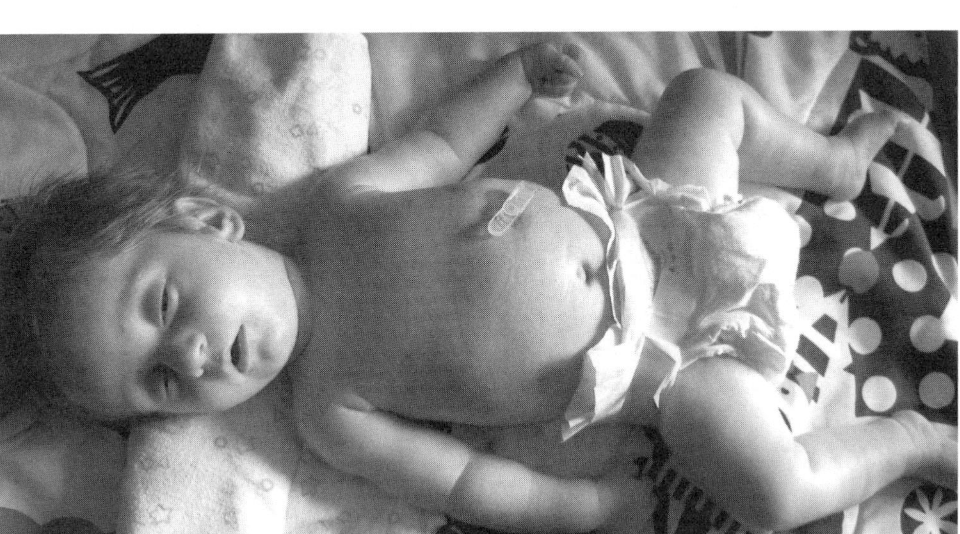

Figure 12-5 Infant with Prader-Willi syndrome. Note the low muscle tone, small mandible, downturned mouth, and gastrostomy "button." The use of a g-tube allows infants with significant feeding difficulties to get expressed human milk through the tube, allowing unpressured development of oral feeding at breast.

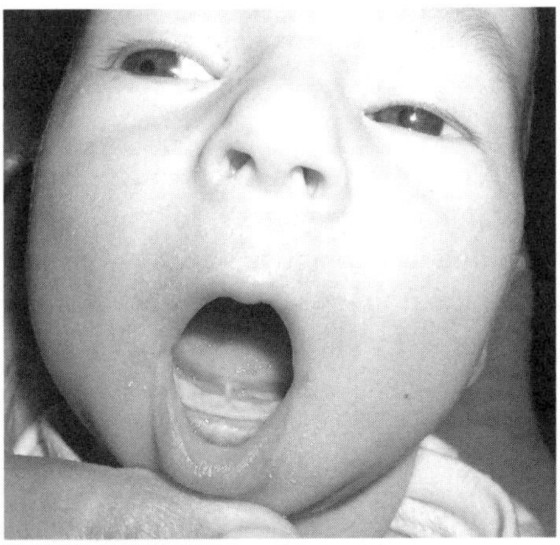

Figure 12-6 This infant with Prader-Willi syndrome has ankyloglossia (tongue-tie) as well as hypotonia, making oral feeding even more problematic.

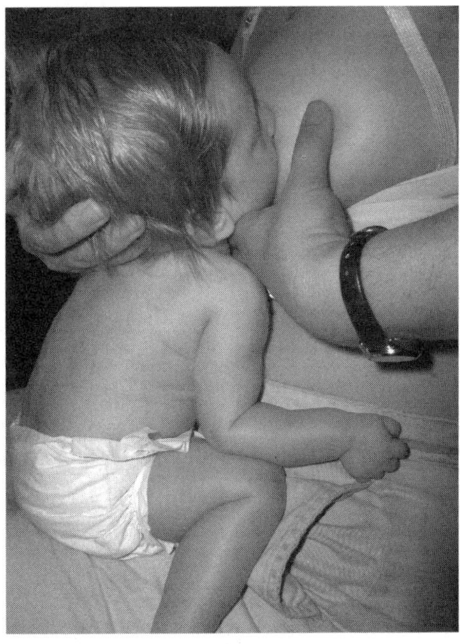

Figure 12-7 Straddle position with jaw support and mild head extension.

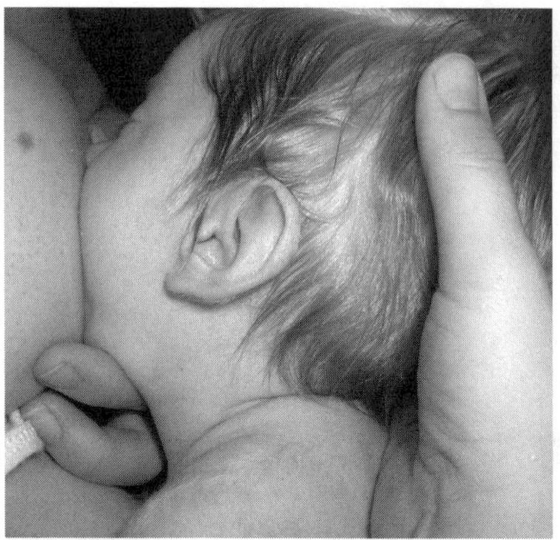

Figure 12-8 Close-up view of jaw support.

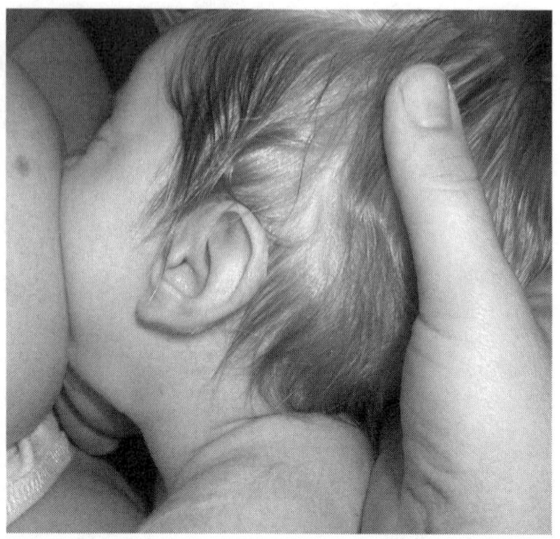

Figure 12-9 Sublingual support and massage can be substituted for jaw support. Light pressure or circular massage is concentrated on the underside of the chin, rather than on the jaw bone, supporting tongue movements during sucking.

can further impact feeding. Children with PWS require fewer calories for their weight and age and are at extreme risk of obesity. Exclusive human milk feeding and growth hormone supplementation may be helpful in achieving a healthy weight. Nutritionists may need education about normal intakes of breastfed infants to avoid overfeeding, especially when the infant is fed via gastrostomy tube (Holm & Pipes, 1976).

The loss of small bits of DNA from the chromosomes (deletions) can cause significant issues. *Williams syndrome* (7q11.23–) causes infants to have feeding difficulties and reduced growth, with cognitive strengths (memory and music) and weaknesses (visual-spatial processing and fine motor delays). Growth retardation is usually greater when the maternal chromosome 7 has the deletion because the paternal area involved seems to be imprinted. Infants and children with Williams syndrome are reluctant to eat and may feed better if music is played during their feedings.

Phelan-McDermid syndrome (22q13–) causes hypotonia, developmental disability, reduced sleep requirement, and extremely delayed or absent speech (**Figure 12-10**). The same neurological dysfunction that leads to speech difficulty contributes to feeding difficulties in newborns with this syndrome. Swallowing may be particularly problematic for infants with Phelan-McDermid syndrome, and they should be allowed to self-pace their feedings.

Cri du chat (cat-cry) syndrome (5p–) causes a malformed larynx and epiglottis that cause a characteristic cry, reduced birth weight with a round face and small head (microcephaly), small jaw (micrognathia), hypotonia, and severe developmental delay. Speech is generally more delayed than receptive language (understanding). Breastfeeding is possible, and therapy should be initiated early if there are sucking or swallowing problems (Cerruti Mainardi, 2006). Distractibility (Clarke & Boer, 1998) may add to the challenge of feeding these infants. Feeding with head extension in prone positions that supply good support can help ease the respiratory symptoms while allowing the infant better jaw contact with the breast. Short, frequent feedings may help these infant consume sufficient calories before their respiratory reserve is depleted.

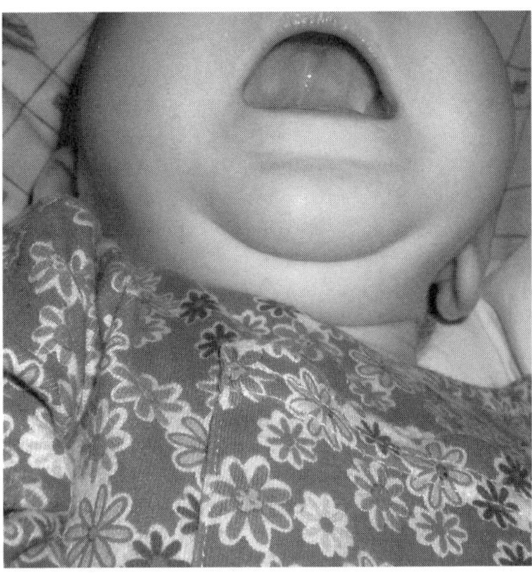

Figure 12-10 Low-set prominent ears and an unusual palate in an infant with Phelan-McDermid syndrome. This infant's habitual posture was with one arm held across the body's midline. Growth had been slow in the early months (approximately 1 pound per month), and hypotonia was diagnosed at birth. Weight loss at 4–5 months of age was initially attributed to breastfeeding. The physician was receptive to the lactation consultant's suggestion that the problem was global, and the child was rapidly diagnosed and provided with a gastrostomy tube and appropriate therapy.

Kabuki syndrome (genetic cause unknown) causes eyes that resemble those of traditional Japanese Kabuki actors, with long palpebral fissures and a lower lid that is everted at the lateral corner (**Figure 12-11**). A high arched palate and poor oral motor function, hypotonia and poor growth during infancy, and persistence of fetal finger pads may be seen in infants with this syndrome. Joint hypermobility is evident in infancy. Tactile defensiveness and dyspraxia may occur, and defects are common in multiple organ systems (Adam & Hudgins, 2005). The use of firm touch during positioning for breastfeeding may help these infants tolerate touch better, and keeping the feeding position as similar as possible from feeding to feeding may help compensate for the reduced motor planning (Chapter 11). Holding the baby very close during feeding may help to increase stability and maintain latch. Side-lying or upright positioning may be helpful if there are swallowing difficulties, and breast compression can improve the baby's milk transfer. Preparatory oral stimulation immediately before feeding can improve muscle tone and oral motor endurance. Gastrostomy tube feeding may be required while the baby learns to breastfeed, which can take several months.

The feeding difficulties in many of these syndromes result from low muscle tone and difficulty coordinating the movements of feeding, swallowing, and breathing. Low muscle tone makes every feeding movement weaker and more effortful, reducing the amount of milk transferred and increasing fatigue. Less coordinated and skillful tongue movements, weaker jaw opening and closing, less ability to maintain and increase negative pressure in the mouth with the tongue and to resist it with the cheeks and lips, and poorer ability to

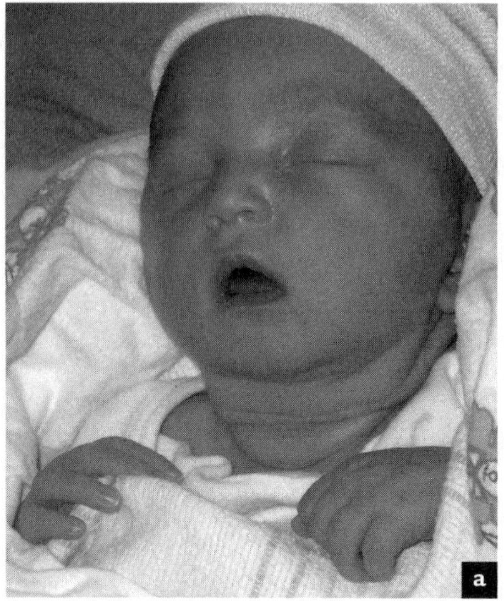

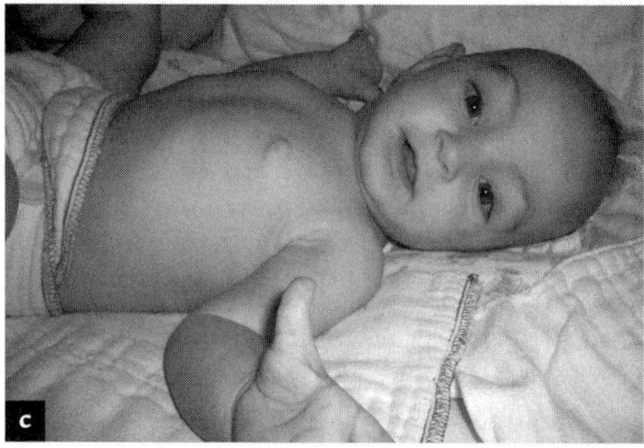

Figure 12-11 Exclusively breastfed infant with Kabuki syndrome. Note the signs of hypotonia (mouth hanging open, soft facial creases), joint hypermobility (hitchhiker thumb), long lateral palpebral fissures (eye slits), and arched, sparse eyebrows.

swallow safely are commonly seen. Nevertheless, the authors have worked with infants with these diagnoses who breastfed exclusively or partially. Each infant's feeding skills should be assessed and feeding should be supported by modifying techniques and expectations while providing facilitative techniques for improving muscle tone and developing missing skills. A team approach is ideal, with a lactation consultant and a feeding therapist working together.

It is generally helpful to research syndromic conditions to have an idea how the infant may be impacted. The Online Mendelian Inheritance in Man database (http://www.ncbi.nlm.nih.gov/omim) is a compendium of human genes and genetic disorders that includes clinical synopses. Many disorders have support organizations whose websites contain accurate but less technical information that may be useful in planning a strategy for helping affected infants to feed. General textbooks on newborn diseases or pediatric neurology can provide useful background information and are often available in libraries or on the Internet. Lactation consultants and therapists should carefully examine materials and websites before referring parents to them for feeding information because some are unduly dismissive of breastfeeding and others contain outdated or commercially slanted information. It can also be valuable to network with colleagues through local or international professional associations and online networking lists, such as Lactnet (http://community.lsoft.com/archives/LACTNET.html), to communicate with peers who have had direct experience with these uncommon disorders.

It is important to note that there is marked variability of severity even within the same diagnosis. Such is the nature of a syndrome. Each infant should be assessed as an individual and not have breastfeeding arbitrarily ruled out due to the diagnosis. Breastfeeding seems to improve the neurological maturation of infants over time. General movement quality, a sensitive indicator of neurological condition, is significantly improved over their own baseline measurements in infants who are exclusively breastfed for at least 6 weeks (Bouwstra et al., 2003). Breastfeeding promotes normal development of tongue movements and optimally shapes the oral cavity (Palmer, 1998), provides immune cross talk between mother and infant from saliva entering the nipple, and is a normalizing experience for both mother and child. Infants with severe feeding difficulties who receive their nutrition by tube can practice oral feeding at the breast. If aspiration is a significant risk, the breast can be expressed before the feeding to minimize milk flow (Narayanan, Mehta, Choudhury, & Jain, 1991), though there is less risk of aspiration during breastfeeding and less risk of aspirating human milk. Moreover, safer swallowing occurs during bottle feeding with human milk than with formula or water (Mizuno, Ueda, Kani, & Kawamura, 2002). Reclined maternal positions with the infant prone also improve coordination of swallowing and breathing.

Special growth charts are available for several syndromic conditions, including Down syndrome and cri du chat syndrome. The use of these special charts allows the infant to be compared with peers and avoids parental anxiety and excessive supplementation. Infants with very significant feeding problems may benefit from the placement of a gastrostomy tube, allowing human milk to be delivered into the stomach while the infant practices oral feeding at the breast. If a feeding tube is used, the infant should be offered the breast immediately before, during, or just after the tube feeding to reinforce the relationship between suckling and satiety.

Rare syndromes may not be diagnosed until the infant fails to thrive. Careful monitoring of early growth with early referral to a lactation consultant can help protect maternal milk production. It may be difficult to differentiate between the effects of suboptimal weight gain on the infant's energy and feeding skills and the effects of a neurological condition. Infants who are underfed due to structural, management, or maternal issues are likely to conserve energy by suppressing movement and sleeping more. Their muscle tone may seem low at first, but when the feeding problem is addressed and they begin to gain weight, energy and activity improve markedly. In contrast, children with neurological disorders do not perk up the same way. Signs of neurological deficit include rapid fatigue without changes in respiratory pattern or other signs of cardiorespiratory stress; floppiness, especially when combined with unusual positioning of the head, arms, or legs; or poor quality of movements. *Dysphagia* (difficulty swallowing) is much more common in infants with neurological conditions and may lead to feeding refusal. Some infants with genetic conditions just look unusual, with subtly *dysmorphic* (unusually shaped) facial features. Areas that are particularly sensitive to genetic influences include:

- The philtrum, or ridge between the nose and the mouth
- The spacing between the eyes, or *hypertelorism* (unusually widely spaced eyes, which can be associated with a submucous cleft palate or genetic conditions) (**Figure 12-12**)
- The length of the eye slit (short or long *palpebral fissures*)
- The shape of the skull: *dolichocephaly* or *scaphocephaly* (disproportionately long, narrow skull) or *brachycephaly* (unusually flat skull)
- The nose (depressed nasal bridge is a common feature of genetic disorders)
- The palate (generally high arched and abnormally shaped)
- The mandible, which may be short due to intrauterine positioning, normal inheritance, or genetic disorder
- The ears, which are generally low set and unusually shaped and are sometimes pitted (*ear pits*) or have extra fleshy protuberances (*preauricular tags*) near the tragus (ear flap) (**Figures 12-13 and 12-14**)

Lactation consultants can help determine whether a breastfeeding problem exists, or if there is suspicion of a more global infant feeding problem, and communicate these findings to the infant's healthcare provider so the infant can be carefully examined. Infants with hypotonia of unknown origin are generally examined by a neurologist and a geneticist. Infants whose feeding skills seem intact but who are failing to gain weight are generally first seen by a gastroenterologist to rule out malabsorption syndromes.

Neuromuscular Junction Issues

Myasthenia gravis (MG) is an autoimmune process in which antibodies attack the acetylcholine (ACh) receptor, causing skeletal muscle weakness and fatigue, especially with repeated activity. These immunoglobulin G (IgG) antibodies transfer through the placenta (Shehata & Okosun, 2004), though only a minority of infants are symptomatic (Tellez-Zenteno, Hernandez-Ronquillo, Salinas, Estanol, & da Silva, 2004). In one large Italian study of mothers with MG, all breastfed their unaffected infants (Batocchi et al., 1999). Although maternal immunosuppressant medications may transfer through milk, several studies have demonstrated no adverse effects of maternal ingestion of cyclosporine on their breastfed infants (Moretti et al., 2003;

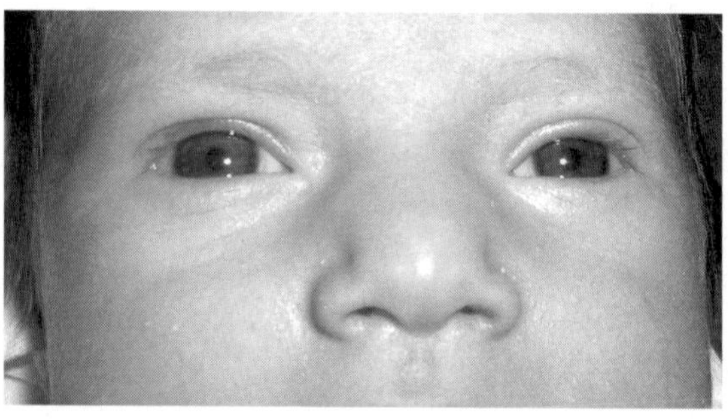

Figure 12-12 Hypertelorism (widely spaced eyes) and paranasal bulging increase suspicion of palate abnormalities.

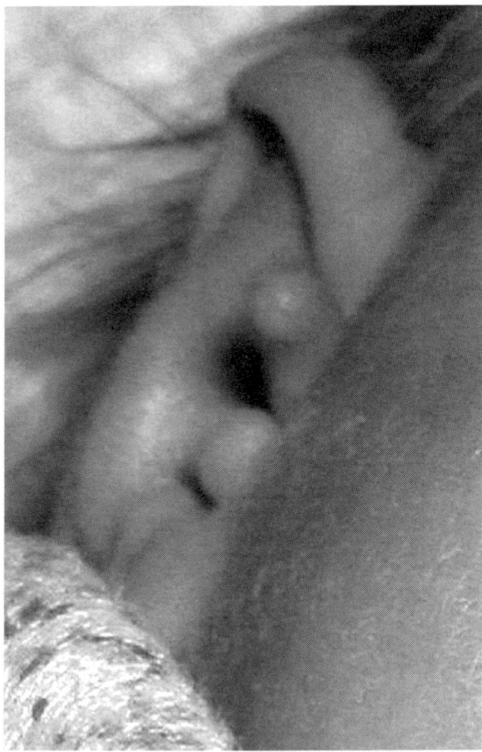

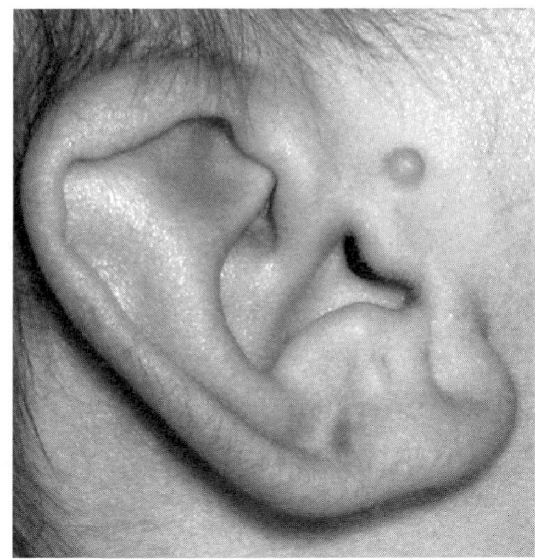

Figure 12-13 (Left) Preauricular tags.

Figure 12-14 (Top) Ear pits and small preauricular tag in an infant with Beckwith-Weidemann syndrome.

Munoz-Flores-Thiagarajan, Easterling, Davis, & Bond, 2001; Nyberg, Haljamae, Frisenette-Fich, Wennergren, & Kjellmer, 1998).

Signs of neonatal MG evolve over the first few hours of life and include hypotonia and feeding difficulties and, rarely, ventilator dependence. Anticholinesterase medications improve symptoms in most affected infants (Ciafaloni & Massey, 2004).

Feeding issues for affected infants include rapid muscle fatigue and hypotonia. Gavage (nasogastric or orogastric tube) feeding is generally required until treatment is effective, but the infant may be put to the breast for very short feedings if the maternal and infant conditions permit.

Effect of Neurological Disorders on Feeding

Some of the issues affecting feeding skills in infants with neurological conditions include muscle tone differences, cognitive deficits that impede learning, coordination difficulties, impeded function of specific nerves or neuromuscular units, and lack of appropriate alertness or energy for feeding.

The brain directs muscle activity, and the nerves serve as the messengers of the brain's directions, so any dysfunction in either or both leaves the muscles less able to perform work. Coordination and rhythm are vital to the effectiveness of feeding movements (Lau & Schanler, 1996), so even the correct movements performed without proper timing can be ineffective, just as a familiar melody played without regard to the proper duration of each note can become unrecognizable. This is a familiar phenomenon to anyone who has observed a child just learning to play a musical instrument. It takes so long for a beginner to recognize the note on the paper, play that note, and move on to the next one that the timing of the melody becomes distorted and the song becomes unrecognizable. This is recognized as a problem in feeding; Palmer's Neonatal Oral-Motor Assessment Scale (NOMAS) includes a category for disorganized sucking, which is defined by deficiencies in rate and rhythm (Palmer & VandenBerg, 1998). Moreover, computer modeling of breastfeeding shows that optimal timing in the suction cycle of the wave-like tongue movements increases milk flow (Zoppou, Barry, & Mercer, 1997).

The Reciprocal Nature of Muscle Activity

Muscles work in pairs, flexing (making the angle between two bones smaller) and extending (making the angle between two bones larger). For example, when a baby bends at the hips, the belly muscles will contract while the back muscles extend. If the tone in the back extensors is higher than normal, the baby may have difficulty not only flexing at the hips, but even maintaining the hips at neutral. An extensor pattern may also translate into a feeding difficulty as overfiring extensors call other muscles into the pattern, pulling back the baby's shoulders and upper spine. This makes it difficult for the baby to be in the workable ear–shoulder–hip aligned configuration and makes attaching to the breast a challenge by retracting (pulling back) the tongue.

Physical and/or occupational therapy can help normalize tone with preparatory handling techniques and by positioning the baby in supportive, pattern-interrupting ways to help reduce the effects of abnormally high tone.

Increased Effort with High and Low Tone

The muscular system is a miracle of balance—flex and extend, contract and release, shorten and lengthen. Moreover, this shortening and lengthening happens in a very controlled manner on either side of a joint. Any time muscle tone is out of balance between reciprocal (antagonist) muscles, or a group of synergistic muscles, the ease of movement is reduced, work increases, and energy expenditure increases. If tone is out of balance toward the high side (*hypertonia*), movement can be restricted as muscle groups are caught (stuck), unable to release extension so contraction can occur on the opposite side of the joint.

This is one reason we encourage mothers to be comfortable while they nurse; not only does it feel better to be comfortable, it is also more sustainable because increased tension wastes energy. Ergonomic use of the body reduces the risk of injury and increases ease of movement. Use of large muscles for holding the baby is easier than stressing smaller muscles. Encouraging mothers to use gravity and their trunk to support the baby's weight rather than their relatively weaker wrists can be important in preventing exacerbation of repetitive stress injuries, such as carpal tunnel syndrome.

Being out of balance the other way is also challenging. Low tone (*hypotonia*) may mean that muscles lack the power to achieve the necessary range of movement; for example, a baby with low tone in the jaw muscles may be unable to open his or her mouth enough to latch well. In addition, these restrictions of movement range may lead to the baby recruiting other muscles to join in assisting the action. This can be challenging because the muscles joining in may not be efficiently designed for this new role. The effect of this is familiar to most lactation consultants when watching a baby with a structural tongue limitation. A baby with a restrictive lingual frenulum, unable to latch deeply enough to feed with stability and power, compensates for the instability of a shallow latch by using the muscles of the upper lip. This is not only painful for mom, but also tiring for the baby because the upper lip muscles are better at the subtle movements of speech than the power movements of repetitive feeding. In a similar fashion, muscles recruited to compensate for lack of range of motion caused by neurological limitations can rapidly fatigue.

Early Intervention Referral

Infants with neurological conditions are often diagnosed in the postpartum unit, but sometimes breastfeeding difficulties are the first manifestation of altered development. Early intervention programs provide free or subsidized evaluation and treatment for infants who are experiencing, or are at high risk for, developmental delay. An Internet search using the keywords "early intervention [*county or locality name*]" will generally yield local information and contacts. Generally, physicians, parents, and other healthcare personnel (including lactation consultants) can refer infants by contacting the local coordinator or agency. The family is assigned a case coordinator, the parents are interviewed, and the child is tested by specialists in cognitive, language, and motor development. If therapy is prescribed for a child younger than age 3, it is usually provided in the family home.

Where bottle feeding has been the cultural norm, the lactation consultant may be the first to point out the need to provide therapy or assistance to the infant. Poor recognition of incoordination among sucking, swallowing, and breathing during bottle feeding allows infants with feeding problems to go undiagnosed. If caregivers lay the infant down, actively insert the artificial nipple, and invert the bottle so the milk flows rapidly into the baby's mouth (as recommended in bottle and formula manufacturers' literature and websites), it is possible to miss the baby's inability to initiate and follow through with normal feeding subskills like wide gaping, tongue depression and extension, tongue grooving around the teat, and rhythmic tongue and jaw movements to transfer milk. The more passive, or reactive, nature of standard bottle feeding, and the acceptance of rapid, gulpy feeds with milk loss and/or vomiting as normal, can conspire to mask baby's difficulty with normal, active feeding skills. The physiological challenges presented by bottle feeding, including lack of standardization of nipple flow rates, high flow rates that compromise respirations, and the lack of conformity to the infant's anatomy, may negatively impact acquisition and maintenance of normal feeding skills. Consequently, abnormal compensatory movements may develop and override normal skill development.

The lactation consultant may be the first, or only, person to suggest that the baby has a feeding issue. The issue may be temporary, or it may have its basis in static or progressive neurological deficits. Parents can be reassured that the recommendation for early intervention evaluation does not imply a lifelong challenge for the baby. If breastfeeding were the cultural norm, all babies having trouble achieving the norm would be evaluated and supported toward that norm. Because some healthcare professionals still consider breastfeeding disposable as long as the baby can bottle feed, even poorly, early intervention may not have been suggested before. Parents will need extra support regarding the simple normalcy of breastfeeding—they are not following some maternal agenda for a feeding style, but they simply want their baby to achieve normal developmental milestones. Dialogue with parents about the simple normality of feeding at the breast is critical. They need information and support to understand that their baby is not being asked to work toward something too challenging for some (like marathon running), but simply to the norm (like walking).

Supportive Techniques

For infants with hypotonia, particular attention should be paid to support and alignment at the breast. Judicious, short-term swaddling in body flexion (with hips and knees flexed, hand brought to midline, and shoulders gently forward) may help floppy infants to use their tongue and jaw more skillfully. Hypotonic infants who have difficulty maintaining attachment or have wide jaw excursions can benefit from chin and jaw support. The *Dancer hand position* (McBride & Danner, 1987) consists of using the webbing between the thumb and first finger to support the infant's jaw while the thumb and first finger support the cheeks. Generally when cheek support is given, forward traction is applied toward the lips (see photos in Chapter 13). Using feeding positions that avoid lifting the breast (bringing the baby to where the nipple naturally falls) reduce the strain on the baby's tongue and jaw that results if the baby needs to stay attached against gravity.

Those with weak tongue movements may be assisted by *sublingual support,* where the feeder places a fingertip under the baby's chin on the soft tissue behind the jaw bone (**Figure 12-15**). Gentle upward pressure is provided to assist tongue movements, and gentle forward traction may help as well. As always, the effect of these interventions needs to be carefully observed. Jaw and cheek support in bottle feeding infants may increase the bolus size. Although it is unlikely that the same is true for breastfeeding infants, the infant should be observed for any difficulty coordinating swallowing and breathing.

Positioning

Infants with hypotonia and reduced energy and alertness may feed better in more upright positions (**Figure 12-16**), such as the straddle or more vertical versions of the clutch hold

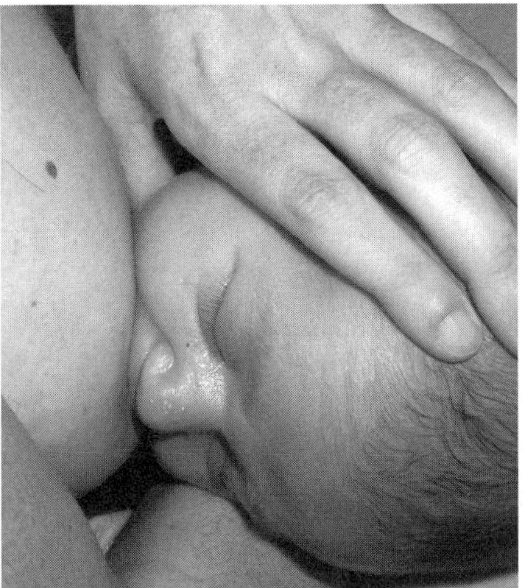

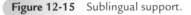

Figure 12-15 Sublingual support.

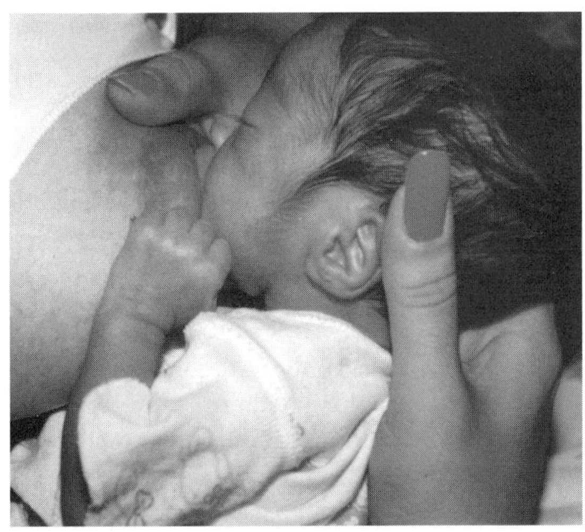

Figure 12-16 Preterm infants with low muscle tone may benefit from upright positioning.

(**Figure 12-17**). Optimal support is important for stability in these infants with reduced postural stability. When using side-lying, mother may want to lay the infant's head on her upper arm and use her lower arms to keep the infant snuggled against her body for positional stability (**Figure 12-18**). See Chapter 13 for more on therapeutic positioning.

Head positioning for neurologically impaired infants during feeding is controversial. For healthy, full-term infants, the ideal head position during breastfeeding is one of mild extension to bring the jaw forward, increase tongue and jaw contact with the breast, and open the airway for reduced resistance to airflow for unstressed breathing. Radiological evidence has shown that head extension facilitated correct sucking and swallowing when feeding with a modified bottle in an infant with structural disabilities (Takagi & Bosma, 1960). Therapists have long been taught to use a neutral head position or chin tuck in feeding neurologically impaired infants. It is believed that the slight chin tuck mechanically improves the safety of swallowing because flexion narrows the airway and raises the larynx. There is evidence that chin tuck during swallowing reduces the number of aspirations in adults with surgical or age-related swallowing problems (Rasley et al., 1993; Shanahan, Logemann, Rademaker, Pauloski, & Kahrila, 1993), but the maneuver was less effective in younger patients and those whose swallowing problems did not stem from overflow from the valleculae. The anatomy of the newborn airway offers protection against aspiration from this mechanism due to the apposition of the soft palate and epiglottis during sucking. Additionally, infants with respiratory instability are less likely to time their swallows appropriately. In newborns, and particularly in preterm infants, overflexion of the neck may result in the occlusion of the pharyngeal airway by the larynx (Ardran & Kemp, 1968).

Lactation consultants working with neurologically impaired infants need to weigh these competing concerns and observe the results of any intervention particularly carefully. Because aspiration can occur without coughing in young infants (Arvedson, Rogers, Buck, Smart, & Msall, 1994), careful assessment of the coordination of swallowing sounds and observation of the infant's respiratory sounds for wet or congested qualities is necessary when feeding neurologically impaired infants. Cervical auscultation is particularly useful for this purpose (Chapter 1).

Interaction of Birth Interventions with Neurological Issues

Any motor pattern or state condition that interferes with the baby's ability to be in a quiet alert state, with relaxed but ready musculature and neuromotor responses, can inhibit a baby's ability to successfully go through the instinctive feeding sequence. Some babies have temporary but significant challenges due to labor or delivery medications or procedures. In the first 48 hours, frequency of feeding helps calibrate future milk production, with 13–16 breastfeeding sessions on the second day of life creating a significantly increased milk production even 6 weeks later in multiparous women, versus the commonly recommended 8–12 feedings (Chen, Nommsen-Rivers, Dewey, & Lonnerdal, 1998). Newborn babies need frequent and untimed access to the breast to receive adequate amounts of colostrum, which provides irreplaceable immunological protection and trophic functions to prepare the gut for larger volumes of mature milk. If the baby is either too irritable or too overwhelmed and shuts down, feeding can be difficult. Restoring skin-to-skin positioning with mom is sometimes enough to restore normal feeding behavior within 15–30 minutes. Hospital routines that expect newborns to interval feed like older babies can disrupt the important calibration and learning period of the first few days.

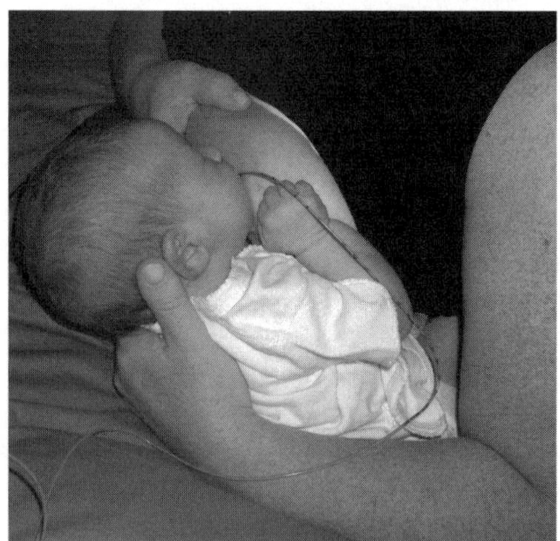

Figure 12-17 Sitting clutch; note that the infant's knees and hips are flexed. If mother reclines, this position becomes more ergonomic. A 5-French feeding tube is providing additional milk.

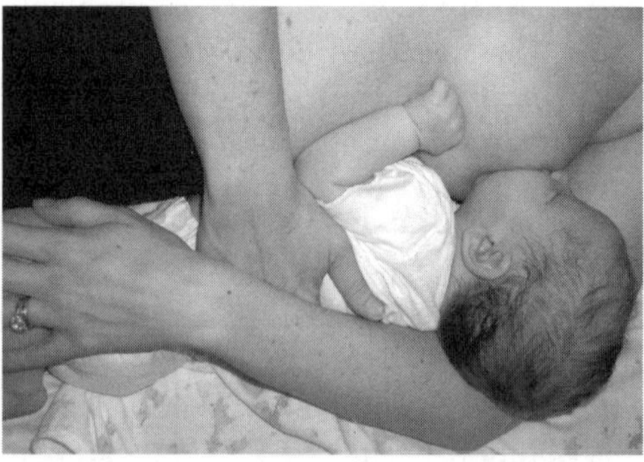

Figure 12-18 Providing optimal support in side-lying.

The low volume and high viscosity of colostrum facilitates practicing the coordination of sucking, swallowing, and breathing with a low risk of aspiration. This practice is especially important for neurologically impaired infants who may have a greater risk of aspiration when the milk volume and flow increase (Arvedson et al., 1994; Stevenson & Allaire, 1991).

Healthy, unmedicated babies will show interest in and initiate feeding when they are ready and need not be rushed, especially if they have been kept skin to skin with their mother since birth. Neurologically impaired infants who are also under the influences of medications, procedures, or separation from their mother are likely to be more disorganized from these interventions than neurotypical infants.

Preparatory Handling

For disorganized or challenged infants, it can be helpful to position or move them in certain ways before the breast is even presented. Babies with tonal issues can be assisted toward the middle of the tone or state continuum by being in positions that either enhance or calm the effects of tone outside the functional middle of the continuum.

Hypertonia

A baby with high tone might need to be wrapped in a blanket, providing full body support for the head, neck, trunk, and limbs, and rocked gently through the air from head to feet (**Figure 12-19**).

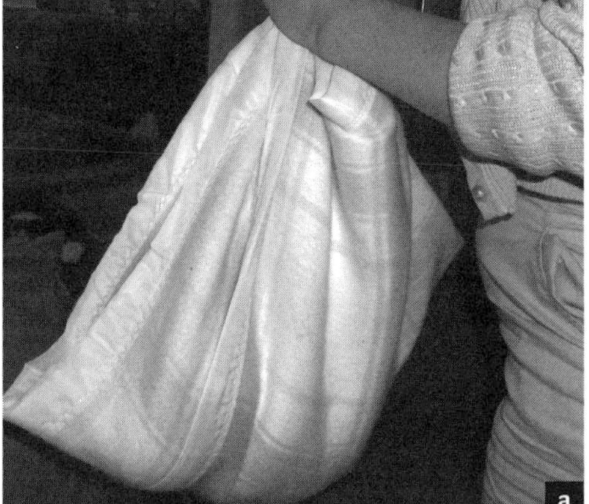

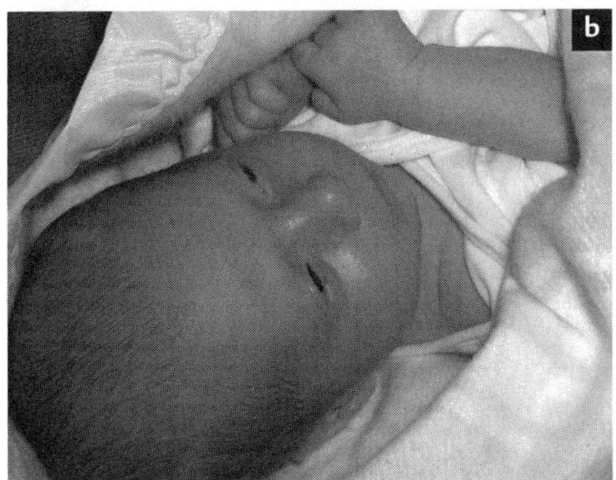

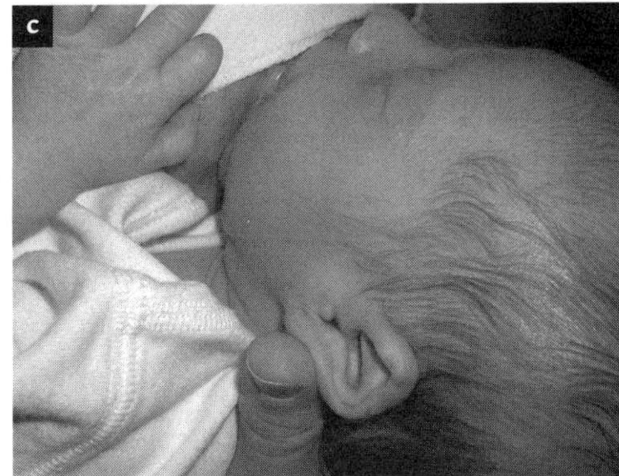

Figure 12-19 Using a blanket swing to relax a stressed, arching infant into flexion, improving neurobehavioral organization and allowing attachment.

This can be relaxing, lowering higher tone toward the middle norm and allowing the baby to move the head and neck more independently from the trunk and limbs. It may also calm an overstimulated or overstressed baby.

Babies can also be calmed by placing them in the colic hold, draped over the forearm with the baby's belly along the forearm muscle of the person holding the baby, with baby's legs and arms allowed to relax around the sides and down around the holder's arm, and the baby's head resting at the side of the widest part of the forearm (**Figure 12-20**).

By switching arms, the holder has the baby over the other forearm, baby's legs on either side of the palm, and the holder's other hand supporting the baby's forehead. The infant can be offered a finger to suck in this position (charm hold, Chapter 13), which can help bring the tongue forward in the mouth and give the lactation consultant another perspective on the tongue's tone, range of motion, and strength.

Hypotonia

A baby with lower tone can be assisted to sit on an adult knee and be gently but arrhythmically bounced or leaned forward and back to stimulate *equilibrium reactions* (righting responses)—attempts to maintain posture despite movement away from a stable center (**Figure 12-21**). Movements that stimulate equilibrium reactions increase alertness and/or tone so the baby can better move the neck and jaws in the instinctive feeding initiation sequence pattern. Babies with suitable neck strength can be supported in a standing position with their feet on a sitting adult's thighs. Most infants placed in this position will

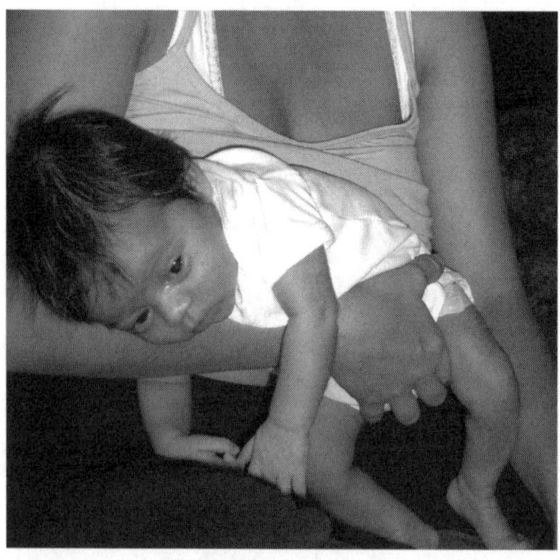

Figure 12-20 Colic hold.

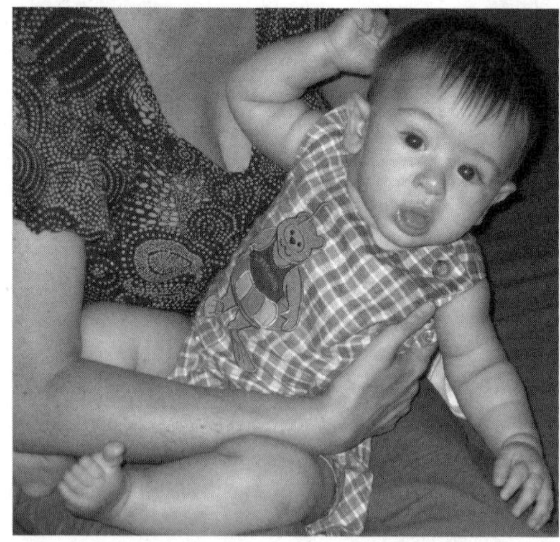

Figure 12-21 Stimulating equilibrium reactions by tilting the baby backward slightly.

enjoy repeatedly pushing down with their feet by extending and flexing their knees (**Figure 12-22**). The proprioceptive input of bouncing or jumping on a slightly resilient surface is believed to improve muscle tone and motor performance in hypotonic children.

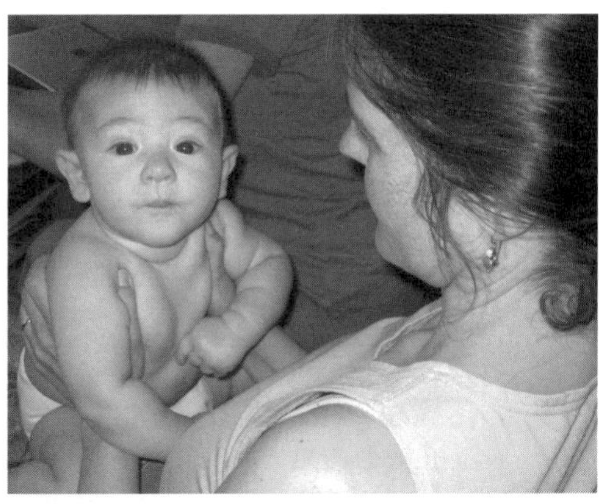

Figure 12-22 Preparatory handling with an infant.

These movements and positions are simple, brief, and may help improve readiness and capabilities for normal latching and feeding in babies who are temporarily or mildly affected by tone or state issues. Babies with severe or ongoing issues may benefit from referral to early intervention (occupational, physical, or speech-language therapists) or to private practice speech or feeding therapists, osteopathic physicians, chiropractors, or other bodywork practitioners, in addition to continuing work with the lactation consultant. Team communication and sharing of perspectives and skills is vital to optimizing normal feeding skills in infancy and beyond.

Alertness

Cerebral depression causes reduced alertness and a lower level of consciousness that can range in severity from coma to an increased proportion of the day spent in sleep. As mentioned earlier in the chapter, anticonvulsants prescribed for neonatal seizures can further sedate the infant. In a neonatal intensive care environment, compromised infants may withdraw from the constant overstimulation, increasing their unavailability for feeding.

Removing aversive stimuli as much as possible and providing organizing stimulation (cuddling, skin-to-skin contact, gentle rocking or swaying) may help infants who are shut down to feel safe. It is generally helpful to watch for behavioral signs of light sleep (squirming, mouthing, sucking, rapid eye movements) and place the depressed infant to breast as soon as these signs occur. Skin-to-skin care (Kangaroo Mother Care) can help to take advantage of briefer periods of alertness by keeping the baby close to the breast and in a more organized state.

In general, arrhythmic vestibular stimulation is alerting, and rhythmic stimulation is organizing. Compromised or preterm infants may find any movement stressful and disorganizing. Skin-to-skin contact with mom without stroking or maternal movement may help a stressed infant become available for feeding. Sensitive observation of the infant will allow stimulation to be withdrawn if the baby shows stress signals.

Sucking Issues in Neurologically Impaired Infants

Infants with neurological deficits may use a disorganized, up and down piston-like movement of the entire tongue during sucking. Sucking pressure can be absent in infants with severe neurological issues (Mizuno et al., 2006). Infants with neurological challenges generally are able to improve their feeding skills (McBride & Danner, 1987), and depending on the severity of their condition, many will learn to breastfeed. Improvement in feeding skills is a good prognostic indicator for future neurological functioning (Mizuno & Ueda, 2005). Breastfeeding can be initiated while the infant is still being gavage (tube) fed, and the gavage feedings can be reduced or eliminated as the baby becomes able to meet his or her nutritional needs at breast. Counseling mom to maintain her supply at a higher level than needed can be helpful for her infant with imperfect sucking skills, as long as the rapid milk flow does not compromise coordination of swallowing and breathing. Sometimes stimulating a swallow by introducing a little bit of milk into the mouth by breast compression or with a periodontal syringe, eyedropper, or tube can lead to stimulation of the central pattern generator for sucking and initiate the suck–swallow–breathe sequence (**Figure 12-23**). Before giving any milk, ensure that the infant is ready to handle the flow (is at least attempting to suck) and keep the bolus small. A squirt of milk that a healthy infant could tolerate might frighten or destabilize a neurologically impaired baby.

If maternal milk production is low or the infant is weak and requires more reward for the effort, additional milk can be given through a tube at breast. Several commercial devices exist for this purpose, including the Lact-Aid Nursing Trainer System, the Supply Line, and the Medela Supplemental Nursing System (SNS) (**Figures 12-24 and 12-25**.) Getting the flow correct is important. Too high a flow can stress the infant's cardiorespiratory system by forcing frequent swallows, suppressing breathing, and reducing blood oxygen levels. Fast flow can also stress the ability to coordinate the swallow correctly and increase the risk of aspiration. Too low a flow fails to provide consistent sensory input for continued sucking efforts and may lead to a spiral of increasing fatigue, poorer feeding, and weight loss.

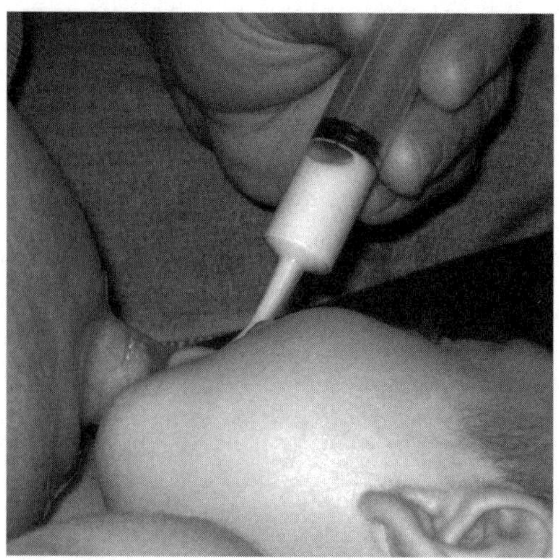

Figure 12-23 Providing an instant reward for mouthing the breast with a curved tip (periodontal) syringe.

Except in situations where the feeder is attempting to jump-start the sucking sequence by delivering a small bolus of milk, the infant should ideally be in control of milk delivery, either actively by pulling milk from the device or with the mother coordinating delivery of supplement with the infant's sucking efforts (**Figure 12-26**). In addition to the danger of aspiration, the infant does not learn as well if milk flow is not contingent on his or her efforts. Infants with cognitive impairments especially require consistency in cueing and oral motor movements required to move milk.

There is a fine balance between rewarding an infant's continued attempts to breastfeed and reinforcing dysfunctional sucking behaviors. Occasionally, motivation may be more important than stimulating correct suckling. Neurologically impaired infants in the author's practice have responded to a nipple shield repeatedly filled with expressed milk with a curved tip syringe or butterfly tubing and syringe. Despite the use of a tongue thrusting pattern, several infants were able to remove milk from the prefilled teat before they were able to transfer milk from the breast (**Figure 12-27**). The experience of obtaining milk from the breast provided positive feedback that led to further attempts at breastfeeding. Tongue movements gradually improved with the use of facilitative techniques and the infants' own experimentation.

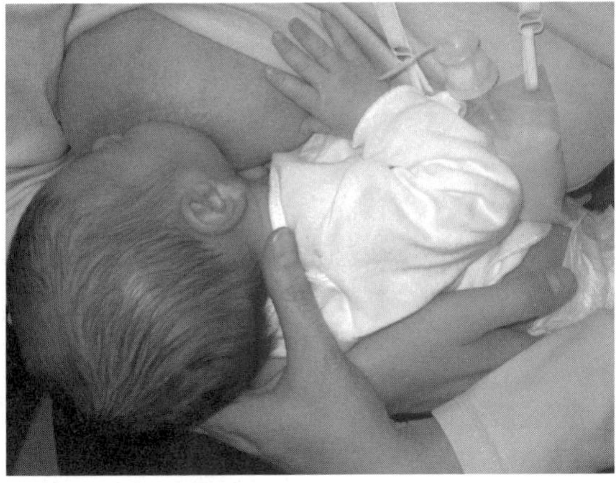

Figure 12-24 The Lact-Aid nursing trainer provides additional milk at breast, and is easy to clean and assemble.

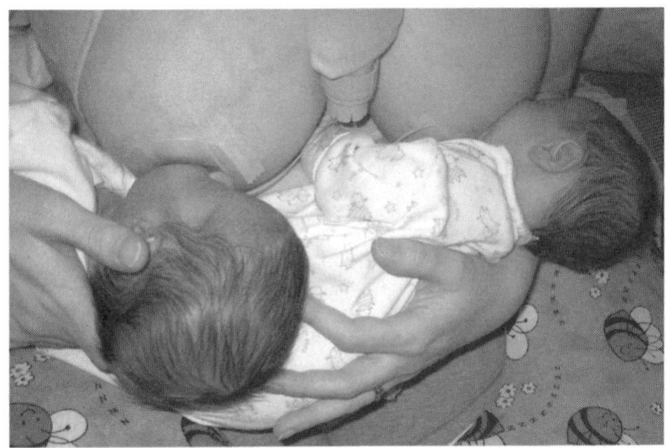

Figure 12-25 The supplemental nursing system has two tubes, and can be used with twins as well as singletons.

Why Some Babies Need Supplementing, Even Though Mom Is Making Sufficient Milk

Daly, Owens, and Hartmann (1993) found that breastfeeding infants will remove an average of 76% of the stored milk from the breast. Infants with sucking problems, particularly tongue-tied or neurologically impaired infants in the author's practice, have been able to remove between 10% and 60% of the milk their mother can subsequently pump. Supplementing at breast generally increases the amount of milk that inefficient infants are able to receive from the breast. This can be demonstrated by weighing the filled

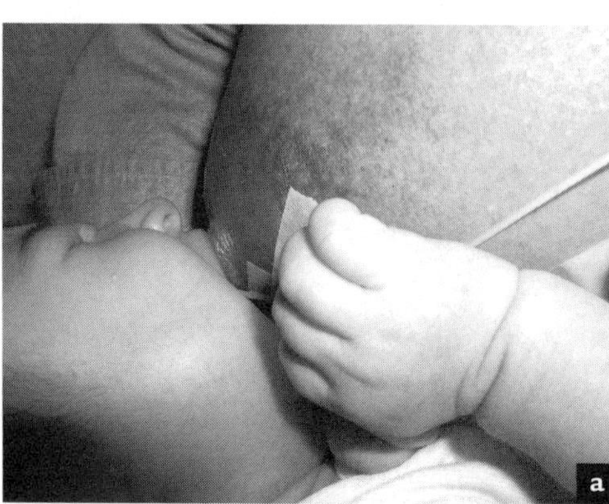

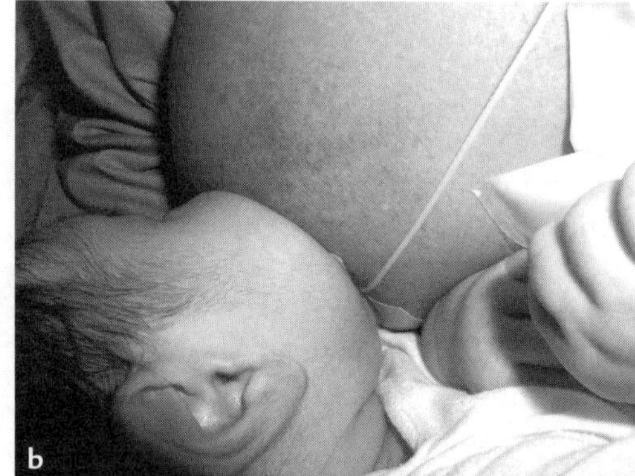

Figure 12-26 (Top left and right) Latching on with a Lact-Aid tube. Placing the tube at the center of the lower lip helps ensure proper tube placement without disrupting latch mechanics.

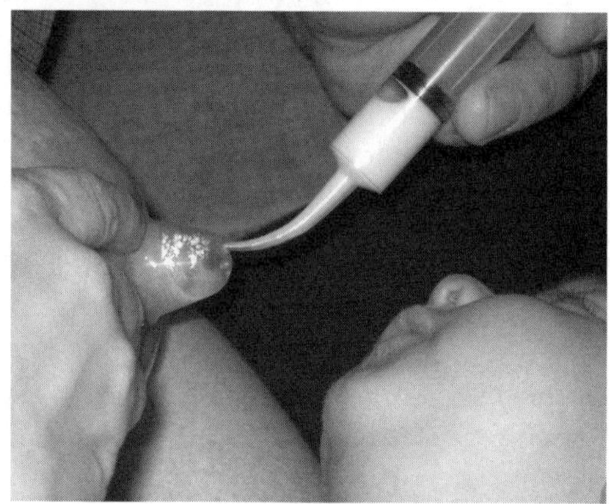

Figure 12-27 (Right) Prefilling a nipple shield allowed this infant to transition back to breast after recovery from neonatal encephalopathy.

supplementer and the baby separately before and immediately after feeding on a scale designed to detect milk intake from the breast. These scales are generally accurate to a few grams, allowing a good estimation of milk intake. Feeding promptly after weighing, and reweighing immediately after feeding, reduces the impact of *insensible water loss* (water vapor lost through normal metabolism and respiration). If the baby is an ineffective feeder, there may be more milk removed from the breast using the supplementer (the baby will have gained more than the supplementer lost) than without it. If the entire milk intake came from the device, then the infant might have been sucking the tube alone (which is obvious by the sound of air being drawn into the mouth and the baby's pursed lips). If straw drinking was not occurring, and little milk was taken from the breast, maternal milk production may be very low. Efforts should be made to increase milk removal to stimulate increased supply.

Some infants' feeding attempts are particularly flow dependent—when the flow of milk subsides, they seem to give up and stop working. Supplementing at breast with a tube feeding device can provide continuous flow to infants for whom breast compression is insufficient. Infants with limited endurance can benefit from supplementation at breast, allowing them to feed in a reasonable time frame and allowing the mother time for milk expression to help protect or increase her supply.

There are two types of supplementer devices: those that require suction (negative intra-oral pressure) and those that are active, or feeder controlled. A periodontal syringe or syringe attached to tubing is an example of an active supplementation device. Obviously, active supplementation is required in infants with overt clefts who cannot create negative pressure in their mouths. Active supplementation also works well with infants who lack energy due to underfeeding. Active supplementation must be performed carefully to avoid exacerbating any underlying condition that led to the infant being unable to feed well. For example, cardiac and respiratory problems that cause an increased respiratory rate or increased work of breathing leave less time for swallowing. Pushing an infant with one of these issues to swallow more frequently can easily reduce the respiratory rate below that needed to maintain oxygenation. The feeder generally waits for the infant to initiate a sucking burst and then supplies small boluses with each suck. If the baby loses milk from the lips or shows signs of flow intolerance, the bolus size is reduced and/or the flow is slowed; if the baby shows impatience (tugging, squirming, lack of swallowing), the flow is increased. The infant is allowed to pace the feeding; the feeder stops delivering milk during respiratory pauses. If the infant is not self-pacing, the feeder observes for increased respiratory rate or stress signs (Chapter 8 and Chapter 11), and the flow is interrupted until recovery occurs.

The Lact-Aid Nursing Trainer, the Supply Line, Medela's SNS, and devices assembled by placing a feeding tube in a container of milk all require negative intraoral pressure. When the infant sucks, milk is drawn out of the breast. If a full mouthful comes from the breast, little or no milk is removed from the supplementer. If only a partial mouthful is removed from the breast, milk flows through the tube to fill the mouth. Flow from the device can be controlled in several ways: crimping the tube in a slot in the commercial devices or lifting the tube out of the supplement stops the flow of milk; lifting the container increases the influence of gravity and increases the speed of the flow; a larger diameter tube increases flow; and for a twin tube device like the SNS, venting the device by opening the second tube increases the flow as well. Taping the venting tube to the container with the opening pointing toward the ceiling can help keep air moving in and prevent milk from moving out. More details on individual devices and nuances of using them can be found in Genna (2009).

Tube devices can make attachment more challenging. Holding or taping the tube where the center of the baby's lower lip will touch it during latch can improve tube placement, bringing it in midline on the tongue, under the nipple. When the tube is placed at the upper lip, mother may pay attention to ensuring that the upper lip covers the tube and may allow the lower lip to slide up to the base of the nipple. This is opposite to the optimal latch, which is obtained when the lower lip and tongue tip are as far from the nipple as possible.

Another challenge of tube devices is that some infants will straw drink and remove milk only from the tube. Withdrawing the tube slightly, so that it no longer extends to the nipple tip or beyond, can reduce this behavior. Infant feeding involves learning, and it is important to provide the right lesson. If supplementation at breast is not leading to correct sucking that removes milk from the breast, it might not be the right intervention. The infant should be assessed again, and other interventions (or a different supplementer device) could be considered.

If feedings are prolonged even with a supplementer device, tube placement in the infant's mouth should be checked, and the tubing should be examined to ensure there are no crimps or clogs. Powdered formula use is a common cause of clogged tubing, and the Lact-Aid Nursing Trainer comes with a filter to strain out lumps during filling. Rubbing the tubing between the thumb and forefinger may soften lumps or release crimps and improve flow. If the infant is getting sufficient milk at breast with the supplementer, but the feeding is long (more than 30–45 minutes), mother can be counseled to use the device every other feeding, and use a faster alternate feeding method in between, to help preserve the dyad's energy and maintain time for milk expression. Milk removal is vital to continued production, and for some dyads, less time at breast and more time spent pumping is the best use of their energy until the baby's skills improve.

Weaning from Supplementers

As the infant shows improved ability to transfer milk from the breast, the mother can be counseled to gradually reduce either the amount of supplement in the container or the proportion of the feeding times when the device is used. Leaving the tube closed off at the beginning of the feeding when the milk ejection is strongest, or offering the device only with the second breast if *paired feedings* (both breasts) are given, are ways to achieve this. Generally the infant will be able to feed at the breast alone at the first morning feeding, or whenever the breast is more full, and will gradually progress to more and more feedings without the device.

Oral Motor Dysfunction and Facilitative Techniques

Specific facilitative techniques are typically used to assist infants with abnormalities in oral motor skills. While these do not necessarily correct the compensatory sucking strategies, they can help the infant achieve more functional feeding. Facilitations should be based on a firm understanding of the normal activity of each structure.

Jaw

The mandible is the moveable part of the jaw. The mandibular gum ridge should be aligned parallel to the maxillary gum ridge; the jaw opening should be smooth and symmetrical, and the gape should be large. Impaired nerve transmission can cause unequal jaw opening, as can positional asymmetries, such as torticollis, from restrictive in utero position. Tongue-tie is often associated with an insufficient gape, perhaps due to traction on the hyoid bone.

Excessive jaw excursions during breastfeeding may be the result of hypotonia, in which case *jaw support* may be helpful. Poor control of the jaw in a neurologically impaired infant may result in slippage of the jaw, providing poor stability for tongue movements (Morris & Klein, 2001), leading to decreased milk transfer and fatigue.

A more common cause of excessive jaw excursions that interrupt attachment to the breast is *ankyloglossia* (tongue-tie). Failure of the anterior tongue to maintain contact with the breast when the posterior tongue depresses enlarges the oral cavity and requires a larger jaw excursion to create sufficient negative pressure to pull milk from the nipple. The excessive jaw excursion may overcome the ability of the lips to seal on the breast, causing repeated loss of attachment. The cheeks may not be capable of resisting the negative pressure in the front of the mouth, and they may collapse. Dimpling of the cheeks in a full-term infant during breastfeeding is an indication that this may be occurring (**Figure 12-28**).

Increasing the depth of attachment will generally improve sucking dynamics by sharing the work of maintaining latch better among the tongue and lips.

Some infants with neurological impairments will move the jaw sideways (lateral *deviations*) or in a circle (*rotary movements*) instead of straight up and down. Lateral deviations may occur in torticollis; rotary movements are normal during chewing, but they do not occur developmentally in a younger infant. Rotary movements may be compensatory for poor tongue mobility or coordination. Jaw support might stabilize the jaw sufficiently for these infants to breastfeed, while therapy addresses the nerve and/or muscular imbalances behind the abnormal movement pattern.

Tongue

Many healthy infants with abnormal tongue movements are attempting to compensate for tongue-tie. Infants with neurologically based sucking difficulties often display a disorganized, up and down piston-like tongue movement or a forceful outward movement of the tongue (thrust). There is generally poor tone and poor central grooving of the tongue. There may be difficulty organizing and initiating sucking movements, and tremors of the jaw and tongue are typically observed (McBride & Danner, 1987). Tremors associated with neurological issues will generally be observed near the beginning of the feed and will be frequent and persistent, whereas fatigue tremors in tongue-tied infants are more likely to occur later in the course of the feeding. Poor central grooving can lead to difficulty making the lateral (side) edges of the tongue contact the palate for safe bolus handling, leading to milk spillage over the tongue, which further challenges swallowing.

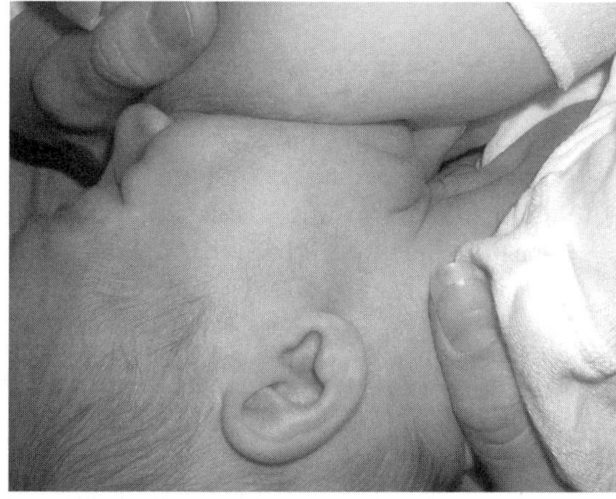

Figure 12-28 Excessive jaw excursions cause flattening or dimpling of the cheeks and loss of attachment.

Specific oral exercises may be helpful to increase awareness of oral structures and movements and prepare the baby for feeding. Whether nonspeech exercises can change tongue movements for speech is a current subject of debate in the speech pathology field (Wilson, Green, Yunusova, & Moore, 2008). Though the quality of existing studies is not ideal, several studies and analyses showed sufficient positive effects of prefeeding stimulation and oral support in preterm infants to support their use at this time (Boiron, Da, Roux, Henrot, & Saliba, 2007; Daley & Kennedy, 2000; Fucile & Gisel, 2010; Fucile, Gisel, & Lau, 2005). Preterm infants share many of the difficulties of neurologically impaired infants, especially impaired reflexes, muscle tone, alertness, and neurological status. Correcting feeding may have a major impact on speech, since the tongue movements used in feeding are used in speech as well (Hiiemae & Palmer, 2003).

Lips

The tongue provides most of the anterior seal between the breast and mouth; the lips are more relaxed, and the orbicularis oris muscle (the circular muscle surrounding the lips) is much less active than the mentalis muscle during breastfeeding (Jacinto-Gonçalves, Gavião, & Berzin, 2004). Fixing of the orbicularis oris may occur when a hypotonic infant attempts to overuse this muscle to improve stability (**Figure 12-29**).

If significant spilling occurs from the lips (**Figure 12-30**), perioral tapping or circular massage just outside of the vermillion border of the lips may temporarily increase tone and help improve lip seal. Infants with swallowing difficulties may deliberately spill milk from the lips. Tongue mobility and grooving should also be assessed in infants who are spilling milk, as should the flow of milk they are being challenged with. It is easy to change flow from the breast—partial pumping or pressure on the breast with a hand to occlude some ducts both slow flow so babies with swallowing difficulties can practice oral feeding. As always, the results of any intervention need to be observed before that intervention is repeated or taught to the infant's parent.

Excessive sweeping movements of the lips may be seen as a compensation for tongue-tie and are usually associated with large sucking blisters and friction calluses along the upper lip. These are often found in midline on the upper lip, but, in the author's experience, they can occur across the skin of both the upper and lower lips in infants with extreme stability difficulties. If the upper labial frenum is also tight, maintaining attachment may be challenging, and dividing both the labial and the lingual frenulum will produce better improvements in feeding (L. Dahl and L. Kotlow, personal communications, 2010).

Cheeks

Full-term infants have a large fat pad in each cheek to form borders for tongue movements that help to keep the tongue in midline during sucking and help to increase the bulk of the cheeks to help them stay rounded during the negative pressure phase of sucking. In hypotonic infants, the cheek muscles may not have sufficient tone to resist negative pressure of normal jaw opening during sucking and may collapse. Cheek support from a fingertip on each cheek

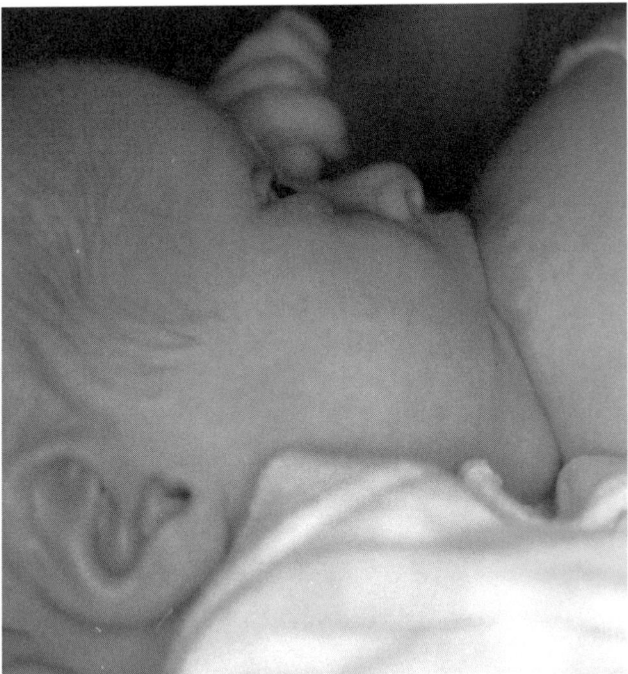

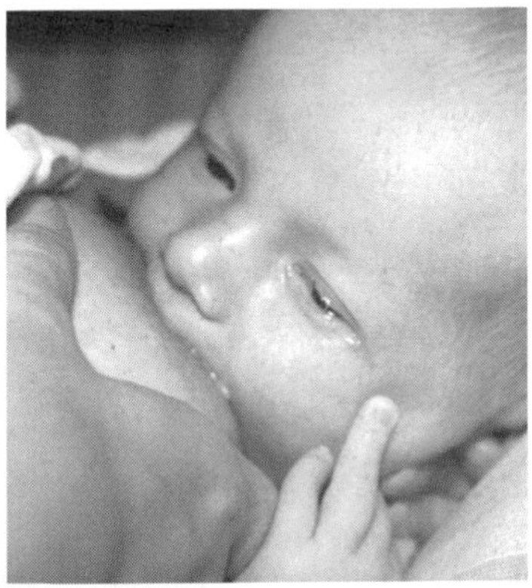

Figure 12-29 (Left) Lip fixing at breast. This is easier to see with the narrower latch on a Haberman feeder teat in Plate 3.

Figure 12-30 (Top right) Spilling milk from the upper lip.

with gentle forward traction (toward the angle of the lips) can be helpful for a baby whose tongue has difficulty remaining in midline or for babies who repeatedly fall off the breast. Biological nurturing (Colson, de Rooy, & Hawdon, 2003) positions may also help redirect gravitational forces to help the baby stay on the breast rather than pulling the baby away.

Palate, Velum, and Pharynx

The hard palate is immobile and plastic, and it is shaped by tongue movements (**Figure 12-31**). The more abnormal the hard palate shape, the more likely the tongue movements are to be abnormal (**Figure 12-32**). Interventions should be directed to improving tongue function. A very abnormal palate shape may be the result of a genetic disorder.

Like all bony structures, the palate is subject to *Wolff's law,* the understanding that bones adapt to the loads placed on them. When muscle power or range are affected by neurological compromise—yielding high, low, or vacillating tone—the bones these muscles attach to adapt to these abnormal stresses. In the case of the palate, tone issues affecting the tongue have an impact on the hard palate. In utero sucking and swallowing movements work to sculpt the palate, but when range of motion, power, or sustained rhythms are compromised, the palate may not be lowered and widened to its most effective feeding configuration. (The same law applies when tongues are mechanically restricted by ankyloglossia.) A limited or weak tongue can cause palatal adaptation toward a higher, narrower palate.

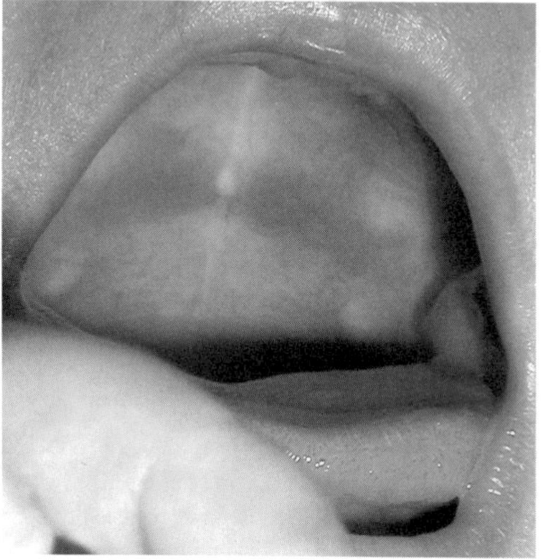

Figure 12-31 Normal palate.

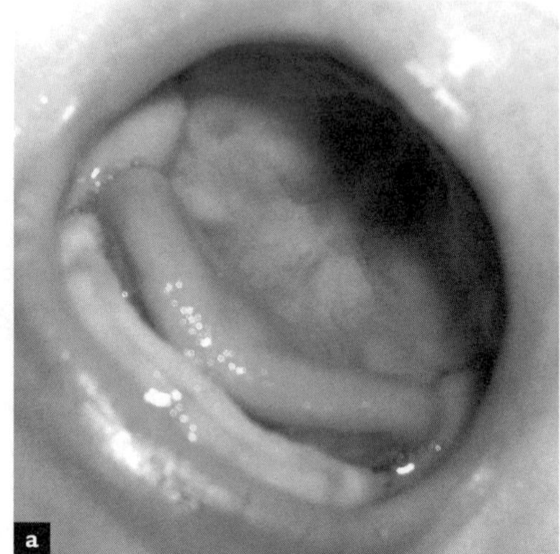

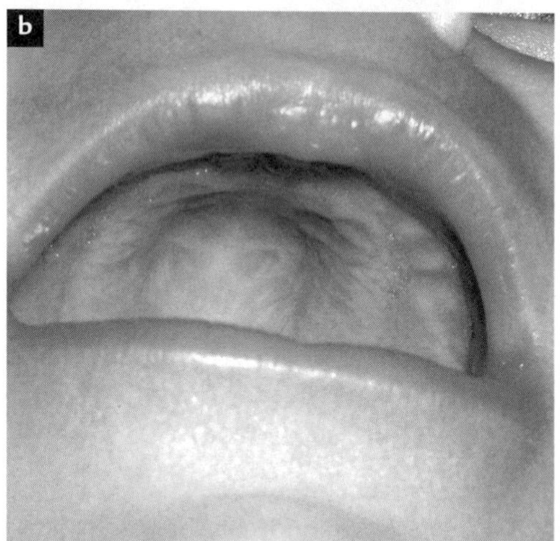

Figure 12-32 (Right) High, narrow palate shapes associated with ankyloglossia (tongue-tie). Note the reduced tongue elevation in part A and the reduced gape in part B.

The limited tongue movements lead to a constellation of feeding challenges practitioners may have noted. This constellation may include the inability to extend, lateralize, or stabilize the tongue; tongue humping or bunching; tongue asymmetry; and concomitant difficulties with the rhythmic, easy interplay of negative pressure and positive pressure that produces efficient, comfortable milk transfer and swallowing, respectively.

The soft palate (*velum*) moves in concert with tongue movements, dropping to seal against the tongue during sucking and raising to meet the walls of the pharynx to seal the nasal airway during swallowing. Signs of soft palate dysfunction include milk dripping from the nose during sucking, feeding-induced apnea (nasopharyngeal backflow of milk triggers apnea in young infants), nasal regurgitation after or between feedings, and short sucking bursts with harsh or wet respiratory sounds during pauses. In infants with neurological issues, velopharyngeal inadequacy can be due to poor coordination and timing between the soft palate and the pharyngeal muscles, so that the nasal cavity is not fully sealed during swallowing or not sealed at the right time to keep milk out. Severe gastroesophageal reflux can be associated with nasal regurgitation as well.

Upright feeding positions can be helpful for infants with poor swallowing due to soft palate dysfunction, as can pacing of the feed (**Figure 12-7**). Aspiration, penetration, and nasopharyngeal backflow were more likely to occur after several sequential swallows (Newman, Keckley, Petersen, & Hamner, 2001). Therefore, limiting an infant with swallowing problems to a few sucks before briefly interrupting the feeding can reduce the risk of milk entering the airway. Exercises that facilitate tongue grooving may help improve swallowing by increasing bolus control (Morris & Klein, 2001). Information on velopharyngeal inadequacy due to anatomic issues is provided in Chapter 8.

Helping Infants Who Feed Ineffectively

If the infant is unable to feed orally, the mother should be encouraged to express milk for tube feedings. Sufficient milk production is most likely when the pump kit fits well (the nipples have room to expand in the nipple tunnel during pumping), expression is initiated within 6 hours of birth, both breasts are pumped simultaneously (Jones, Dimmock, & Spencer, 2001) about eight times in 24 hours (Hill, Aldaq, & Chatterton, 2001), and pumping is preceded by very brief breast massage. Manual expression of milk is effective as well, perhaps even more effective than mechanical pumps for the removal of colostrum (Ohyama, Watabe, Hayasaka, Saito, & Mizuguchi, 2007). Expressing by hand before or after using a mechanical pump in the first few days postpartum markedly increases milk production in mothers of nonnursing infants (Morton et al., 2009). Colostrum can be manually expressed into a teaspoon and fed directly to the infant, or it can be expressed into a medicine cup for feeding with a syringe or eyedropper or swabbing into the NPO infant's mouth (mouth care). If an electric pump is used in the first days of life, a very small collection container should be used to avoid wasting colostrum. A spare Ameda silicone diaphragm can be upended in the top of any standard collection bottle and can be used as a feeding cup (**Figure 12-33**), or a sterile

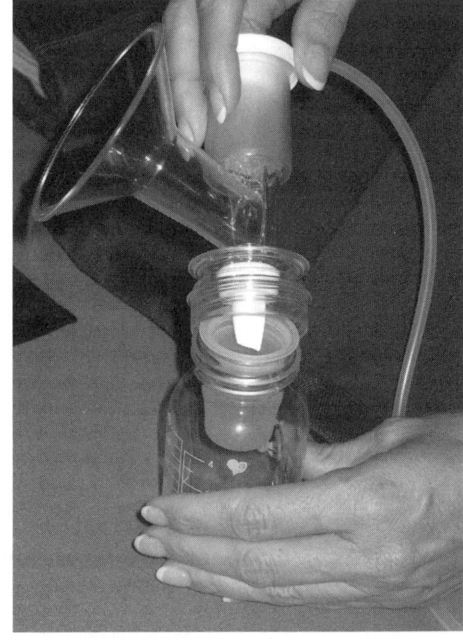

Figure 12-33 Using an Ameda diaphragm as a colostrum collector.

colostrum container with a lid, such as Snappies, can be used if the colostrum is to be stored. See Genna (2009) for information on specific products.

When infants breastfeed ineffectively despite intervention, it may be helpful to provide brief feeds at breast for practice while supplying the bulk of the baby's nutrition another way. Limiting the time at breast until the infant can transfer significant amounts of milk helps preserve the energy of both mother and baby and allows time for milk expression to maintain production, but it may lead to flow preference and breast refusal. Rather than prescribing a set time limit for breastfeeding, mothers should be taught to recognize effective feeding by the infant's lower suck–swallow ratio, slower sucking speed, open eyes, and intent expression. *Breast compression* (alternate massage) can help increase milk flow to the infant. When the baby stops swallowing, mother gently squeezes the breast (far enough from the baby's mouth to avoid disrupting the latch), holds the compression during sucking bursts, and releases it during respiratory pauses (**Figure 12-34**). Some inefficient infants respond to having their cheek or chin tickled to initiate a sucking burst, and others respond to the delivery of a small bolus of milk through a tube or periodontal (curved tip) syringe, but these techniques must be used judiciously and with careful observation of the infant's respiratory pattern. They are appropriate for infants with low energy reserves or reduced alertness who have normal cardiorespiratory function. Preterm and neurologically impaired babies and infants with cardiorespiratory issues are at high risk of hypoxia if their feeding is not self-paced.

Alternative Feeding

Bottle Feeding

Babies are less likely to refuse to breastfeed when they are not frustrated at breast and when alternate feeding maintains active infant participation and as many breastfeeding-appropriate behaviors as possible (**Figure 12-35**). When using a bottle for a breastfed infant, a nipple with a cylindrical teat and a wider base is usually preferable (Kassing, 2002) (**Figure 12-36**). A shorter or softer teat may be helpful for infants with a hypersensitive gag reflex or those who cannot get their lips well back on the wide base of the teat otherwise. It is also helpful to have a bottle design that allows for horizontal holding of the bottle so flow can be initiated and more directed by the baby (**Figure 12-37**). Bottles that must be tipped up high for milk to flow, especially ones with anything other than a quite slow flow, can encourage a baby to become a reactive feeder, thus making transition to breast much more difficult as initiating skills and patience are extinguished.

The teat can be held across the infant's upper and lower lips with the tip at the philtrum (the ridge between nose and upper lip) to cue a wide gape, and the infant can be snuggled onto the bottle as it is tipped into the mouth (**Figures 12-38 and 12-39**). Infants who are very passive can be encouraged to gradually take more control, so that eventually they gape, lunge, and orally grasp the bottle teat the same way they do at the breast. The bottle can be tipped so the first few sucks deliver little or no milk to preserve the infant's patience in working for the milk ejection at the breast. Swallowing air is not a big concern—during a

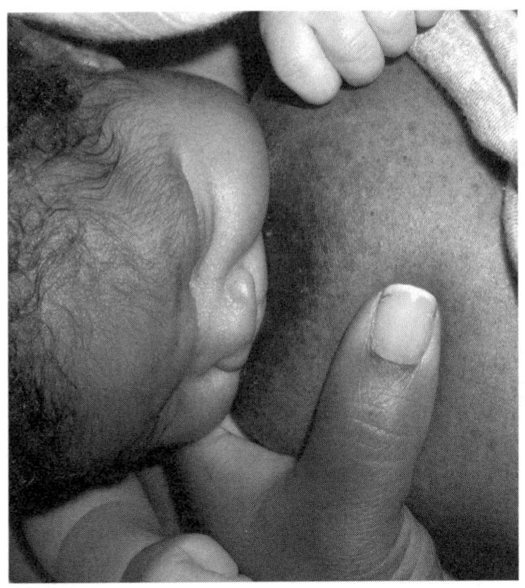

Figure 12-34 When breast compression is used, the fingers should be far enough away from baby's mouth to avoid disrupting the attachment.

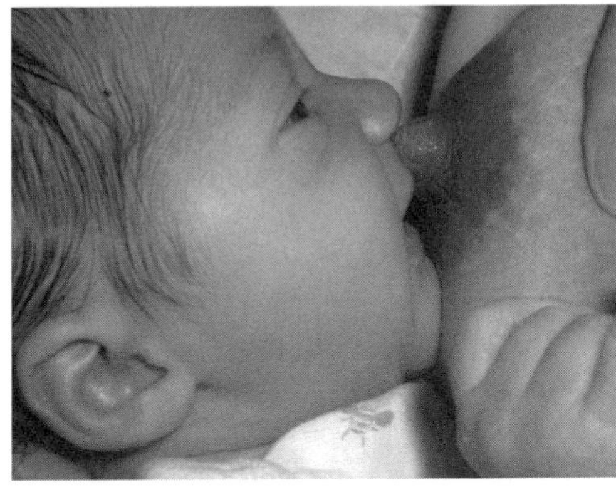

Figure 12-35 Instinctive position for attaching to breast. Note where breast touches infant's face.

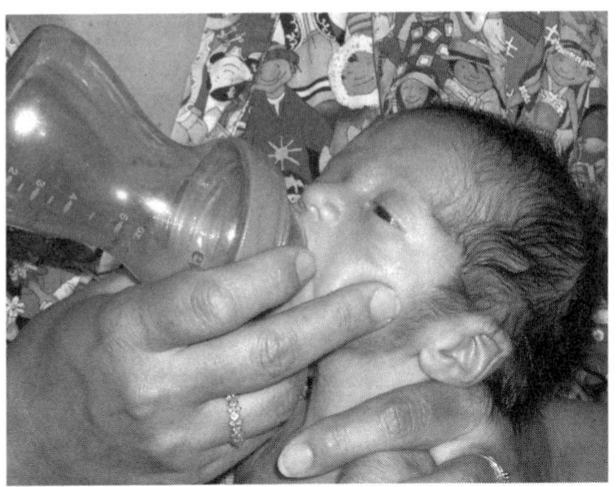

Figure 12-36 Providing cheek and jaw support during bottle feeding with a wide-based teat.

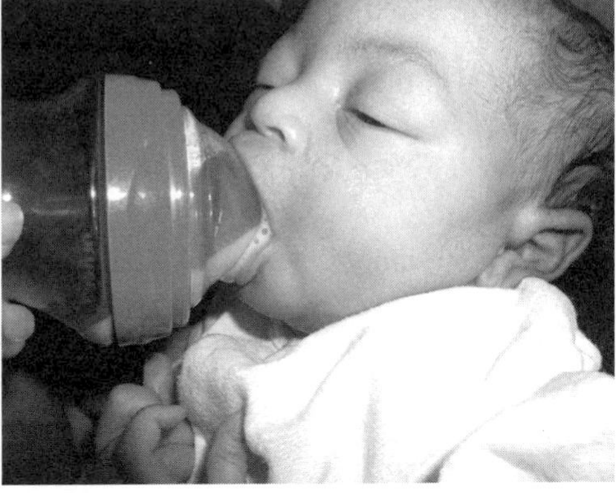

Figure 12-37 Horizontal positioning of the bottle reduces flow, but this infant is still having difficulty, indicated by the spillage at the lips.

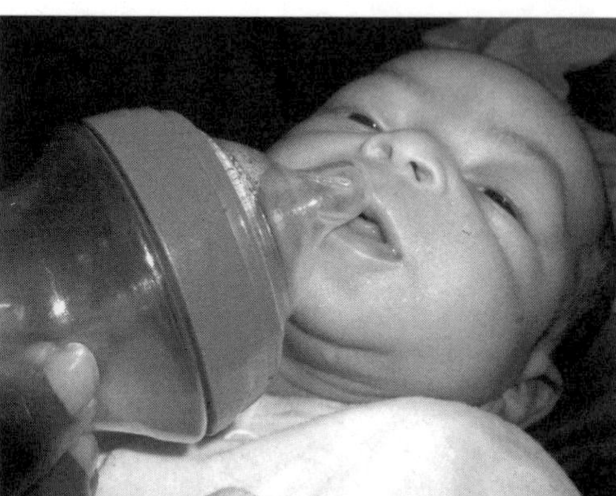

Figure 12-38 The bottle is removed from the mouth and rested at the philtrum. The infant will gape when ready to feed again.

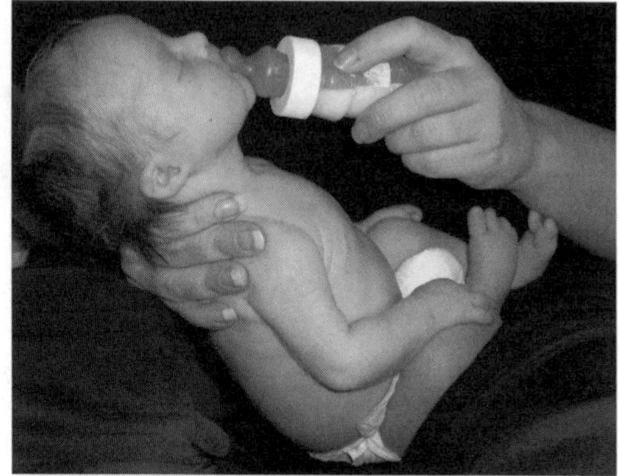

Figure 12-39 Bottle nipple is held across both lips to stimulate maximal gape response. The infant is supported with hips flexed against the feeder's thighs and hand in a slightly upright position to increase alertness and improve stability and muscle tone.

controlled swallow, the soft palate pushes air out of the nose, whereas gulping due to fast flow results in air swallowing.

Similar methods can be used for fingerfeeding—the feeder should stimulate a wide gape, touch the tongue tip with the back of the first or second interphalangeal joint (knuckle), and encourage the infant to pull the finger deeply into the mouth and start sucking properly before allowing milk to be transferred. Alternate feeding can be performed against or near the bare breast to help the infant associate the breast with feeding.

Fingerfeeding

There is little published research on fingerfeeding of newborns, though it is recommended by respected clinicians as an alternative to cup feeding for infants who are unable to breastfeed (Marmet, Shell, & Aldana, 2000; Newman, 1990, 1996). Substitution of fingerfeeding for bottle feeding in preterm infants with developing or faulty sucking techniques in a hospital in Perth, Australia, increased the rate of breastfeeding on discharge from 44% to 71% (Oddy & Glenn, 2003).

Fingerfeeding reinforces the contingent nature of feeding (Bovey, Noble, & Noble, 1999). Done properly, it puts the infant in control. The choice of feeding tool is determined first by the infant's capabilities and needs and then the parent's abilities and preferences. A baby with some oral motor competency can use the Hazelbaker FingerFeeder (Hygeia Inc.). The Hazelbaker container rests in the feeder's hand, and a soft, flexible tube can be held to the finger with the thumb or taped to the finger (**Figure 12-40**). The top of the container contains a valve, so the infant needs to draw milk from the tube by forming negative pressure in the mouth. The container is soft enough to allow the feeder to squeeze it to supplement the infant's efforts.

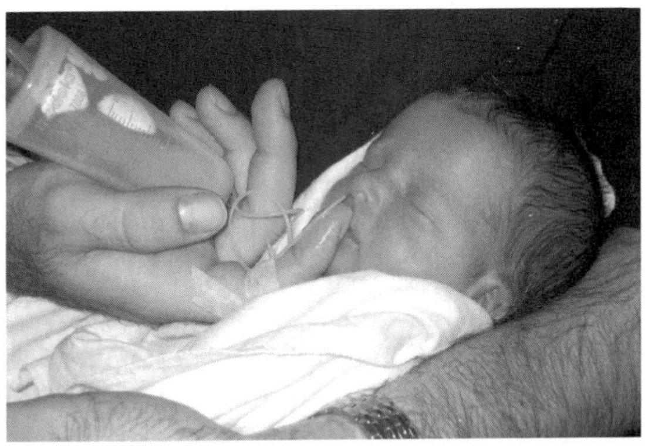

Figure 12-40 Hazelbaker FingerFeeder used by the father of a preterm infant. Note the use of a large finger and the position of the finger across the lips to stimulate gape.

Whichever device is chosen, the tube is placed either atop or beside an adult finger. A large finger, such as the index finger or middle finger, is preferred for better modeling of the mouth position on the breast. The finger is held pad side up to better conform to the palate. The feeder should stimulate the infant's gape response and encourage a wide gape to preserve this breastfeeding behavior. To stimulate the gape response, the feeder can cross the nail side of the finger across the infant's lips, with the second knuckle bent and the fingertip at the infant's philtrum. When the infant opens wide, the finger is slid along the palate until it reaches the junction of the hard and soft palates. The infant will quickly learn to assist with the tongue in pulling the finger into the mouth. This skill can later be generalized to breastfeeding.

When the infant sucks, a small bolus (0.5–1.0 cc) is delivered to the infant. If milk spills from the corner of the baby's lips, the respiratory rate increases markedly; or if the baby shows any stress signs (splayed fingers or widened eyes), the milk flow is slowed. Ideally, feeding should proceed at a pace that allows a 1:1 suck–swallow ratio during sucking bursts, particularly at the beginning of the feeding. Feeding should follow the normal burst–pause pattern of a 3–5 second respiratory break after a sucking burst of 5–20 sucks, depending on the infant's maturity and aerobic capacity. Devices with which the infant self-paces (Hazelbaker FingerFeeder) should be used only when the infant has sufficient feeding competence to move milk from the device reliably. Devices that are designed for supplementing at the breast (Lact-Aid, Supply Line, and SNS) are useful for fingerfeeding if a slow flow is needed, such as for an infant with a respiratory issue that causes reduced aerobic capacity. These devices might not supply sufficient flow or might require too much work for preterm or ill infants. As always, careful assessment of the results of any intervention and its appropriateness for each individual dyad is imperative.

Very fine control of milk delivery can be achieved with a periodontal syringe, a curved tip syringe commonly used by dentists to irrigate the mouth. Fine control is particularly important for very preterm infants or infants with swallowing difficulties who need practice in swallowing tiny boluses presented at longer intervals, because control of swallowing is better during isolated rather than sequential swallows (Chi-Fishman & Sonies, 2000).

Curved-tip (periodontal) syringes are not soft and flexible like supplementer tubes and therefore should be introduced against the feeder's finger after the baby has grasped the finger to the junction of the hard and soft palate. The feeder should keep the syringe tip pressed against the finger toward the front of the baby's mouth to avoid poking the oral mucosa with the stiff tip.

Fingerfeeding for Oral Motor Facilitation. Fingerfeeding can be used during oral stimulation to couple milk flow with improved tongue movements. It is especially useful to help reduce tongue tip elevation (the firm tactile input helps the infant realize that food sources go on top of the tongue) and to reduce tongue retraction and posterior elevation. To reduce tongue retraction, a small amplitude circular massage can be performed on the posterior tongue with the (trimmed) nail side of the finger to stimulate extension. Milk is not delivered while the tongue is retracted; it is delivered when the tongue tip is over the anterior gum ridge.

To reduce posterior elevation, the feeder can angle the fingertip downward against the humped posterior tongue to provide counter-pressure, or a gentle forward stroking motion can be used (like smoothing out the humped tongue as if it were a wrinkle in a piece of fabric). Sublingual pressure can be provided at the same time to increase the forward traction on the tongue (**Figure 12-41**). Some degree of posterior tongue elevation is normal during sucking, so the feeder should not attempt to cause the infant to flatten the tongue completely.

Oral Stimulation

In studies of fetal amniotic fluid swallowing, perioral self-stimulation usually preceded swallowing (Miller, Sonies, & Macedonia, 2003). Hand-to-mouth movements are part of the newborn breast-seeking (self-attachment) behavior (Matthiesen, Ransjo-Arvidson, Nissen, & Uvnas-Moberg, 2001). Preterm infants in neonatal intensive care incubators

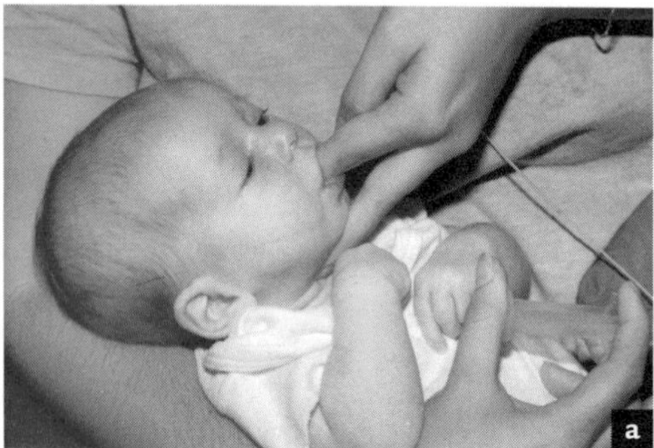

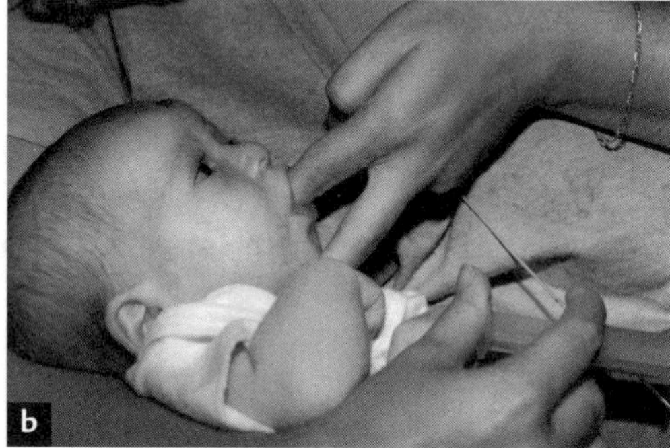

Figure 12-41 Fingerfeeding with sublingual pressure. When the infant humps the posterior tongue, the feeder provides counter-pressure.

benefit from perioral stimulation and show faster maturation of feeding skills (Fucile, Gisel, & Lau, 2005). Earlier experience with oral feeding (Bromiker et al., 2005) and constant skin-to-skin care (Kangaroo Mother Care) (Cattaneo et al., 1998; Penalva & Schwartzman, 2006) also improve the feeding abilities of preterm infants (**Figure 12-42**).

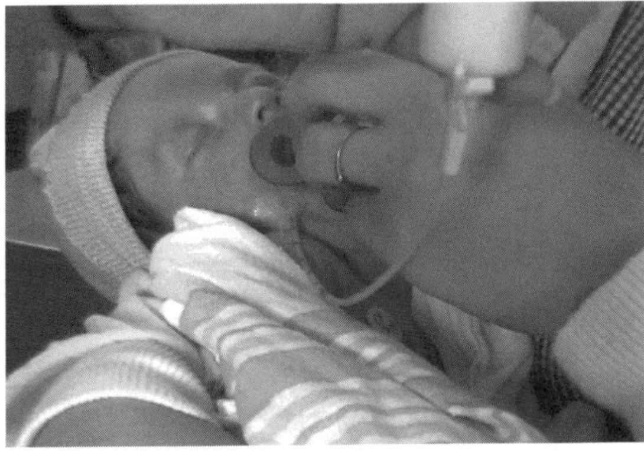

Figure 12-42 Preterm, neurologically impaired infant receiving gavage feeding after feeding at breast but transferring little milk. Sucking on the breast or pacifier during gavage feedings facilitates the transition to oral feeding.

For infants with impaired oral reflexes and feeding problems, gentle oral stimulation before feeding decreased oral motor dysfunction and improved milk transfer at breast and bottle in a blinded but uncontrolled experiment (Rendon-Macias et al., 1999). Simply stimulating the infant to open the mouth and suck a clean or gloved adult finger may stimulate the infant's central pattern generator for sucking and promote feeding behaviors. This mechanism may underlie the success of suck training (Marmet & Shell, 1984). Bovey et al. (1999) recommend observing for specific motor deficits and targeting these rather than using stereotyped interventions.

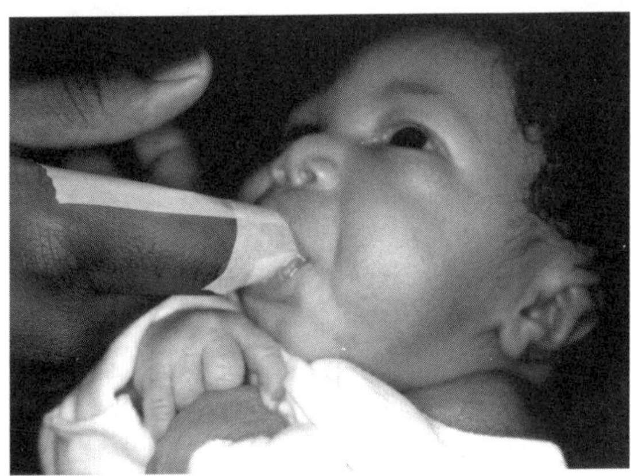

Figure 12-43 Infant enjoying fingerfeeding.

Infants have a strong drive to suck. In addition to providing food, sucking helps improve neurobehavioral organization and relieves pain. As long as the infant is in control of whether or not a finger enters the mouth and how long it stays, and appropriate infection control is used (hand washing in all cases, and the use of a glove or finger cot if not a member of the infant's household), oral exercises are unlikely to do harm (**Figure 12-43**). It is important to model sensitivity to and respect for the infant in all interactions and actively instruct the parents in how to read and respond to the infant's cues. Stress signs in neurologically impaired infants can be far more subtle than in typical infants. Subtly tightening the orbicularis oris muscle to purse the lips, lifting a finger or two, closing the eyes, or subtle changes in respiratory pattern or other autonomic functions mean the infant is overstimulated and needs a break (**Figures 12-44 and 12-45**).

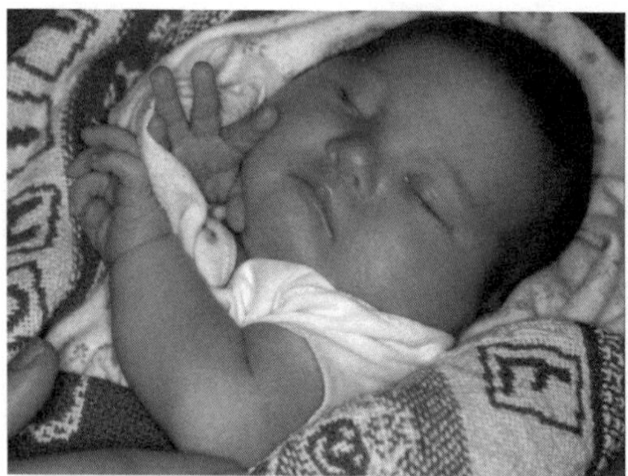

Figure 12-44 Infant with Down syndrome warding off stimulation.

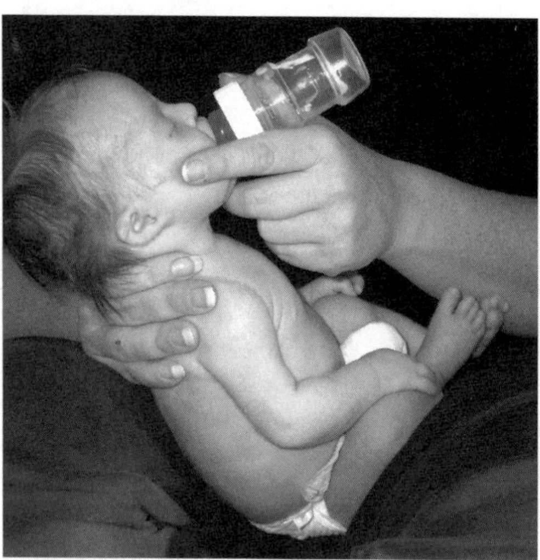

Figure 12-45 Cheek and jaw support during bottle feeding for an infant with Down syndrome and significant hypotonia.

Books on feeding issues for speech and occupational therapists are fertile sources for oral motor facilitation information, but many are based on the US *cultural* norm of bottle feeding. Lactation consultants and therapists working with breastfeeding infants can modify these exercises to compensate for the differences in muscle activation, movements, and cueing required for the *biological* norm of breastfeeding. Briefly, encouraging a large gape, stimulating the tongue to depress and extend as the mouth opens, increasing midline tongue grooving and wave-like movements from anterior to posterior, decreasing tongue humping (excessive posterior elevation), and strengthening lip tone without encouraging pursing are all goals compatible with normal feeding.

Ideally, the infant will be an active participant in the exercise, and it will be enjoyable for both the infant and the adult. Smiling, making eye contact, and making amusing sounds to go along with the touch stimuli can increase enjoyment for infants who tolerate multimodal stimulation. Those who are easily overstimulated may prefer a quieter voice and less eye contact. Infants with low alertness or energy may not respond immediately and may benefit from being primed for oral stimulation by gentle massage near the temporomandibular joint (TMJ) and stroking of the cheeks from the TMJ to the corner of the lips. Low-energy infants may not open the mouth spontaneously at first. Gently running a finger across the lips until they relax (**Figure 12-46**), slipping a finger under the lip to massage the outer surfaces of the gums until the baby opens the mouth (**Figure 12-47**), stroking the hard palate until the tongue makes an attempt to grasp the finger (**Figure 12-48**), and then presenting the finger to suck may allow a low-energy infant to wake up and participate.

The timing of oral exercises needs to be individualized. Cognitively impaired infants may have more difficulty generalizing learning. This may make it more difficult for them to transfer newly learned tongue movements from the finger to the breast if the exercises

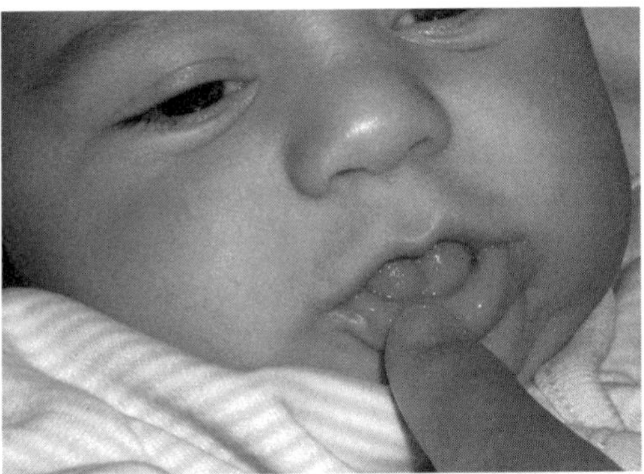

Figure 12-46 Touch to the lips encourages the infant to open the mouth.

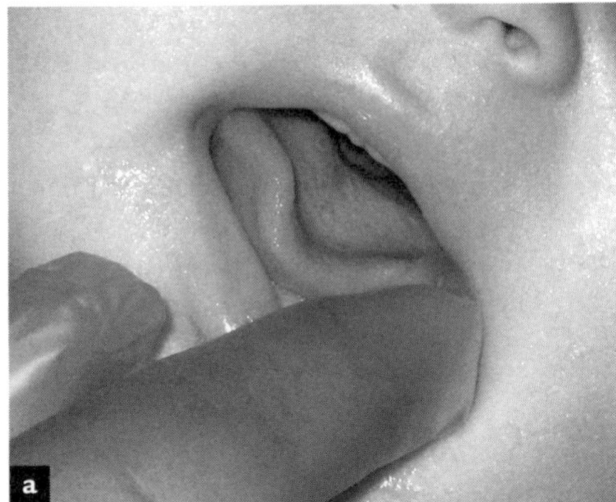

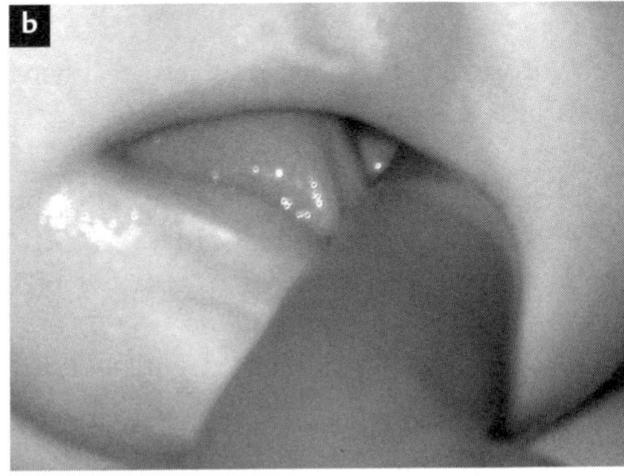

Figure 12-47 (Above) Stimulating the transverse tongue reflex, which causes the tongue to lateralize when the side of the gum is stroked.

are not temporally associated with feeding. Neurologically impaired infants are also more likely to become disorganized by stimulation, which negatively impacts feeding skills. Careful observation of the infant for alert times between feedings, starting the exercise before the infant shows feeding behaviors or cues, or doing the exercise after feeding from one breast and before offering the second (for infants who need paired feedings) are all possible timing strategies for infants who do not tolerate a brief facilitation break before feeding.

Basic Suck Training

In this method by Marmet and Shell (1984), the rooting reflex is stimulated by stroking the cheek toward the lips with a fingertip, then the lips are brushed to induce the infant to open the mouth. The gums are massaged, first the outside of the lower gums, then the tooth-bearing surfaces, then the outsides of the upper gums and their tooth-bearing surfaces. The finger is slid into the mouth with the pad side up, and the posterior hard palate and tongue are alternately rubbed, giving downward and forward pressure to the tongue. Alternatively, the finger can be inserted with

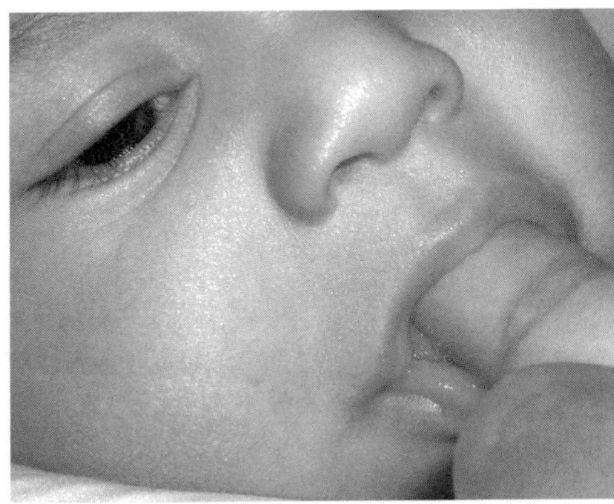

Figure 12-48 The finger pad is up and deep in the mouth, with the fingertip at the junction of the hard and soft palates.

the pad side toward the tongue and behind the humped posterior tongue, which is gently pulled forward with the fingertip. Milk is supplied when the tongue is correctly positioned over the lower gum. The authors recommend using the suck training technique before each feeding until the infant's suckling pattern is corrected.

The Oral Stimulation Program for Infants with Neurologically and Medically Based Sucking Disabilities

This program, created by Rendon-Macias and colleagues (1999), started with the infant's head extended, and the rooting reflex was gently stimulated by light fingertip touch to the cheeks and lips. The upper lip and anterior surface of the gum was massaged using a small circular motion for 5 minutes, then a 1 cm circular motion was used at the lateral gums and inner surfaces of the cheek. Gentle pressure was applied to the lower lip, and then firm pressure was placed on the hard palate to stimulate sucking. In older infants, a drop of honey was then placed on the palate (human milk should be substituted in infants younger than age 1 year to avoid the risk of botulism), and the infant was given a pacifier continuously between feedings.

The authors reported that "the application of positive oral tactile stimuli with the removal of harmful stimuli, induced the recovery of oral reflexes in the infants in our study" (Rendon-Macias et al., 1999, p. 326).

Oral Motor Preparatory Stimulation for Hypotonic Infants

Babies who do not gape widely can be stroked or massaged in small spirals all along the edge of the jawline, starting just in front of the baby's ear and working simultaneously down both sides of the jaw to the tip of the chin. This can cue the baby that these long muscles need to wake up and provide the power for a wide gape and the opening and closing of the mouth we see in babies who latch and feed well. This can be repeated two or three times and need not take more than a few seconds.

Speech-language therapists suggest following the jaw massage with several gentle compressions in the middle of each cheek. Gentle compression in the center of each cheek with the thumb and middle finger of one hand provides sensory stimulation to the sides of the tongue as it gently meets the fat pad of each cheek. This can help bring the tongue forward in the mouth in preparation for latching on to the breast. Finally, and also briefly, the baby's lower lip can be gently flipped or stroked downward, providing the baby with the same sensation that initiates seeking as the baby's chin touches mom's breast—gentle neck extension, wide gaping, tongue movement down and forward over the alveolar gum ridge, and overall readiness to draw breast tissue deep into the baby's mouth for effective and comfortable nursing.

Stimulating Central Grooving of the Tongue

Side Sweep. After stimulating the infant to open wide, place the finger flat on the front half of the tongue in midline. Pause. Then sweep the finger along the tongue from the center to one side, pause, sweep back to the center, pause, then sweep to the opposite side, pause, then sweep back to center. This stimulates the transverse intrinsic muscle layer that runs from side to side in the tongue, which contracts to form the central groove.

Slide Back. After stimulating mouth opening with a finger to the philtrum, slide the fingertip along the tongue in midline from the tip to about halfway back. Repeat several times as tolerated.

Stroking the Tongue. This exercise not only supports central grooving, but also helps reduce tongue retraction. The infant is stimulated to open wide, and a finger is placed on the middle of the tongue in midline. The fingertip is pressed down on the tongue in midline and slides along the tongue as it is withdrawn from the mouth. The infant can be told "tongue down" while the stroke is occurring.

Stimulating Wavelike Tongue Movements

Walking Back on the Tongue. The infant is stimulated to open the mouth by a touch to the philtrum or upper lip. The fingertip is placed on the tongue, just beyond the tongue tip, and wiggled in place to provide vibration to the tongue. The finger slides back a few millimeters, and vibration is repeated. This is repeated all along the front half of the tongue, stopping short of stimulating the gag reflex.

This exercise is meant to stimulate sequential muscle contraction of the tongue from front to back, in the direction of the wavelike movements of normal swallowing. If a mechanical vibrator is used, it should be held in the adult's hand so the vibration is transferred through the finger. The First Years sells vibrating teething toys for infant use; they can be used for this exercise, or they can be given to infants so they can mouth them and increase oral tone.

Wiggle Worm. Joan Dietrich Comrie, CCC-SLP, uses the following exercise to stimulate normal tongue tone and movements. The infant is stimulated to open the mouth, and the finger pad (up to the second joint) is placed on the tongue in midline. The tongue is stroked from anterior to posterior with firm but gentle downward pressure, like kneading bread dough.

Sequential Stimulation of Feeding-Related Reflex Movements

When infants do not seem to make the correct sequence of movements to attach to the breast, this sequence is sometimes helpful. For infants suspected of autistic spectrum disorders or other infants who are easily overwhelmed by sensations, it is helpful to engineer the environment to reduce the sensory load before using the exercise (lower lights, turn off noise sources, and perhaps undress or swaddle the infant below the waist).

Hold a finger across the infant's lips, with the nail side of the finger at the philtrum and the second joint right below the center of the lower lip. When the infant opens the mouth (gapes), the fingertip touches the front of the lower gum ridge until the tongue is extended and depressed. The tongue tip is then gently tickled with the fingertip until the tongue grasps the finger and the infant begins to pull the finger into the mouth. The feeder may continue the motion until the finger pad is on the posterior hard palate, at or near the junction of the soft palate. The palate can be stimulated by wiggling the fingertip on the palate to start the sucking reflex. Milk is then delivered from the feeding device as in normal fingerfeeding. When the infant begins to perform more of the feeding sequence without the individual stimulation steps (searches for the finger with the lips and tongue and draws it in and immediately begins sucking), the infant is placed at breast in the instinctive position and is encouraged to gape by placing a finger on the philtrum, if the baby does not respond to the breast with this behavior. Drops of milk can be expressed onto the nipple for the infant to smell, and a curved tip syringe can be used to deliver a bit of milk to reward any attempt to close the mouth on the areola. These inducements can be withdrawn as the infant becomes more skilled at breastfeeding.

The lactation consultant may encounter infants exhibiting a variety of problems that may interfere with their ability to breastfeed. Interventions that may help the infant to breastfeed can be employed when the basis of the problem is understood and appropriate techniques are chosen. Until oral motor evaluation and facilitation become a standardized part of lactation consultant training, each consultant will need to decide which of these techniques fit her expertise and comfort level. Unless the lactation specialist is also a therapist, infants who are having difficulty feeding should be referred for evaluation, particularly when the difficulty occurs during both breastfeeding *and* bottle feeding. The lactation consultant is a specialist in normal feeding and can provide valuable input to the other members of the feeding team.

Dysphagia and the Neurologically Involved Baby

Infants with neurological deficits are at greater risk for dysphagia. Full-term infants may suffer from neurologically based or structurally based swallowing difficulties, whereas for very low birth weight infants, dysphagia may be among their residual disabilities.

The videofluoroscopic swallow study (VFSS) was developed to study the oropharyngeal phases of the swallow in adults and has been generalized to children (Arvedson & Brodsky, 2002). The VFSS is conducted by a speech-language pathologist (SLP) and radiologist. In some institutions, an occupational therapist may carry out the study or be present to assist with positioning. A clinical assessment, including a thorough history, is always performed before requesting a VFSS. Postural and flow rate adjustments should be part of the clinical assessment to determine if these will improve feeding safety. Infant endurance, medical condition, cognitive abilities, and level of alertness are prerequisites.

The VFSS allows the therapist to observe the infant or child's oropharyngeal structures during bottle feeding. Healthcare providers have frequently not evaluated feeding skills at the breast in neurologically impaired infants, nor have they included breastfeeding in therapeutic goals. There have been some reports at feeding conferences that SLPs are including breastfeeding in addition to bottle feeding during VFSS. One SLP has been using barium contrast in human milk in a supplementer used at breast. The difficulty in performing VFSS during breastfeeding lies in positioning mother and infant in a way that allows imaging without disrupting attachment. When a breastfeeding infant is evaluated using a bottle, an accurate picture of the infant's ability to control flow and transfer milk may not be obtained due to differences in flow patterns and volume of milk delivered per bolus. Research comparing respiration and heart rate in preterm infants who served as their own controls showed less disruption of either rate while breastfeeding (Meier, 1988; Meier & Anderson 1987). Furthermore, infants who were bottle fed different fluids had safer swallowing and better coordination of sucking, swallowing, and breathing with human milk versus formula or water (Mizuno, Ueda, & Takeuchi, 2002). With this information in mind, the infant's breastfeeding abilities deserve evaluation. Ultrasound is becoming an important diagnostic tool to study the oral preparatory and oral phases of the swallow and may provide another modality that is more accurate for breastfeeding infants (Geddes, Chadwick, Kent, Garbin, & Hartmann, 2010; Weber, Woolridge, & Baum, 1986; Yang, Loveday, Metreweli, & Sullivan, 1997).

Fiberoptic endoscopic evaluation of swallowing (FEES) does not observe the actual swallow, but it can identify residue from dyed food in the airway immediately after the swallow. There are some reports of FEES being used during breastfeeding, though they are not documented in the literature. The main challenge would be getting the coloring agent into the baby's mouth along with the breast, again this could theoretically be done with a lactation aid or nursing supplementer.

Options when aspiration is diagnosed include changing positions (prone feeding on a reclining mother works well for improving swallowing during breastfeeding), pacing the feeding, thickening, and limiting oral feeding and substituting tube feedings. Thickening human milk is problematic due to its enzyme content and requires that milk come from a container other than the breast. Coordination of swallowing and breathing is likely to be best during breastfeeding, and human milk is a biocompatible fluid that is less irritating to the human airway than other substances. Experiences at the breast should not be discontinued unless significant sequelae of aspiration are occurring. Techniques to decrease or minimize flow are possible to allow the infant to be at the breast when alternate means of feeding are deemed necessary due to risk of aspiration. Sucking for comfort at the freshly expressed breast helps to preserve immunological communication between infant saliva and the maternal enteromammary system, and it preserves at least part of a relationship that was important to both mother and child.

Infants and children with neurologically based feeding problems require periodic monitoring for changes in ability. With a degenerative neurological disorder, swallowing ability will quite probably deteriorate over time. A child with mild cerebral palsy or prematurity may continue to improve. Each infant or child should be approached as an individual with strengths and weaknesses. The mother should be assisted to breastfeed, whether exclusively or in combination with alternative feeding methods.

Postural Support

In addition to supportive positioning and preparatory handling, certain postural modifications may help infants with dysphagia. Some infants handle flow best when side-lying, others when their head is elevated relative to the rest of the body, as in a sitting football hold or a straddle position. Prone positioning with the mother reclining may be the most helpful position for breastfeeding infants with swallowing difficulty. Pacing, or regulating, an infant by breaking the suction when signs of stress occur during feeding can be done at the breast. The mother should be instructed to insert her finger between the gums to break suction. Because breaking the suction and removing the breast from the infant's mouth can make it difficult for the infant to reorganize, it should be carried out when the infant is experiencing a problem, but not on a frequent basis throughout the feeding. One mother sang out "one, two, three" to let her infant know that the pause was temporary. If the preterm or neurologically impaired infant requires frequent pacing at the breast due to incoordination of sucking, swallowing, and breathing, another option is to have the mother express her breasts until the first (and usually strongest) milk ejection subsides prior to breastfeeding. This reduces the active flow of the breast, when babies typically experience difficulty with bolus control, but it can have the unwanted effect of increasing milk production, which itself increases flow. Pressing on the breast with the side of the hand to block off some ducts is another way to temporarily reduce flow, especially during the first and strongest milk ejection. Signs of difficulty necessitating a break include nasal flaring, rapid respirations, frequent swallows without breathing pauses, gulping, choking, coughing, or stridor. For further suggestions and information on improving flow control issues, see Chapter 6.

Feeding Environment

A quiet feeding environment with low lights may assist a neurologically immature or involved infant by facilitating organization and a quiet alert state. Picking the infant up and maintaining containment by holding him or her in flexion against the mother's or assistant's body will ease the transition from the sleeping surface to where the feeding will take place (Waitzman, 2002). Some feeding therapists find that rocking a full-term or older infant from head to toe at the rate of one rock per second helps reinforce the rhythm of suck-swallow-breathe. Other therapists have used classical music that has that same one beat per second rhythm (Morris & Klein, 2001). Rocking and music may be too much stimulation for preterm infants, however, and is generally not recommended for that population.

Gastroesophageal Reflux

Gastroesophageal reflux (GER) is a normal occurrence in infants younger than age 1 year, with regurgitation resolving by 6–7 months in 71% of infants, and breastfed infants improving sooner (Campanozzi et al., 2009). Campanozzi and colleagues' prospective study showed that short, frequent feeds, appropriate positioning for feeding, and burping after feeds reduced symptoms in 72% of infants. According to Rudolf (2006), GER is not a disease in itself, but the consequences of reflux can contribute to disease. Reflux takes place when the strength of the lower esophageal sphincter is overcome by increased abdominal or thoracic pressure (Bibi et al., 2001). Infants who are at greater risk for developing gastroesophageal reflux disease (GERD) have diagnoses of prematurity, congenital heart disease, esophageal atresia, tracheoesophageal fistula, brainstem tumors, airway anomalies, or neurological impairment. GER affects the esophageal phase of the swallow and can be present with or without oropharyngeal dysphagia.

GERD can damage the lining of the esophagus and predisposes the infant to aspiration by damaging the recurrent laryngeal nerve (Suskind et al., 2006). GER can be the cause or contribute to the severity of respiratory disease, including allergies and asthma. When the infant or child has labored breathing from asthma or bronchopulmonary dysplasia (respiratory disease seen in premature infants), thoracic pressure increases. Some of the signs and symptoms of GERD include vomiting, gagging, choking, apnea, halitosis, frequent swallowing, burping, stridor, coughing, hiccoughing, gurgly respirations, irritability, torticollis (Sandifer syndrome), back arching, sleep disturbances, recurrent respiratory infections, feeding refusal, and acute life-threatening events (Arvedson & Brodsky, 2002).

The gastroenterologist uses a variety of tests to diagnose GER. Recent studies report pH testing is more effective when combined with impedance probe monitoring, which has the ability to detect nonacidic refluxate and the movement of the bolus through the esophagus (Wenzl, 2003; Wenzl et al., 2001). Endoscopy is another method for evaluating the presence of GERD. Esophagogastroscopy is used for visualizing the mucosa around the esophagus, larynx, and airway, and it can be used to determine if esophagitis or other erosive effects of GERD are taking place (Arvedson & Brodsky, 2002). Ultrasonography has recently been shown helpful in diagnosing GERD in infants and children (Hashemi, Mehdizadeh, & Shakiba, 2009; Koumanidou, Vakaki, Pitsoulakis, Anagnostara, & Mirilas, 2004) and has the advantage of being noninvasive.

Gastroenterologists have treated GERD with both surgery and medications. Studies report that both H2 receptor antagonists and proton pump inhibitors allow the esophageal mucosa to heal and decrease the GER symptoms in infants and children. Antacids and motility drugs are still being used but are reported to have more limited effectiveness. Surgical treatment is considered when medications have proven ineffective or when there are life-threatening complications. A fundoplication is the procedure commonly performed to treat GERD. This procedure involves wrapping the fundus of the stomach around the distal esophagus. A gastrostomy tube may also be placed to prevent complications sometimes seen with the fundoplication procedure, for non-oral feedings when the infant or child has severe symptoms, or to supplement oral feedings. Outcomes of the surgical procedures have been varied, and the selection of patients based on symptoms influences success (Arvedson & Brodsky, 2002; Richards, Milla, Andrews, & Spitz, 2001; Wales et al., 2002).

Feeding therapists have treated GERD in infants by thickening feedings, providing small and frequent feedings, and positioning the infant with the bed elevated after feedings

(Arvedson & Brodsky, 2002; Khoshoo, Ross, Brown, & Edell, 2000; Wolf & Glass, 1992). Arvedson and Brodsky report that thickening may worsen symptoms if the patient has delayed gastric emptying from dysmotility.

McPherson, Wright, and Bell (2005) reviewed a number of methods for managing reflux. They summarized the outcomes of studies that employed various methods for treating the symptoms of vomiting and regurgitation. They reported mixed outcomes regarding treatment of symptoms when carob bean gum thickener was used and a decrease in symptoms when rice cereal was used. In studies that measured improvement through pH probe monitoring to test for acidity, thickening with carob bean gum showed mixed improvement, and thickening with rice cereal showed no improvement. Regarding positioning, when pH was tested with infants in seats positioned at 60 degrees their symptoms worsened, and when infants were placed in beds with the head elevated to 30 degrees they showed no improvement. The authors stated that these various studies primarily focused on formula-fed infants, and reported outcomes were insufficient for application to breastfed infants. In addition, they stated that no strategies were offered for supporting breastfeeding while the infant was being treated.

Several studies revealed difficulties with absorption of calcium, iron, and zinc due to the fiber content of many thickeners mixed with formula (Bosscher, Van Caillie-Bertrand, & Deelstra, 2001; Bosscher et al., 2000; Corvaglia et al., 2006). Human milk was found to have better bioavailability of those minerals when mixed with starch-based thickeners (Bosscher, Lu et al., 2001; Bosscher, Van Caillie-Bertand & Deelstra 2001; Bosscher, Van Dyck, Van Cauwenberg, & Deelstra, 2001); however, a study of preterm infants who were fed breastmilk thickened with a starch-based product found no evidence of decrease in reflux episodes (Corvaglia et al., 2006). Thickeners can cause other adverse effects. Recently, 15 cases of necrotizing enterocolitis (NEC) occurred in preterm infants given SimplyThick from one manufacturing plant, leading the FDA to warn not to feed this product to preterm infants (U.S. Food and Drug Administration, 2011).

Feeding teams should make every effort to maintain breastfeeding infants at the breast. In addition to H2 receptor antagonist or proton pump inhibitors (medications that reduce stomach acid release), strategies that seem useful clinically include short frequent feedings, holding the infant upright for 20 minutes after a feeding, and nonnutritive sucking after feeding to help stimulate esophageal peristalsis. It is important to prevent or treat injury to the esophageal mucosa and vocal fold area that can further stress swallowing and feeding.

Conclusion

Infants with neurological deficits may present with significant feeding challenges. A combination of compensatory strategies and gentle facilitation techniques have been covered that can be employed to help infants with neurological problems achieve normal feeding. Each infant should be evaluated as an individual, and not as a diagnosis, though knowledge of the mechanisms of neurological disorders is helpful in creating strategies to assist feeding. Infants with significant impairments benefit from the input of a feeding team and early intervention specialists. Ideally, the lactation consultant will continue to participate on the child's team to provide expertise in normal feeding.

References

Adam, M. P., & Hudgins, L. (2005). Kabuki syndrome: A review. *Clinical Genetics, 67*(3), 209–219.

Ardran, G. M., & Kemp, F. H. (1968). The mechanism of changes in form of the cervical airway in infancy. *Medical Radiography and Photography, 44*(2), 26–38.

Arvedson, J. C., & Brodsky, L. (2002). *Pediatric swallowing and feeding: Assessment and management* (2nd ed.). Albany, NY: Singular Thomson Learning.

Arvedson, J., Rogers, B., Buck, G., Smart, P., & Msall, M. (1994). Silent aspiration prominent in children with dysphagia. *International Journal of Pediatric Otorhinolaryngology, 28*(2–3), 173–181.

Ashwal, S. (1999). Congenital structural defects. In K. F. Swaiman & S. Ashwal (Eds.), *Pediatric neurology: Principles and practice* (3rd ed., pp. 234–300). St. Louis, MO: Mosby.

Astley, S. J., & Clarren, S. K. (2001). Measuring the facial phenotype of individuals with prenatal alcohol exposure: Correlations with brain dysfunction. *Alcohol and Alcoholism, 36*(2), 147–159.

Bahi-Buisson, N., Poirier, K., Boddaert, N., Fallet-Bianco, C., Specchio, N., Bertini, E., Caglayan O., . . . Chelly, J. (2010). GPR56-related bilateral frontoparietal polymicrogyria: Further evidence for an overlap with the cobblestone complex. *Brain, 133*, 3194–3209.

Bahi-Buisson, N., Poirier, K., Boddaert, N., Saillour, Y., Castelnau, L., Philip, N., Buyse G., . . . Chelly, J. (2008). Refinement of cortical dysgenesis spectrum associated with TUBA1A mutations. *Journal of Medical Genetics, 45*, 647–653.

Batocchi, A. P., Majolini, L., Evoli, A., Lino, M. M., Minisci, C., & Tonali, P. (1999). Course and treatment of myasthenia gravis during pregnancy. *Neurology, 52*(3), 447–452.

Bertrand, J., Floyd, L. L., & Weber, M. K. (2005). Guidelines for identifying and referring persons with fetal alcohol syndrome. *Morbidity and Mortality Weekly Report, Recommended Reports, 54*(RR-11), 1–14.

Bibi, H., Khvolis, E., Shoseyov, D., Ohaly, M., Ben Dor, D., London, D., & Ater, D. (2001). The prevalence of gastroesophageal reflux in children with tracheomalacia and laryngomalacia. *Chest, 119*(2), 409–413.

Boiron, M., Da, N. L., Roux, S., Henrot, A., & Saliba, E. (2007). Effects of oral stimulation and oral support on non-nutritive sucking and feeding performance in preterm infants. *Developmental Medicine and Child Neurology, 49*, 439–444.

Bosscher, D., Lu, Z., Van Caillie-Bertrand, M., Robberecht, H., & Deelstra, H. (2001). A method for in vitro determination of calcium, iron and zinc availability from first-age infant formula and human milk. *International Journal of Food Science and Nutrition, 52*(2), 173–182.

Bosscher, D., Van Caillie-Bertrand, M., & Deelstra, H. (2001). Effect of thickening agents, based on soluble dietary fiber, on the availability of calcium, iron, and zinc from infant formulas. *Nutrition, 17*(7–8), 614–618.

Bosscher, D., Van Caillie-Bertrand, M., Van Dyck, K., Robberecht, H., Van Cauwenberg, R., & Deelstra, H. (2000). Thickening infant formula with digestible and indigestible carbohydrate: Availability of calcium, iron, and zinc in vitro. *Journal of Pediatric Gastroenterology and Nutrition, 30*(4), 373–378.

Bosscher, D., Van Dyck, K., Van Cauwenberg, R., & Deelstra, H. (2001). In vitro availability of calcium, iron, and zinc from first-age infant formulae and human milk. *Journal of Pediatric Gastroenterology and Nutrition, 32*(1), 54–58.

Bouwstra, H., Boersma, E. R., Boehm, G., Dijck-Brouwer, D. A., Muskiet, F. A., & Hadders-Algra, M. (2003). Exclusive breastfeeding of healthy term infants for at least 6 weeks improves neurological condition. *Journal of Nutrition, 133*(12), 4243–4245.

Bovey, A., Noble, R., & Noble, M. (1999). Orofacial exercises for babies with breastfeeding problems? *Breastfeeding Review, 7*(1), 23–28.

Bromiker, R., Arad, I., Loughran, B., Netzer, D., Kaplan, M., & Medoff-Cooper, B. (2005). Comparison of sucking patterns at introduction of oral feeding and at term. *Acta Paediatrica, 94*(2), 201–204.

Campanozzi, A., Boccia, G., Pensabene, L., Panetta, F., Marseglia, A., Strisciuglio, P., Barbera, C., . . . Staiano, A. (2009). Prevalence and natural history of gastroesophageal reflux: Pediatric prospective survey. *Pediatrics, 123*, 779–783.

Cattaneo, A., Davanzo, R., Worku, B., Surjono, A., Echeverria, M., Bedri, A., Haksari, E., . . . Tamburlini, G. (1998). Kangaroo mother care for low birthweight infants: A randomized controlled trial in different settings. *Acta Paediatrica, 87*(9), 976–985.

Cerruti Mainardi, P. (2006). Cri du chat syndrome. *Orphanet Journal of Rare Diseases, 1*, 33.

Chapman, N. H., Estes, A., Munson, J., Bernier, R., Webb, S. J., Rothstein, J. H., Minshew, N. J., . . . Wijsman, E. M. (2011). Genome-scan for IQ discrepancy in autism: Evidence for loci on chromosomes 10 and 16. *Human Genetics, 129*, 59–70.

Chen, D. C., Nommsen-Rivers, L., Dewey, K. G., & Lonnerdal, B. (1998). Stress during labor and delivery and early lactation performance. *American Journal of Clinical Nutrition, 68*(2), 335–344.

Chi-Fishman, G., & Sonies, B. C. (2000). Motor strategy in rapid sequential swallowing: New insights. *Journal of Speech, Language, and Hearing Research, 43*(6), 1481–1492.

Ciafaloni, E., & Massey, J. M. (2004). The management of myasthenia gravis in pregnancy. *Seminars in Neurology, 24*(1), 95–100.

Clarke, D. J., & Boer, H. (1998). Problem behaviors associated with deletion Prader-Willi, Smith-Magenis, and cri du chat syndromes. *American Journal of Mental Retardation, 103*(3), 264–271.

Cole, N. W., Pfeifer, H. H., & Thiele, E. A. (2010). Initiating and maintaining the ketogenic diet in breastfed infants. *ICAN: Infant, Child, and Adolescent Nutrition, 2*, 177–180.

Colson, S. D., de Rooy, L., & Hawdon, J. M. (2003). Biological nurturing increases duration of breastfeeding for a vulnerable cohort. *MIDIRS Midwifery Digest, 13*, 92–97.

Corvaglia, L., Ferlini, M., Rotatori, R., Paoletti, V., Alessandroni, R., Cocchi, G., & Faldella, G. (2006). Starch thickening of human milk is ineffective in reducing the gastroesophageal reflux in preterm infants: A crossover study using intraluminal impedance. *Journal of Pediatrics, 148*(2), 265–268.

Cusco, I., Medrano, A., Gener, B., Vilardell, M., Gallastegui, F., Villa, O., Gonzalez, E., . . . Perez-Jurado, L. A. (2009). Autism-specific copy number variants further implicate the phosphatidylinositol signaling pathway and the glutamatergic synapse in the etiology of the disorder. *Human Molecular Genetics, 18*, 1795–1804.

Daley, H. K., & Kennedy, C. M. (2000). Meta analysis: Effects of interventions on premature infants feeding. *Journal of Perinatal and Neonatal Nursing, 14*, 62–77.

Daly, S. E., Owens, R. A., & Hartmann, P. E. (1993). The short-term synthesis and infant-regulated removal of milk in lactating women. *Experimental Physiology, 78*(2), 209–220.

Dapretto, M., Davies, M. S., Pfiefer, J. H., Scott, A. A., Sigman, M., Bookheimer, S. Y., & Iacoboni, M. (2006). Understanding emotions in others: Mirror neuron dysfunction in children with autism spectrum disorders. *Nature Neuroscience, 9*(1), 28–30.

Fucile, S., & Gisel, E. G. (2010). Sensorimotor interventions improve growth and motor function in preterm infants. *Neonatal Network, 29*, 359–366.

Fucile, S., Gisel, E. G., & Lau, C. (2005). Effect of an oral stimulation program on sucking skill maturation of preterm infants. *Developmental Medicine and Child Neurology, 47*(3), 158–162.

Geddes, D. T., Chadwick, L. M., Kent, J. C., Garbin, C. P., & Hartmann, P. E. (2010). Ultrasound imaging of infant swallowing during breast-feeding. *Dysphagia, 25*, 183–191.

Genna, C. W. (2009). *Selecting and using breastfeeding tools improving care and outcomes*. Amarillo, TX: Hale.

Gohlke, J. M., Griffith, W. C., & Faustman, E. M. (2005). A systems-based computational model for dose-response comparisons of two modes of action hypotheses for ethanol-induced neurodevelopmental toxicity. *Toxicological Sciences, 86*(2), 470–484.

Gressens, P. (2005). Neuronal migration disorders. *Journal of Child Neurology, 20*(12), 969–971.

Grigorenko, E. L., Han, S. S., Yrigollen, C. M., Leng, L., Mizue, Y., Anderson, G. M., Mulder, E. J., . . . Bucala, R . (2008). Macrophage migration inhibitory factor and autism spectrum disorders. *Pediatrics, 122*, e438–e445.

Guerrini, R. (2005). Genetic malformations of the cerebral cortex and epilepsy. *Epilepsia, 46*(Suppl. 1), 32–37.

Hashemi, H., Mehdizadeh, M., & Shakiba, M. (2009). Diagnostic efficacy of distal esophagus ultrasonography in diagnosis of gastroesophageal reflux disease in children. *Research Journal of Biological Sciences, 4*, 71–76.

Hiiemae, K. M., & Palmer, J. B. (2003). Tongue movements in feeding and speech. *Critical Reviews in Oral Biology and Medicine, 14*, 413–429.

Hill, P. D., Aldaq, J. C., & Chatterton, R. T. (2001). Initiation and frequency of pumping and milk production in mothers of non-nursing preterm infants. *Journal of Human Lactation, 17*(1), 9–13.

Holm, V. A., & Pipes, P. L. (1976). Food and children with Prader-Willi syndrome. *Archives of Pediatrics and Adolescent Medicine, 130*, 1063–1067.

Jacinto-Gonçalves, S., Gavião, M. B., & Berzin, F. (2004). Electromyographic activity of perioral muscle in breastfed and non-breastfed children. *Journal of Clinical Pediatric Dentistry, 29*(1), 57–62.

Jones, E., Dimmock, P. W., & Spencer, S. A. (2001). A randomised controlled trial to compare methods of milk expression after preterm delivery. *Archives of Disease in Childhood, Fetal Neonatal Edition, 85*, F91–F95.

Kassing, D. (2002). Bottle-feeding as a tool to reinforce breastfeeding. *Journal of Human Lactation, 18*(1), 56–60.

Kato, M., & Dobyns, W. B. (2003). Lissencephaly and the molecular basis of neuronal migration. *Human Molecular Genetics, 12*(Spec. No. 1), R89–R96.

Khoshoo, V., Ross, G., Brown, S., & Edell, D. (2000). Smaller volume, thickened formulas in the management of gastroesophageal reflux in thriving infants. *Journal of Pediatric Gastroenterology and Nutrition, 31*(5), 554–556.

Kim, H. I., Palmini, A., Choi, H. Y., Kim, Y. H., & Lee, J. C. (1994). Congenital bilateral perisylvian syndrome: Analysis of the first four reported Korean patients. *Journal of Korean Medical Science, 9*(4), 335–340.

Knickmeyer, R. C., & Baron-Cohen, S. (2006). Fetal testosterone and sex differences in typical social development and in autism. *Journal of Child Neurology, 21*(10), 825–845.

Koumanidou, C., Vakaki, M., Pitsoulakis, G., Anagnostara, A., & Mirilas, P. (2004). Sonographic measurement of the abdominal esophagus length in infancy: A diagnostic tool for gastroesophageal reflux. *AJR American Journal of Roentgenology, 183*, 801–807.

Kuzniecky, R., Andermann, F., & Guerrini, R. (1993). Congenital bilateral perisylvian syndrome: Study of 31 patients. The CBPS Multicenter Collaborative Study. *Lancet, 341*(8845), 608–612.

Lau, C., & Schanler, R. J. (1996). Oral motor function in the neonate. *Neonatal Gastroenterology, 23*(2), 161–178.

LeBouder, E., Rey-Nores, J. E., Raby, A. C., Affolter, M., Vidal, K., Thornton, C. A., & Labeta, M. O. (2006). Modulation of neonatal microbial recognition: TLR-mediated innate immune responses are specifically and differentially modulated by human milk. *Journal of Immunology, 176*, 3742–3752.

Ludington-Hoe, S. M., Cong, X., & Hashemi, F. (2002). Infant crying: Nature, physiologic consequences, and select interventions. *Neonatal Network, 21*(2), 29–36.

Mandelli, M., Tognoni, G., & Garattini, S. (1978). Clinical pharmacokinetics of diazepam. *Clinical Pharmacokinetics, 3*(1), 72–91.

Marmet, C., & Shell, E. (1984). Training neonates to suck correctly. *The American Journal of Maternal Child Nursing, 9*(6), 401–407.

Marmet, C., Shell, E., & Aldana, S. (2000). Assessing infant suck dysfunction: Case management. *Journal of Human Lactation, 16*(4), 332–336.

Matthiesen, A. S., Ransjo-Arvidson, A. B., Nissen, E., & Uvnas-Moberg, K. (2001). Postpartum maternal oxytocin release by newborns: Effects of infant hand massage and sucking. *Birth, 28*(1), 13–19.

McBride, M. C., & Danner, S. C. (1987). Sucking disorders in neurologically impaired infants: Assessment and management. *Clinical Perinatology, 14*(1), 109–130.

McGirt, M. J., Leveque, J. C., Wellons, J. C., III, Villavicencio, A. T., Hopkins, J. S., Fuchs, H. E., & George, T. M. (2002). Cerebrospinal fluid shunt survival and etiology of failures: A seven-year institutional experience. *Pediatric Neurosurgery, 36*(5), 248–255.

McPherson, V., Wright, S. T., & Bell, A. D. (2005). Clinical inquiries. What is the best treatment for gastroesophageal reflux and vomiting in infants? *Journal of Family Practice, 54*(4), 372–375.

Meier, P. (1988). Bottle- and breast-feeding: Effects on transcutaneous oxygen pressure and temperature in preterm infants. *Nursing Research, 37*(1), 36–41.

Meier, P., & Anderson, G. C. (1987). Responses of small preterm infants to bottle and breast-feeding. *American Journal of Maternal Child Nursing, 12*(2), 97–105.

Miller, J. L., Sonies, B. C., & Macedonia, C. (2003). Emergence of oropharyngeal, laryngeal and swallowing activity in the developing fetal upper aerodigestive tract: An ultrasound evaluation. *Early Human Development, 71*(1), 61–87.

Mizuno, K., Aizawa, M., Saito, S., Kani, K., Tanaka, S., Kawamura, H., . . . Doherty, D. (2006). Analysis of feeding behavior with direct linear transformation. *Early Human Development, 82*(3), 199–204.

Mizuno, K., & Ueda, A. (2005). Neonatal feeding performance as a predictor of neurodevelopmental outcome at 18 months. *Developmental Medicine and Child Neurology, 47*, 299–304.

Mizuno, K., Ueda, A., Kani, K., & Kawamura, H. (2002). Feeding behaviour of infants with cleft lip and palate. *Acta Paediatrica, 91*(11), 1227–1232.

Mizuno, K., Ueda, A., & Takeuchi, T. (2002). Effects of different fluids on the relationship between swallowing and breathing during nutritive sucking in neonates. *Biology of the Neonate, 81*(1), 45–50.

Moretti, M. E., Sgro, M., Johnson, D. W., Sauve, R. S., Woolgar, M. J., Taddio, A., . . . Ito, S. (2003). Cyclosporine excretion into breast milk. *Transplantation, 75*(12), 2144–2146.

Morris, S. E., & Klein, M. D. (2001). *Prefeeding skills* (2nd ed.). San Diego, CA: Academic Press.

Morton, J., Hall, J. Y., Wong, R. J., Thairu, L., Benitz, W. E., & Rhine, W. D. (2009). Combining hand techniques with electric pumping increases milk production in mothers of preterm infants. *Journal of Perinatology, 29*, 757–764.

Moster, D., Lie, R. T., Irgens, L. M., Bjerkedal, T., & Markestad, L. (2001). The association of Apgar score with subsequent death and cerebral palsy: A population based study in term infants. *Journal of Pediatrics, 138*(6), 798–803.

Moster, D., Lie, R. T., & Markestad, L. (2002). Joint association of Apgar scores and early neonatal symptoms with minor disabilities at school age. *Archives of Disease in Childhood, Fetal and Neonatal Edition, 86*(1), 16–21.

Munoz-Flores-Thiagarajan, K. D., Easterling, T., Davis, C., & Bond, E. F. (2001). Breast-feeding by a cyclosporine-treated mother. *Obstetrics and Gynecology, 97*(5 Pt. 2), 816–818.

Narayanan, I., Mehta, R., Choudhury, D. K., & Jain, B. K. (1991). Sucking on the "emptied" breast: Non-nutritive sucking with a difference. *Archives of Disease in Childhood, 66*(2), 241–244.

Newman, J. (1990). Breastfeeding problems associated with the early introduction of bottles and pacifiers. *Journal of Human Lactation, 6*(2), 59–63.

Newman, J. (1996). Decision tree and postpartum management for preventing dehydration in the "breastfed" baby. *Journal of Human Lactation, 12*(2), 129–135.

Newman, L. A., Keckley, C., Petersen, M. C., & Hamner, A. (2001). Swallowing function and medical diagnoses in infants suspected of dysphagia. *Pediatrics, 108*(6), 106.

Niemitz, E. L., & Feinberg, A. P. (2004). Epigenetics and assisted reproductive technology: A call for investigation. *American Journal of Human Genetics, 74*(4), 599–609.

Nyberg, G., Haljamae, U., Frisenette-Fich, C., Wennergren, M., & Kjellmer, I. (1998). Breast-feeding during treatment with cyclosporine. *Transplantation, 65*(2), 253–255.

Oddy, W. H., & Glenn, K. (2003). Implementing the Baby Friendly Hospital Initiative: The role of finger feeding. *Breastfeeding Review, 11*(1), 5–10.

Ohyama, M., Watabe, H., Hayasaka, Y., Saito, K., & Mizuguchi, H. (2007). Which is more effective, manual or electric expression in the first 48 hours after delivery in a setting of mother-infant separation? A preliminary report. *Breastfeeding Medicine, 2*(3), 179.

Palmer, B. (1998). The influence of breastfeeding on the development of the oral cavity: A commentary. *Journal of Human Lactation, 14*(2), 93–98.

Palmer, M. M., & VandenBerg, K. A. (1998). A closer look at neonatal sucking. *Neonatal Network, 17*(2), 77–79.

Pavone, L., Rizzo, R., & Dobyns, W. B. (1993). Clinical manifestations and evaluation of isolated lissencephaly. *Child's Nervous System, 9*(7), 387–390.

Penalva, O., & Schwartzman, J. S. (2006). Descriptive study of the clinical and nutritional profile and follow-up of premature babies in a kangaroo mother care program. *Jornal de Pediatria, 82*(1), 33–39.

Poirier, K., Saillour, Y., Bahi-Buisson, N., Jaglin, X. H., Fallet-Bianco, C., Nabbout, R., . . . Chelly, J. (2010). Mutations in the neuronal ss-tubulin subunit TUBB3 result in malformation of cortical development and neuronal migration defects. *Human Molecular Genetics, 19*, 4462–4473.

Rasley, A., Logemann, J. A., Kahrilas, P. J., Rademaker, A. W., Pauloski, B. R., & Dodds, W. J. (1993). Prevention of barium aspiration during videofluoroscopic swallowing studies: Value of change in posture. *American Journal of Roentgenology, 160*(5), 1005–1009.

Rendon-Macias, M. E., Cruz-Perez, L. A., Mosco-Peralta, M. R., Saraiba-Russell, M. M., Levi-Tajfeld, S., & Morales-Lopez, M. G. (1999). Assessment of sensorial oral stimulation in infants with suck feeding disabilities. *Indian Journal of Pediatrics, 66*(3), 319–329.

Richards, C. A., Milla, P. J., Andrews, P. L., & Spitz, L. (2001). Retching and vomiting in neurologically impaired children after fundoplication: Predictive preoperative factors. *Journal of Pediatric Surgery, 36*(9), 1401–1404.

Rudolf, C. D. (2006). *The impact of GERD on feeding in infants with neurodevelopmental disorders*. Presented at Pediatric Dysphagia Series: Exploring the Brain-Gut Feeding Connection, Conference session, Cincinnati Children's Hospital Medical Center.

Shanahan, T. K., Logemann, J. A., Rademaker, A. W., Pauloski, B. R., & Kahrila, P. J. (1993). Chin-down posture effect on aspiration in dysphagic patients. *Archives of Physical Medicine and Rehabilitation, 74*(7), 736–739.

Shehata, H. A., & Okosun, H. (2004). Neurological disorders in pregnancy. *Current Opinions in Obstetrics and Gynecology, 16*(2), 117–122.

Siegel, B. (1996). *World of the autistic child: Understanding and treating autistic spectrum disorders.* New York, NY: Oxford University Press.

Stevenson, R. D., & Allaire, J. H. (1991). The development of normal feeding and swallowing. *Pediatric Clinics of North America, 38*(6), 1439–1453.

Streissguth, A. P., Barr, H. M., & Martin, D. C. (1983). Maternal alcohol use and neonatal habituation assessed with the Brazelton scale. *Child Development, 54*(5), 1109–1118.

Suskind, D. L., Thompson, D. M., Gulati, M., Huddleston, P., Liu, D. C., & Baroody, F. M. (2006). Improved infant swallowing after gastroesophageal reflux disease treatment: A function of improved laryngeal sensation? *Laryngoscope, 116*(8), 1397–1403.

Takagi, Y., & Bosma, J. F. (1960). Disability of oral function in an infant associated with displacement of the tongue: Therapy by feeding in the prone position. *Acta Paediatrica Supplementum, 49*(Suppl. 123), 62–69.

Tanoue, Y., & Oda, S. (1989). Weaning time of children with infantile autism. *Journal of Autism and Developmental Disorders, 19*(3), 425–434.

Tellez-Zenteno, J. F., Hernandez-Ronquillo, L., Salinas, V., Estanol, B., & da Silva, O. (2004). Myasthenia gravis and pregnancy: Clinical implications and neonatal outcome. *BMC Musculoskeletal Disorders, 5*, 42.

Thach, B. T. (2001). Maturation and transformation of reflexes that protect the laryngeal airway from liquid aspiration from fetal to adult life. *American Journal of Medicine, 111*(Suppl. 8A), 69–77.

U.S. Food and Drug Administration. (2011). *FDA warns not to feed SimplyThick to premature infants.* Retrieved from http://www.fda.gov/ForConsumers/ConsumerUpdates/ucm256250.htm

Volpe, J. J. (2001). Neurobiology of periventricular leukomalacia in the premature infant. *Pediatric Research, 50*(5), 553–562.

Waitzman, K. A. (2002). *Developmental care/feeding readiness.* Presented at Neonatal CORE, TriHealth Hospitals, Cincinnati, Ohio.

Wales, P. W., Diamond, I. R., Dutta, S., Muraca, S., Chait, P., Connolly, B., & Langer, J. C. (2002). Fundoplication and gastrostomy versus image-guided gastrojejunal tube for enteral feeding in neurologically impaired children with gastroesophageal reflux. *Journal of Pediatric Surgery, 37*(3), 407–412.

Weber, F., Woolridge, M. W., & Baum, J. D. (1986). An ultrasonographic study of the organisation of sucking and swallowing by newborn infants. *Developmental Medicine and Child Neurology, 28*, 19–24.

Wenzl, T. G. (2003). Evaluation of gastroesophageal reflux events in children using multichannel intraluminal electrical impedance. *American Journal of Medicine, 115*(Suppl. 3A), 161–165.

Wenzl, T. G., Schenke, S., Peschgens, T., Silny, J., Heimann, G., & Skopnik, H. (2001). Association of apnea and nonacid gastroesophageal reflux in infants: Investigations with the intraluminal impedance technique. *Pediatric Pulmonology, 31*(2), 144–149.

Williams, D. L., Goldstein, G., & Minshew, N. J. (2006). The profile of memory function in children with autism. *Neuropsychology, 20*(1), 21–29.

Wilson, E. M., Green, J. R., Yunusova, Y., & Moore, C. A. (2008). Task specificity in early oral motor development. *Seminars in Speech and Language, 29*, 257–266.

Wolf, L. S., & Glass, R. P. (1992). *Feeding and swallowing disorders in infancy: Assessment and management.* Austin, TX: Pro-Ed.

Yang, W. T., Loveday, E. J., Metreweli, C., & Sullivan, P. B. (1997). Ultrasound assessment of swallowing in malnourished disabled children. *British Journal of Radiology, 70*, 992–994.

Zoppou, C., Barry, S. I., & Mercer, G. N. (1997). Comparing breastfeeding and breast pumps using a computer model. *Journal of Human Lactation, 13*(3), 195–202.

CHAPTER

13

Therapeutic Positioning for Breastfeeding

Chele Marmet and Ellen Shell

The Importance of Positioning

Supportive positioning facilitates breastfeeding and, when necessary, helps to compensate for special problems. Although older, healthy babies can breastfeed in a variety of positions of their own invention, including practically standing on their heads, young babies and those with special problems need positional stability. Mothers and babies instinctively adopt a great variety of positions, but common to all effective positions is stability.

A newborn's natural posture is physiologic flexion. The baby is most stable in a prone position on a supportive surface and can even move forward in a coordinated pattern (Widstrom et al., 1987). When the baby is supine, limb movements often elicit a startle reflex, interfering with controlled mobility. Normal neuromuscular development increases stability in the *proximal* (central) parts of the body (hips and trunk). When this proximal base of stability is established, the baby has greater mobility and more refined distal control, including control of the mouth and tongue (Morris & Klein, 1987). Refined oral-motor skills rely on a proximal base of stability from the neck and shoulder girdle, which in turn are dependent on trunk and pelvic stability (Wolf & Glass, 1992). Even the structures of the face and oral cavity need stability in order to function. Bosma (1972) describes the tongue's contact with the cheeks, hard and soft palate, alveolar ridge, and lips as providing stability for the tongue. He posits that the buccal fat pads and other subcutaneous oral fat deposits provide a functional "exoskeleton" to support oral, pharyngeal, and temporomandibular joint stabilization for refined mandibular movement.

It is vital to have a basic understanding of neonatal neuromotor development and the relationships between proximal stability and distal mobility in order to analyze which position(s) will be therapeutic for a complex breastfeeding situation.

Neuromotor and physiologic relationships are complex; however, the key to these concepts is simple. What begins at the hips ends at the lips (stability), so that what begins at the lips (breastfeeding) ends up on the hips (weight gain).

Achieving optimal latch and positioning is usually the first and often the only treatment needed to facilitate suck and correct most breastfeeding problems. Therapeutic positioning is often an important piece of the treatment plan for sore nipples, breast refusal, milk supply issues, or anatomical variations of mother or baby. Additionally, therapeutic positions assist in correcting or compensating for suckling problems (Marmet & Shell, 1993; Snyder, 1995).

Regardless of the breastfeeding position chosen, if the baby is gaining weight and thriving, and breastfeeding is comfortable for mother and infant, no intervention is needed. Because of variations in the size, shape, physical abilities, and preferences of mothers and infants, no one position is correct for all breastfeeding dyads (Cioni, Ferrari, & Prechtl, 1989). Likewise, Blair, Cadwell, Turner-Maffei, and Brimdyr (2003) found that no one group of attributes (head position, body position, or breastfeeding dynamic) was more related to the level of pain experienced by the mother than another. The researchers concluded that no one aspect of positioning is more crucial than another. Successful intervention requires recognition of the need for special positioning as well as the ability to create dyad-specific positions when required.

Naming Positions

Names chosen for positions in this chapter most frequently describe the baby's position in space, but some were chosen because they reflect the mother's relationship to the baby (Marmet & Shell, 1993). Descriptive names with universal appeal have been selected so they are easy to remember and are translatable to other cultures and languages. Standardized naming of positions creates a common vocabulary so that verbal and written information can readily be exchanged. The intention is not to create a body of jargon, but to facilitate clear and accurate communication between professionals, with parents, and in charting. In some cases, both descriptive and medical names are available for positions (e.g., top-breast-lying-down versus Sims; reclining versus modified semi-Fowler). When working with a mother, however, descriptive terms are easier for her to understand and remember.

The Importance of Skin-to-Skin Contact

Mammals are preprogrammed with neurobehaviors to expect a specific habitat or place during the newborn period (Alberts, 1958). For humans, this habitat is skin to skin, heart to heart with their mothers—warm, safe, and close to the breast for feeding. Harlow's famous primate studies of attachment describe the infant as "actively seeking to adhere to as much skin surface on the mother's body as possible" (1958/1971, pp. 1–25). This is the basis of healthy development (Schore, 2001a). Likewise, when a human baby is in his or her habitat, skin to skin with the mother, preprogrammed neurobehaviors naturally play out in breastfeeding, which stimulates mother's milk release and production. Rey and Martinez reported in 1983 that Kangaroo Mother Care (continuous skin-to-skin contact) was superior to incubator care for stable preterm infants, and hundreds of research articles have since validated their findings (Anderson, Marks, & Wahlberg, 1986; Anderson, Moore, Hepworth, & Bergman, 2003; Browne, 2004; Charpak, de Calume, & Ruiz, 2000; World Health Organization, 2003).

On the other hand, animal and human research reveals protest-despair behavior as a universal mammalian response to separation from the correct habitat (mother). When a newborn is separated from his or her habitat (mother), the newborn exhibits a hyperarousal response. The sympathetic autonomic nervous system is suddenly and significantly activated, increasing the heart rate and blood pressure (Christensson, Cabrera, Christensson, Uvnas-Moberg, & Winberg, 1995). The newborn's distress "is expressed in crying, then screaming" (Schore, 2001b, p. 210). Human babies separated from their mothers make 10 times as many cry signals as babies in skin-to-skin care (Rosenblum & Andrews, 1994). Anderson's (1988) research has led her to suggest that crying in protest is detrimental for the infant because it impairs lung functioning, jeopardizes the closure of the foramen ovale in the heart, increases intracranial pressure, and initiates a cascade of stress reactions that put the infant at risk for poor adaptation to extrauterine life. If there is prolonged separation and the crying of protest fails to elicit maternal care, despair occurs. Then the baby exhibits disassociation, conserves energy, and, to foster survival, will feign death, a passive state of profound detachment where blunting endogenous opiates are elevated and the heart rate and blood pressure are decreased. Human magnetic resonance imaging research of the developing brain provides evidence of "toxic neurochemistry" caused by abuse and neglect (Schore, 2001b, p. 210).

The beginning of all positioning is ideally skin to skin. Harlow (1958/1971), in discussing his cloth versus wire mother monkey studies, said that

> we were not surprised to discover that contact comfort was an important basic-affectional variable but we did not expect it to overshadow so completely the variable of nursing; indeed, the disparity is so great as to suggest that primary function of nursing is that of insuring frequent and intimate body contact of the infant with the mother. (p. 36)

Similarly, Montegue (1971) stated that the skin is the largest organ system of the body and perhaps, other than the brain, the most important. Of all of the human organs, the skin is the most sensitive organ and also the first medium of communication. The sense of touch is essential not only for the baby, but also for the mother, so it is critical to foster skin-to-skin contact between the mother and infant.

Some breastfeeding experts have reported when helping mothers with breastfeeding problems that just placing the mother and baby in unclothed, chest-to-chest contact and allowing time for them to relax together leads to the baby self-attaching and breastfeeding well. When infants are stressed, they cannot access their feeding and growth responses. Difficulty latching to the breast and disorganized sucking behavior may result. Is it possible that continuous skin-to-skin contact of the baby and mother may reboot the neurobehavioral programming into the feeding mode and remove the negative stress patterns that had been interfering with breastfeeding? Though skin-to-skin contact will not correct all breastfeeding problems, it is certainly the correct habitat for babies and provides a strong foundation during the process of correcting whatever problems exist.

It seems prudent to extrapolate that regardless of the variety of positions utilized, keeping the mother and young baby skin to skin as much of the time as possible is ideal. A carrier that keeps the baby skin to skin with mother, except for changing, bathing, and occasional attention from other family members, such as the carrier used traditionally by the Basque community in Spain (Crawford, 1994), may be an ideal tool for universal use.

If skin-to-skin care cures breastfeeding problems, then we may ask why it is necessary to labor over specific positions. The answer is that even with an all-natural birth and no separation, breastfeeding difficulties still occur in a small percentage of term babies.

Therapeutic Positions for Treatment

Alteration in positioning for breastfeeding can be an effective compensatory strategy for sucking problems, anatomical variations, and neurological deficits. Consider the following issues when choosing a therapeutic position: the mother's and baby's general anatomy and health status, the relationship of the breast and baby in space, and the specific breastfeeding issues involved. For example, a mother with long forearms, carpal tunnel syndrome, and large breasts with a 35-week premature baby might need very different modifications than a reference-sized mother with reference-sized breasts and a term infant with a bubble palate (Marmet & Shell, 1993; Snyder, 1995, 1997). As with all interventions, careful evaluation of the effectiveness of positioning suggestions is required.

Hand Position on the Base of the Baby's Head

If the position requires the mother's hand to hold the baby's head, her thumb and first finger wrap around the base of the skull (occiput) just under the ears (**Figure 13-1**). Placing the hand higher on the back of the baby's head can interfere with the baby's ability to latch, especially when the baby is experiencing problems. The heel of the mother's hand and her pinky and ring fingers rest on the shoulders, supporting the back and neck. By providing support for the head, stability is achieved in the back, neck, and shoulders, thus protecting the neck.

Baby Sitting (Mother Sitting)

It is possible that sitting-upright positions might be a good choice for many compromised babies. Research indicates that premature babies in Kangaroo Mother Care are best kept in upright positions (World Health Organization, 2003). Clinical experience has provided evidence that an upright position of the infant helps correct some breastfeeding problems.

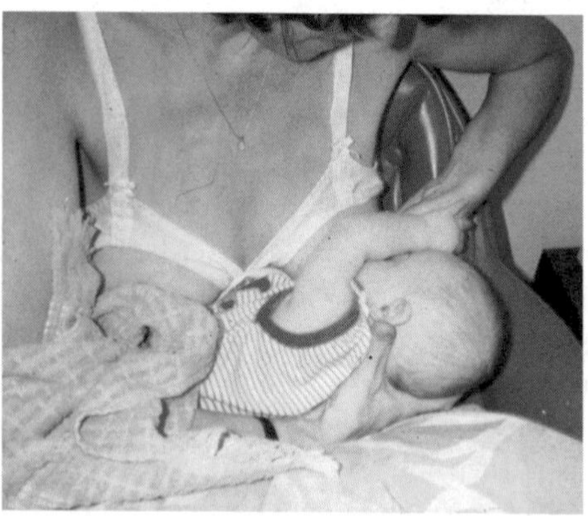

Figure 13-1 Thumb and first finger wrap around the neck at or just under the ears, giving support at the base of the occiput.

Straddle Sit, Side-Saddle Sit, and Clutch-V Position

Maternal comfort and infant muscle tone determine which of these three positions is chosen, though the straddle sit and side-saddle sit require tone that is typically not found until a baby is older than 6 weeks. Some mothers like to use a combination of these at different feedings.

The most common reasons for selecting sitting positions are as follows:

- To assist babies with consistent tongue elevation, upright positions may work with gravity to bring the tongue down.
- For a baby with a cleft palate, velopharyngeal inadequacy, or repeated ear infections, especially if on artificial infant milk supplements, vertical positions help prevent milk from entering the nasopharynx and eustachian tubes.
- Bringing the baby into a more upright position can help improve alertness and give support for improved sucking in some neurologically impaired infants.

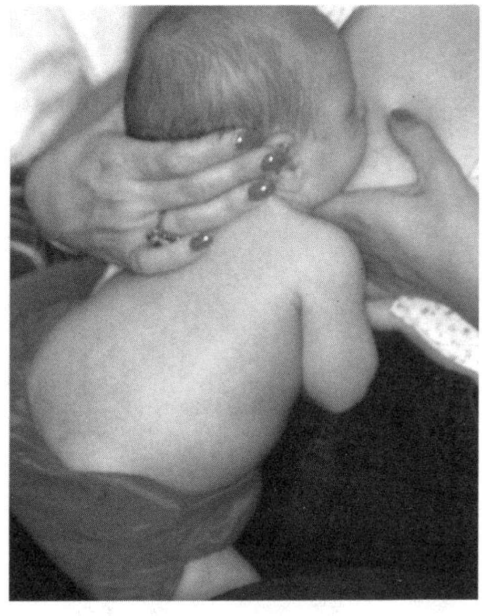

Figure 13-2 (Above) Straddle sit.

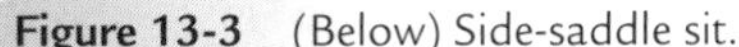

Figure 13-3 (Below) Side-saddle sit.

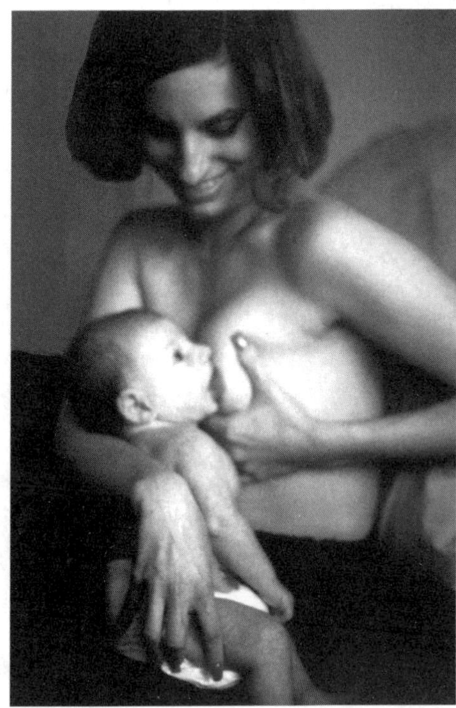

Straddle Sit. In a straddle sit position (**Figure 13-2**), the baby's legs straddle one of the mother's legs. If needed, a pillow or rolled blanket can be used to prevent excessive head extension in the infant.

Side-Saddle Sit. The baby sits on the mother's leg in a side-saddle position, with his chest to her chest (**Figure 13-3**). Neurotypical babies approximately 4 months and older can rotate at the hips to face the mother while maintaining shoulder and ear alignment. A younger baby's whole body must be angled to face the mother and maintain alignment of the ears, shoulders, and hips.

Clutch-V Position. This position provides physiologic flexion along with vertical positioning. Starting from a clutch position (where the baby's body and legs form an L at the mother's side), elevate the baby's shoulders so the baby is flexed at the hips into a V position (**Figure 13-4**). Depending on issues such as the size and the shape of the mother and baby, the baby's legs may either be flexed as in the fetal position or extended up the back of the chair.

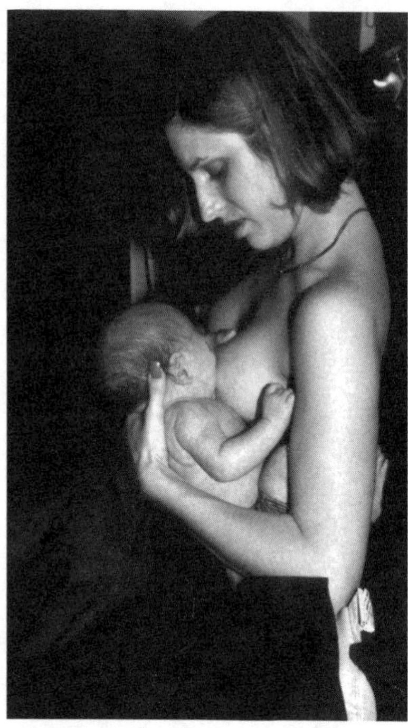

Figure 13-4 Clutch-V position.

Mother Sitting (Baby in Other Positions)

Physiologic Flex

When to use: Physiologic flexion is helpful for calming an extremely fussy baby and reducing arching in hypertonic infants.

Description: The baby's arms and legs are placed in physiologic flexion and held in this curled up position against the mother's trunk (**Figure 13-5**).

Fake Position

When to use: This position is helpful for a baby who is having difficulty breastfeeding on one breast but does well on the other. This position tricks the baby into thinking he or she is on the preferred side and can accommodate an ear infection or a unilateral structural problem, such as torticollis, vocal fold paralysis, or respiratory malformations that are more severe on one side.

Description: After breastfeeding the baby on the preferred breast in the preferred position, slide the baby across to the other breast, keeping the baby's head and body in the same position and plane (**Figure 13-6**). If the baby has difficulty with skin contact, the

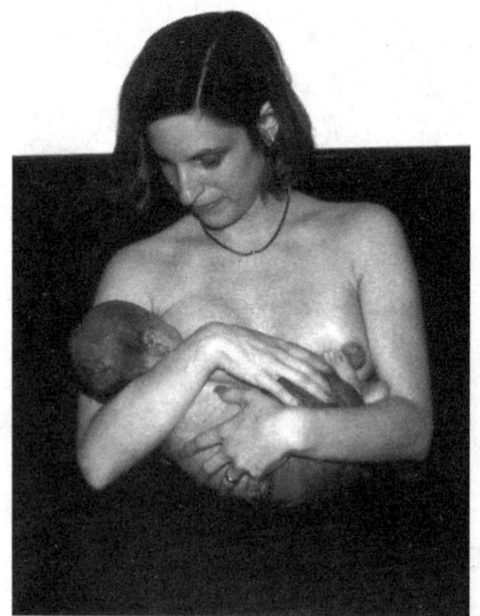

Figure 13-5 Physiologic flex.

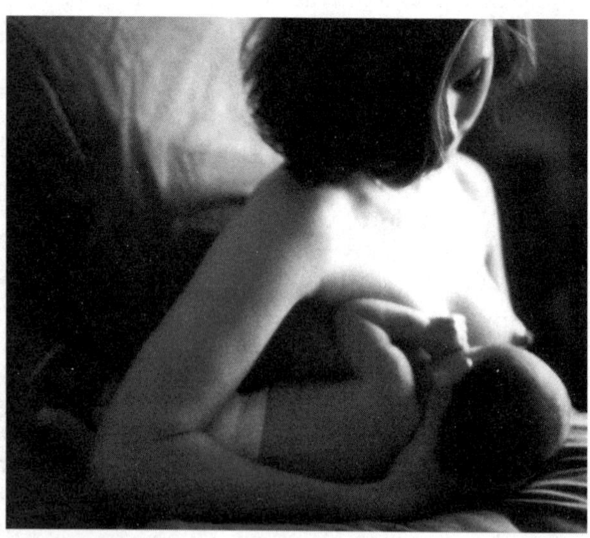

Figure 13-6 Fake position.

baby's body may need to rest on pillows rather than across the mother's lap. It is relatively easy to slide a pillow with the baby on it to the other breast.

Baby Prone Positions (Mother Supine)

Robin's 1934 study indicated immediate improvement in oral and pharyngeal function, including reduced symptoms of upper respiratory obstruction, with prone or partially upright (orthostatic) feeding positions. Sick babies bottle feeding in prone position showed better oxygenation and higher sucking pressures than when supine (Mizuno, Inoue, & Takeuchi, 2000). Prone positions seem helpful for breastfeeding-compromised babies. Breastfed preterm babies had better oxygenation than when they bottle-fed (Meier & Anderson, 1987). Breastfeeding in any position is likely better for compromised babies than bottle feeding.

Vertical, Horizontal, and Diagonal Prone Positions

When to use: The vertical, horizontal, and diagonal prone positions can be used interchangeably:

- Prone positioning works with gravity to bring the tongue forward.
- A baby with a short tongue, tongue held in a retracted position, or with a tongue-tie can improve tongue contact with the breast using gravity.
- Prone positions may help infants who have difficulty handling milk flow.

Description: In all prone positions the mother is supine and the baby is prone, and they are chest to chest. The mother can control the baby's head with her hand at the forehead or at the base of the skull. If desired, a rolling latch can also be employed, but it is often not as effective in this position (Curley et al., 2005). Well-placed, firm pillows facilitate the mother's comfort and her ability to assist the baby with latch. A pillow or two under the mother's head, but not under her shoulders, allows her to see the baby. A pillow along each side of the mother provides elevation and support for her arms, and pillows under her bent knees helps avoid a backache.

Vertical Prone. The baby is prone and vertical to the mother (**Figure 13-7**).

Horizontal Prone. The baby is prone and horizontal to the mother (**Figure 13-8**).

Diagonal Prone. The baby is prone and diagonal to the mother (**Figure 13-9**).

Other Prone Positions

Prone Suck Training/Fingerfeeding Charm Hold. Suck training in the prone position is also beneficial for babies with a retracted tongue, a short tongue, or a tight frenulum. The chest is supported by the mother's arm or hand while her other hand supports the forehead so her first or second finger can reach the mouth for suck training (Marmet & Shell, 1984). The hand is curved, giving the baby an air pocket for breathing (**Figure 13-10**). It works like a charm!

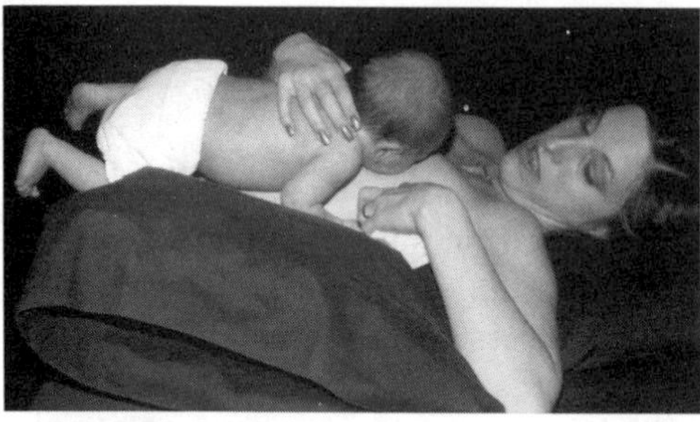

Figure 13-7 Vertical prone.

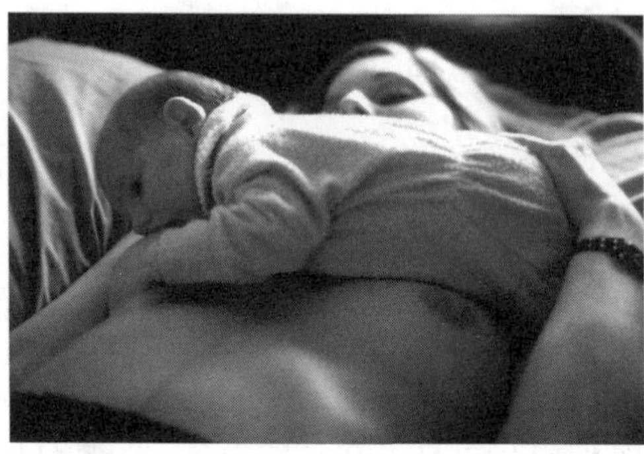

Figure 13-8 Horizontal prone.

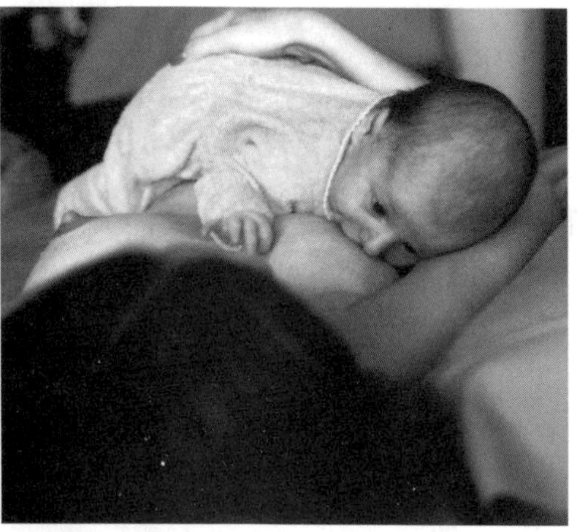

Figure 13-9 Diagonal prone.

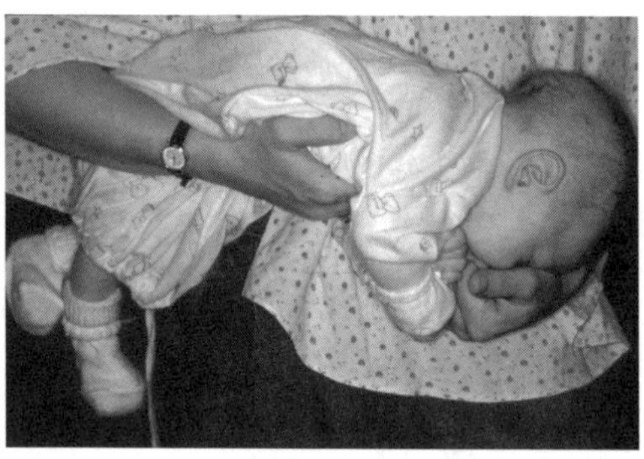

Figure 13-10 Prone suck training/fingerfeeding charm hold.

Over-the-Shoulder Prone Position

When to use: This position is especially useful when the mother has nipple or areolar injury or infection, and the pressure points from suckling need to be changed dramatically to allow healing to occur.

Description: The baby kneels on the bed and leans over the mother's shoulder to reach the breast (**Figure 13-11**). Older babies may prefer sitting at the mother's shoulder and bending over it to reach the breast.

Floating Prone Position

When to use: This position is particularly helpful when repeated unsuccessful breastfeeding attempts have left the baby frustrated and refusing to try again. If the sucking problem has been corrected and the baby is still rejecting the breast, this position often does the trick because the baby does not have the same negative associations in this position.

Except for the head, the baby is positioned away from the mother's body. It often helps to explain to the mother that the baby is not rejecting her, but is instead rejecting the method of feeding that he could not make work. When the baby is successfully breastfeeding, the breast will become the baby's favorite food delivery system as designed, and the baby is then usually willing to use other positions.

Description: The baby is placed prone on a pillow that is next to the mother's side so the baby's body floats on the pillow while only his head rests on the mother's breast (**Figure 13-12**). It may be necessary to place a cloth on the mother's breast so the baby's face touches cloth, not skin. Only mouth-to-breast contact is mandatory. The mother can support the baby's head at the base of the skull (occiput) with her hand, but she may need to use a cloth between her hand and the baby's head.

Lateral Prone Position

When to use: Although it is especially useful for a baby with a receding chin, this position is particularly comfortable when resting or sleeping for dyads with or without breastfeeding problems.

Description: The baby is lateral to the mother and in an angled prone position. For the mother's right breast, the baby is placed on his left side on the mother's right arm, which is on a pillow. Then the whole baby is rolled forward against the mother's body so that he is no longer perpendicular to the bed but is at a 30- to 45-degree angle in an angled-prone position. The baby's head is at breast level, and his mouth is just below the nipple so that latch can occur. The mother's right arm cradles her baby, while pillows cradle her (**Figure 13-13**).

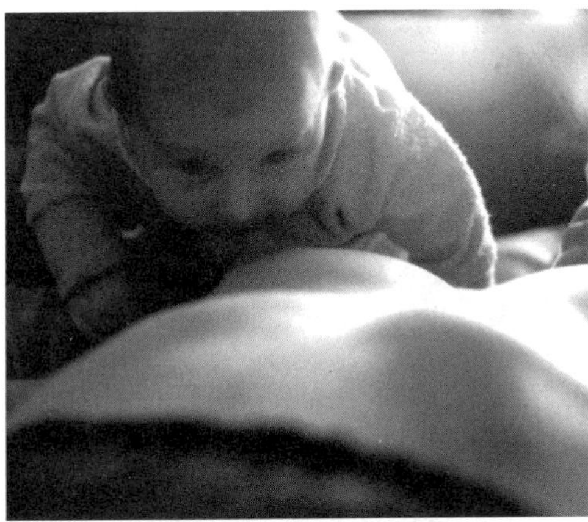

Figure 13-11 Over-the-shoulder prone position.

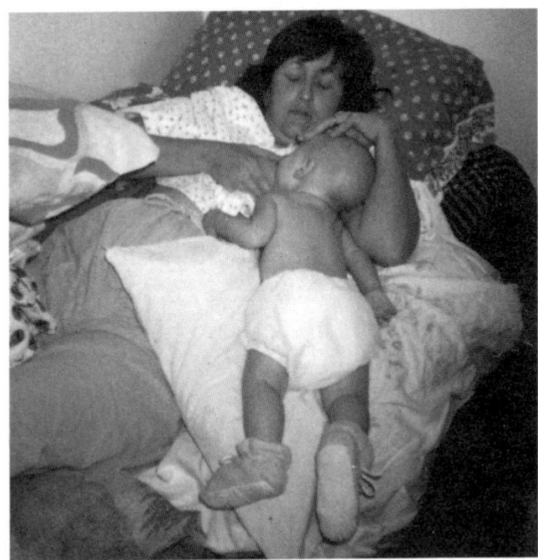

Figure 13-12 Floating prone position.

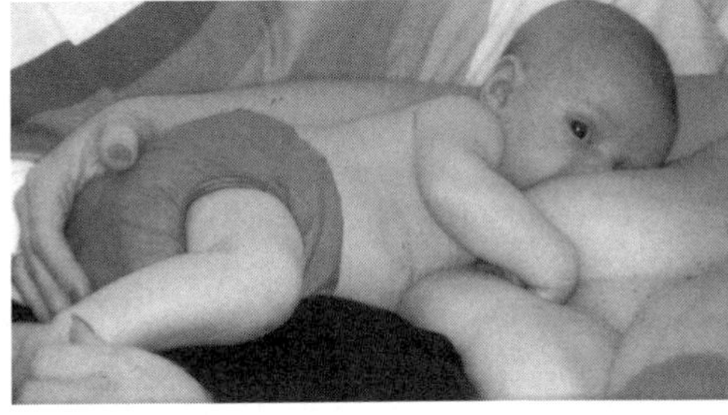

Figure 13-13 Lateral prone position.

Kneeling Prone Position

When to use: This position is useful for infants with a receding chin or a mother with abdominal surgery.

Description: The baby is placed kneeling at the mother's side facing her, next to her breast. Then the baby's chest is brought forward to latch so the chest and head are almost prone. The mother needs to be sure the baby's knees don't slip away from her body. With the baby kneeling next to the mother's left breast and the baby's mouth centered just above her nipple, the mother controls her baby's head with her left hand at the base of the baby's occiput, while her left arm supports the baby's back, thus keeping the baby tucked tightly next to her. The mother's right hand is free to control the left breast. Initially the mother can drop the head onto her breast as soon as the baby is ready to latch. Within a few tries, the baby often self-attaches. The ease with which babies adapt to this position amazes mothers and healthcare professionals alike, but the baby feels right at home in this almost fetal position. Placing a small pillow to the side of the baby's head, after the baby is breastfeeding well, will usually allow the mother to relax her hold on the baby's head and rest her hand (**Figure 13-14**).

Mother Reclining Positions (Modified Semi-Fowler)

If mother scoops up the baby's buttocks with her elbow and reclines to allow gravity to hold the baby against her, she may not need pillows to support her arm.

The reclining angle for these positions is approximately 45 degrees but may vary depending on the amount of compensation that is needed. It is easy to help a mother into a reclining position in an adjustable hospital bed. This is known as a semi-Fowler position when the patient is using a hospital bed. The mother is semireclining with bent knees so that her body, upper and lower legs, and feet form a W shape. When using a standard bed, pillows support the mother's lower back and bent knees. It also helps to brace the mother's feet against a pillow or rolled blanket so they do not slide. In a recliner chair, the mother's knees may need to be bent and supported with pillows depending on the shape of the chair. In a regular chair or sofa, the mother sits nearer the edge and leans back onto sufficient pillows behind her pelvis to support her reclining position. Her shoulders then rest on the chair back, and her feet rest on a footstool that is nearly chair height so her knees are bent. A very tall mother may find a lower footstool sufficient. Pillows can be used under her knees if desired, but this usually is not necessary; however, arm support is often helpful. In all of these variations, pillows can be used to support the mother's arms.

Reclining Straddle Sit (Baby Semiprone)

When to use: This is used for infants with receding chins when the mother needs or wants to sit.

Description: For the right breast, the baby is placed facing the mother, straddling her right leg, and is leaned forward into a semiprone position. A small rolled towel is placed between the baby's chest and the mother to keep the baby's head from overextension (**Figure 13-15**).

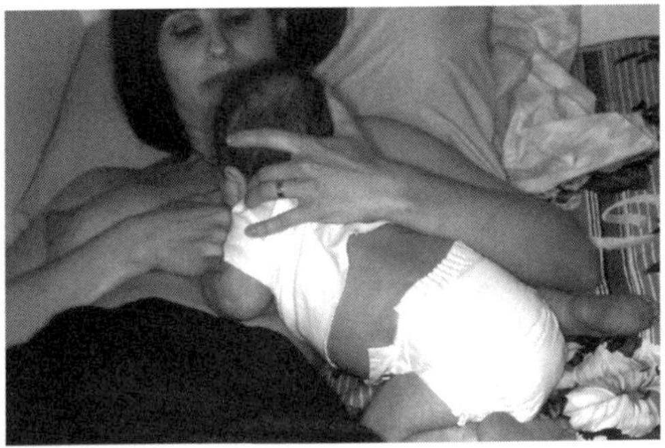

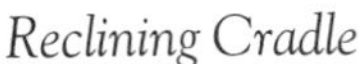

Figure 13-14 Kneeling prone position.

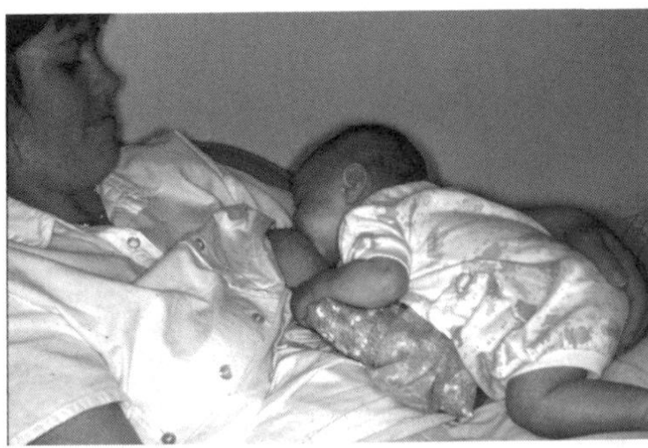

Figure 13-15 Reclining straddle sit.

Reclining Cradle

When to use: This is a very comfortable position after a cesarean birth because a pillow can cover the incision area to protect it.

Description: The baby is in a cradle position (**Figure 13-16**).

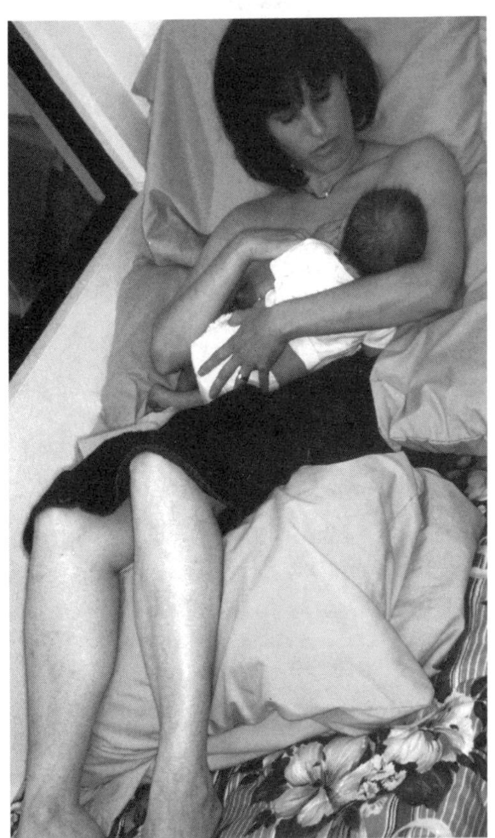

Figure 13-16 Reclining cradle.

Reclining Sit

When to use: This position is for temporary use as sore nipples heal, especially with older infants.

Description: The baby is sitting next to the mother's side, facing the mother, in a semi-prone position by leaning forward (**Figure 13-17**). Care must be taken to ensure good alignment of the baby's ears, shoulders, and hips.

Dancer Hand Positions

All three Dancer hand positions make the oral cavity smaller to help increase intraoral (negative) pressure (Marmet & Shell, 1993; Chapter 12). This is helpful for infants with a poor seal or weak suck; babies who fall off the breast if not held in place; or babies with neuromotor problems, including high tone or low tone (e.g., Down syndrome).

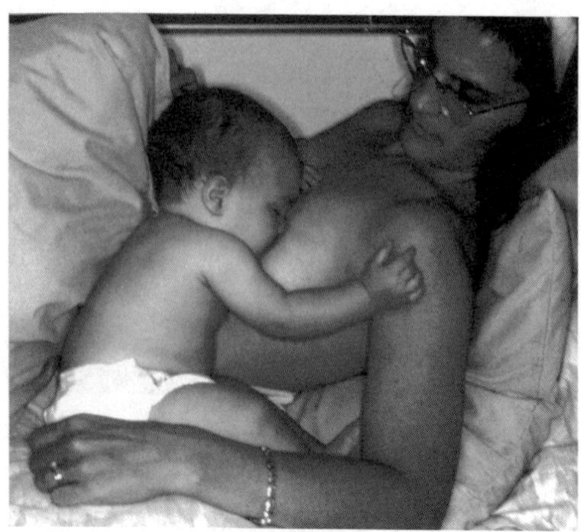

Figure 13-17 Reclining sit.

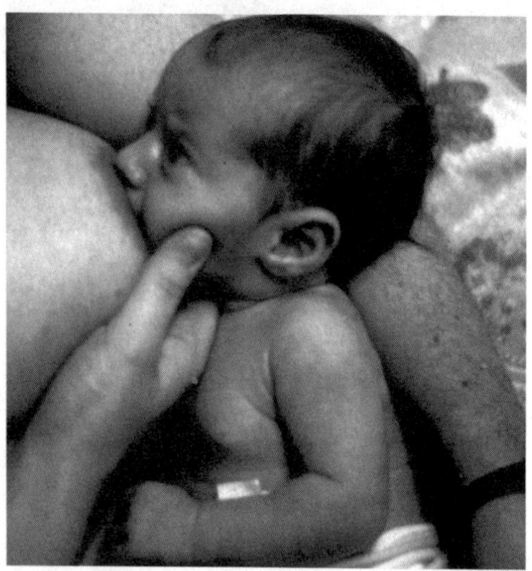

Figure 13-18 Classic Dancer hand position.

Classic Dancer Hand Position

When to use: This position is for infants with excessive jaw excursions in addition to low intraoral pressure (**Figure 13-18**) (Danner & Cerutti, 1989).

Description: The hand provides a sling to support the baby's mandible while simultaneously putting pressure with the index finger and thumb into the baby's buccal muscle (check cavities).

Three-Finger Dancer Suck Training Position

When to use: This position is used for suck training with or without supplementation when a baby needs jaw support and help increasing his intraoral pressure.

Description: This position can be accomplished in two ways: using a thumb and two fingers, or using three fingers (**Figure 13-19**). The mother's hand size, finger length, and manual dexterity will determine which digits she uses to apply pressure to the baby's cheeks over the buccinators and to support the mandible (chin). An additional finger is used in the baby's mouth for the suck training.

Two-Finger Dancer Hand Position

When to use: When jaw support is not needed, two fingers can be used to decrease intraoral space.

Description: During suck training, eliminate the finger on the chin, leaving two fingers for pressure points on the buccal muscles. When the baby is at the breast, two hands are used to provide the pressure points (**Figure 13-20**).

Modifications for Specific Problems

Receding Chin Prone Positions

A baby with a receding chin (overbite or retrognathia) is easily identified by looking at the baby in profile (**Figures 13-21 and 13-22**). If the mandible is significantly less prominent

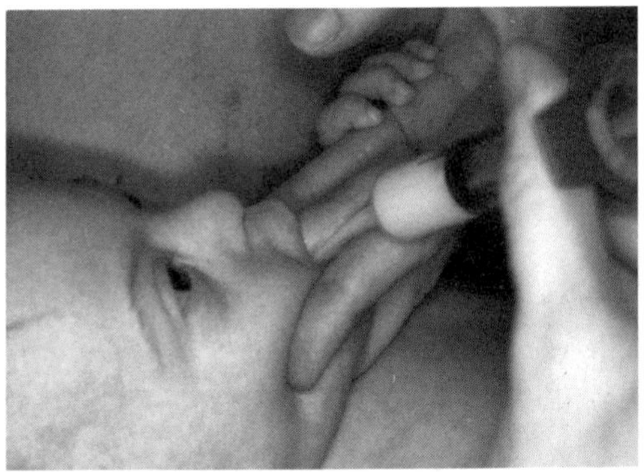

Figure 13-19 Three-finger Dancer supplementation with a periodontal syringe.

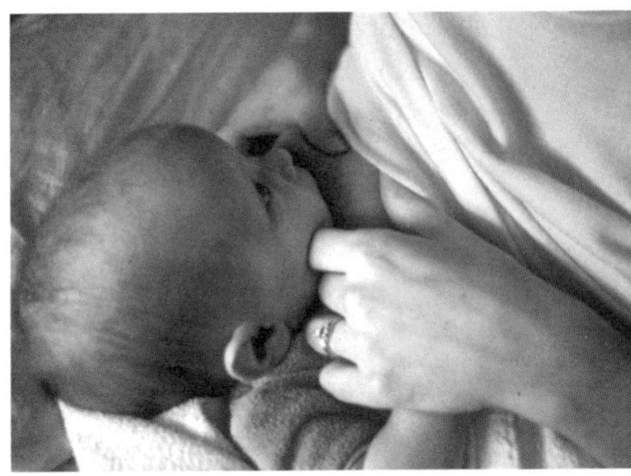

Figure 13-20 Two-finger Dancer.

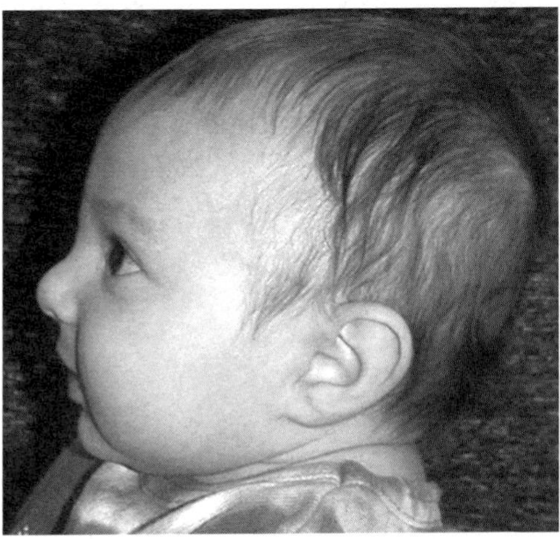

Figure 13-21 (Above) Normal chin.

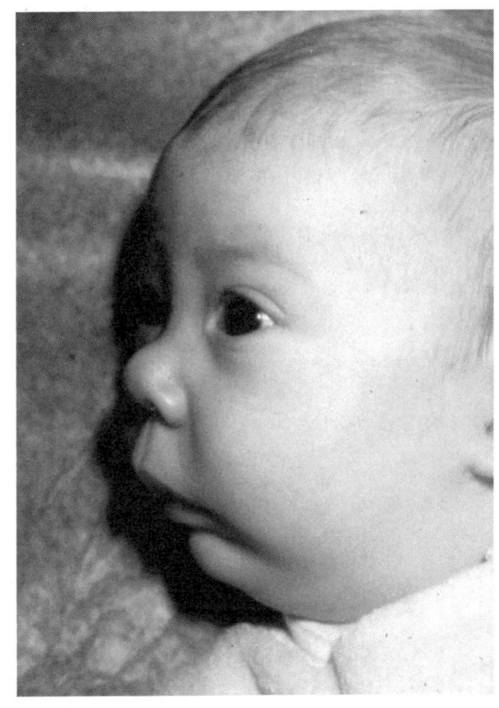

Figure 13-22 (Right) Receding chin.

than the maxilla, then the baby has a receding chin. Restoring maternal nipple comfort and promoting effective infant milk transfer are goals of positioning strategies. Lateral prone, kneeling prone, and mother reclining with the baby in the straddle sit semiprone position are particularly effective.

The mandible grows quickly during the first 3 months of life, so most retrognathic babies can breastfeed in basic positions by 3 months of age.

Note: Another very rare malalignment of the mandible is a protruding chin (underbite or prognathic mandible). The positional treatment is the opposite of the treatment for the receding chin; the baby can be placed in a semisupine position with the mother sitting and leaning forward.

Cradle Prone (Pierre Robin Position)

When to use: This position is particularly helpful for a baby with Pierre Robin sequence. It helps bring the tongue forward while using pillows to position the baby, thus freeing the mother's hands to support her breasts and manipulate feeding tools used at the breast (e.g., periodontal syringe). It may also be useful for situations other than Pierre Robin that require the mother's hands to be free while feeding the baby. The semiprone position helps keep the baby latched during this process.

Description: The mother sits upright or very slightly reclining (no more than 70 degrees) to bring the baby partially prone. The baby is propped on pillows on his or her side as if in a cradle position, but not cradled in the mother's arms (**Figure 13-23**). Instead, the baby is leaned forward so the chest is supported by the mother's chest, halfway between prone and perpendicular in a spatial sense. If the baby is being supplemented at breast with a periodontal syringe or feeding tube device, the mother may angle him slightly away from her body temporarily to view the mouth for supplementation.

All Fours Position (Hands and Knees)

When to use: This is an awkward and uncomfortable position, though it is excellent for temporary use to clear plugged ducts and may help the rare baby who cannot tolerate skin-to-skin contact.

Description: The baby is supine on a supportive surface. The mother is on her hands and knees with her breast hanging down to the baby's mouth (**Figure 13-24**).

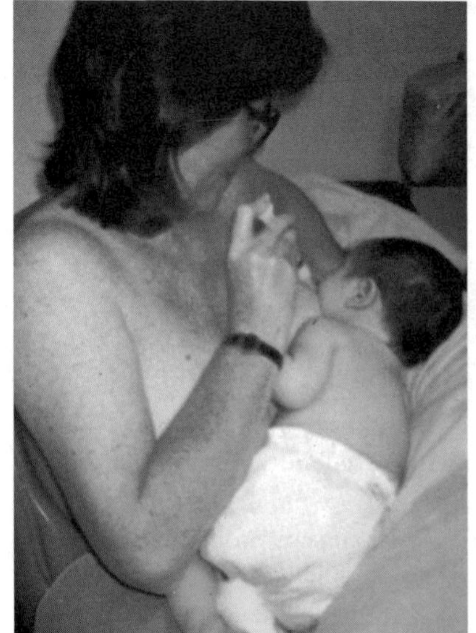

Figure 13-23 Cradle prone.

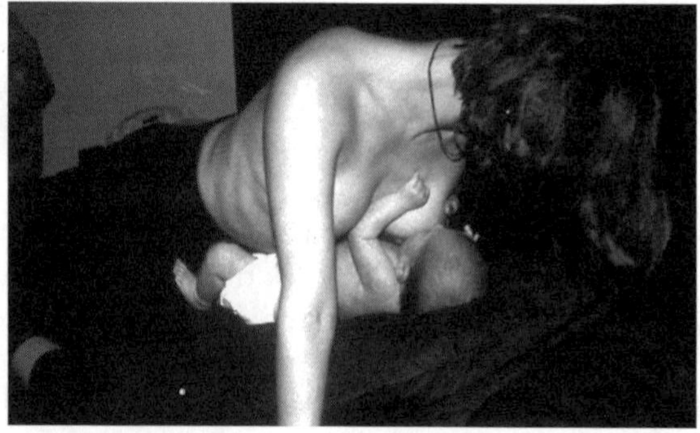

Figure 13-24 All fours position (hands and knees).

Upside Down

When to use: Like the kneeling prone position, this unusual position is terrific if a mother has sore nipples.

Description: Both the mother and baby lie on their sides, but the baby is upside down in relation to the mother, with the feet pointing toward the mother's head (**Figure 13-25**).

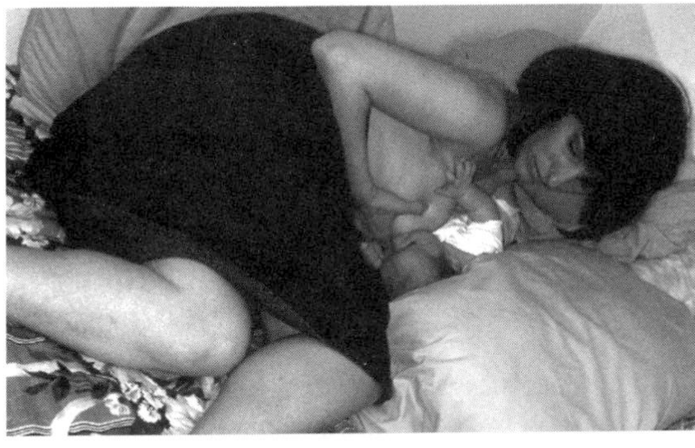

Figure 13-25 Upside down.

Hip Dysplasia Positions

Infants who have hip dysplasia, and are consequently put into a cast or brace, breastfeed well in a straddle sit position (**Figure 13-26**). A cradle or transition hold can also be utilized with pillow support between the legs to blunt the weight and the awkwardness of the cast or brace. Because these babies cannot mold their bodies to their mothers' bodies, the mother usually has to compress her breast with her finger to make an air pocket.

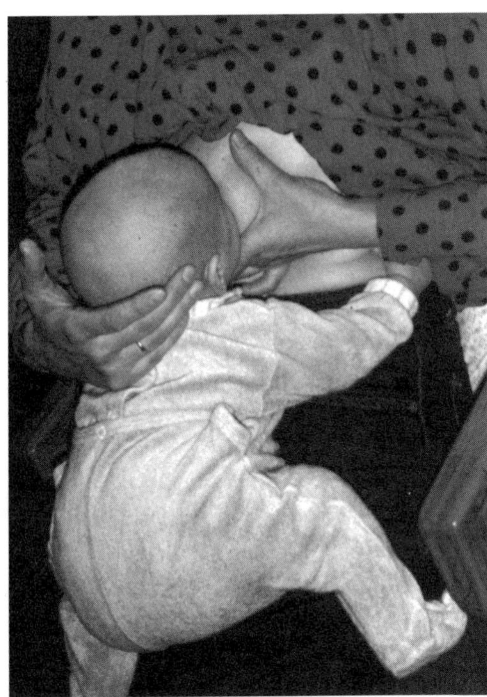

Figure 13-26 Hip dysplasia.

Modified Cradle Position to Accommodate Large Breasts

If a mother's breasts are too large to allow her arm to support her baby in front of her body, it may be helpful to approximate the position of the baby in the cradle hold using pillows to support and control the baby's head and body (**Figure 13-27**). If the breast is so

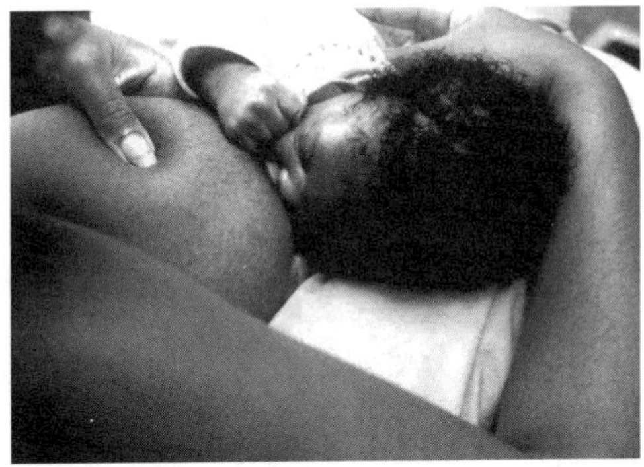

Figure 13-27 Modified cradle position for large breasts.

pendulous that the baby cannot access the nipple while on the mother's lap, a rolled hand towel or cloth diaper can lift the breast to improve access. Variations in mother's or baby's anatomy may require positioning adaptations. The infant's body can be pressed against the mother's breast to provide stability (body part to body part) (Morris & Klein, 1987). Other positions can also be modified with these principles.

Positions for Multiples

Breastfeeding twins simultaneously can allow substantial savings of maternal time and energy. With more than two babies, most mothers find that planning and record keeping is necessary to be sure each baby gets fed. With triplets, she may feed the first two together, each on one breast for their full feeding, then offer both breasts to the third baby. The babies are rotated at each feeding so they change breasts and each has a turn at solitary and paired (two-breasted) feedings. Mothers of multiples usually need a great deal of help in the early days. Learning to dance with more than one partner requires extra time and extra practice.

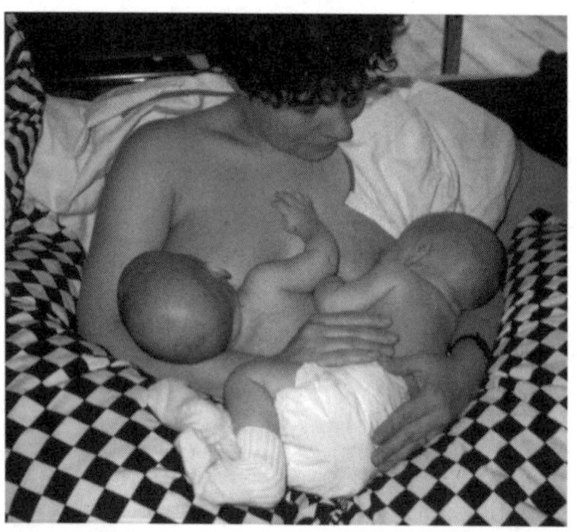

Figure 13-28 Double cradle position.

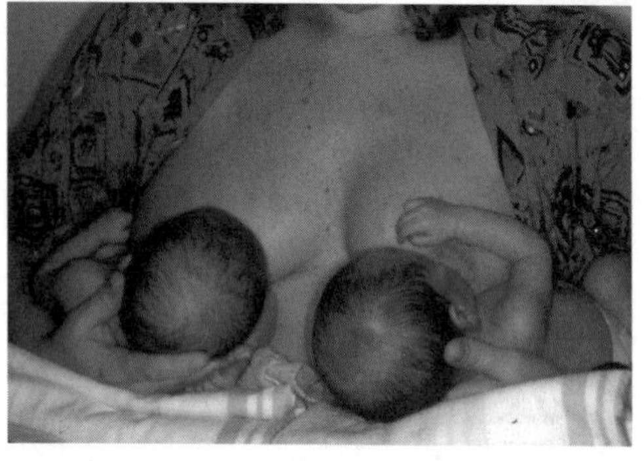

Figure 13-29 Double clutch position.

Double Cradle Position

The mother places the first twin across her trunk, supporting the infant on one arm. Then the second baby is cradled in the other arm on top of or behind the sibling. The baby in the mother's right arm latches to her right breast, and the baby in her left arm latches to her left breast (**Figure 13-28**).

Double Clutch Position

For this position, both babies are in a clutch position, each under one of the mother's arms (**Figure 13-29**).

Parallel Position (Cradle–Clutch Position)

When the twins are young, one twin can be placed in a cradle position and the other in a clutch position (**Figure 13-30**). As the babies get bigger, the baby in the clutch position has his legs wrapped around his mother or off to the side, so the twins' legs are parallel to each other.

Double V Hold

This position works especially well for mothers with long torsos. The babies' bodies are each a side of a V shape they form together in their mother's arms and lap (**Figure 13-31**).

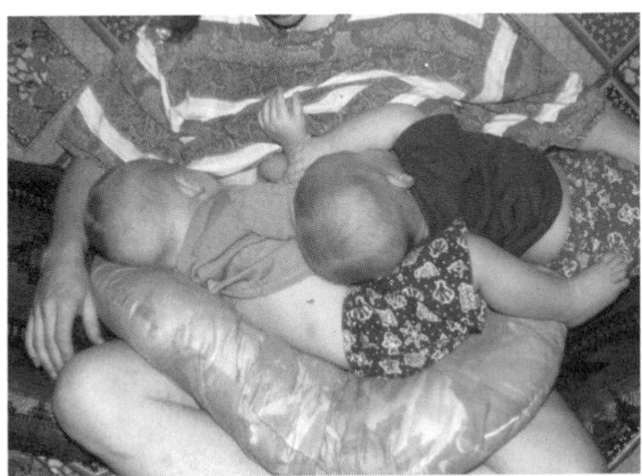

Figure 13-30 Parallel position.

Conclusion

When the lactation consultant has a firm understanding of normal suckling, the infant's feeding neurobehavior and instinctive feeding position, and issues that can make feeding difficult, therapeutic positions can be developed to help compensate for challenges. The therapeutic positions reviewed in this chapter were developed by the authors from their long experience working with infants who have feeding challenges.

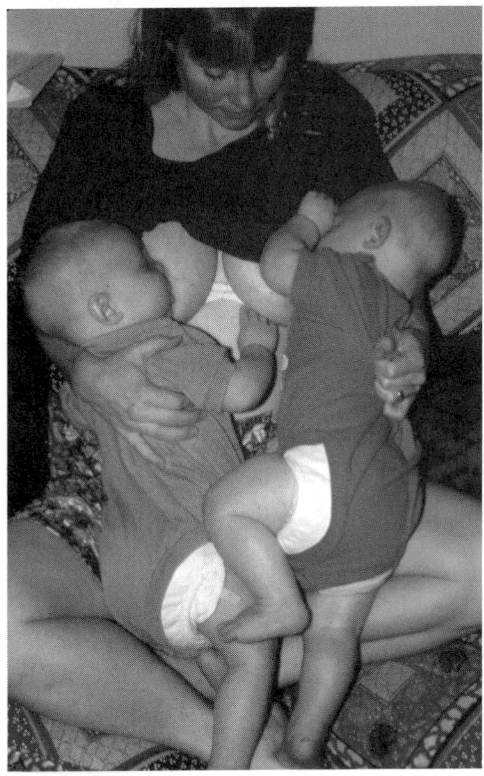

Figure 13-31 Double V hold.

References

Alberts, J. R. (1958). Learning as adaption of the infant. *Acta Paediatrica, 397*(Suppl.), 77–85.

Anderson, G. C. (1988). Crying, foramen ovale shunting, and cerebral volume. *Journal of Pediatrics, 113*(2), 411–412.

Anderson, G. C., Marks, E. A., & Wahlberg, V. (1986). Kangaroo care for premature infants. *American Journal of Nursing, 86*(7), 807–809.

Anderson, G. C., Moore, E., Hepworth, J., & Bergman, N. J. (2003). Early skin-to-skin contact for mothers and their healthy newborn infants. *Cochrane Collaboration Systematic Review* (CD003519). Oxford: Update Software.

Blair, A., Cadwell, K., Turner-Maffei, C., & Brimdyr, K. (2003). The relationship between positioning, breastfeeding dynamic, the latching process and pain in breastfeeding mothers with sore nipples. *Breastfeeding Review, 11*(2), 5–10.

Bosma, J. F. (1972). Form and function in the infant's mouth and pharynx. In J. F. Bosma (Ed.), *Oral sensations and perceptions in the mouth of the infant* (pp. 3–29). Springfield, IL: Charles C. Thomas.

Browne, J. V. (2004). Early relationship environments: Physiology of skin-to-skin contact for parents and their preterm infants. *Clinics in Perinatology, 31*(2), 287–298.

Charpak, N., de Calume, Z. F., & Ruiz, J. G. (2000). The Bogota declaration on kangaroo mother care: Conclusions at the second international workshop on the method. Second International Workshop of Kangaroo Mother Care. *Acta Paediatrica, 89,* 1137–1140.

Christensson, K., Cabrera, T., Christensson, E., Uvnas-Moberg, K., & Winberg, J. (1995). Separation distress call in the human infant in the absence of maternal body contact. *Acta Paediatrica, 84,* 468–473.

Cioni, G., Ferrari, F., & Prechtl, H. F. (1989). Posture and spontaneous motility in full-term infants. *Early Human Development, 18*(4), 247–262.

Crawford, C. J. (1994). Parenting practices in the Basque country: Implications of infant and childhood sleeping location for personality development. *Ethos, 22*(1), 42–84.

Curley, M. A. Q., Hibberd, P. L., Fineman, L. D., Wypig, D., Shih, M.-C., Thompson, J. E., . . . Arnold, J. H. (2005). Effect of prone positioning on clinical outcomes in children with acute lung injury. *Journal of the American Medical Association, 294*(2), 229–237.

Danner, S., & Cerutti, E. R. (1989). *Nursing your baby with Down syndrome.* Rochester, NY: Childbirth Graphics.

Harlow, H. F. (1971). The nature of love. In A. Montegue (Ed.), *Touching: The human significance of skin* (pp. 1–25). New York, NY: Harper and Row. (Reprinted from *The American Psychologist, 13,* 673–685.)

Marmet, C., & Shell, E. (1984). Training neonates to suck correctly. *MCN. The American Journal of Maternal Child Nursing, 9*(6), 401–407.

Marmet, C., & Shell, E. (1993). *Lactation forms: A guide to lactation consultant charting.* Encino, CA: Lactation Institute.

Meier, P., & Anderson, G. (1987). Responses of small preterm infants to bottle- and breast-feeding. *MCN. The American Journal of Maternal Child Nursing, 12,* 97–105.

Mizuno, K., Inoue, M., & Takeuchi, T. (2000). The effects of body positioning on sucking behaviour in sick neonates. *European Journal of Pediatrics, 159*(11), 827–831.

Montegue, A. (1971). *Touching: The human significance of skin.* New York, NY: Harper & Row.

Morris, S. E., & Klein, M. D. (1987). *Pre-feeding skills.* Tucson, AZ: Therapeutic Skill Builders.

Rey, E. S., & Martinez, H. G. (1983). *Manejo racional del niño prematuro.* In *Curso de medicina fetal* (pp. 137–151). Bogotá, Colombia: Universidad Nacional.

Robin, P. (1934). Glossoptosis due to atresia and hypotrophy of the mandible. *American Journal of Diseases of Children, 48,* 541.

Rosenblum, L. A., & Andrews, M. W. (1994). Influences of environmental demand on maternal behavior and infant development. *Acta Paediatrica, 397*(Suppl.), 57–63.

Schore, A. N. (2001a). Effects of a secure attachment relationship on right brain development, affect regulation, and infant mental health. *Infant Mental Health Journal, 22,* 7–66.

Schore, A. N. (2001b). The effects of early relational trauma on right brain development, affect regulation, and infant mental health. *Infant Mental Health Journal, 22*(1–2), 201–269.

Snyder, J. (1995). *Variation in infant palatal structure.* Encino, CA: Lactation Institute.

Snyder, J. B. (1997). Bubble palate and failure to thrive: A case report. *Journal of Human Lactation, 13*(2), 139–143.

Widstrom, A. M., Ransjo-Arvidson, A. B., Christensson, K., Mathieson, A. S., Winberg, J., & Uvnas-Moberg, K. (1987). Gastric suction in healthy newborn infants: Effects on the circulation and developing feeding behavior. *Acta Paediatrica Scandinavica, 76,* 566–572.

Wolf, L. S., & Glass, R. P. (1992). *Feeding and swallowing disorders in infancy.* Tucson, AZ: Therapy Skills Builders.

World Health Organization. (2003). *Kangaroo mother care: A practical guide.* Geneva, Switzerland: Author.

Additional Resources

Henderson, A., Stamp, G., & Pincombe, J. (2001). Postpartum positioning and attachment education for increasing breastfeeding: A randomized trial. *Birth, 28*(4), 236–242.

Marmet, C., Shell, E., & Aldana, S. (2000). Assessing infant suck dysfunction: Case management. *Journal of Human Lactation, 16*(4), 332–336.

McKenna, J., Thoman, E. B., Anders, T. F., Sadeh, A., Schechtman, V. L., & Glotzbach, S. F. (1993). Infant-parent co-sleeping in an evolutionary perspective: Implications for understanding infant sleep development and the sudden infant death syndrome. *Sleep, 16*(3), 263–282.

CHAPTER

14

Counseling Mothers of Infants with Feeding Difficulties

Nancy Williams

Parenting, and perhaps mothering in particular, is generally experienced as both more joyous and more complicated and overwhelming than the parent imagined, expected, or could possibly have anticipated. This is true even for experienced parents who add to their families, because each baby is a unique individual who must teach the mother and father how to parent him or her. For parents who face feeding difficulties, prematurity, disabilities, and the like, the most intense experience of their lifetime may be encompassed in caring for this child. Few parents are prepared in advance for the unique challenges incurred by a baby with special needs, even if they are relatively simple feeding problems that are time limited. How much more so for the family whose baby has a myriad of problems or whose feeding difficulties will not be easily resolved with time and a bit of creativity and patience!

Bringing a new child into the family is often an enormous opportunity for marital bonding, and fortunately so, because with this child comes increased stress on the marital unit as well. For a single mother, these stresses may spill over into whatever relationships exist within her home. If she is alone, she will also be faced with isolation and little or no respite from the demands of her infant. The tasks before her are daunting.

Westerners live in a world that is fast paced, driven by material need and a desire to achieve. This is often not conducive to the demands of motherhood, especially where an infant is demanding special attention, even above the expected. This adds to the complexity of the new roles and tasks before the parents. It is important for lactation consultants to have some understanding of the maternal context for this baby in order to provide optimum care to each dyad.

As lactation care providers, we must realize that some of our prescriptions involve a great deal of time and energy. Depending on the baby's capabilities, it may be that feeding takes up such a large portion of the day that there isn't time for anything else. Our plan may simply be impossible for a mother, depending on her resources and support, maturity, experience, obligations to other children or work outside the home, and so on. It is important for us to continually check in with her and to devise our care plan in conjunction with her stated goals, desires, and capabilities. The likelihood of success is much higher when she buys in by helping to create the plan.

It may also be appropriate in some instances to help her to sort through exactly where her stressors lie. Commonly, those around her may offer confusing information that point to her attempts to breastfeed as the reason why she is tired, overwhelmed, and so forth. In reality, it is often the normal demands of mothering a small child (or children) coupled with the feeding difficulties that exist apart from breastfeeding. For women who are also trying to juggle jobs, partner issues, or other problems, it may be necessary to assist her in assessing what can be let go or put on hold during this most intense time of need on the part of her little one. It is not unusual to discover that her stress becomes compounded, emotionally as well as physically, following weaning—particularly a weaning that was imposed on the mother by either subtle or overt pressure. This would be true even in the case of an older baby. Weaning—complete or partial—should take place only when the mother and baby are ready. With feeding disorders, readiness on either or both parts may come early out of exhaustion, resignation, or a whole host of reasons not truly associated with lactation problems.

Adult Development

Clearly, a woman experiences monumental psychological upheaval as she makes the transition into motherhood. Many of these changes are positive and may be capitalized on by lactation consultants and others who care for the dyad. Recent animal studies suggest that rather than diminished cognitive abilities in the period following birth, women may be at a lifetime peak in problem-solving abilities. Researchers have suggested that comparing a brain of a nonmother to that of a new mother is comparing apples to oranges (Kinsley & Lamber, 2006). It is important to note that the process of birth and the transformation of becoming a mother results in profound changes in brain function.

Erikson, in his classic work on psychosocial development (1968), described stages of change through crisis throughout the life span. His model helps us to understand the psychological tasks a woman is undertaking concurrent with assuming her new role as a mother. When motherhood arrives, a woman biologically will be in one of three Eriksonian developmental stages. If she is still an adolescent, she will be in the throes of learning her Identity versus Role Confusion. If she is a young adult, she will be struggling with Intimacy versus Isolation. For an older primipara, the challenge lies in Generativity versus Self-Absorption/Stagnation. Each of these stages offers ample opportunity to embrace this motherhood experience and to experience great emotional and cognitive growth as a result. Failure to do so often results in a stunting of development and a state of being somewhat stuck in an unnecessarily immature state. Recognition by healthcare providers of the differing needs in each developmental state may help to provide optimal care.

Having some grasp of this can be helpful for the lactation consultant as she assesses how best to teach and plan for the mother's care. The consultant should acknowledge that her own developmental experiences may implicitly affect treatment situations. For example, a lactation consultant who is working on Generativity may find herself tempted to inappropriately mother the mother in ways that are not productive.

Maternal Adequacy

Very few experiences facilitate adult development as thoroughly and profoundly as becoming a parent. We learn to live outside of ourselves, find a stronger voice, care about the world differently, and mature quickly. This author conducted a survey while preparing for a presentation several years ago and asked both men and women how parenthood had changed them. Although many ideas were brought forth, the one answer given by each and every respondent was, "I'm not as selfish."

If feeding difficulties arrive with the first baby, the new mother has yet to begin this process, identity change, and the new lesson in stepping outside of herself. In their seminal work on the acquisition of the parental role, authors Bocar and Moore (1987) describe a predictable sequence of behaviors and internal states that define the development of an emerging new identity with the advent of the first baby. Initially, parents find themselves in what has been called the Formal Stage, where they want rules and proscriptions for everything involved in baby care. Given that feeding or other difficulties add several levels of complexity to the situation, first-time parents may need assistance with opposing tasks—learning what needs to be done while at the same time learning to take command of their situation and become their child's advocate. They may find themselves clinging to the Formal Stage, finding comfort in the promises given by books and professionals yet being forced to move quickly to more maturity as parents while they seek to understand the needs of this child and possibly be called upon to advocate for him within the complicated context of the medical system.

It stands to reason that if feeding difficulties first present with a second or subsequent baby, the mother may have already developed a depth of maturity and comfort with her role. In terms of acquiring her parental role, it is likely that she will have arrived at Bocar and Moore's Personal Stage, that is, assuming Mother as her identity by developing a unique set of behaviors and attitudes that are appropriate for her, leading to confidence and competence. However, she also has a conflict because her other child (or children) needs her energies, obligating her to perform a juggling act with her time and attention. Understanding the mountain of demands being placed on this mother is vital while developing interventions and care plans.

In most normal situations, mothers are encouraged to bond primarily through their baby's attaching behaviors and cues. Infants teach parents how to care for them and engage their unique personality and needs. Occasionally this may go awry because a baby may not display the usual cues and seems to overtly reject the mother. Many mothers whose babies arch their back, scream, and push away from the breast (or arms and cradling) perceive that their babies do not like them. Persistent and patient parents learn how to help the baby settle into the arms or at breast, but sometimes they may need some teaching and encouragement from the lactation consultant. Educating them on the baby's cognitive immaturity, which precludes rejection, can be helpful. Above all, healthcare providers should not participate in negative interpretations of a baby's behavior with comments about stubbornness, anger, laziness, being a bad baby, and the like.

Understanding differing stages and experiences allows the lactation consultant to modify her teaching and support in a way that individualizes and makes relevant what she is trying to accomplish. Each mother and her needs are unique, and she needs to be cared for with understanding and creativity that acknowledges a given situation.

Resistance

It is very rewarding to offer educational support to the new dyad and to watch them succeed. It is equally or more discouraging when things do not go well. One possible reason that often leaves medical personnel scratching their heads is resistance.

Resistance can be a compensatory protective means of coping with something that is beyond us. It allows us to feel some modicum of control in an otherwise out-of-control situation. An important thing to remember in the presence of this resistance is that we need to take great care in including parents in the decisions, rather than telling them what to do. This allows them to feel more control.

Understanding the normal course of a crisis may be helpful. Although Kübler-Ross's (1969) model was intended for dying patients, many people have applied it to grief, loss, and crisis in general. One often observes the parents of babies with special needs exhibiting these predictable patterns, which include denial, anger, bargaining, depression, and finally acceptance. It is noteworthy to add that these may not manifest themselves in any linear fashion. It is also possible to return to a state, such as denial, long after one believes it to have resolved. Due to the intensity of the emotional response to crisis, it is often difficult for the parents to think clearly and make rational decisions. Hence it is all the more important for the lactation consultant to offer information and guidance gently but firmly as parents sort through advice and directions that seemingly come from all sides. It is also helpful to explain to parents that they won't always feel the way they do right now and to normalize their reaction to such a difficult experience. Our job as caring helpers is to support them in ways that leave them stronger as a result of their crisis, rather than in a more dependent or weakened state.

Therefore, when there is a problem or some deviation from the expectation of the parents, it becomes difficult, at best, to move toward acceptance of the situation. Many levels of resistance and confusion may be at play. The mother may have brought baggage to this experience from previous births, losses, or parenting, not to mention her own childhood.

Other common components to crisis include ambivalence and detachment. The parents are a bundle of tangled, unnamed negative emotions. This often causes them to swing back and forth in their thoughts, feelings, plans, and decisions. Lactation consultants may use this to their advantage in recognizing that a decision to give up breastfeeding may indeed be immediately reversible or changed in the near future. Gentle, respectful sharing of information on the ramifications of a decision to wean can be helpful. Detachment, similar to denial, is a defense mechanism often seen in the wake of shock. This protects one from the searing pain of feeling the totality of whatever loss is occurring. Sometimes the parents may present with a very flat affect while in the process of detaching from the situation. The danger lies in parents not being able to move back to engagement, which healthcare providers can help to guard against. When parents are detached, it may be somewhat more difficult for the healthcare providers to enter into a caring relationship. Recognizing this phenomenon for what it is may allow the lactation consultant to carefully confront it a bit and move forward.

Attachment

The primary psychological task of any newborn, according to Erickson (1968), is to learn to trust. The baby is hardwired to engage in all manner of attachment-seeking behaviors. It is the baby who will inspire the parent to respond with bonding behaviors. He smells nice, and she pulls him closer for a whiff. He is soft, and she runs her hands along his skin. He scans his horizon, and she responds with a gaze that he can lock onto. He smiles, and she returns his happy countenance. He whimpers, and she picks him up. He mouths his hands, and she feeds him. He cries, and she relieves his discomfort.

The attachment that forms during the first 3 years, with great emphasis placed on the foundational first year, will serve as the basis for the relationships formed by this baby throughout his life span. The classic work of Ainsworth, Blehar, Waters, and Wall (1978) clearly demonstrated that whatever "attachment style" formed in the first year was still being evidenced decades later as spouses and other adult relationships were sought and constructed. Bowlby (1982) was able to demonstrate the need for young children to have continual access to the primary caretaker, absent of significant separations. Bergman (2001) admonishes us to "never separate a mother and baby."

Consequently, the mother–baby relationship being forged is exceedingly important. Additionally, we know that a secure attachment is responsible for helping the child to learn empathy and general social skills (including language) and for helping to build proper synaptic structures in the brain, particularly to develop the orbitofrontal area of the brain that connects thought and emotion, allowing us to make thoughtful responses to a situation, rather than to simply react. Poorly attached children fail to learn emotional regulation—that is, the ability to calm and soothe themselves—and cannot cope and move forward when things are not going well. In short, the emotional abilities seen in babies who fail to attach are so limited as to be crippling throughout life.

In the case of an infant who is not able to cue correctly and elicit proper responses, there is some risk that the normal course of attachment and bonding may be disrupted. This will likely result in one of two dysfunctional extremes: overcompensating in the form of enmeshment and overprotection; or parental self-protection and withdrawal, resulting in disengagement. Parents who fail to bond experience deficits in their parenting abilities and in the relationship itself. It is not only the infant who loses when bonding and attachment fail.

When dealing with problems of any kind during the newborn period, some parents find themselves at a loss as to how to bond with the baby, particularly if the baby's attaching behaviors are somehow compromised. It is not unusual for a parent to globalize and feel incompetent and inadequate to the whole of parenting. The converse may also be true wherein parents understand that this particular child will need something from them that they had not imagined, and they step up to fulfill that need, adding to their feeling of parental power.

Birth Resolution

In the past 15 years, it has become increasingly common for women to experience a myriad of birth interventions. A woman may often find herself without knowledge or power in making decisions and choices about her baby's birth. The overall effect of this may be that she misses out on the empowerment inherent in a birth of her design as she takes on her new role as mother. If she is to advocate for her child within the medical establishment, this may have disastrous consequences.

If she has had a cesarean or other highly medicalized birth, it is also likely that she will be experiencing pain or psychological discomfort that will make it more difficult to meet the needs of a difficult-to-feed infant. Surely she will benefit from our best helping skills and is likely to experience breastfeeding success, despite obstacles in initiation.

Fostering Attachment

Many parents may be appreciative of encouragement and instruction for deliberately engaging in reparative attachment behaviors. Because it is the baby who usually drives this process, when the process is short-circuited, it will likely require some compensatory effort on the part of the parents. Soliciting the parents' responses in this way will have the added bonus of creating a feeling of importance in an otherwise powerless situation.

It would be a mistake to assume that because bonding got off to a slow start, or even experienced complete disruption in the early days, all is lost. Although there is a very real risk that the family could continue down a path of disconnection, it is likely that with good support the family can make up for lost time and develop solid attachments. For parents who themselves demonstrate secure attachment styles (Ainsworth et al., 1978), this task will likely be an easy transition with a bit of reassurance from the healthcare team.

When working with families who are not as fortunate in their own upbringings and backgrounds, didactic instruction on basics—such as the importance of eye contact, skin-to-skin contact, availability, engaging facial animation, and so forth—are important. Parents can be taught to be deliberately compensatory in their own bonding behaviors to assist the baby. Maybe even more important are referrals to support groups such as La Leche League, where mothers have ample opportunities to observe mother–baby interactions and vent when they feel frustration, fear, or other unexpected emotions.

Oxytocin, the hormone responsible for bonding, milk ejection, and satisfaction, may have been inhibited at crucial times. Normally, there is a significant burst at the time of birth. This is initiated as the baby's head creates pressure on the vaginal walls, which is obviously absent during a cesarean delivery. Additionally, epidural anesthesia is known to inhibit oxytocin release. There is evidence that the pain of labor, which causes endorphin release, also contributes to attachment. Attachment researchers are continuing to question the ramifications of violating the design of biology in this regard.

Many women find their birth experiences to be singularly dissatisfying, even to the point of mourning plans that went awry. A mother may be puzzled about what went wrong, or she may experience feelings of failure and inadequacy that threaten to invade her perception of her newly developing mothering skills. It is possible that she feels bitter disappointment as she contemplates the reality of her experience alongside her hopes and dreams for birth.

Conversely, it is possible that, given her approach to life in general, she is perfectly happy with allowing others to make decisions about her birth, which follows into her mothering. She may then have difficulty following through and think that caring for this baby might better be performed by experts. A passive style such as this can be challenging for the lactation consultant who may be encouraging her to come into a more empowered place. The consultant must realize that for some, this process is substantially protracted.

Imperfect Baby

First responses to birth anomalies often create yet another mix of confusing emotions. It is normal to see parents swing from one emotional extreme to another as they navigate this aspect of the situation. Unfortunately, they may also be subject to the unhelpful advice and opinions of people around them.

During the immediate crisis, it is crucial for healthcare providers to be as clear and repetitive as possible, in anticipation of the likelihood that the parents cannot take in everything that is being shared. A simplified explanation of all things medical allows the parents to grasp the situation more thoroughly. Having a written summary of care plans, referrals, and the like will be most helpful. It may also be advantageous to include other family members or support people in teaching times so that others can help relay information later and encourage the parents to share tasks when appropriate.

Teen Mothers

Although in many respects teen mothers have the same needs and goals as any mother, there are some unique needs within this population that must be considered during teaching and development of care plans.

It is common to note that the average teen mother has both high energy and multitasking abilities. This is fortunate because it is also generally true that she is under a great deal of both internal and external pressure to fulfill several roles at once. She is now a mother, student, family member, girlfriend or wife, social teen, and possibly an employee. She has not been given any extra hours in her day, yet she often finds herself trying to accomplish more than is possible.

Often one observes that not only are her financial resources quite limited—an important consideration when advising on pumps, supplementers, and the like—but also due to her immaturity she may simply not have the patience for a difficult feeding regimen. She may also be expected to return to school by 2 weeks postpartum, regardless of the baby's status. Because mother-baby attachment issues are potentially more critical for this dyad, it is important to weigh these aspects and try to simplify her tasks as much as possible. A back-to-basics approach may be best, limiting interventions as much as possible. Utilizing peers and adult mentors are both creative ways to provide ongoing support for breastfeeding.

It would likely be a significant mistake to assume that because a mother is young she is incapable of learning about the care of her baby. Allison was barely 16 when her son was born, aspirating meconium during birth:

> I checked the machines he was hooked up to, making sure his oxygen saturation levels and heart and breathing rates were what the nurses expected them to be. They were. I would pad down the hallway, back into my room, rubbing my soft, wrinkled tummy and pull out my new breast pump. (Crews, 1999)

Teens are more likely to birth by cesarean and are statistically more likely to give birth to premature or anomalous infants. They are also more likely to bottle feed, theoretically because of the multitude of barriers against obtaining help and information regarding breastfeeding. The genuine caring assistance of a lactation consultant may be exactly what she needs to defy the statistics and become a successful breastfeeder, despite any problems getting started.

One potentially positive aspect of working with teens is that they may be exquisitely aware of their need for teaching and support. They usually respond well to adults who do not condescend to them but rather offer genuine caring. Including the teen's parents in teaching time is often best, in order to enlist their support and to detour incorrect information. Additionally, the lactation consultant can model an attitude that promotes the new young mother's need to occupy her new role.

Advice of Outsiders

Under the best of circumstances, new parents find themselves bombarded with advice and suggestions. Usually this is well intended, though sometimes family members attempt to exert control over the new parents or the situation. Although advice givers are sometimes knowledgeable and can offer positive suggestions, this is not always the case. Add to that the fact that some personality types are more susceptible to advice, possibly seeking out multiple opinions, and it can be a very frustrating situation for the healthcare providers.

Bear in mind that if this is a first baby, the parents are looking for the rules that will help them to succeed. It can be very positive to include extended family members in care plan formation and discussion and to validate their concerns and ideas when possible, while at the same time empowering the parents to do what they think is best.

It is also an unfortunate possibility that family and friends will withdraw in the face of a disabled or critically ill infant. Such an event exacerbates the pain of parents who are already struggling to cope. Encouragement, comfort, and referrals to support groups can be very helpful.

Family of Origin Issues

During times of stress, families may be tempted to revert to unhealthy patterns of communicating and interacting. Long-buried wounds may once again rise to the surface. Inabilities to work together, pushing buttons, and other problems may add to an already difficult situation. Due to the emotional vulnerability of the parents, hypersensitivity may cause new conflicts to erupt.

Conversely, many families find new strengths when they are stressed. The abilities to share time, energy, and even monetary resources are often discovered for possibly the first time. A new bonding among extended family members tends to take place if the members allow it. The lactation consultant may find herself in a unique role as facilitator as the family looks to her for help, information, and support.

Grief and Coping Skills

Feeding problems are generally perceived as crisis situations, even in the mildest of circumstances. Inherent in any crisis is a feeling of loss, leading to grief. Grief is among the most complex of experiences, with tangled webs of emotion. It is important to note that grief also provides a rich opportunity for personal growth and development. When one survives a crisis with the support of caring people, one often comes out the other side with greater knowledge, strength, compassion, and a multitude of positive developments.

Further, as previously mentioned, grief has a somewhat predictable course, including the roller coaster ride of emotions that are a conglomerate of positives (hope) and negatives (despair). Old losses may reassert their presence in the form of newly provoked pain. Over time, the intensity that the mother may be feeling will diminish. Educating her about this fact will give her something to cling to on her bad days and something to look forward to overall. Bear in mind that the unfolding of grief cannot be hurried, and the parents should expect it to take time. Healthcare providers will sometimes confuse normal, healthy grieving with the abnormal state of depression. It is important to encourage the parents to allow the grieving process to proceed, and let them know that it has its own pace and there is nothing wrong with them. Encouraging the use of antidepressants or other medications to alleviate symptoms of normal sadness may be in error and may, in fact, prolong the natural course of mourning.

A healthy acceptance of whatever situation the parents are facing is not to be confused with resignation. Acceptance includes an embracing of the baby, a celebration of the positive aspects of the situation, and a powerful moving forward. In the event of the death of the infant, acceptance is still the goal. Resignation connotes a loss of power and an inability to see anything worth celebrating.

In the case of a baby with feeding difficulties, the parents will most likely experience what is referred to as ambiguous grief. On the one hand, they have a surviving baby, with many capabilities and lovable qualities. Well-meaning people will often point this out, claiming that there is nothing to be sad about. The reality, however, is that the mother may indeed experience strong grief for the loss of her expectations, whatever they may have been. Disappointing birth experiences or, worse, traumatic births, as well as any fears for her baby's future, may accompany and intensify such grief. Add to that exhaustion, hormonal shifts, confusing medical advice, and so forth, and the potential for a negative state becomes significant.

Grief is a multifaceted, complex experience. In addition to sadness about the situation, many people find themselves isolated in misunderstanding. Well-meaning people may suggest that there is everything to be thankful for, nothing to complain about, and that it is time to move on. After all, the baby is alive, healthy, beautiful, or some other positive adjective. The fact that the mother may be mourning the loss of her expectation of a warm, smooth breastfeeding experience is minimized by those who are telling her what to be thankful for.

It will be important for healthcare providers and other caring people to encourage the parents to take care of each other and themselves. This may be very challenging if feeding regimens allow for little time away. The requirements of constant pumping, feeding, washing equipment, and so forth, all while healing from birth, seemingly do not allow for self-care. The reality is that if self-care is not built into the care plan, most parents will not manage the long haul. Extended family members and friends may be recruited for help with the mundane: cooking, cleaning, taking care of the car, caring for other children, and so forth. Although this is a gift to any new parents, it becomes crucial for parents who have more than their share of challenges. Religious groups can be called upon to offer such assistance, as well. The added benefit of eliciting help from others is that it is often an opportunity for reestablishing or strengthening important emotional ties with the parents. This will support the grieving process and provide practical care and help.

Substance Abuse

In some instances, the feeding difficulties presented in the infant are a result of substance use in one or both parents. Or there may be no direct relationship, yet the baby is born to a parent with addictive patterns already in place.

Lactation consultants have many resources to turn to for their own education and would do well to have handouts or other information available for clients. Although there may be room for professional disagreement about minimal use of some substances, such as alcohol or nicotine, there is consensus that most street drugs are generally incompatible with breastfeeding. Still, some mothers may be able to use "pump and dump" information or, better still, be encouraged toward sobriety on behalf of their baby.

Possibly a more immediate concern with these families is whether the parents are functioning well enough to care for a baby. This can be explored with the help of the lactation consultant, including reviewing the facts of safe cosleeping and other issues about which there may be concerns. Note that the lactation consultant may not be hearing the entire accurate picture from a family that has substance abuse at its center, and the lactation consultant may want to carefully offer information based on her hunches, even if those hunches are not verbally validated.

Substance users will many times increase patterns of usage in times of stress and crisis. Lactation consultants should be alert to this possibility. Good referrals for programs, therapy, or other positive support would be in order.

Lactation Consultants' Feelings and Responsibilities

Lactation consultants may also have very strong emotions in situations where breastfeeding goals are not met. Many consultants entered this profession because of the great satisfaction we know when we watch a successfully nursing dyad, accompanied by joy when we observe the relieved look of the mother as the baby finally latches nicely. Consequently, when our best efforts fail to yield the desired result, we may wonder what we could have done differently as we feel frustration, anger, confusion, puzzlement, and much more. Out of our own pain, we may be tempted to withdraw from the mother or try to affix inappropriate blame. If we are clear and aware of our own process, allowing us to stay connected, we may be invited to enter into the mother's grief, providing support and walking with her down a lonely road. It is not an easy one for the consultant to walk either, despite its privilege. In the end, we may find that we have grown personally and developed new counseling skills as well!

These counseling skills–active listening and reflecting feelings as the mother explores her situation, asking good open-ended questions leading to choices and decision making, and educating her about real options and possibilities–will help to see the mother through the immediate future and down the road. This is time consuming, involving a commitment to the well-being of the family that transcends what we often are doing for breastfeeding support. The rewards to everyone are well worth the cost, however.

Of course it is also the responsibility of the lactation consultant to do her best to ensure that the milk supply is protected during the period when the baby is unable to feed at the breast. Keeping up to date on promoting and maintaining a good supply is crucial, especially as reproductive technology helps mothers with hormonal issues to have babies that they then wish to breastfeed. Clearly we need some counseling abilities and problem solving abilities to address milk production issues and help the mother and infant breastfeed. **Figure 14-1** provides an overview of the hierarchy of feeding choices.

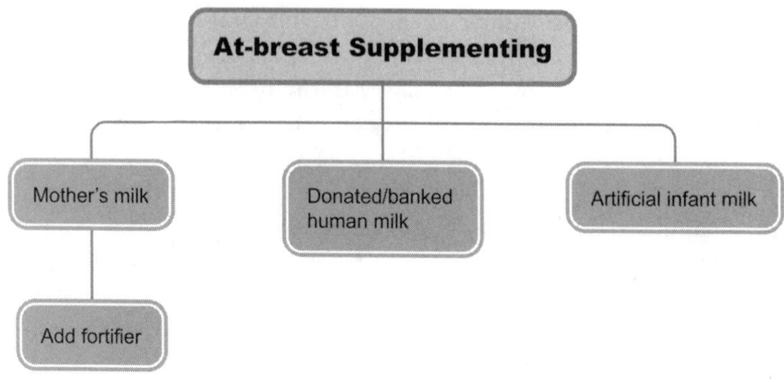

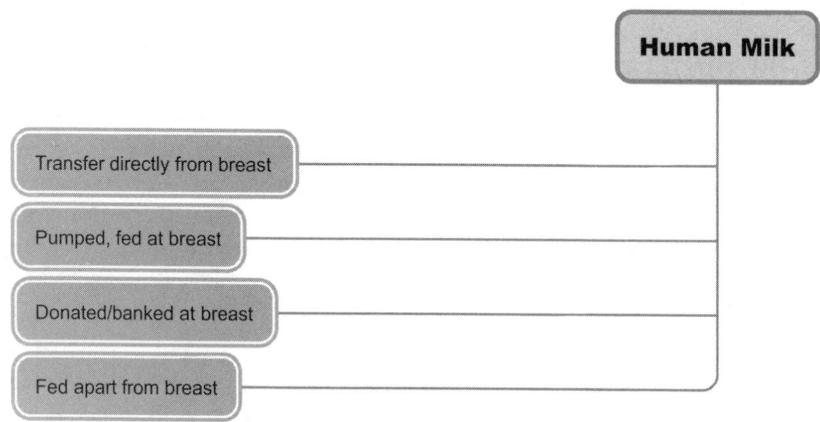

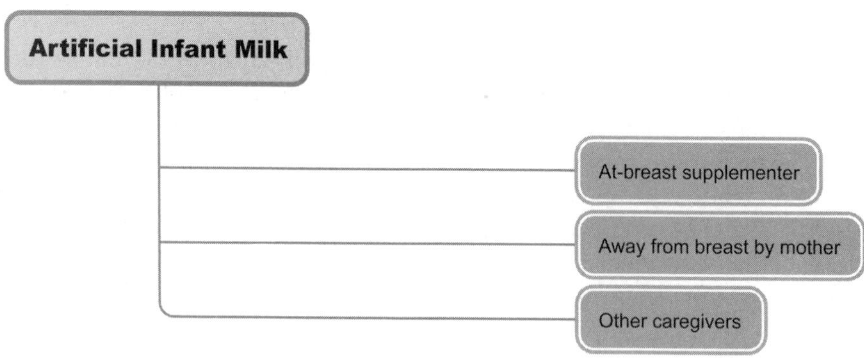

Figure 14-1 Hierarchy of optimal feeding.

The Importance of Listening

Developing listening skills brings many benefits to professional helpers. Active listening (i.e., restating and rephrasing the client's statements) can sometimes feel so simplistic as to be questionable. The client shares that she "has to wean the baby." We reply, "You have to wean the baby." As we do so, we have time to gather ourselves from what may have been an unexpected remark, we make sure that we are on the same page with the client and that we stay on it if she goes in an unexpected direction, and it also encourages her to elaborate. Her next statement may be, "Well, yes, because my husband says my breasts are his."

Reflective listening, wherein we explore with her the emotional aspects of her experience, is optimum for creating a connection with her. She states, "I've had it with pumping 10 times a day, then feeding, cleaning parts, and then starting over." We may reply, "It sounds like you are feeling overwhelmed, exhausted, and frustrated." The client then experiences us as understanding her situation more fully and trusts us enough to move to a deeper place of communication. Further, she begins to understand her own tangled mass of feelings that are driving her to making a possibly regrettable decision. Making the effort to understand another person on this level is a true gift.

One of the best ways to help someone grasp concepts is by asking them, in the form of an open-ended question, to think it through. Closed-ended questions such as "Do you want to breastfeed?" don't necessarily elicit much information and actually have a tendency to shut down further discussion. Asking "Why don't you want to breastfeed?" implies judgment, puts the client on the defensive, and probably does not have a good answer anyway. All of these nonproductive ways of asking can be developed into good questions that make the mother think. "What are the factors that are causing you to want to wean?" "How did you reach this decision?" "Where do you imagine yourself in the future?" As she formulates responses to these questions, she is obligated to weigh her positions in a new way, often leading to a different conclusion.

Finally, after trust has been established and we have developed a caring relationship with the mother, a tall order to be sure given the time constraints, we may be able to confront her with new information that she has not factored in to her decision making.

> Client: My baby has had so much to deal with since the surgery. My family all think that it would just be easier to wean so the baby and I would both be less stressed.
>
> Lactation consultant: I've heard you talk about the pressure you are feeling. I'm so impressed at the skills you've already developed as Andrew's mother. I'm wondering what you think about your family's advice. Perhaps you would like to hear about some of the long-term effects of weaning a baby of this age. May I share that with you?

Notice that the information is presented in a way that respects the mother's autonomy and is sandwiched in with praise and validation.

These families are truly in need of the gift of time. Many lactation consultants, especially when working in the context of a hospital or clinic, find themselves feeling pushed and harried to see every client, finish paperwork, and so forth. Yet grief can't and won't be hurried. These special circumstances will require the lactation consultant to set aside other demands and give this family as much as they need.

Sometimes we become uncomfortable with a developing dependence on us as the parents look more and more to us beyond the scope of breastfeeding assistance. Some dependence is normal during a crisis. If lactation consultants can accept this without fostering an unhealthy growth of neediness, this can be a positive experience, opening the door to more teaching and help. We may become quite bonded to this mother, which is rewarding in and of itself.

Helping the Bottle Feeding Mother Nurse Her Baby

There are times when, despite the best efforts of parents, healthcare providers, and other support people, breastfeeding is deemed to be impossible. Fortunately, this is largely avoidable with skilled help and good information. Nonetheless it does occur, to the dismay of all involved.

The process of breastfeeding is a complex, multilevel experience. It is much more than simply a way of getting nutrition from the mother to the baby, though often it is simplified to terms such as that. In addition to feeding, however, mother and baby will provide mutual comfort and cuddling, entertainment, relational behaviors, warmth, and immunological and hormonal support appropriate for each of them. Consequently, with the loss of breastfeeding comes the threat of much more than compromised nutrition.

Many mothers are able to give pumped milk in a bottle, by cup, or using some other method, even if transfer directly from the breast is impossible. Although this is far from ideal, it is also far from the least favorable option, which is to feed artificial infant milk from a bottle.

Much of this can be ameliorated by assisting the mother in learning to nurse her bottle-fed baby. Educating her on the importance of skin-to-breast contact, holding the baby for the entirety of each and every feeding, allowing him to pacify at breast if he is able, and so forth can restore some of what might otherwise be lost.

This teaching will promote the bonding and attachment needs of the dyad. So much is now known about the critical need for mother and baby to be together, to spend time skin to skin, and to have the time and supportive context for falling in love. With these challenging situations, such a necessary experience can potentially short circuit. Therefore, it is incumbent on us to do our best to provide the necessary teaching and support to restore these relational abilities.

Conclusion

A lactation consultant who is faced with assisting the families of babies with feeding difficulties has her work cut out for her! This may be the most time consuming, sometimes painful, and challenging work that she may be fortunate enough to be engaged in. If she is able to open herself up to the possibilities of both sadness and fear, as well as being a conduit for hope and healing, she may also experience more joy in these situations than any other.

References

Ainsworth, M., Blehar, M., Waters, E., & Wall, S. (1978). *Patterns of attachment: A psychological study of the strange situation.* Hillsdale, NJ: Erlbaum.

Bergman, Nils. (Producer). (2001). *Kangaroo mother care II: Restoring the original paradigm* [Motion picture]. Available from Nils Bergman, 8 Francis Rd., Pinelands 7405, South Africa, or http://www.kangaroomothercare.com

Bocar, D., & Moore, K. (1987). *Acquiring the parental role: A theoretical perspective* (La Leche League International, Lactation Consultant Series, Unit 16). Garden City Park, NY: Avery.

Bowlby, J. (1982). *Attachment and loss* (Rev. ed., Vol. 1). New York, NY: Basic Books.

Crews, A. (1999). *When I was garbage.* Retrieved from http://www.girl-mom.com

Erikson, E. (1968). *Identity: Youth and crisis.* New York, NY: Norton.

Good Mojab, C. (2002). Helping breastfeeding mothers grieve. Retrieved from http://home.comcast.net/~ammawell/helping_mothers_grieve.html

Kinsley, C., & Lamber, K. (2006, January). The maternal brain. *Scientific American,* 72–79.

Kübler-Ross, E. (1969). *On death and dying.* New York, NY: Touchstone.

Additional Resources

Ainsworth, M. (1967). *Infancy in Uganda: Infant care and the growth of love.* Baltimore, MD: Johns Hopkins University Press.

Bartlik, B., Greene, K., Graf, M., Sharma, G., & Melnick, H. (1999). *Examining PTSD as a complication of infertility.* Retrieved from http://www.medscape.com/viewarticle/719243

Crain, W. (2011). Erikson and the eight stages of life. In W. Crain (Ed.), *Theories of development: Concepts and applications* (6th ed., pp. 281–305). New York, NY: Prentice Hall.

Herforth, D. (1986). *Counseling grieving families* (La Leche League International, Lactation Consultant Series, Unit 12). Garden City Park, NY: Avery.

Hummel, P. (2003). Parenting the high-risk infant. *Newborn and Infant Nursing Reviews, 3*(3), 88–92.

Kluger-Bell, K. (1998). *Unspeakable losses: Understanding the experience of pregnancy loss, miscarriage, and abortion.* New York, NY: W. W. Norton.

Kohn, I., Moffitt, P.-L., & Wilkins, I. A. (2000). *A silent sorrow: Pregnancy loss—guidance and support for you and your family.* London, England: Routledge.

Parker, D., & Williams, N. (2006). *Teens and breastfeeding* (2nd ed., La Leche League International, Lactation Consultant Series Two, Unit 3). Garden City Park, NY: Avery.

Tagliaferre, L. (2001). *Recovery from loss: A personalized guide to the grieving process.* Gainesville, FL: Center for Applications of Psychological Type.

Vidyashanker, C. (2003). Postnatal depression linked to poor growth of infants. *Archives of Disease in Childhood, 88,* 34–37.

Williams, N. (1997). Maternal psychological issues in the experience of breastfeeding. *Journal of Human Lactation, 13,* 57–60.

Williams, N. (2002). Supporting the mother coming to terms with persistent insufficient milk supply: The role of the lactation consultant. *Journal of Human Lactation, 18,* 262–263.

Williams, N. (2004). When the blues arrive with baby. *New Beginnings, 21*(3), 84–88.
Worden, J. W. (2002). *Grief counseling and therapy: A guide for the mental health professional.* New York, NY: Springer.
Wright, H. N. (1993). *Recovering from the losses of life.* Grand Rapids, MI: Fleming H. Revell.
Wright, H. N. (2003). *The new guide to crisis and trauma counseling.* Ventura, CA: Regal Books.

Index

B

L

M

T

U

V

W

Z